Characterizing the HIV/AIDS Epidemic in the Middle East and North Africa

Characterizing the HIV/AIDS Epidemic in the Middle East and North Africa

TIME FOR STRATEGIC ACTION

Laith J. Abu-Raddad, Francisca Ayodeji Akala,
Iris Semini, Gabriele Riedner, David Wilson,
and Ousama Tawil

THE WORLD BANK
Washington, D.C.

ISBN: 978-0-8213-8137-3
eISBN: 978-0-8213-8138-0
DOI: 10.1596/978-0-8213-8137-3

Cover design by Naylor Design.

Library of Congress Cataloging-in-Publication Data

Characterizing the HIV/AIDS epidemic in the Middle East and North Africa : time for strategic action / Laith Abu-Raddad . . . [et al.].
    p. ; cm.
  Includes bibliographical references.
  ISBN 978-0-8213-8137-3
  1. AIDS (Disease)—Middle East. 2. AIDS (Disease)—Africa, North. I. Abu-Raddad, Laith.
II. World Bank.
  [DNLM: 1. Acquired Immunodeficiency Syndrome—epidemiology—Africa, Northern.
2. Acquired Immunodeficiency Syndrome—epidemiology—Middle East. 3. HIV Infections—epidemiology—Africa, Northern. 4. HIV Infections—epidemiology—Middle East. 5. HIV Infections—transmission—Africa, Northern. 6. HIV Infections—transmission—Middle East.
7. Health Planning—Africa, Northern. 8. Health Planning—Middle East. 9. Health Policy—Africa, Northern. 10. Health Policy—Middle East. 11. Risk Factors—Africa, Northern. 12. Risk Factors—Middle East. WC 503.4 JA2 C469 2009]
  RA643.86.M628C53 2009
  614.5'9939200956—dc22

                                                                                    2009041797

Contents

Acknowledgments

This report presents the findings of the synthesis of existing data and other information on the HIV/AIDS (human immunodeficiency virus/acquired immunodeficiency syndrome) epidemics in the Middle East and North Africa (MENA) made up of countries covered by the World Bank, the Joint United Nations Programme on HIV/AIDS (UNAIDS) MENA Regional Support Team (RST), and the Eastern Mediterranean Regional Office (EMRO) of the World Health Organization (WHO). The synthesis supports countries to better define their epidemic ("know your epidemic") in order to plan and implement more strategic actions to prevent or reduce further transmission of the infection and to also mitigate the impact of the infection on those already infected and affected.

The report is a joint interagency effort between the World Bank MENA Region, UNAIDS MENA RST, and WHO/EMRO. The team was led by Francisca Ayodeji Akala (Task Team Leader and Senior Public Health Specialist, World Bank) and includes Laith J. Abu-Raddad (Principal Investigator of the scientific study; World Bank Consultant; Director of Epidemiology, Biostatistics and Biomathematics Research Core; Assistant Professor in Public Health at Weill Cornell Medical College, Qatar), Iris Semini (UNAIDS MENA RST), Gabriele Riedner (WHO/EMRO), David Wilson (World Bank), Ousama Tawil (UNAIDS MENA RST), Hamidreza Setayesh (UNAIDS MENA RST), Fatou Fall (World Bank), and Juliana Victor-Ahuchogu (World Bank). The report was prepared under the guidance of Akiko Maeda, World Bank MENA, Health, Nutrition, and Population Sector Manager. The peer reviewers of the report are Jody Kusek (World Bank), Partricio Marquez (World Bank), Barbara O. de Zalduondo (UNAIDS), Robert Lyerla (UNAIDS), Ying Lo-Ru (WHO), and Yves Souteyrand (WHO). We appreciate their time and efforts in providing useful comments that were helpful in strengthening the final report.

We would like to specially acknowledge the valuable scientific contributions to this project of Nahla Hilmi (Research Assistant and World Bank consultant) and Manal Benkirane (Research Assistant and UNAIDS consultant). Nahla was instrumental in conducting systematic literature reviews and epidemiological analyses. Manal provided epidemiological summaries and translations of French language data and documents.

This project could not have been conducted without the support of organizations and agencies at the international and national levels in providing documents, other data sources, and input for the purpose of this synthesis. In particular, we thank the UNAIDS MENA RST and WHO/EMRO for providing hundreds of documents and other data sources to be investigated for this project. Among the many colleagues who provided data, documents, or input are Ahmad Sayed Alinaghi (Iranian Research Center for HIV/AIDS, the Isalmic Republic of Iran), Ramzi Alsalaq (Fred Hutchinson Cancer Research Center), Alia Al-Tayyib (Colorado Department of Public Health), Rhoda Ashley Morrow (University of Washington), Ruanne Barnabas (Fred Hutchinson Cancer Research Center), Veronique Bortolotti (WHO/EMRO), Hiam Chemaitelly (Weill Cornell Medical College, Qatar), Jesus M. García Calleja (WHO), Jocelyn DeJong (American University of Beirut), Paul Drain (University of Washington), Golda El-Khoury (United Nations Children's Fund [UNICEF]), Majdi Al-Touhki (World Bank),

Ali Feizzadeh (UNAIDS/Iran), Sarah Hawkes (London School of Hygiene and Tropical Medicine), Joumana Hermez (WHO/EMRO), Rachel Kaplan (University of California, Los Angeles), Adnan Khan (Research and Development Solutions), Hamida Khattabi (WHO/EMRO), Laura Koutsky (University of Washington), Abdalla Ismail (WHO/Somalia), Wadih Maalouf (United Nations Office on Drugs and Crime), Carla Makhlouf Obermeyer (WHO), Yolisa Sarah Mashologu (WHO/EMRO), Willi McFarland (University of California, San Francisco), Dewolfe Miller (University of Hawaii), Ghina Mumtaz (Weill Cornell Medical College, Qatar), Agnes Nabaloga (World Bank), Yaa Oppong (World Bank), Assad Rahal (National AIDS Program/Jordan), Marian Schilperoord (United Nations High Commissioner for Refugees), George Schmid (WHO), Joshua Schiffer (Fred Hutchinson Cancer Research Center), Sharif Sawires (University of California, Los Angeles), Cherif Soliman (Family Health International), Anna Wald (University of Washington), Helen Weiss (London School of Hygiene and Tropical Medicine), Najin Yasrebi (UNICEF), Saman Zamani (Kyoto University), and Hany Ziady (WHO/EMRO).

We greatly appreciate and thank all the researchers, research participants, and data contributors who contributed to the body of evidence, data, and research that were reviewed and synthesized for this work: the most comprehensive research work on HIV/AIDS in MENA since the beginning of the epidemic.

Executive Summary

Despite a fair amount of progress on understanding human immunodeficiency virus (HIV) epidemiology globally, the Middle East and North Africa (MENA) region is the only region where knowledge of the epidemic continues to be very limited, and subject to much controversy. It has been more than 25 years since the discovery of HIV, but no scientific study has provided a comprehensive data-driven synthesis of HIV/AIDS (acquired immunodeficiency syndrome) infectious spread in this region. The region continues to be viewed as the anomaly in the HIV/AIDS world map and "a real hole in terms of HIV/AIDS epidemiological data."[1]

This report addresses this dearth of strategic information on HIV infections in MENA through a joint effort of the World Bank, the MENA Regional Support Team (RST) of the Joint United Nations Programme on HIV/AIDS (UNAIDS), and the Eastern Mediterranean Regional Office (EMRO) of the World Health Organization (WHO). It builds on a series of publications by the World Bank that focuses on different aspects of HIV/AIDS epidemic and response. In 2003, the World Bank, in collaboration with UNAIDS and WHO/EMRO, issued the *HIV/AIDS in the Middle East and North Africa: The Cost of Inaction* report, which provided an analysis of the vulnerability factors in MENA along with an economic analysis of the impact based on the limited HIV data recognized at the time. In 2005, the World Bank issued the *Preventing HIV/AIDS in the Middle East and North Africa: A Window of Opportunity to Act* report, which provided an analysis of a prevention strategy for HIV in MENA. The current report provides the first comprehensive scientific assessment and data-driven epidemiological synthesis of HIV spread in MENA since the beginning of the epidemic. It is based on a literature review and analysis of thousands of widely unrecognized publications, reports, and data sources extracted from scientific literature or collected from sources at the local, national, and regional levels.

For the purpose of an epidemiologically relevant classification, the MENA population has been divided into different risk classes. The first class includes the **priority groups** that are at the highest risk of HIV infection. These groups include injecting drug users (IDUs), men who have sex with men (MSM), and female sex workers (FSWs). The second class includes the **bridging populations**, such as clients of sex workers, who experience an intermediate risk of HIV infection and provide links between priority groups and the general population. The **general population**, the third risk class, experiences the lowest risk of HIV infection and includes most of the population in any community. It also includes the **vulnerable populations** that are generally at low risk of HIV infection, such as prisoners, youth, and mobile populations, but are vulnerable to practices that may put them at higher risk of HIV infection.

This report covers all countries that are included in the definition for the Middle East and North Africa Region at the World Bank, UNAIDS MENA RST, and WHO/EMRO. Explicitly, this report includes data on Afghanistan, Algeria, Bahrain, Djibouti, the Arab Republic of Egypt, the Islamic Republic of Iran, Iraq, Jordan, Kuwait, Lebanon, Libya, Morocco, Oman, Pakistan, Qatar, Saudi Arabia, Somalia, Sudan, the Syrian Arab Republic, Tunisia, the United Arab Emirates, West Bank and Gaza (Occupied Palestinian Territories), and the Republic of Yemen.

---

[1] Bohannon, "Science in Libya."

KEY FINDINGS

HIV epidemics in MENA

HIV infection has already reached all corners of MENA and the majority of HIV infections are occurring in the existing sexual and injecting drug risk networks. The region as a whole is failing to control HIV spread along the contours of risk and vulnerability despite promising recent efforts. Priority populations, including IDUs, MSM, and FSWs, are documented to exist in all MENA countries. IDUs and MSM and their sexual partners, along with commercial sex networks, are the MENA populations most impacted by HIV/AIDS. In this sense, MENA is not an anomaly to the global HIV transmission patterns apart from the general population epidemics in sub-Saharan Africa.

There is substantial heterogeneity in HIV spread across MENA and different risk contexts are present throughout the region. However, the HIV epidemic in MENA can be roughly classified, in terms of the extent of HIV spread, into two groups. The first is the group of considerable HIV prevalence, which includes Djibouti, Somalia, and Southern Sudan, and is labeled here as the **Subregion with Considerable Prevalence**. The second group, which includes the rest of the MENA countries, has a more modest HIV prevalence and is labeled here as the **Core MENA Region**. Because the latter group consists of most of the MENA countries, HIV epidemiology here represents the main patterns found in MENA.

HIV epidemic typology in the Core MENA Region

Two epidemiologic patterns describe HIV epidemiology in this group of MENA countries. The first is the pattern of **exogenous HIV exposures** among the nationals of these countries, or HIV infections among their sexual partners upon their return. This pattern exists in all MENA countries at some level or another, but appears to be also the dominant pattern in several MENA countries. The weak surveillance systems of priority populations prevent us from conclusively stating whether this is indeed the dominant or only epidemiologic pattern in these countries. HIV could be spreading among some of the priority groups, or within pockets of these populations, without public awareness

of this endemic spread. However, there is no evidence to date that such considerable endemic transmission exists in these countries.

The second pattern in several MENA countries is that of concentrated HIV epidemics among priority populations. A concentrated epidemic is defined as an epidemic with an HIV prevalence consistently exceeding 5% in a priority population. There is already documented evidence for concentrated epidemics among IDUs in several MENA countries and considerable evidence suggesting concentrated epidemics among MSM. There is no evidence for the existence of major concentrated epidemics among FSWs. All evidence indicates no HIV epidemic among the general population.

HIV epidemic typology in the Subregion with Considerable Prevalence

Djibouti, parts of Somalia, and Southern Sudan are in a state of generalized HIV epidemics. A generalized HIV epidemic is defined as an epidemic with an HIV prevalence consistently exceeding 1% among pregnant women. Most HIV infections in these countries, however, are concentrated in priority groups and bridging populations. HIV dynamics are focused around commercial sex networks in settings where the size of the commercial sex network is large enough to support an epidemic with a prevalence exceeding 1% in the population.

There is no evidence of sustainable general population HIV epidemics in this group of MENA countries. Nevertheless, Southern Sudan is of particular concern. There are insufficient data to satisfactorily characterize HIV epidemiology in this part of Sudan, and it could be already in a state of general population HIV epidemic.

HIV spread and risk behavior by risk group

Injecting drug users

Injecting drug use is a persistent and a growing problem in MENA, with 0.2% of the total MENA population, almost a million people, injecting drugs. MENA is a major source, route, and destination for the global trade in illicit drugs.

HIV has already established itself among a number of IDU populations in MENA, while it is still at low or nil prevalence in other populations. Levels of HIV prevalence among populations where the infection is already established are comparable to those observed in other regions.

Levels of risk behavior practices, such as using nonsterile injecting equipment, are generally high, confirming the potential for further HIV spread among IDUs. Levels of hepatitis C virus (HCV), a marker of using nonsterile injecting equipment, are in the intermediate to high range, also confirming the potential for further HIV spread. IDUs are sexually active and report high levels of sexual risk behavior, indicating substantial overlap of risks among the three priority groups of IDUs, MSM, and FSWs. Levels of comprehensive HIV knowledge among IDUs vary across the region, with both high and low levels being reported in different settings.

The IDU risk context suggests the possibility of further concentrated HIV epidemics among IDUs in MENA over the next decade. The low or nil HIV prevalence in a number of IDU populations appears to reflect lack of HIV introduction into these populations, or that is has only recently been introduced, or the nature injecting network structure among the IDUs.

There is an urgent need for HIV surveillance to better understand transmission dynamics, risk behavior practices, and population estimates so that this information can be used to plan and implement more effective prevention and care services for IDUs. There is an opportunity to prevent IDU epidemics in MENA through needle exchange programs, access to frequent testing, prevention of heroin uptake, safe sex messages, and condom distribution.

Men who have sex with men
MSM are the most hidden and stigmatized risk group of all HIV risk groups in MENA. Nevertheless, homosexuality is prevalent at levels comparable to those in other regions, with a few percentage points of the male population engaging in homosexual contacts.

HIV is spreading among MSM, with apparently a rapidly rising epidemic in at least one country (Pakistan). HIV prevalence among MSM is already at considerable levels in several other countries, but data are still too limited to confirm the trend.

MSM report high levels of sexual risk behavior, such as multiple sexual partnerships of different kinds, low condom use, and high prevalence of sex work. MSM risk behaviors overlap considerably with heterosexual sex and injecting drug risk behaviors. Prevalence levels of sexually transmitted infections (STIs) other than HIV are substantial, suggesting epidemic potential for HIV. Levels of comprehensive HIV knowledge among MSM vary across the region with, both high and low levels being reported in different settings.

The MSM risk context suggests the possibility of concentrated HIV epidemics among MSM in MENA over the next decade. Indeed, MENA may already be in a stage of concentrated HIV epidemics among MSM in several countries, but definitive and conclusive data are lacking to support this possibility.

There is urgent need for HIV surveillance to better understand the transmission dynamics among MSM so that this information can be used to plan and implement more effective prevention and care services for this population group in MENA. Expansion of prevention and treatment efforts for MSM, such as condom distribution, counseling, HIV testing, HIV and STI treatment, and social and medical services, is key to preventing considerable HIV epidemics among MSM.

Commercial sex networks
Commercial sex is prevalent all over MENA, although levels are rather low in comparison to other regions. Economic pressure, family disruption or dysfunction, and political conflicts are major pressures for commercial sex in this region. Roughly 0.1% to 1% of women appear to exchange sex for money or other commodities, and a few percentage points of men report sexual contacts with FSWs. Accordingly, commercial sex networks are the largest of the three priority group networks in MENA.

HIV prevalence continues to be at low levels among FSWs in most countries, although at levels much higher than those in the general population. HIV spread does not appear to be well established in many commercial sex networks in the region. In three countries, however, namely Djibouti, Somalia, and Sudan, HIV prevalence among some FSW groups has reached high levels, indicating concentrated HIV epidemics in at least parts of these countries. Nevertheless, HIV prevalence among FSWs in these countries is at lower levels than those found in hyperendemic HIV epidemics in sub-Saharan Africa.

FSWs report considerable levels of sexual risk behavior, including roughly one client per calendar day; low levels of condom use, particularly in areas of concentrated HIV epidemics among FSWs; anal and oral sex in addition to vaginal sex; having clients or sexual partners who inject drugs; and injecting drugs themselves. Considerable levels of STI prevalence other than HIV are found among FSWs. STD (sexually transmitted disease) clinic attendees repeatedly report acquiring STDs through paid sex. Levels of comprehensive HIV knowledge among FSWs vary across the region, with both high and low levels being documented in different settings.

There is a potential for further HIV spread among FSWs, but probably not at high levels in most countries, except possibly for Djibouti, Somalia, and Sudan. Near universal male circumcision, with its efficacy against HIV infection, and the rather lower risk behavior compared to other regions, may prevent massive or even concentrated HIV epidemics among FSWs from materializing in most countries in MENA for at least a decade, if ever, should these conditions persist.

Yet, HIV prevalence among FSWs will be at levels much higher than those of the general population. Subgroups within FSWs may be particularly at high risk of HIV, such as those who inject drugs, have clients who inject drugs, female IDUs who exchange sex for money or drugs, as well as FSWs with low socioeconomic status who have poor HIV knowledge or are not able to afford or negotiate condom use.

FSWs need prevention and care services not only because of HIV infection, but also because of the considerable levels of other STIs in their population. Dedicated STI services for FSWs need to be established, and in settings where they are already established, they need to be expanded.

Potential bridging populations

A sizable fraction of MENA populations belong to what could be labeled as *potential bridging populations*, such as clients of sex workers, other sexual partners of priority populations, truck drivers, fishermen, and military personnel. Evidence on HIV prevalence, other STI prevalence, sexual risk behavior measures, and drug-injecting practices among potential bridging populations remains rather limited. Existing evidence suggests considerable levels of sexual risk behavior among potential bridging populations, but still limited HIV prevalence, except possibly for Djibouti, Somalia, and Sudan.

The limited HIV prevalence among potential bridging populations is probably a consequence of the low HIV prevalence among FSWs and the high coverage of male circumcision among men. In this sense, these populations are not key contributors to the dynamics of HIV infectious spread in MENA and are not effectively bridging populations capable of spreading the infection further to the general population.

An important characteristic of HIV in MENA is the role of the sexual partners of priority populations: they are shouldering a sizable proportion of HIV disease burden, but they rarely transmit the infection further. Women are especially vulnerable because most risk behaviors are practiced by men. HIV prevention efforts in MENA should address this key vulnerability.

General population

HIV prevalence in the general population is at very low levels in all MENA countries, apart from Djibouti, Somalia, and Sudan. There is no evidence of a substantial HIV epidemic in the general population in any of the MENA countries.

Sexual behavior data in the general population in MENA remain rather limited. Existing evidence suggests that sexual risk behaviors are present, but at rather low levels in comparison to other regions. However, levels of sexual risk behavior appear to be increasing, particularly among youth, though probably not to a level that can support an HIV epidemic in the general population. Available sexual risk behavior measures suggest limited potential for a sustainable HIV epidemic in the general population in at least the foreseeable future, if ever, should these conditions persist.

STI prevalence data, including herpes simplex virus type 2 (HSV-2), human papillomavirus (HPV), syphilis, gonorrhea, and chlamydia, indicate low prevalence of these infections among the general population in MENA in comparison to other regions. Unsafe abortions are also at low levels in MENA compared to other regions. These proxy measures of sexual risk behavior imply low levels of risk behavior in the general population and further indicate limited potential for a sustainable HIV epidemic in this part of the population.

Male circumcision is almost universal in MENA and is associated with a strong biological efficacy against HIV infection. This further indicates limited potential for a sustainable HIV epidemic in the general population.

In the other regions around the world, there is no evidence for a sustainable general population HIV epidemic apart from parts of sub-Saharan Africa. It is inconceivable that the MENA region will be the exception to this pattern after consistently very low HIV prevalence in the general population for over two decades since the virus' introduction into MENA in the 1980s. Considering all the evidence reviewed for this report, it is unlikely that the HIV epidemic in MENA will take a course similar to that in sub-Saharan Africa if the existing social and epidemiological context in the region remains largely the same. At most, the region may face up to a few percentage points prevalence in the population of several of its countries. **Still, this would be an immense disease burden and subsequent economic burden in a region that is mostly unprepared for such an epidemic.**

A major unknown in the understanding of the HIV epidemiology in the general population in MENA is that of the levels of recent increases, and future trends, in risk behaviors, particularly among youth. If the increases in risk behavior are substantial, this could put some aspects of the analytical view of the dynamics in question. The trajectory of the HIV epidemic may be different and possibly result in substantial HIV epidemics in MENA populations. Studying the levels of risk behaviors and STI incidence among youth should be a priority for scientific research in MENA.

RECOMMENDATIONS

The recommendations provided here focus on key strategies related to the scope of this report and its emphasis on understanding HIV epide-

miology in MENA as a whole. The recommendations are based on identifying the status of the HIV epidemic in MENA, through this synthesis, as a **low HIV prevalence setting with rising concentrated epidemics among priority populations**. General directions for prevention interventions as warranted by the outcome of this synthesis are also discussed briefly, but are not delineated because they are beyond the scope of this report. This report was not intended to provide intervention recommendations for each MENA country.

Recommendation 1: Increase and expand baseline and continued surveillance

The analytical insights drawn here from a synthesis of thousands of studies and data sources indicate that there is no escape from the necessity of developing robust surveillance systems to monitor HIV spread among priority populations. Inadequate and limited HIV epidemiological and methodological surveillance continue to be one of the most pervasive problems in this region. Effective and repeated surveillance of IDUs, MSM, and FSWs is key in MENA countries to definitively conclude whether HIV spread is indeed limited in priority populations, and to detect epidemics among these groups at an early stage.

Surveillance work should include the mapping of risk and vulnerability factors, risk behavior measures, population size estimations, and, importantly, measurements of HIV prevalence and risk biomarkers, such as STI and HCV prevalence levels. This would offer a window of opportunity to target prevention at an early phase of an epidemic. Monitoring recent infections and examining the nature of exposures could also be useful in detecting emerging endemic transmission chains within MENA populations.

An approach of integrated biobehavioral surveillance surveys (IBBSS) among representative priority populations should be the main component of surveillance efforts, rather than reliance on facility-based surveillance using convenient population samples that are not capturing the dynamics of HIV transmission in MENA. Resources should not be wasted on surveillance among low-risk populations while overlooking HIV spread in priority populations.

Recommendation 2: Expand scientific research and formulate evidence-informed policies

The data synthesis in this report highlights the large gap in methodological scientific research in relation to HIV and other STI epidemiology in MENA. The limited human and financial resources are key challenges in most countries, and these constraints are preventing the region from formulating effective and evidence- informed policies.

The first research priority should be to conduct repeated, multicenter IBBSS studies on priority groups to monitor trends, combining HIV sero-surveillance with STI, HCV, and risk behavior surveillance. These studies also need to explore the network structures among these risk groups, including both sexual and injecting drug networks.

The second priority is research on mapping and size estimation of hard-to-reach priority populations, which are essential for the quantitative assessments of HIV epidemiology and trends, and would help in planning sufficient and more effective prevention strategies and programs.

The third priority is to conduct multicenter cohort or cross-sectional studies among vulnerable populations, such as the youth, to assess trends of HIV and other STI incidence, other infectious disease incidence such as HCV, sexual and injecting drug use risk behaviors, and drivers of risky behavior. With the high rates of population mobility in MENA, it is also a priority to assess levels of risk behavior and infection among migrants because data on this population remain limited, although the socioeconomic context of migration in this region may predispose this population to risky behavior practices.

The fourth priority is to conduct mathematical modeling and cost-effectiveness studies to explore the full range of the complex HIV dynamics and predict intervention impacts in MENA. These studies would build inferences and suggest policy recommendations by using the individual and population level data that will become increasingly available over the next few years from surveillance studies on priority populations.

Recommendation 3: Focus on risk and vulnerability, not on law enforcement

The HIV transmission patterns delineated in this report show that HIV spread is merely a reflection of existing contours of risk and vulnerability in the societies in which it is spreading. HIV cannot be addressed fundamentally except by addressing the underlying causes of these risks and vulnerabilities. HIV spread is not a question of law enforcement to prevent risky behavior. Repressive measures will only complicate prevention efforts and push risky behavior further underground, making it even more difficult to reach these groups with programs. This would not change the vulnerability settings but would deprive MENA governments and their partners from the ability to prevent the epidemic and administer prevention interventions as needed. The "security" approach to HIV policy has already led to documented failures in controlling HIV spread in MENA countries.

Policies, programs, and resources continue to be diverted from where they are needed. The mandatory testing of many population groups at low risk of HIV infection, such as the general population, which is the practice in the region, is disconnected from the epidemiological reality of HIV infection in the region. Some of this testing may also violate basic human rights and is likely not effective from a public health perspective. Efforts need to be prioritized to the contours of risk and vulnerability and focus on priority groups. Recognizing the settings of risks, and implementing effective, evidence- informed interventions, is the only available path for controlling HIV spread in MENA.

Recommendation 4: Strengthen civil society contributions to HIV efforts

A structural weakness of the HIV response in MENA is the meager contribution of nongovernmental organizations (NGOs), community organizations, and people living with HIV (PLHIV) groups in the formulation, planning, and implementation of the response. Strengthening civil society contributions to HIV efforts is essential given the epidemiological reality of HIV transmission being concentrated among largely hidden and stigmatized priority populations, as documented by this synthesis.

There is no escaping the fact that grassroots NGOs need to be developed within the MENA region to support the HIV response. NGOs may be able to help governments deal with priority groups indirectly, thereby avoiding cultural sensitivities in explicit outreach efforts for stigmatized populations. Discreet interventions for HIV prevention have already proven effective in a number of MENA countries.

Recommendation 5: An opportunity for prevention

There is still an open window of opportunity for MENA to control the HIV epidemic. HIV programs involving the general population should stress stigma reduction, while prevention efforts should be focused on priority populations that are at increased risk of HIV infection. Interventions need to capitalize on the strengths represented by cultural traditions, as well as be culturally sensitive, while fostering effective responses to the epidemic. Access to testing, care, and treatment services must be expanded substantially. To impede future HIV transmission, it is imperative to remove all barriers to HIV testing and diagnosis, particularly among priority groups.

There is a need to invest in a comprehensive analysis of the current gaps in the HIV response as well as the promising opportunities. This can be accomplished by combining transmission mode analysis in each country with the mapping of current interventions, including a taxonomy of prevention.

Although countries need to address the structural factors that drive risky behavior practices, the priority in the public health sector should be on addressing the direct factors that put individuals at risk of HIV exposure. Since almost all infections occur when an infected individual shares body fluids with an uninfected individual, prevention programs must focus on addressing the situations in which this is happening. Careful analysis of transmission patterns must be conducted to inform policy decisions.

Beyond doubt, *harm reduction* should be at the core of intervention policy, although targeted prevention should go further than harm reduction. The concept of harm reduction should be applied not only to IDUs, but should also be considered for MSM and FSWs. Harm reduction is the most direct and effective strategy to stem the tide of HIV, considering that addressing the root causes of risks and vulnerabilities might be a much more challenging task. The Islamic Republic of Iran has already paved the way by showing how harm reduction can be implemented within the cultural fabric of MENA and in consonance with religious values.

BIBLIOGRAPHY

Bohannon, J. 2005. "Science in Libya: From Pariah to Science Powerhouse?" *Science* 308: 182–84.

Key Definitions and Abbreviations

KEY DEFINITIONS

Bridging populations

Bridging populations are populations at intermediate risk of exposure to HIV and provide links between the high-risk priority populations and the low-risk general population. Conventionally, bridging populations include groups such as truck drivers, military personnel, sailors, and sexual partners of IDUs, FSWs, and MSM.

General population

The general population is the part of the population that is at relatively low risk of HIV exposure and encompasses most of the population in any community. It is strictly defined here as the total population not belonging to priority or bridging populations.

Priority populations

Priority populations are populations that experience the highest probability of being exposed to HIV infection. Priority populations include IDUs, MSM (including MSWs), and FSWs.

Vulnerable populations

Vulnerable populations form a subset of the general population and generally are at low risk of HIV exposure but are vulnerable to practices that may put them at a higher risk of HIV infection. Vulnerable populations include prisoners, youth, and mobile populations. Once these vulnerable populations adopt higher-risk practices, they become part of the priority or bridging populations.

ABBREVIATIONS

AIDS	Acquired immunodeficiency syndrome
ANC	Antenatal clinic
ART	Antiretroviral therapy
ARV	Antiretroviral
ASR	Age-standardized rates
DHS	Demographic and Health Survey
ELISA	Enzyme-linked immunoassay
EMRO	Eastern Mediterranean Regional Office (World Health Organization)
FBO	Faith-based organization
FHI	Family Health International
FSW	Female sex work(er)
GFATM	Global Fund to Fight AIDS, Tuberculosis, and Malaria
GONGO	Government organized nongovernmental organizations
GST	Group of sustainable transmission
GUD	Genital ulcer disease
HBV	Hepatitis B virus
HCV	Hepatitis C virus

HCWs	Health care workers
HIV	Human immunodeficiency virus
HPV	Human papillomavirus
HSV-1	Herpes simplex virus type 1
HSV-2	Herpes simplex virus type 2
HSW	*Hjira* sex worker
IARC	International Agency for Research on Cancer
IEC	Information, Education, and Communication
IBBSS	Integrated biobehavioral surveillance survey
ICPS	International Centre for Prison Studies
IDPs	Internally displaced persons
IDU	Injecting drug use(r)
INCAS	Iranian National Center for Addiction Studies
IOM	International Organization for Migration
KAP	Knowledge attitudes and practices
MENA	Middle East and North Africa
MENAHRA	MENA Harm Reduction Association
MeSH	Medical subheading
M&E	Monitoring and evaluation
MMT	Methadone maintenance treatment
MOH	Ministry of health
MSM	Men who have sex with men
MSW	Male sex work(er)
NGO	Nongovernmental organization
NSNAC	New Sudan National AIDS Council
NSP	National strategic plan
NSP	Needle and syringe program
OST	Opioid substitution therapy
PITC	Provider initiated testing and counseling
PLHIV	People living with HIV
PMTCT	Prevention of mother-to-child transmission
PRB	Population Reference Bureau
RSA	Rapid situation assessment
RST	Regional Support Team
RTI	Reproductive tract infection
SAR	South Asia Region
SNAP	Sudan National AIDS Programme
STD	Sexually transmitted disease
STI	Sexually transmitted infection
TB	Tuberculosis
UN	United Nations
UNAIDS	Joint United Nations Programme on HIV/AIDS
UNDP	United Nations Development Programme
UNFPA	United Nations Population Fund
UNHCR	United Nations High Commissioner for Refugees
UNICEF	United Nations Children's Fund
UNODC	United Nations Office on Drugs and Crime
UNRWA	United Nations Relief and Works Agency for Palestine Refugees in the Near East
USAID	United States Agency for International Development
VCT	Voluntary counseling and testing
WBA	Western blot assays
WHO	World Health Organization

Characterizing the HIV/AIDS Epidemic in the Middle East and North Africa: Why and How?

BACKGROUND AND RATIONALE FOR THIS REPORT

The human immunodeficiency virus (HIV) pandemic continues as one of the most devastating health crises ever. The Joint United Nations Programme on HIV/AIDS (UNAIDS) and the World Health Organization (WHO) estimate that 35,000 (24,000–46,000) people were infected with HIV within the UNAIDS definition of the Middle East and North Africa (MENA) region[1] in 2008.[2] This brings the total number of people living with HIV (PLHIV) in MENA to 310,000 (250,000–380,000).[3] It is also estimated that 20,000 (15,000–25,000) people died of HIV-related causes in 2008.[4] In appendix A, table A.1 lists the estimated number of PLHIV in a number of MENA countries.

Despite much progress on understanding HIV epidemiology globally, MENA stands out as the only region where knowledge of the epidemic continues to be very limited and subject to much controversy.[5] More than 25 years since the discovery of the HIV virus, no scientific study has provided a comprehensive data-driven synthesis of the HIV infectious spread in this region. The region continues to be viewed as the anomaly in the HIV/AIDS (acquired immunodeficiency syndrome) world map and "a real hole in terms of HIV/AIDS epidemiological data."[6]

This report addresses this dearth of strategic information on HIV infections in MENA through a joint effort by the World Bank, the MENA Regional Support Team (RST) of UNAIDS, and the Eastern Mediterranean Regional Office (EMRO) of WHO. It builds on a series of publications by the World Bank that focus on different aspects of the HIV/AIDS epidemic and response. In 2003, the World Bank, in collaboration with UNAIDS and WHO/EMRO, issued the *HIV/AIDS in the Middle East and North Africa: The Cost of Inaction* report, which provided an analysis of the vulnerability factors in MENA along with an economic analysis of the impact based on the limited HIV data at the time. In 2005, the World Bank issued the *Preventing HIV/AIDS in the Middle East and North Africa: A Window of Opportunity to Act* report, which provided an analysis of a prevention strategy for HIV in MENA. This current report provides the first comprehensive scientific assessment and data-driven epidemiological synthesis of HIV spread in MENA since the beginning of the epidemic. It is based on a literature review and the analysis of thousands of widely unrecognized publications, reports, and data sources extracted from the scientific literature or collected from sources at the local, national, and regional levels.

---

[1] Excluding Afghanistan, the Islamic Republic of Iran, and Pakistan.
[2] UNAIDS and WHO, *AIDS Epidemic Update 2009.*
[3] Ibid.
[4] Ibid.
[5] Obermeyer, "HIV in the Middle East."

[6] Bohannon, "Science in Libya."

Just as in other regions, MENA has several vulnerability factors for HIV. The process of modernization, including mass education and urbanization, known to occur with the abandonment of traditional patterns of behavior,[7] continues in MENA at full throttle. Most countries are experiencing diverse influences including changing family structures, exposure to different cultures, openness of the market, tourism, and enhanced communication and technology, such as satellite television and the Internet.[8] There is a sociocultural transition leading to more tolerance and acceptance of behaviors such as premarital and extramarital sex and increased opportunities for sexual partnerships beyond traditional forms.[9] The cultural tradition of balancing premarital chastity with early marriage is no longer the norm.[10] Social and gender tensions have been exacerbated by the clashing forces of traditional culture and modern culture.[11] There are numerous strains in preserving traditional values during the modernization of society, leading to a communication discrepancy as well as social tension at the community and family levels.

The social determinants of health in terms of political conflict, limited resources, and gender inequity continue to challenge the region.[12] Denial that HIV exists or is an important challenge remains widespread. Priority groups, including injecting drug users (IDUs), female sex workers (FSWs), and men who have sex with men (MSM), are highly stigmatized and lack access to comprehensive and confidential services. Community organizations serving at-risk populations are emerging, but are insufficient to meet current needs and are not well coordinated. Health promotion approaches remain didactic and prescriptive, are divorced from behavioral theory, and are nonparticipatory. There is a lack of evidence-based policies that can guide effective interventions. HIV response in MENA is an amalgam of moralism, pragmatism, and political and regime sensitivities. In the absence of data-driven policies, the HIV response will continue to be beset by numerous challenges.

MENA is distinctively characterized by a "tidal wave" youth bulge; one-fifth of the population, 95 million people,[13] is in the 15–24 years age group,[14] the normal age range of initiation of sexual activities.[15] Extensive levels of migration, displacement, and mobility exist in MENA, which has the highest number of refugees and internally displaced persons in the world.[16] MENA is flooded with inexpensive drugs due to high levels of heroin production in Afghanistan and major drug trade routes that pass through the region.[17] MENA suffers from the high prevalence of unnecessary medical injections and blood transfusions, the reuse of needles and syringes, occupational injuries of health care workers (HCWs), and skin scarifications,[18] suggesting a potential for considerable parenteral HIV transmissions beyond injecting drug use.

The apparent lack of HIV data has fueled an intense, but unnecessary, polemical debate on the status of the epidemic in MENA.[19] Some argued that adherence to cultural values provides "cultural immunity" against HIV spread and that MENA is immune to HIV through its fabric of "moral prophylaxis," including strong prohibitions against premarital and extramarital sex, homosexuality, and alcohol and drug use.[20] Meanwhile, others argued that there is a public health crisis "behind the veil" and that the failure to combat the disease stems from cultural traditions slowing, if not freezing, the ability of MENA societies to deal with the epidemic.[21] This

[7] Carael, Cleland, and Adeokun, "Overview and Selected Findings."

[8] Busulwa, "HIV/AIDS Situation Analysis Study"; Mohammad et al., "Sexual Risk-Taking Behaviors"; Abukhalil, "Gender Boundaries and Sexual Categories in the Arab World."

[9] Busulwa, "HIV/AIDS Situation Analysis Study."

[10] Mohammad et al., "Sexual Risk-Taking Behaviors."

[11] Abukhalil, "Gender Boundaries and Sexual Categories in the Arab World."

[12] Shaar and Larenas, "Social Determinants of Health."

[13] Assaad and Roudi-Fahimi, "Youth in the Middle East and North Africa."

[14] UNAIDS, "Notes on AIDS in the Middle East and North Africa"; Roudi-Fahimi and Ashford, Sexual & Reproductive Health.

[15] Roudi-Fahimi and Ashford, Sexual & Reproductive Health.

[16] UNAIDS, "Notes on AIDS in the Middle East and North Africa."

[17] UNODC, World Drug Report.

[18] Khawaja et al., "HIV/AIDS and Its Risk Factors in Pakistan"; World Bank Group, World Bank Update 2005; Yerly et al., "Nosocomial Outbreak"; Khattab et al., "Report on a Study of Women Living with HIV"; Burans et al., "Serosurvey of Prevalence of Human Immunodeficiency Virus"; Zafar et al., "Knowledge, Attitudes and Practices"; Hossini et al., "Knowledge and Attitudes"; Yemen MOH, National Strategic Framework; Kennedy, O'Reilly, and Mah, "The Use of a Quality-Improvement Approach."

[19] Obermeyer, "HIV in the Middle East."

[20] Khawaja et al., "HIV/AIDS and Its Risk Factors in Pakistan"; Gray, "HIV and Islam;" Lenton, "Will Egypt Escape the AIDS Epidemic?"

[21] Kelley and Eberstadt, "Behind the Veil"; Kelley and Eberstadt, "The Muslim Face of AIDS."

view also stresses that if leaders continue to ignore the problem, HIV/AIDS could debilitate or even destabilize some of MENA societies by its drastic effects on morbidity, mortality, and economic productivity among the 15 to 49 years age group.[22] Neither of these views has been substantiated by the epidemiological data synthesized in this report and both are far from the reality of HIV spread in MENA.

Objective and scope of report

The main objective of this report is to address the dearth of strategic information on HIV in MENA by delineating an evidence-based and data-driven overview of HIV epidemiology and an integrated analysis of HIV transmission trends and dynamics in this region. This report describes the major characteristics and the levels of HIV spread in diverse groups of MENA populations. It also identifies priority population groups with elevated HIV prevalence or risk factors and examines the major explanations for such variations in HIV transmission. The synthesis explores the epidemic potential for further HIV spread by contrasting HIV transmission, risk patterns, and trends in different HIV risk groups.

The ultimate goal of this synthesis is to provide the scientific evidence necessary for strategic prioritization; resource allocation and coverage; and effective, high-quality interventions. To this end, the authors have critically reviewed and interpreted data and studies on HIV/AIDS, sexual and injecting drug risk behaviors, vulnerability settings, sexually transmitted infections (STIs), and hepatitis C virus (HCV).

This report is concerned with an overview of HIV epidemiology in the region as a whole as opposed to country-level analyses. It is not part of the scope of this report to provide intervention recommendations for each MENA country.

CONCEPTUAL FRAMEWORK AND RESEARCH METHODOLOGY

This report uses an evidence-based and data-driven approach to characterize HIV epidemiology and dynamics in the MENA region. The theme of this approach is the synthesis and integrated analysis of multiple sources of data, examined side by side, including biological data, risk behavior data, and proxy measures. The authors examined information collected by different methods, by different groups, and in different populations, and corroborated the conclusions across datasets, thereby minimizing the impact of potential biases that can exist in a single study, dataset, or line of evidence. This approach is especially suited for MENA considering the lack of representation and methodological rigor in a large number of studies.

Conceptual framework for HIV epidemiology

The risk of HIV infection depends on the transmission mode, HIV prevalence, and the behavioral attributes of the population. Human populations exhibit widely variable sexual and injecting drug risk behaviors, a heterogeneity in risk conventionally conceptualized in terms of three population groupings[23] (figure 1.1). The first is the core group, which experiences the highest risk of exposure to HIV. The high-risk core population typically includes IDUs, MSM, and female and male sex workers (MSWs). The second group is the bridging population, which experiences an intermediate risk of exposure and provides links, such as through the clients of sex workers, between the high-risk core group and the third group, which is the low-risk general population.

The general population encompasses most of the population in any community as well as the vulnerable populations, who are generally at a low risk of HIV infection, such as prisoners, youth, and mobile populations, but who are also vulnerable to practices that may put them at higher risk of HIV infection. Once these vulnerable populations adopt higher-risk practices, they become part of the core or bridging populations. Different risk groups for different modes of HIV transmission can overlap, providing opportunities for an infection in one risk group to seed an epidemic in another group. The size and pattern of the epidemic also depend on the manner of mixing between the different risk groups, HIV prevalence in

---

[22] Kelley and Eberstadt, "Behind the Veil"; Kelley and Eberstadt, "The Muslim Face of AIDS."

[23] Low et al., "Global Control."

Figure 1.1 Heterogeneity in Risk of Exposure to a Sexually Transmitted Infection

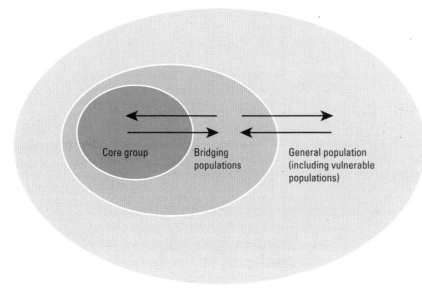

Core group

Bridging populations

General population (including vulnerable populations)

Source: Authors.

the different risk groups, and size of the different risk groups.

The heterogeneity in the spread of HIV or other STIs' spread can be understood analytically in terms of the basic reproductive number (R_0): the number of secondary infections that an index case would generate upon entrance into an infection-free population.[24] For an infection to spread, R_0 needs to be larger than one (figure 1.2, panel A). If $R_0 < 1$, the number of secondary infections each index case produces is on average less than one and the infection cannot sustain itself and dies out (figure 1.2, panel B). R_0 for a specific population depends on the risk behavior attributes of this population and duration of infection, as well as the transmission probability per coital act. The last can be influenced by a number of biological factors such as stage of HIV infection,[25] male circumcision status,[26] and coinfections.[27]

Since sexual risk behavior and injecting drug use are characterized by substantial heterogeneity, each risk group in the population has its own R_0. HIV or other STIs can be sustainable

and endemic in some risk groups (such as FSWs) while being below the sustainability threshold in other groups.[28] In the latter groups, STIs can still spread, but the transmission chains are not sustainable and eventually face "dead ends." This variability in risk leads to the group of sustainable transmission (GST)[29] concept, where the GST for a specific STI is the population where the infection's transmission chains are sustainable ($R_0 > 1$). The size of the GST in any community determines the potential size of the STI epidemic, and different STIs have different GST sizes (see appendix B, table B.1).

HIV spreads most rapidly in the high-risk core populations due to the higher levels of risk behavior, implying an R_0 considerably larger than one. Therefore, IDUs, MSM, and FSWs are normally the groups that first experience the burden of the HIV epidemic (figure 1.3). Subsequently, HIV spreads to the bridging populations (sexual partners of core populations). Bridging groups may or may not pass the infection to the general population. If bridging populations do pass the infection to the general population, then the levels of risk behavior in the latter population would determine the potential for a general population HIV epidemic. If the levels of risk are sufficiently high, such that $R_0 > 1$, then the infectious transmission chains are sustainable among the general population irrespective of further sexual contacts with core and bridging populations (figure 1.3, panel A). HIV will remain endemic in the general population even if all sexual contacts with core and bridging populations are protected or stopped. This is what has occurred in parts of sub-Saharan Africa, resulting in massive HIV epidemics.

On the other hand, if $R_0 < 1$, the HIV transmission chains are not sustainable, and the waves of HIV spread in the general population would stop shortly after entering this population

[24] Anderson and May, *Infectious Diseases of Humans.*

[25] Wawer et al., "Rates of HIV-1 Transmission."

[26] Auvert et al., "Randomized, Controlled Intervention Trial"; Bailey et al., "Male Circumcision for HIV Prevention"; Gray et al., "Male Circumcision for HIV Prevention."

[27] Abu-Raddad et al., "Genital Herpes"; Abu-Raddad, Patnaik, and Kublin, "Dual Infection with HIV and Malaria."

[28] Boily and Masse, "Mathematical Models"; Brunham and Plummer, "A General Model"; Yorke, Hethcote, and Nold, "Dynamics and Control."

[29] Abu-Raddad et al., "Genital Herpes"; Boily and Masse, "Mathematical Models"; Brunham and Plummer, "A General Model."

(figure 1.3, panel B). It is then unlikely that the HIV spread in the whole population would reach the massive scale it reached in sub-Saharan Africa, and the dynamics of HIV will be concentrated in the core and bridging populations, as is the case in Asia.[30] HIV infection could not then be endemic in the general population and would die out if all sexual contacts with core and bridging populations are protected or stopped. Figure 1.3 shows a schematic diagram contrasting a general population HIV epidemic versus a concentrated HIV epidemic in the core populations.

As shown below in our discussion of HIV spread in the different risk groups in MENA, the role of the general population in the HIV epidemics in MENA is very limited. HIV dynamics are mostly concentrated in the core populations of IDUs, MSM, and FSWs; therefore, these core populations are labeled in this report as *priority populations* to signify that these are the groups where curtailing HIV spread to below sustainability ($R_0 < 1$) would control the HIV epidemic in the whole population. Priority populations are the key populations for focusing HIV prevention efforts.

The conceptual framework delineated above will be adapted to help understand the dynamics of HIV infectious spread in MENA and the prospects for HIV infection expansion in different populations. The priority (core), bridging, and general populations will be defined within the context of MENA and the levels of risk will be delineated by the synthesis approach. This assessment will help facilitate a qualitative determination of the epidemic potential for each risk group and the potential for sustainable transmission in the general population. The synthesis also facilitates a determination of the phases of the HIV epidemics in MENA

Figure 1.2 Schematic Diagram of the Concept of R_0

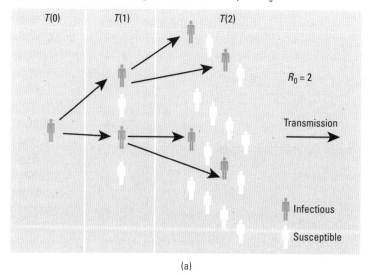

(a)

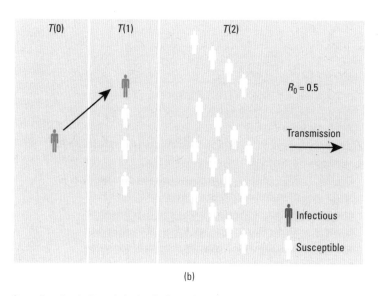

(b)

Source: Reproduced with permission from Dr. Ruanne Barnabas, Fred Hutchinson Cancer Research Center, Seattle, Washington, USA.

Note: If $R_0 > 1$, the infection's transmission chains in the population are sustainable and the infection would spread. If $R_0 < 1$, the infection's transmission chains are not sustainable and the infection does not have the "critical mass" to spread in the population. T(i) denotes the generation number of infection transmission.

and the degree of HIV penetration in the populations where it is self-sustainable.

One of the challenges of behavioral research in MENA is desirability bias.[31] Although such bias is documented in all regions for both sexual behavior[32] and injecting drug use,[33] the higher

[30] Commission on AIDS in Asia, *Redefining AIDS in Asia*.

[31] Lee and Renzetti, "The Problems of Researching Sensitive Topics."
[32] Lee and Renzetti, "The Problems of Researching Sensitive Topics"; Caldwell and Quiggin, "The Social Context of AIDS"; Wadsworth et al., "Methodology of the National Survey."
[33] Latkin and Vlahov, "Socially Desirable Response Tendency."

Figure 1.3 Two Patterns of HIV Infectious Spread in a Population

Flow of HIV infection in a general population HIV epidemic

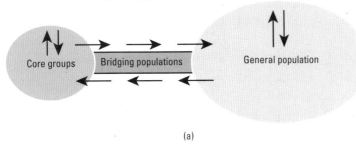

(a)

Flow of HIV infection in a concentrated HIV epidemic

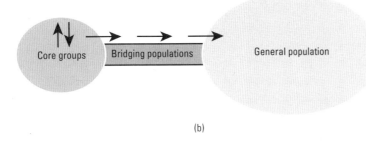

(b)

Source: Authors.

sensitivity of sexual and injecting attitudes and practices in conservative cultures, such as in MENA, adds a further limitation to behavioral research.[34] Individuals may find it difficult to report their true risk practices. Furthermore, it is often not possible to ask explicit questions about sexual behavior, particularly to women. Asking a general question such as "did you have a sexual contact" may lead to an affirmative answer for the wrong reason, because what is defined for these women as a sexual contact may be merely kissing.[35] Hence, in addition to reviewing HIV biological measures and risk behavior measures, this report also reviews the evidence for biological markers of risk behavior, including HCV infection prevalence for injecting drug users and STI prevalence, such as that of herpes simplex virus type 2 (HSV-2), for the sexually active populations. These proxy measures can gauge different aspects of the levels of risk behavior in the population and complement and validate reported levels of risk behavior.

---

[34] Tehrani and Malek-Afzalip, "Knowledge, Attitudes and Practices."
[35] Hajiabdolbaghi et al., "Insights from a Survey of Sexual Behavior."

Countries covered in this report

This report covers all countries that are included in the definition for the MENA Region at the World Bank, the UNAIDS MENA Regional Support Team (RST), and the Eastern Mediterranean Regional Office (EMRO) of WHO. Explicitly, this report includes data on Afghanistan, Algeria, Bahrain, Djibouti, the Arab Republic of Egypt, the Islamic Republic of Iran, Iraq, Jordan, Kuwait, Lebanon, Libya, Morocco, Oman, Pakistan, Qatar, Saudi Arabia, Somalia, Sudan, the Syrian Arab Republic, Tunisia, the United Arab Emirates, the West Bank and Gaza, and the Republic of Yemen. Considering similarity in the cultural context and geographic proximity, data were also occasionally included for Israel (mainly among Israeli Arabs), Mauritania, and Turkey, when appropriate, bearing in mind that there are still differences in the epidemiological context between these countries and MENA countries.

Reflecting the availability of data at the country level, this report included more data from some countries than others. It is by no means an attempt to single out specific countries as opposed to others. The scale of HIV efforts is highly heterogeneous in the region and the level of willingness to share or report confidential data varies from one country to another.

Research methodology

The research methodology consists of an evidence-based epidemiological synthesis and analysis to characterize HIV epidemiology and assess HIV epidemic potential. This is achieved by identifying, collecting, reviewing, and analyzing extensive literature to establish the epidemiological risk factors, determine the nature and phases of HIV epidemics, delineate the populations affected, analyze proxy measures, and understand the vulnerabilities and drivers of the epidemic in the MENA context.

Identified and reviewed data sources

In preparing this report, the following publications, reports, and data sources were identified and reviewed, and their evidence synthesized:

1. Scientific literature identified through a Medline (PubMed) search for the topics covered in this project using a strategy with both free text and medical subheadings (MeSH). No language or year limitation was imposed. The literature review included searches for HIV infectious spread, sexual behavior, HSV-2 prevalence, human papillomavirus (HPV) and cervical cancer prevalence, bacterial STI prevalence, and HCV prevalence. The details of the search criteria are listed in appendix B. More than 3,900 literature sources were examined in this search.

2. Scientific literature on HIV, STIs, and HCV in peer-reviewed publications published in local and regional research journals not indexed in PubMed, but identified through the use of Google Scholar.

3. Thousands of country-level reports and datasources, governmental studies and publications, nongovernmental organizations' (NGOs) studies and publications, and other institutional reports related to HIV in MENA. These reports were obtained from their sources or through contacts facilitated by UNAIDS, WHO, and the World Bank.

4. Hundreds of international organizations' reports and databases, covering a multitude of issues related to HIV infectious spread such as point-prevalence surveys; vulnerabilities; social studies; cervical cancer incidence and mortality rates at surveillance sites and at country levels; injecting drug use prevalence and trends and drug trade patterns; imprisonment rates; demographic and socioeconomic trends; and migration, refugees, and internally displaced persons. The organizations from which data were obtained include UNAIDS, WHO, the World Bank, the United Nations Children's Fund (UNICEF), the United Nations Office on Drugs and Crime (UNODC), the International Agency for Research on Cancer (IARC), the International Organization for Migration (IOM), the International Centre for Prison Studies (ICPS), the Office of the UN High Commissioner for Refugees (UNHCR), the Population Reference Bureau (PRB), and Family Health International (FHI).

5. Demographic and Health Survey (DHS) reports of MENA countries including Egypt, Jordan, Mauritania, Morocco, Sudan, Tunisia, and the Republic of Yemen. The utility of these reports was determined in terms of measures such as HIV knowledge, prevalence of symptoms of sexually transmitted diseases (STDs), and condom use among other behavioral and demographic measures.

6. An extensive WHO/EMRO database of notified HIV/AIDS cases and surveillance reports.

7. Consultations with key experts, public health officials, researchers, and academics in the region and beyond.

Nature of HIV/AIDS epidemiological evidence in MENA

This synthesis has highlighted the following characteristics of existing HIV/AIDS epidemiological evidence:

1. There is actually a considerable amount of epidemiological data on HIV/AIDS in MENA, contrary to the widely accepted perception of very limited data.

2. In addition to large sums of data published in peer-reviewed scientific literature, there are hundreds of studies that have never been published in scientific publications and are not easily or widely accessible. A large sum of data and studies continue to be disseminated within small circles at the national and regional levels in the form of confidential and nonconfidential reports, unpublished data, and news articles.

3. Data are fragmented, amorphous, and lack integration. The nature of evidence is best exemplified by *shattered glass*. Thousands of studies and point-prevalence surveys are fragmented and distributed among a multitude of stakeholders at the local, national, and regional levels with no coherent synthesis, analysis, or integration.

4. Large sums of data have never been methodically studied or analyzed. Valuable data such as HIV, STI, and HCV point-prevalence surveys among different general population groups, vulnerable population groups, and priority groups can be found in hundreds

of periodic country reports and case notifications.

5. The large sums of available data are not necessarily representative of the populations that they are supposed to represent and are often not collected using standard and accepted surveillance methodologies. A large fraction of data originates from facility-based surveillance on convenient samples of the population. It is often not clear whether internationally accepted ethical guidelines for human subject research were strictly followed while conducting the studies.

Limitations of this synthesis

Epidemiologic evidence in MENA varies substantially in quality. Although the quality of point-prevalence surveys in MENA has been steadily improving, a proportion of the data reported here are gleaned from point-prevalence surveys not conducted using standard methodology and internationally accepted guidelines for HIV sentinel surveillance and population-based surveys. In this report, an HIV point-prevalence survey refers to a measurement of HIV prevalence: the proportion of a population infected in a population sample consisting of a number of individuals identified with a common attribute. Although limited-quality point-prevalence surveys provide useful data, they may not be representative of the populations they are supposed to represent.[36] In this regard it must be stressed that all data reported here for any population group represent only the population sample on which the study was conducted. **The reported measures should not be generalized to represent the whole population group in any given country. Whenever data are cited in this report, the citation refers to a very specific, studied population sample.**

This report found that scientific papers published in peer-reviewed publications provided the best empirical evidence. Reports and studies on HIV not published in scientific journals tended to vary in quality and value, with the best reports and studies conducted or commissioned by international organizations such as UNAIDS, WHO, and the World Bank. Many MENA countries report their notified HIV/AIDS cases and other HIV-related data to the WHO/EMRO Regional Database on HIV/AIDS, but the representativeness of these data could not be evaluated because countries did not report consistently over time and a description of data collection methodologies was not usually included in their reports.

The authors of this report elected to use all available data sources in the synthesis while paying special attention to data sources that may be questionable on methodological grounds. The synthesis factored in the limited representation of some of the data in the analyses and conclusions. The different data sources, irrespective of their representativeness or reliability, have generally converged on a consistent picture of HIV epidemiology that is delineated throughout this report.

BIBLIOGRAPHY

Abukhalil, A. 1997. "Gender Boundaries and Sexual Categories in the Arab World." *Fem Issues* 15: 91–104.

Abu-Raddad, L. J., A. S. Magaret, C. Celum, A. Wald, I. M. Longini, S. G. Self, and L. Corey. 2008. "Genital Herpes Has Played a More Important Role Than Any Other Sexually Transmitted Infection in Driving HIV Prevalence in Africa." *PLoS ONE* 3: e2230.

Abu-Raddad, L. J., P. Patnaik, and J. G. Kublin. 2006. "Dual Infection with HIV and Malaria Fuels the Spread of Both Diseases in Sub-Saharan Africa." *Science* 314: 1603–6.

Anderson, R. M., and R. M. May. 1991. *Infectious Diseases of Humans: Dynamics and Control*. Oxford: Oxford University Press.

Assaad R., and F. Roudi-Fahimi. 2007. "Youth in the Middle East and North Africa: Demographic Opportunity or Challenge?" Population Reference Bureau, Washington, DC.

Auvert, B., D. Taljaard, E. Lagarde, J. Sobngwi-Tambekou, R. Sitta, and A. Puren. 2005. "Randomized, Controlled Intervention Trial of Male Circumcision for Reduction of HIV Infection Risk: The ANRS 1265 Trial." *PLoS Med* 2: e298.

Bailey, R. C., S. Moses, C. B. Parker, K. Agot, I. Maclean, J. N. Krieger, C. F. M. Williams, R. T. Campbell, and J. O. Ndinya-Achola. 2007. "Male Circumcision for HIV Prevention in Young Men in Kisumu, Kenya: A Randomised Controlled Trial." *Lancet* 369: 643–56.

Bohannon, J. 2005. "Science in Libya: From Pariah to Science Powerhouse?" *Science* 308: 182–84.

Boily, M. C., and B. Masse. 1997. "Mathematical Models of Disease Transmission: A Precious Tool for the

---

[36] Pisani et al., "HIV Surveillance."

Study of Sexually Transmitted Diseases." *Can J Public Health* 88: 255–65.

Brunham, R. C., and F. A. Plummer. 1990. "A General Model of Sexually Transmitted Disease Epidemiology and Its Implications for Control." *Med Clin North Am* 74: 1339–52.

Burans, J. P., M. McCarthy, S. M. el Tayeb, A. el Tigani, J. George, R. Abu-Elyazeed, and J. N. Woody. 1990. "Serosurvey of Prevalence of Human Immunodeficiency Virus amongst High Risk Groups in Port Sudan, Sudan." *East Afr Med J* 67: 650–55.

Busulwa, R. 2003. "HIV/AIDS Situation Analysis Study." Conducted in Hodeidah, Taiz, and Hadhramut, Republic of Yemen.

Caldwell, C., and P. Quiggin. 1989. "The Social Context of AIDS in Sub-Saharan Africa." *Population and Development Review* 15: 185–234.

Carael, M., J. Cleland, and L. Adeokun. 1991. "Overview and Selected Findings of Sexual Behaviour Surveys." *AIDS* 5 Suppl 1: S65–74.

Commission on AIDS in Asia. 2008. *Redefining AIDS in Asia: Crafting an Effective Response*. New Delhi, India: Oxford University Press. Presented to Ban Ki-moon, UN Secretary General, on March 26, 2008.

Gray, P. B. 2004. "HIV and Islam: Is HIV Prevalence Lower among Muslims?" *Soc Sci Med* 58: 1751–56.

Gray, R. H., G. Kigozi, D. Serwadda, F. Makumbi, S. Watya, F. Nalugoda, N. Kiwanuka, L. H. Moulton, M. A. Chaudhary, M. Z. Chen, N. K. Sewankambo, F. Wabwire-Mangen, M. C. Bacon, C. F. M. Williams, P. Opendi, S. J. Reynolds, O. Laeyendecker, T. C. Quinn, and M. J. Wawer. 2007. "Male Circumcision for HIV Prevention in Men in Rakai, Uganda: A Randomised Trial." *Lancet* 369: 657–66.

Hajiabdolbaghi, M., N. Razani, N. Karami, P. Kheirandish, M. Mohraz, M. Rasoolinejad, K. Arefnia, Z. Kourorian, G. Rutherford, and W. McFarland. 2007. "Insights from a Survey of Sexual Behavior among a Group of At-Risk Women in Tehran, Iran, 2006." *AIDS Educ Prev* 19: 519–30.

Hossini, C. H., D. Tripodi, A. E. Rahhali, M. Bichara, D. Betito, J. P. Curtes, and C. Verger. 2000. "Knowledge and Attitudes of Health Care Professionals with Respect to AIDS and the Risk of Occupational Transmission of HIV in 2 Moroccan Hospitals." *Sante* 10: 315–21.

Kelley, L., and N. Eberstadt. 2005a. "Behind the Veil of a Public Health Crisis: HIV/AIDS in the Muslim World." National Bureau of Asian Research (NBR) Special Report, Seattle, Washington.

———. 2005b. "The Muslim Face of AIDS." *Foreign Policy* 149: 42–48.

Kennedy, M., D. O'Reilly, and M. W. Mah. 1998. "The Use of a Quality-Improvement Approach to Reduce Needlestick Injuries in a Saudi Arabian Hospital." *Clin Perform Qual Health Care* 6: 79–83.

Khattab, H. A. S., M. A. Gineidy, N. Shorbagui, and N. Elnahal. 2007. "Report on a Study of Women Living with HIV." Egyptian Society for Population Studies and Reproductive Health.

Khawaja, Z. A., L. Gibney, A. J. Ahmed, and S. H. Vermund. 1997. "HIV/AIDS and Its Risk Factors in Pakistan." *AIDS* 11: 843–48.

Latkin, C. A., and D. Vlahov. 1998. "Socially Desirable Response Tendency as a Correlate of Accuracy of Self-Reported HIV Serostatus for HIV Seropositive Injection Drug Users." *Addiction* 93: 1191–97.

Lee, R. M., and C. M. Renzetti. 1990. "The Problems of Researching Sensitive Topics." *American Behavioral Scientist* 33: 510–28.

Lenton, C. 1997. "Will Egypt Escape the AIDS Epidemic?" *Lancet* 349: 1005.

Low, N., N. Broutet, Y. Adu-Sarkodie, P. Barton, M. Hossain, and S. Hawkes. 2006. "Global Control of Sexually Transmitted Infections." *Lancet* 368: 2001–16.

Mohammad, K., F. K. Farahani, M. R. Mohammadi, S. Alikhani, M. Zare, F. R. Tehrani, A. Ramezankhani, A. Hasanzadeh, and H. Ghanbari. 2007. "Sexual Risk-Taking Behaviors among Boys Aged 15–18 Years in Tehran." *J Adolesc Health* 41: 407–14.

Obermeyer, C. M. 2006. "HIV in the Middle East." *BMJ* 333: 851–54.

Pisani, E., S. Lazzari, N. Walker, and B. Schwartlander. 2003. "HIV Surveillance: A Global Perspective." *J Acquir Immune Defic Syndr* 32 Suppl 1: S3–11.

Roudi-Fahimi, F., and L. Ashford. 2008. *Sexual & Reproductive Health in the Middle East and North Africa: A Guide for Reporters*. Population Reference Bureau, Washington, DC.

Shaar, A. N., and J. Larenas. 2005. "Social Determinants of Health." Palestine Country Paper, World Health Organization.

Tehrani, F. R., and H. Malek-Afzalip. 2008. "Knowledge, Attitudes and Practices concerning HIV/AIDS among Iranian At-Risk Sub-Populations." *Eastern Mediterranean Health Journal* 14.

UNAIDS (Joint United Nations Programme on HIV/AIDS). 2008. "Notes on AIDS in the Middle East and North Africa." RST, MENA.

UNAIDS, and WHO (World Health Organization). 2009. *AIDS Epidemic Update 2009*. Geneva.

UNODC (United Nations Office on Drugs and Crime). 2007. *World Drug Report*. New York.

Wadsworth, J., J. Field, A. M. Johnson, S. Bradshaw, and K. Wellings. 1993. "Methodology of the National Survey of Sexual Attitudes and Lifestyles." *J R Stat Soc Ser A Stat Soc* 156: 407–21.

Wawer, M. J., R. H. Gray, N. K. Sewankambo, D. Serwadda, X. Li, O. Laeyendecker, N. Kiwanuka, G. Kigozi, M. Kiddugavu, T. Lutalo, F. Nalugoda, F. Wabwire-Mangen, M. P. Meehan, and T. C. Quinn. 2005. "Rates of HIV-1 Transmission per Coital Act, by Stage of HIV-1 Infection, in Rakai, Uganda." *J Infect Dis* 191: 1403–9.

World Bank Group. 2005. "*World Bank Update 2005: HIV/AIDS in Pakistan*." Washington, DC.

Yemen MOH (Ministry of Health). Unknown. *National Strategic Framework for the Control and Prevention of HIV/AIDS in the Republic of Yemen*.

Yerly, S., R. Quadri, F. Negro, K. P. Barbe, J. J. Cheseaux, P. Burgisser, C. A. Siegrist, and L. Perrin. 2001. "Nosocomial Outbreak of Multiple Bloodborne Viral Infections." *J Infect Dis* 184: 369–72.

Yorke, J. A., H. W. Hethcote, and A. Nold. 1978. "Dynamics and Control of the Transmission of Gonorrhea." *Sex Transm Dis* 5: 51–56.

Zafar, A., N. Aslam, N. Nasir, R. Meraj, and V. Mehraj. 2008. "Knowledge, Attitudes and Practices of Health Care Workers regarding Needle Stick Injuries at a Tertiary Care Hospital in Pakistan." *J Pak Med Assoc* 58: 57–60.

Chapter 2

Injecting Drug Users and HIV

This chapter focuses on the biological evidence for the extent of human immunodeficiency virus (HIV) spread among injecting drug users (IDUs), the behavioral evidence for risky injection and sexual practices among this population group, and the context of injecting drug use in the Middle East and North Africa (MENA).

HIV PREVALENCE AMONG IDUs

Injecting drug use is one of the leading modes of HIV transmission and accounts for about 10% of HIV/AIDS (acquired immunodeficiency syndrome) cases worldwide.[1] HIV has been documented among IDUs in at least half of the MENA countries,[2] and there is robust evidence of concentrated epidemics among IDUs in the Islamic Republic of Iran and Pakistan.[3] IDU has been documented as the dominant transmission mode in the Islamic Republic of Iran (more than 67% of cases)[4] and Libya (as much as 90%).[5] Of the 570 new infections reported in 2000 in Libya, almost all were among IDUs.[6] IDU is also a significant mode of transmission for HIV in Afghanistan,[7] Bahrain,[8]

Kuwait,[9] Oman,[10] Pakistan,[11] and Tunisia.[12] IDU has also contributed substantially to the epidemics in Algeria and Morocco.[13]

Table 2.1 contains the results of available HIV point-prevalence surveys of IDUs in MENA. HIV prevalence varies across and within countries, and observed levels of prevalence are not dissimilar to those observed in other regions.[14] The data suggest that HIV prevalence among IDUs in MENA countries is in the low to intermediate range compared to other countries around the world.[15] Globally, HIV prevalence ranges at the country level from below 0.01% in eight countries to 72.1% in Estonia.[16]

In what appears to be the first HIV incidence study in MENA, HIV incidence was measured among IDUs in detention in the Islamic Republic of Iran and found to be at a very high level of 16.8% per person-year.[17]

HIV biological data suggest that HIV has established itself among at least a number of IDU populations in several MENA countries.

---

[1] UNAIDS and WHO, *AIDS Epidemic Update 2003.*
[2] UNAIDS and WHO, *AIDS Epidemic Update 2002.*
[3] UNAIDS, "Notes on AIDS in the Middle East and North Africa."
[4] Iran Center for Disease Management, "AIDS/HIV Surveillance Report."
[5] UNAIDS and WHO, *AIDS Epidemic Update 2001.*
[6] Ibid.
[7] Todd et al., "HIV, Hepatitis C, and Hepatitis B."
[8] Al-Haddad, Baig, and Ebrahim, "Epidemiology of HIV and AIDS in Bahrain."

[9] UNAIDS and WHO, *AIDS Epidemic Update 2005.*
[10] Ibid.
[11] Shah et al., "An Outbreak of HIV Infection"; UNAIDS and WHO, *AIDS Epidemic Update 2005;* Rai et al., "HIV/AIDS in Pakistan"; Bokhari et al., "HIV Risk in Karachi and Lahore, Pakistan."
[12] UNAIDS and WHO, *AIDS Epidemic Update 2003;* UNAIDS and WHO, *AIDS Epidemic Update 2007.*
[13] Ibid.
[14] Aceijas et al., "Global Overview."
[15] Mathers et al., "Global Epidemiology."
[16] Ibid.
[17] Jahani et al., "HIV Seroconversion."

Table 2.1 HIV Prevalence among IDUs in MENA

Country	Surveys' results for HIV prevalence among IDUs
Afghanistan	0.0% (World Bank 2008) 3.0% (Todd et al. 2007; Sanders-Buell et al. 2007) 3.4% (Mathers et al. 2008)
Algeria	11.0% (self-reported; Mimouni and Remaoun 2006; Algeria MOH [unknown])
Bahrain	0.0%–2.3% (Aceijas et al. 2004) 21.1% (Al-Haddad et al. 1994) 0.3% (Mathers et al. 2008)
Egypt, Arab Republic of	0.15% (drug addicts; Watts et al. 1993) 0.0% (El-Ghazzawi, Hunsmann, and Schneider 1987) 0.0% (Baqi et al. 1998) 0.0% (Aceijas et al. 2004) 0.0% (Saleh et al. 2000; El-Ghazzawi et al. 1995) 0.6% (Egypt MOH and Population National AIDS Program 2006) 2.55% (Mathers et al. 2008)
Iran, Islamic Republic of	1.2% (Khani and Vakili 2003) 4.0% (Ministry of Health and Medical Education of Iran 2004) 0.9% (injecting and noninjecting drug users; Alizadeh et al. 2005) 7.0% (incarcerated IDUs; Rahbar, Rooholamini, and Khoshnood 2004) 0.0% (treatment center; Rahbar, Rooholamini, and Khoshnood 2004) 63.0% (up to, in prisons; UNAIDS and WHO 2003) 30.0% (local prison; Nassirimanesh 2002) 6.9% (incarcerated IDUs; Rahbar, Rooholamini, and Khoshnood 2004) 22.0% (newly admitted IDUs to prison; Farhoudi et al. 2003) 24.0% (resident incarcerated IDUs in prison; Farhoudi et al. 2003) 24.4% (incarcerated IDUs; Jahani et al. 2009) 0.8% (Khani and Vakili 2003) 15.2% (Zamani et al. 2005) 23.2% (Zamani et al. 2006) 5.4% (noninjecting drug users; Zamani et al. 2005) 72.0% (a rural population of highly selected IDUs; Mojtahedzadeh et al. 2008) 1.4% (mainly noninjecting drug users; Talaie et al. 2007) 15.0% (Mathers et al. 2008)
Iraq	0.0% (prior to occupation; Aceijas et al. 2004)
Jordan	4.2% (Aceijas et al. 2004)
Kuwait	0.0% (Aceijas et al. 2004)
Lebanon	7.8% (Aceijas et al. 2004) 0.0% (Mishwar 2008)
Libya	0.5% (UNAIDS 2002b) 59.4% (Groterah 2002) 49.0% (up to; UNAIDS and WHO 2003) 22.0% (Mathers et al. 2008)
Oman	5.0% (Aceijas et al. 2004; Tawilah and Tawil 2001) 12.0% (IDUs under treatment; Oman MOH 2006) 18.0% (IDUs outside of prison and not under treatment; Oman MOH 2006) 27.0% (incarcerated IDUs; Oman MOH 2006) 11.8% (Mathers et al. 2008)
Morocco	6.5% (self-reported; Mathers et al. 2008) 1.6% (Alami 2009) 0.0% (Morocco MOH 2007)
Pakistan	0.0% (Iqbal and Rehan 1996) 0.0% (Kuo et al. 2006) 0.0% (Khawaja et al. 1997) 0.63% (Altaf et al. 2004)

Table 2.1 *(Continued)*

Country	Surveys' results for HIV prevalence among IDUs
	1.77% (Khawaja et al. 1997)
	0.4% (Parviz et al. 2006)
	9.7% (Shah et al. 2004)
	9.3% (Sindh AIDS Control Program 2004; Ur Rehman, Emmanuel, and Akhtar 2007)
	26.3% (Pakistan National AIDS Control Program 2005b)
	24.0% (Achakzai, Kassi, and Kasi 2007)
	0.5% (Bokhari et al. 2007)
	23.1% (UNAIDS and WHO 2005; Rai et al. 2007; Bokhari et al. 2007)
	10.8% (average of different cities with a range of 0.3%–25.4%; Pakistan National AIDS Control Program 2005a)
	15.8% (average of different cities with a range of 0%–51.8%; Pakistan National AIDS Control Program (2006–07)
	20.8% (average of different cities with a range of 12.3%–28.5%; Pakistan National AIDS Control Program 2008)
	2.6% (Platt et al. 2009)
	0.0% (Platt et al. 2009)
	10.8% (Mathers et al. 2008)
Saudi Arabia	0.15% (Njoh and Zimmo 1997b)
	0.14% (Mathers et al. 2008)
Sudan	0.0% (Mathers et al. 2008)
Syrian Arab Republic	0.3% (Aceijas et al. 2004)
	0.5% (51% of sample are IDUs; Syria Mental Health Directorate 2008)
Tunisia	0.3% (Aceijas et al. 2004; Mathers et al. 2008)
Turkey	2.65% (Mathers et al. 2008)

HEPATITIS C PREVALENCE AS A PROXY MARKER OF RISKY BEHAVIOR AMONG IDUs

HIV is only one of several blood-borne infections that can be transmitted through IDU. Hepatitis C virus (HCV) is a classical infection transmitted predominantly through percutaneous exposures and therefore can be used as a proxy of risky drug-injecting practices. IDUs form the leading risk group for HCV infection.[18] HCV, however, is about six times as infectious as HIV through the parenteral route.[19] Substantial presence of HCV infection in an IDU population does not necessarily imply that HIV is destined to have substantial prevalence in this population. Nevertheless, a high HCV prevalence in an IDU population suggests the potential for HIV transmission along the same route that HCV has traveled because both infections share the same transmission mode.

Table 2.2 describes the results of the available HCV point-prevalence surveys of IDUs in MENA. HCV prevalence levels are generally in the inter-mediate to high range compared to those reported in other regions.[20] This confirms the potential for HIV to spread if HIV enters IDU networks and suggests that the use of nonsterile injecting equipment is a common practice. Recent and rapidly growing HIV epidemics documented among IDUs in Pakistan,[21] following many years of low HIV prevalence,[22] validate this conjecture. It bears notice that there is low awareness of HCV infection in MENA despite its seriousness. Only 20% of IDUs in Pakistan were aware of the existence of HCV, but 85% knew of the existence of HIV.[23]

PREVALENCE OF DRUG INJECTION

The prevalence of IDU in MENA, at 0.2% of the population, is in the intermediate range compared

---

[18] Ray Kim, "Global Epidemiology."

[19] Goldmann, "Blood-Borne Pathogens and Nosocomial Infections"; Gerberding, "Management of Occupational Exposures."

[20] Sy and Jamal, "Epidemiology of Hepatitis C Virus (HCV) Infection."

[21] Shah et al., "An Outbreak of HIV Infection"; UNAIDS and WHO, *AIDS Epidemic Update 2005*; Rai et al., "HIV/AIDS in Pakistan"; Bokhari et al., "HIV Risk in Karachi and Lahore, Pakistan."

[22] Baqi et al., "HIV Antibody Seroprevalence"; Altaf et al., "Harm Reduction"; Parviz et al., "Background Demographics and Risk Behaviors"; UNODCP, "Baseline Study"; Agha et al., "Socio-Economic and Demographic Factors."

[23] Kuo et al., "High HCV Seroprevalence."

Table 2.2 HCV Prevalence among IDUs in MENA

Country	Survey results for HCV prevalence among IDUs
Afghanistan	36.6% (Todd et al. 2007)
Egypt, Arab Republic of	63.0% (Saleh et al. 2000; El-Ghazzawi et al. 1995)
Iran, Islamic Republic of	30.0% (injecting and noninjecting drug users; Alizadeh et al. 2005) 60.0% (Rahbar, Rooholamini, and Khoshnood 2004) 52.0% (Zamani et al. 2007) 59.4% (incarcerated IDUs; Rahbar, Rooholamini, and Khoshnood 2004) 78.0% (local prison; Nassirimanesh 2002) 47.4% (Khani and Vakili 2003) 45.3% (Zali et al. 2001) 11.2% (Imani et al. 2008) 14.48% (mainly noninjecting drug users; Talaie et al. 2007) 25.4% (Altaf et al. 2009) 19.2% (Altaf et al. 2009)
Lebanon	< 20.0% (Aceijas and Rhodes 2007) 25.0% (HIV infected; Ramia et al. 2004) 49.0% (Mishwar 2008) 80.0% (incarcerated IDUs; Kheirandish et al. 2009) 7.35% (injecting and noninjecting drug users; Mohammad et al. 2003)
Oman	11%–53% (Oman MOH 2006)
Pakistan	88.0% (Kuo et al. 2006) 89.0% (UNODCP and UNAIDS 1999) 60.0% (Achakzai, Kassi, and Kasi 2007) 87.0% (Pakistan National AIDS Control Program 2005c) 91.0% (Pakistan National AIDS Control Program 2005c) 17.3% (Platt et al. 2009) 8.0% (Platt et al. 2009)
Saudi Arabia	69.0% (Iqbal 2000) 75.0% (Njoh and Zimmo 1997a)
Syrian Arab Republic	60.5% (Othman and Monem 2002) 21.0% (self-reported; 51% of sample are IDUs; Syria Mental Health Directorate 2008)
Tunisia	39.7% (HIV infected; Kilani et al. 2007)

to other regions.[24] The prevalence from IDU globally is at 0.363%, with a range from 0.056% in South Asia to 1.5% in Eastern Europe.[25] This translates into 15.9 million people injecting drugs around the world.[26]

Table 2.3 provides estimates of the number of IDUs in a number of MENA countries as extracted from a global review of IDU.[27] In another study, Aceijas et al. estimated that there are 0.3 to 0.6 million IDUs in MENA.[28] Further studies estimate that there are 7,500

(400 in Kabul) IDUs[29] in Afghanistan; 400,000[30] in the Arab world; 112,000,[31] 137,000,[32] at least 166,000,[33] 200,000,[34] 300,000,[35] and 70,000[36] in the Islamic Republic of Iran; and 60,000[37] and 180,000[38] in Pakistan. The average prevalence of IDU has been measured to be 4.7 IDUs per 1,000 men in a number of cities in Pakistan.[39]

[24] Aceijas et al., "Global Overview"; Mathers et al., "Global Epidemiology"; Aceijas et al., "Estimates of Injecting Drug Users."
[25] Mathers et al., "Global Epidemiology."
[26] Ibid.
[27] Mathers et al., "Global Epidemiology"; Aceijas et al., "Estimates of Injecting Drug Users."
[28] Aceijas et al., "Global Overview."

[29] Action Aid Afghanistan, "HIV AIDS in Afghanistan"; World Bank, *HIV/ AIDS in Afghanistan*; Ryan, "Travel Report Summary."
[30] UNODC, *World Drug Report 2004*.
[31] Aceijas et al., "Global Overview."
[32] Gheiratmand et al., "Uncertainty on the Number of HIV/AIDS Patients."
[33] Razzaghi, Rahimi, and Hosseini, *Rapid Situation Assessment*.
[34] Razzaghi et al., "Profiles of Risk."
[35] Wodak, "Report to WHO/EMRO."
[36] Ghys et al., "The Epidemics of Injecting Drug Use and HIV in Asia."
[37] United Nations Drug Control Programme, "Drug Abuse in Pakistan."
[38] Haque et al., "High-Risk Sexual Behaviours."
[39] Pakistan National AIDS Control Program, *HIV Second Generation Surveillance* (Round I).

Table 2.3 Estimates of the Number and Prevalence of IDUs, Selected MENA Countries

Country	IDU estimates			IDU prevalence (%)		
	Low	Middle	High	Low	Middle	High
Afghanistan	22,720	34,080	45,440	0.16	0.24	0.32
	6,870	6,900	6,930	0.05	0.05	0.05
Algeria	26,333	40,961	55,590	0.14	0.22	0.29
Bahrain	337	674	1,011	0.08	0.16	0.24
Egypt, Arab Republic of	56,970	88,618	120,265	0.13	0.21	0.28
Iran, Islamic Republic of	70,000	185,000	300,000	0.17	0.46	0.74
		180,000			0.4	
Iraq	23,115	34,673	46,230	0.19	0.28	0.37
Jordan	3,200	4,850	6,500	0.11	0.16	0.22
Kuwait	2,700	4,100	5,500	0.2	0.3	0.41
Lebanon	2,200	3,300	4,400	0.09	0.14	0.19
Libya	4,633	7,206	9,779	0.15	0.23	0.32
		1,685			0.05	
Morocco		18,500			0.1	
Oman	2,800	4,250	5,700	0.2	0.3	0.4
Pakistan	54,000	462,000	870,000	0.07	0.5	1.12
				0.13	0.14	0.16
Qatar	780	1,190	1,600	0.15	0.22	0.3
Saudi Arabia	15,172	23,600	32,028	0.13	0.2	0.27
Sudan	24,319	37,828	51,337	0.13	0.2	0.28
Syrian Arab Republic	4,000	6,000	8,000	0.04	0.07	0.09
Tunisia	8,462	13,163	17,864	0.14	0.21	0.29
Turkey	66,591	99,887	133,182	0.16	0.23	0.31
United Arab Emirates	3,200	4,800	6,400	0.2	0.3	0.4
Yemen, Republic of	12,710	19,770	26,830	0.15	0.23	0.31

Sources: Adapted from Aceijas et al. (2006), with more recent estimates from Mathers et al. (2008).

In Kabul, Jalalabad, and Mazar-i-Sharif in Afghanistan, the IDU prevalence is estimated at 2.24 IDUs per 1,000 men.[40]

There is evidence of a growing IDU problem in both the Islamic Republic of Iran[41] and Pakistan.[42] The proportion of IDUs out of all drug users in Pakistan appears to have increased from 3% in 1993, to 15% in 2000–01, and to 26% in 2006.[43]

Drug injection is only one component of a wider drug problem in MENA. The Islamic Republic of Iran has the highest rate of heroin and opium dependence (injecting and noninjecting)

in the world (1 in every 17 people).[44] One study estimated that there are 0.5 million heroin addicts in Pakistan.[45] Another study reported an opiate use prevalence of 0.8% in Pakistan compared to 0.6% in the United States and 0.4% in India.[46] The prevalence of drug use in Saudi Arabia is estimated at 0.002% to 0.01%.[47] There are 27,000 drug users in Kuwait,[48] and 7,000, mostly IDUs, in Libya.[49] A study among Egyptian youth found

[40] World Bank, "Mapping and Situation Assessment."
[41] Reid and Costigan, "Revisiting the Hidden Epidemic."
[42] Khawaja et al., "HIV/AIDS and Its Risk Factors in Pakistan."
[43] UNODC, World Drug Report 2007.
[44] Razzaghi et al., "Profiles of Risk"; UNODC, World Drug Report 2005, Volume I: Analysis.
[45] UNODCP, "Global Illicit Drug Trends."
[46] UNODC, World Drug Report 2005, Volume II: Statistics.
[47] Njoh and Zimmo, "The Prevalence of Human Immunodeficiency Virus"; Hafeiz, "Socio-Demographic Correlates."
[48] Jenkins and Robalino, HIV in the Middle East and North Africa.
[49] Ibid.

that 6% of respondents reported that they had ever used drugs.[50] Prevalence of drug use in the West Bank and Gaza was estimated at 0.86%–1.21%, with a total of 35,000–45,000 drug users[51] (including 900–1,400 heroin users[52]).

MENA is flooded with inexpensive drugs due to record levels of heroin production in Afghanistan.[53] Around 92% of the world's supply of heroin in 2006 came from Afghanistan,[54] where it is estimated that 2.9% of all arable land is devoted to opium cultivation.[55] According to the United Nations Office on Drugs and Crime (UNODC),[56] the area under illicit opium poppy cultivation worldwide increased by 33% in 2006, mainly due to the 59% increase in Afghanistan. Afghan opium is increasingly being processed into morphine and heroin before exportation. In 2006, 53% of the opiates that left Afghanistan went via the Islamic Republic of Iran, and 33% left via Pakistan. These are the main routes for drug trafficking in the region. In 2006, 67% of opiate seizures worldwide occurred in the countries neighboring Afghanistan. Almost 30% of the global seizures occurred in the Islamic Republic of Iran alone, compared to 1.8% in the United Kingdom and 1.4% in the United States. MENA is a drug-trafficking destination as well as a route for drug traffic to Africa, Europe, and North America.

The countries surrounding Afghanistan, such as the Islamic Republic of Iran and Pakistan, are experiencing increases in heroin usage with the increased supply. IDU and HIV are known to follow drug-trafficking routes.[57] Opiate consumption is rising in MENA, though it is stable or declining in most other regions including North America, Western Europe, Oceania, and East and Southeast Asia.[58] Increases in drug use have been cited in the West Bank and Gaza since 1994, despite its severe isolation.[59]

Afghanistan, the epicenter of opiate production, has very limited resources to deal with the IDU problem among its population.[60]

FEMALE INJECTING DRUG USERS

The hardest-to-reach population of IDUs in MENA is that of the female IDUs; therefore, knowledge of this risk group is limited.[61] There is a prevailing perception that the IDU problem in MENA is heavily concentrated among men. A study in the Islamic Republic of Iran among nursing students found that males were much more likely to use drugs than females.[62] A study mapping IDU in Pakistan found that only 0.2% of IDUs were females.[63] However, there is also evidence suggesting a considerable injection drug problem among women. Although all IDUs in one study in Oman were males, 25%–58% of them knew of at least one female IDU.[64] Similarly in the Syrian Arab Republic, 48% of IDUs were familiar with at least one female IDU.[65] In the 1999 rapid situation assessment (RSA) in the Islamic Republic of Iran, 6.6% of drug users were women.[66] Another RSA of prisoners estimated that 10%–50% of female inmates had a history of drug use.[67] The number of female IDUs in the Islamic Republic of Iran has been estimated at 14,000.[68] There is a perception that drug dependence among Iranian women has been increasing in recent years.[69] Lastly, in a study of IDUs in Morocco, 16% were females.[70]

INJECTING DRUG USERS AND RISKY BEHAVIOR

This section examines risky behaviors and practices in relation to HIV among IDUs, including the use of nonsterile injecting equipment,

[50] Ibid.
[51] Shareef et al., "Assessment Study."
[52] Shareef et al., "Drug Abuse Situation."
[53] UNODC, World Drug Report 2007.
[54] Ibid.
[55] UNODC, Afghanistan: Opium Survey 2003.
[56] UNODC, World Drug Report 2007.
[57] Beyrer et al., "Overland Heroin Trafficking Routes"; Sarkar et al., "Relationship of National Highway"; Xiao et al., "Expansion of HIV/AIDS in China"; Beyrer, "Human Immunodeficiency Virus (HIV) Infection Rates."
[58] UNODC, World Drug Report 2007.
[59] Shareef et al., "Assessment Study."

[60] Todd, Safi, and Strathdee, "Drug Use and Harm Reduction in Afghanistan."
[61] Day et al., "Patterns of Drug Use."
[62] Ahmadi, Maharlooy, and Alishahi, "Substance Abuse."
[63] Pakistan National AIDS Control Program, HIV Second Generation Surveillance (Round I).
[64] Oman MOH, "HIV Risk."
[65] Syria Mental Health Directorate, "Assessment of HIV Risk."
[66] Razzaghi, Rahimi, and Hosseini, Rapid Situation Assessment.
[67] Bolhari et al., "Assessment of Drug Abuse."
[68] Jenkins, "Report on Sex Worker Consultation in Iran."
[69] Shakeshaft et al., "Perceptions of Substance Use."
[70] Asouab, "Risques VIH/SIDA chez UDI."

frequency of drug injection, network structure, engagement in risky sexual behavior, and other high-risk practices.

Use of nonsterile injecting equipment among IDUs

The key risk behavior that exposes IDUs to HIV infection is the use of nonsterile injecting equipment. Evidence on IDUs in MENA depicts generally a high-risk environment. Several studies have documented relatively high levels of injection equipment reuse, such as the reuse of needles or syringes during last injection, last month, last six months, last year, or during lifetime. Table 2.4 lists prevalence of the use of nonsterile injecting equipment in different studies.

An average of six reuse incidents per person, per month has been reported among IDUs in Oman.[71] Half of the IDUs in one district in the Islamic Republic of Iran used nonsterile injecting equipment on a daily basis.[72] There are also reports of group injecting, such as in Pakistan, where, as reported in two studies, 79.5%[73] and 78%[74] of IDUs reported this practice. Forty percent of IDUs in Afghanistan reported receiving injections by a "street doctor" in the past six months.[75] This practice is associated with higher reuse of injecting equipment.[76]

Use of nonsterile injections appears to be common in MENA, and the cleaning of syringes with bleach is very limited or not done at all.[77] In Pakistan, only 12.2% of IDUs in one study and 30.2% in another study reported using a clean syringe every time they injected drugs.[78] The use of nonsterile equipment varies substantially by socioeconomic status, such as in the Islamic Republic of Iran where it varies between 30% and 100%, with the highest proportion of those reusing injecting equipment among those at the lowest socioeconomic level.[79] Almost one-third of IDUs in

Afghanistan reported using nonsterile injecting equipment.[80] Seventy-eight percent of IDUs in Pakistan reported reusing syringes.[81]

The fraction of drug users who are injecting or reusing injection equipment appears to be increasing in at least some settings. After the 2001 Afghanistan war, levels of needle reuse increased in Pakistan from 56% to 76%, possibly due to changes in drug availability, purity and price, as well as the number of drug addicts.[82] Though the majority of drug users in Pakistan use opiates by inhaling fumes of heroin powder burned on foil (a practice known as "chasing the dragon"),[83] there appears to be a shift toward injecting drugs, possibly due to an increase in heroin quality, which makes it not useful for inhalation, as well as the wider availability of injectable forms and the unavailability or rising cost of other forms of drugs after the Afghanistan war.[84] Changes in drug supply have been associated with increases in IDU in other countries including the Russian Federation, Thailand, and the United States.[85] This highlights the importance of strengthening surveillance systems to monitor changes in risky behavior.

Frequency of drug injection

The higher the frequency of drug injection, the larger the potential for HIV to spread in injecting drug networks. IDUs in MENA appear to inject drugs at a rate of more than once per day. IDUs reported 2.6 injections per day in Afghanistan.[86] Also in Afghanistan, 72% reported injecting drugs at least once a day and two-thirds reported injecting drugs for more than five years.[87] In Egypt, 75.3% of IDUs reported injecting drugs at least once per day.[88] In studies in Pakistan, 89.9%,[89] 67.7%,[90] 58%,[91] and 38%[92] of IDUs

[71] Oman MOH, "HIV Risk."

[72] Razzaghi et al., "Profiles of Risk."

[73] Altaf et al., "High Risk Behaviors."

[74] Emmanuel et al., "HIV Risk Behavior."

[75] World Bank, "Mapping and Situation Assessment."

[76] Pakistan National AIDS Control Program, *HIV Second Generation Surveillance in Pakistan* (Round III).

[77] Oman MOH, "HIV Risk"; Parviz et al., "Background Demographics and Risk Behaviors."

[78] Kuo et al., "High HCV Seroprevalence."

[79] Razzaghi et al., "Profiles of Risk."

[80] World Bank, *HIV/AIDS in Afghanistan.*

[81] Emmanuel et al., "HIV Risk Behavior."

[82] Strathdee et al., "Rise in Needle Sharing."

[83] Ahmed et al., "HIV/AIDS Risk Behaviors."

[84] Altaf et al., "High Risk Behaviors"; Shah and Altaf, "Prevention and Control of HIV/AIDS."

[85] Neaigus et al., "Potential Risk Factors"; Rhodes et al., "Explosive Spread"; Westermeyer, "The Pro-Heroin Effects."

[86] World Bank, "Mapping and Situation Assessment."

[87] Action Aid Afghanistan, "HIV AIDS in Afghanistan."

[88] Elshimi, Warner-Smith, and Aon, "Blood-Borne Virus Risks."

[89] Kuo et al., "High HCV Seroprevalence."

[90] Ibid.

[91] Platt et al., "Prevalence of HIV."

[92] Ibid.

Table 2.4 Levels of Nonsterile Needle or Syringe Use among IDUs in Several MENA Countries

Country	Survey results for use of nonsterile needles or syringes
Afghanistan	50.0% (UNAIDS 2008) 50.4% (Todd et al. 2007) 46.0% (World Bank 2008)
Algeria	41.0% (Mimouni and Remaoun 2006)
Egypt, Arab Republic of	32.2% (Egypt MOH and Population National AIDS Program 2006) 11.0% (Salama et al. 1998) 59.0% (UNAIDS 2008) 55.0% (Elshimi, Warner-Smith, and Aon 2004)
Iran, Islamic Republic of	67.0% (Day et al. 2006) 49.8% (Razzaghi, Rahimi, and Hosseini 1999) 24.8% (Razzaghi, Rahimi, and Hosseini 1999) 48.3% (Zamani et al. 2006) 11.0% (Zamani et al. 2006) 30.6% (Zamani et al. 2005) 30%–100% (Razzaghi et al. 2006) 21.0% (Zamani et al. 2008) 39.9% (Zamani et al. 2008) 35.2%–48.6% (Farhoudi et al. 2003) 73.0% (Mojtahedzadeh et al. 2008) 26.6% (Kheirandish et al. 2009)
Lebanon	33.0% (Ingold 1994) 42.0% (Aaraj [unknown]) 40.0% (Jenkins and Robalino 2003) 64.7% (Hermez [unknown]) (Aaraj [unknown]) 34.2% (Mishwar 2008) 17.0% (Mishwar 2008) 34.2% (Mishwar 2008)
Libya	44.0% (UNAIDS 2008)
Morocco	47.0% (UNAIDS 2008) 72.6% (Asouab 2005; Morocco MOH 2007)
Oman	44%–70% (different groups of IDUs; Oman MOH 2006)
Pakistan	56.8% (Ahmed et al. 2003) 56.0% (Ahmed et al. 2003) 76.0% (Strathdee et al. 2003) 52.0% (Baqi et al. 1998) 47.0% (Parviz et al. 2006) 48.2% (Zafar et al. 2003) 58.7% (Emmanuel et al. 2004) 82.0% (Pakistan National AIDS Control Program 2005b) 23.0% (Pakistan National AIDS Control Program 2005c) 78.1% (Emmanuel and Fatima 2008) 18.0% (Bokhari et al. 2007) 48.0% (Pakistan National AIDS Control Program 2005c) 82.0% (Pakistan National AIDS Control Program 2005c) 72.2% (Afghan refugees; Zafar et al. 2003) 25.2% (Saleem, Adrien, and Razaque 2008) 47.1% (Pakistan National AIDS Control Program 2005a) 21.9% (Pakistan National AIDS Control Program 2006–07) 17.6% (Pakistan National AIDS Control Program 2008) 8.5% (Altaf et al. 2009) 33.6% (Altaf et al. 2009) 41.0% (Platt et al. 2009) 14.0% (Platt et al. 2009)
Syrian Arab Republic	47.0% (UNAIDS 2008) 28.0% (Syria Mental Health Directorate 2008)

reported a daily injection. Also in Pakistan, studies found that IDUs reported a mean of 2,[93] 2.3,[94] 2.3,[95] 2.2,[96] and 2.18[97] injections per day. In Syria, IDUs reported a mean of 41 injections per month.[98]

Network structure among injecting drug users

The social and injecting networks of IDUs play an important role in determining the risk of HIV infection.[99] Collecting data on just a few risky behavior measures, such as the use of nonsterile injecting equipment, is not sufficient to map the risk of HIV exposure. MENA appears to have a diversity of typologies of risk networks across countries and sometimes within any one country.[100] In Lebanon, it appears that IDUs form closed, small networks with injection occurring in private homes and not at shooting galleries.[101] For 56.7% of IDUs, the main partner in injection reuse was a friend, and the average number of partners in syringe reuse was 1.24.[102] Group injecting with nonsterile injecting equipment was reported by 26.7% of IDUs; this was often part of a ritual among friends.[103] A similar pattern was found in Syria[104] and among some of the IDU communities in the Islamic Republic of Iran.[105]

In Syria, a study has found that when the syringe was given to someone else after use, it was given to a friend in 62% of cases, usual sexual partner in 19% of cases, and to an acquaintance in 8% of cases.[106] Among 67% of the study participants, the person who injected the IDU was a friend, among 11% of cases the person was the usual sexual partner, and among 4% of the cases the person was an acquaintance.[107] Injection by a dealer was reported by only 5% of the participants.[108]

A study in two settings in the Islamic Republic of Iran found that the mean size of the injecting drug network in the previous month was 2.1 and 2.6 persons.[109] Most injection equipment reuse occurred between people who knew each other closely, such as friends or spouses.[110] In such circumstances, the injecting network and the social network appear to overlap and HIV cannot easily propagate from one subnetwork to another.

In other parts of MENA, the social and injecting networks are not necessarily overlapping and the reuse of injection equipment can occur between people who are not necessarily socially related, such as in shooting galleries. This has been observed among some IDU communities in the Islamic Republic of Iran[111] and Pakistan.[112] Seventy-three percent of IDUs in one study in Pakistan injected drugs in groups, with 50% of them using nonsterile injecting equipment.[113] In another study in Pakistan, between 79% and 89% of IDUs had their last injection in a park or a street.[114] In further studies in Pakistan, this was also reported by 77.7%,[115] 65.7%,[116] and 82.2%[117] of IDUs, although 72.3%,[118] 64.1%,[119] and 64.4%[120] of these IDUs reported injecting with a friend or an acquaintance. In studies, injection by a "professional" injector or street

[93] Bokhari et al., "HIV Risk in Karachi and Lahore, Pakistan"; Pakistan National AIDS Control Program, "Pilot Study in Karachi & Rawalpindi."

[94] Altaf et al., "High Risk Behaviors"; Pakistan National AIDS Control Program, HIV Second Generation Surveillance (Round I).

[95] Pakistan National AIDS Control Program, HIV Second Generation Surveillance (Round I).

[96] Pakistan National AIDS Control Program, HIV Second Generation Surveillance (Round II).

[97] Pakistan National AIDS Control Program, HIV Second Generation Surveillance (Round III).

[98] Syria Mental Health Directorate, "Assessment of HIV Risk."

[99] Neaigus et al., "The Relevance of Drug Injectors."

[100] Razzaghi et al., "Profiles of Risk."

[101] Mishwar, "An Integrated Bio-Behavioral Surveillance Study."

[102] Aaraj, "Report on the Situation Analysis"; Hermez et al., "HIV/AIDS Prevention among Vulnerable Groups."

[103] Hermez, "HIV/AIDS Prevention through Outreach"; Aaraj, "Report on the Situation Analysis."

[104] Syria Mental Health Directorate, "Assessment of HIV Risk."

[105] Razzaghi et al., "Profiles of Risk."

[106] Syria Mental Health Directorate, "Assessment of HIV Risk."

[107] Ibid.

[108] Ibid.

[109] Zamani et al., "Needle and Syringe Sharing Practices."

[110] Ibid.

[111] Razzaghi et al., "Profiles of Risk."

[112] Emmanuel and Fatima, "Coverage to Curb the Emerging HIV Epidemic."

[113] Ibid.

[114] Pakistan National AIDS Control Program, "Pilot Study in Karachi & Rawalpindi."

[115] Pakistan National AIDS Control Program, HIV Second Generation Surveillance (Round I).

[116] Pakistan National AIDS Control Program, HIV Second Generation Surveillance (Round II).

[117] Pakistan National AIDS Control Program, HIV Second Generation Surveillance (Round III).

[118] Pakistan National AIDS Control Program, HIV Second Generation Surveillance (Round I).

[119] Pakistan National AIDS Control Program, HIV Second Generation Surveillance (Round II).

[120] Pakistan National AIDS Control Program, HIV Second Generation Surveillance (Round III).

doctor at least once in the last month was reported by 42.1%,[121] 27.1%,[122] and 60.6%[123] of IDUs in Pakistan. According to a study conducted in Afghanistan, a large fraction of IDUs reported injecting drugs in open spaces such as in streets or parks.[124]

By reusing injection equipment, street doctors may connect different IDU subnetworks together. Well-connected injecting drug networks are most conducive to HIV spread. This is manifested in the high HIV and HCV prevalence levels among different IDU communities in the Islamic Republic of Iran, Libya, and Pakistan, as delineated above. The social environment and injecting network structure need to be considered in any prevention interventions among IDUs in MENA. Network-level interventions can reinforce individual-level interventions.[125]

Engagement of IDUs in risky sexual behavior

Various studies indicated that the majority of IDUs in MENA are sexually active and engage in risky sexual behavior.[126] Being married (currently or at some point) was reported by 55.5% of IDUs[127] in Egypt; 57%,[128] 52%,[129] and 59%[130] in different studies in the Islamic Republic of Iran; 50%[131] in Pakistan; and 3%–28%[132] in Oman. In Pakistan, 44.7%,[133] 45.24%,[134] and 41.1%[135] of IDUs in

different studies reported current marriage. Multiple sexual partnerships were reported by 73% of IDUs in Egypt,[136] and 24% in Pakistan.[137]

In Afghanistan, IDUs reported multiple,[138] regular, and casual sexual partnerships and contacts with female sex workers (FSWs), and 75% of them at some point had sex with a female.[139] In Egypt, 70.5% of IDUs had sex in the last year.[140] In the Islamic Republic of Iran, one-third of married IDUs had extramarital sex, over half of those divorced or separated had sex after separation, and over 70% of unmarried IDUs reported premarital sex.[141] Also in the Islamic Republic of Iran, 54% of IDUs reported two or more sexual partners in their lifetime,[142] and 57.1% of HIV-positive and 39.4% of uninfected incarcerated IDUs reported more than three lifetime sexual partners.[143] In yet another study in the Islamic Republic of Iran, drug use was associated with premarital and extramarital sex among truck drivers and youth.[144] A recent RSA in the Islamic Republic of Iran has also indicated that 44% of married drug users engage in extramarital sex.[145]

In Lebanon, the average number of sex partners among IDUs in the last year was 2.85, and 34.1% of IDUs reported a casual sexual partner in the past month.[146] Another study reported that 66% of IDUs had one to five sexual partners and 3% had more than five partners.[147] In Morocco, 48.1% of males and 70.1% of females of a group of mainly IDUs reported multiple sexual partners in the last 12 months.[148]

In Oman, 91%–100% of IDUs reported they had sex with two to eight sexual partners in the past month.[149] In Pakistan, 58%–79% of IDUs had sex in the last six months with a nonpaid

[121] Pakistan National AIDS Control Program, *HIV Second Generation Surveillance* (Round I).

[122] Pakistan National AIDS Control Program, *HIV Second Generation Surveillance* (Round II).

[123] Pakistan National AIDS Control Program, *HIV Second Generation Surveillance* (Round III).

[124] World Bank, "Mapping and Situation Assessment."

[125] Neaigus, "The Network Approach."

[126] Egypt MOH and Population National AIDS Program, *HIV/AIDS Biological and Behavioral Surveillance Survey;* Kuo et al., "High HCV Seroprevalence"; Elshimi, Warner-Smith, and Aon, "Blood-Borne Virus Risks."

[127] Egypt MOH and Population National AIDS Program, *HIV/AIDS Biological and Behavioral Surveillance Survey.*

[128] Zamani et al., "High Prevalence of HIV Infection."

[129] Zamani et al., "Prevalence of and Factors Associated with HIV-1 Infection."

[130] Zamani et al., "Prevalence and Correlates of Hepatitis C Virus."

[131] Haque et al., "High-Risk Sexual Behaviours"; Pakistan National AIDS Control Program, "Pilot Study in Karachi & Rawalpindi."

[132] Oman MOH, "HIV Risk."

[133] Pakistan National AIDS Control Program, *HIV Second Generation Surveillance* (Round I).

[134] Pakistan National AIDS Control Program, *HIV Second Generation Surveillance* (Round II).

[135] Pakistan National AIDS Control Program, *HIV Second Generation Surveillance* (Round III).

[136] El-Sayed et al., "Evaluation of Selected Reproductive Health Infections."

[137] Emmanuel et al., "HIV Risk Behavior."

[138] Sanders-Buell et al., "A Nascent HIV Type 1 Epidemic."

[139] World Bank, "Mapping and Situation Assessment."

[140] Egypt MOH and Population National AIDS Program, *HIV/AIDS Biological and Behavioral Surveillance Survey.*

[141] Razzaghi, Rahimi, and Hosseini, *Rapid Situation Assessment.*

[142] Zamani et al., "High Prevalence of HIV Infection."

[143] Rahbar, Rooholamini, and Khoshnood, "Prevalence of HIV Infection."

[144] Tehrani and Malek-Afzalip, "Knowledge, Attitudes and Practices."

[145] Narenjiha et al., "Rapid Situation Assessment."

[146] Aaraj, "Report on the Situation Analysis"; Hermez et al., "HIV/AIDS Prevention among Vulnerable Groups."

[147] Mishwar, "An Integrated Bio-Behavioral Surveillance Study."

[148] Asouab, "Risques VIH/SIDA chez UDI"; Morocco MOH, "Situation épidémiologique actuelle du VIH/SIDA au Maroc."

[149] Oman MOH, "HIV Risk."

partner,[150] and 42%–62% reported having sex with a woman in the last year.[151] Also in Pakistan, individual studies reported that 42.2%,[152] 45.7%,[153] and 37.8%[154] of IDUs had regular female sexual partners in the last six months. A history of a sexually transmitted disease (STD) was reported in different studies to be 66%,[155] 54.1%,[156] and 40%[157] for IDUs. Seven percent of those arrested for drug-related crimes were found positive for syphilis (a sexually transmitted infection [STI]).[158] In Syria, IDUs had a mean number of seven sexual partners over the last 12 months.[159]

Further data in MENA indicate that 44% of IDUs in Algeria either had sex with FSWs or sold sex.[160] Thirty-eight percent of female IDUs in Egypt were previously convicted for prostitution.[161] Seventy-four percent of sex partners of IDUs in one study in the Islamic Republic of Iran were FSWs,[162] and for women who injected drugs in a study in the Islamic Republic of Iran, the most common source of income was sex work.[163] Nine percent of IDUs in one study in Pakistan reported using nonsterile needles or syringes with a sex worker in the last week.[164]

Table 2.5 shows a summary of several other measures of overlapping injecting and sexual risk behaviors among IDUs. The overlap measures include having ever paid for sex and contacting commercial sex workers, engagement in sex work for drugs or money in the last month, having sex with a man or a boy, and condom use.

Other high-risk practices

Other high-risk drug-injection practices have been documented in MENA. Ninety-one percent of IDUs in a study in Pakistan reported deliberately drawing their blood into the syringe when they injected drugs (a practice known as "jerking").[165] This procedure was associated with a sevenfold higher chance of HCV infection, attesting to the danger of this practice for HIV transmission.[166] There is also documented evidence of the commercial sale of blood among IDUs. In a number of studies in Pakistan, 52%,[167] 22%,[168] 30%,[169] 28%,[170] 27%,[171] and 3%[172] of IDUs reported giving blood for profit. This practice led to a large number of HIV infections in China through contaminated blood.[173] Private clinics in Pakistan are known to provide monetary reimbursement for blood donation, thereby creating an incentive for IDUs to give blood.[174] Lastly, there is evidence of at least some mobility among drug users; between 54% and 72% of different IDU groups in Oman reported injecting outside Oman.[175]

KNOWLEDGE OF HIV/AIDS

Levels of HIV/AIDS knowledge among IDUs in MENA appear to be variable. Only 40% of IDUs in Afghanistan[176] and 18.3% of Afghani IDUs in Pakistan[177] reported ever hearing of HIV/AIDS. A report from Egypt indicated a higher level at 43%, but with 40% reporting not knowing that HIV/AIDS can be transmitted through reuse of nonsterile needles.[178] However, almost all IDUs in a different study in Egypt were aware of HIV and some of its transmission modes, but still had

[150] Pakistan National AIDS Control Program, "Pilot Study in Karachi & Rawalpindi."

[151] Bokhari et al., "HIV Risk in Karachi and Lahore, Pakistan."

[152] Pakistan National AIDS Control Program, *HIV Second Generation Surveillance* (Round I).

[153] Pakistan National AIDS Control Program, *HIV Second Generation Surveillance* (Round II).

[154] Pakistan National AIDS Control Program, *HIV Second Generation Surveillance* (Round III).

[155] Kuo et al., "High HCV Seroprevalence."

[156] Ibid.

[157] Haque et al., "High-Risk Sexual Behaviours."

[158] Baqi, "HIV Seroprevalence."

[159] Syria Mental Health Directorate, "Assessment of HIV Risk."

[160] Mimouni and Remaoun, "Etude du Lien Potentiel entre l'Usage Problématique de Drogues et le VIH/SIDA."

[161] Salama et al., "HIV/AIDS Knowledge and Attitudes."

[162] Razzaghi, Rahimi, and Hosseini, *Rapid Situation Assessment*.

[163] Razzaghi et al., "Profiles of Risk."

[164] Mayhew et al., "Protecting the Unprotected."

[165] Kuo et al., High HCV Seroprevalence."

[166] Ibid.

[167] Baqi et al., "HIV Antibody Seroprevalence."

[168] Ibid.

[169] Ahmed et al., "HIV/AIDS Risk Behaviors."

[170] Altaf et al., "High Risk Behaviors."

[171] Platt et al., "Prevalence of HIV."

[172] Ibid.

[173] Lau, Thomas, and Lin, "HIV-Related Behaviours."

[174] Ahmed et al., "HIV/AIDS Risk Behaviors."

[175] Oman MOH, "HIV Risk."

[176] Todd, Safi, and Strathdee, "Drug Use and Harm Reduction in Afghanistan."

[177] Zafar et al., "HIV Knowledge and Risk Behaviors."

[178] Action Aid Afghanistan, "HIV AIDS in Afghanistan."

Table 2.5 Measures of Overlapping Injecting and Sexual Risk Behaviors of IDUs in MENA

Country	Paying for sex and contacting commercial sex workers	Engagement in sex work for drugs or money	Having sex with a man or a boy	Condom use
Afghanistan	69.0% (World Bank 2006) 76.2% (Todd et al. 2007) 48.0% (World Bank 2008)		32.0% (World Bank 2006) 8.3% (Todd et al. 2007) 21.0% (World Bank 2008)	0.0% (ever use; Sanders-Buell et al. 2007) 17.0% (ever use; commercial sex; World Bank 2008)
Algeria		40.0% (Mimouni and Remaoun 2006) 44.0% (Algeria MOH [unknown])		
Egypt, Arab Republic of	13.3% (Egypt MOH and Population National AIDS Program 2006)		9.4% (Egypt MOH and Population National AIDS Program 2006)	34.1% (ever use; regular partners; Egypt MOH and Population National AIDS Program 2006) 12.8% (ever use; nonregular non-commercial partners; Egypt MOH and Population National AIDS Program 2006) 11.8% (ever use; with CSWs; Egypt MOH and Population National AIDS Program 2006) 66.0% (ever use; Elshimi, Warner-Smith, and Aon. 2004) 20.0% (ever use; El-Sayed et al. 2002) 9.0% (always; El-Sayed et al. 2002)
Iran, Islamic Republic of	23.0% (Narenjiha et al. 2005) 9.2%–14.9% (IDU prisoners; Farhoudi et al. 2003) 23.3% (Kheirandish et al. 2009)	28.6% (last month; Eftekhar et al. 2008)	30.0% (Razzaghi, Rahimi, and Hosseini 1999) 13.3% (Narenjiha et al. 2005) 1.6% (IDU prisoners; Farhoudi et al. 2003) 5%–17% (Ministry of Health and Medical Education of Iran 2006; Mostashari, UNODC, and Darabi 2006) 5.0% (Kheirandish et al. 2009)	53.0% (ever use; Zamani et al. 2005) 52.0% (ever use; Narenjiha et al. 2005) 37.0% (last sex; Zamani et al. 2005) 11.3%–12.4% (ever use; IDU prisoners; Farhoudi et al. 2003)
Lebanon	47.1% (Mishwar 2008) 32.9% (last month; Hermez [unknown]; Aaraj [unknown])	33.0% (UNAIDS 2008) 27.1% (Hermez [unknown]; Aaraj [unknown]) 17.0% (Mishwar 2008)	24.7 (Aaraj [unknown])	88.0% (ever use; Aaraj [unknown]) 59.0% (ever use; Ingold 1994) 5.8% (last sex; regular; Hermez [unknown]; Aaraj [unknown]) 34.6% (last sex; casual sex; Aaraj [unknown]; Hermez et al. [unknown]) 39.3% (last sex; commercial sex; Aaraj [unknown]; Hermez et al. [unknown])
Oman		60%–97% (Oman MOH 2006)	12%–25% (always; Oman MOH 2006)	53%–69% (ever use; Oman MOH 2006) 12%–25% (always; Oman MOH 2006)

Table 2.5 *(Continued)*

Country	Paying for sex and contacting commercial sex workers	Engagement in sex work for drugs or money	Having sex with a man or a boy	Condom use
Pakistan	68.9% (Kuo et al. 2006)	5.5% (Emmanuel et al. 2004)	37.4% (Kuo et al. 2006)	40.0% (ever use; Emmanuel and Fatima 2008)
	50.4% (Kuo et al. 2006)	14%–20% (Pakistan National AIDS Control Program 2005b)	14.0% (Haque et al. 2004)	37.5% (ever use; Kuo et al. 2006)
	58.3% (Altaf et al. 2007)	5.3% (Emmanuel and Fatima 2008)	10.8% (Emmanuel et al. 2004)	14.2% (ever use; Kuo et al. 2006)
	49.0% (Haque et al. 2004)	5%–11% (Bokhari et al. 2007)	14.7% (Emmanuel and Fatima 2008)	7.0% (ever use; Parviz et al. 2006)
	42.9% (Strathdee et al. 2003)	19.6% (Pakistan National AIDS Control Program 2006–07)	14.0% (Bokhari et al. 2007)	34.0% (ever use; Altaf et al. 2007)
	20.8% (Emmanuel et al. 2004)	16.8% (Pakistan National AIDS Control Program 2008)		10.0% (ever use; Haque et al. 2004)
	41.0% (Afghani refugees; Zafar et al. 2003)			17%–32% (last sex; FSW; Bokhari et al. 2007)
	13%–28% (Pakistan National AIDS Control Program 2005b)			10%–25% (last sex; sex work; Bokhari et al. 2007)
	12.6% (Emmanuel and Fatima 2008)			7%–13% (last sex; commercial sex; Bokhari et al. 2007)
	30%–34% (Bokhari et al. 2007)			46%–66% (not used last six months; nonpaid partners; Pakistan National AIDS Control Program 2005b)
	18%–23% (with MSWs; Bokhari et al. 2007)			49%–86% (not used last six months; commercial sex; Pakistan National AIDS Control Program 2005b)
	8%–27% (with MSWs; Pakistan National AIDS Control Program 2005b)			25.0% (last sex; regular partner; Pakistan National AIDS Control Program 2005a)
	3.3% (with *hijra*; Emmanuel et al. 2004)			16.5% (last sex; regular partner; Pakistan National AIDS Control Program 2006–07)
	26.6% (Pakistan National AIDS Control Program 2005a)			33.5% (last sex; regular partner; Pakistan National AIDS Control Program 2008)
	12.6% (Pakistan National AIDS Control Program 2006–07)			16.6% (last sex; FSW; Pakistan National AIDS Control Program 2005a)
	17.7% (Pakistan National AIDS Control Program 2008)			20.9% (last sex; FSW; Pakistan National AIDS Control Program 2006–07)
	13.2% (with MSW or *hijra*; Pakistan National AIDS Control Program 2005a)			31.0% (last sex; FSW; Pakistan National AIDS Control Program 2008)
	14.7% (with MSW or *hijra*; Pakistan National AIDS Control Program 2006–07)			12.5% (last sex; man or *hijra*; Pakistan National AIDS Control Program 2005a)
	13.9% (with MSW or *hijra*; Pakistan National AIDS Control Program 2008)			12.9% (last sex; MSW or *hijra*; Pakistan National AIDS Control Program 2006–07)
	24.0% (Platt et al. 2009)			13.8% (last sex; MSW or *hijra*; Pakistan National AIDS Control Program 2008)
	21.0% (Platt et al. 2009)			45.0% (last sex; Platt et al. 2009)
	14.0% (with a transgendered person; Platt et al. 2009)			32.0% (last sex; Platt et al. 2009)
	2.0% (with a transgendered person; Platt et al. 2009)			

(continued)

Table 2.5 *(Continued)*

Country	Paying for sex and contacting commercial sex workers	Engagement in sex work for drugs or money	Having sex with a man or a boy	Condom use
Syrian Arab Republic		47.0% (51% of sample are IDUs; Syria Mental Health Directorate 2008)	5.0% (51% of sample are IDUs; Syria Mental Health Directorate 2008)	39.0% (less than half the time; 51% of sample are IDUs; Syria Mental Health Directorate 2008)
				21.0% (more than half the time; 51% of sample are IDUs; Syria Mental Health Directorate 2008)
				19.0% (consistent; 51% of sample are IDUs; Syria Mental Health Directorate 2008)
				27.0% (less than half the time; commercial sex; 51% of sample are IDUs; Syria Mental Health Directorate 2008)
				5.0% (more than half the time; commercial sex; 51% of sample are IDUs; Syria Mental Health Directorate 2008)
				17.0% (consistent; commercial sex; 51% of sample are IDUs; Syria Mental Health Directorate 2008)

Note: CSW=commercial sex worker; MSW=male sex worker.

several misconceptions.[179] The knowledge level was very high in Lebanon and almost all IDUs were aware of the risk of infection through reuse of nonsterile injecting equipment (95.5%) and unprotected sex (100%).[180] However, despite HIV/AIDS knowledge, a large fraction of IDUs do not feel at risk of HIV infection. According to individual studies, only 33.9%,[181] 31.1%,[182] and 35.9%[183] of IDUs in Pakistan and 27% of IDUs in Syria[184] reported feeling at risk of HIV infection. A more comprehensive study of HIV/AIDS knowledge in MENA can be found in chapter 7.

---

[179] Egypt MOH and Population National AIDS Program, *HIV/AIDS Biological and Behavioral Surveillance Survey.*

[180] Aaraj, "Report on the Situation Analysis"; Hermez et al., "HIV/AIDS Prevention among Vulnerable Groups."

[181] Pakistan National AIDS Control Program, *HIV Second Generation Surveillance* (Round I).

[182] Pakistan National AIDS Control Program, *HIV Second Generation Surveillance* (Round II).

[183] Pakistan National AIDS Control Program, *HIV Second Generation Surveillance* (Round III).

[184] Syria Mental Health Directorate, "Assessment of HIV Risk.

Analytical summary

Injecting drug use is a persistent and a growing problem in MENA, with close to a million people injecting drugs: a population prevalence of 0.2%. MENA is a major source, route, and destination for the global trade in illicit drugs.

There is considerable evidence on HIV prevalence and risky behavior practices among IDUs in MENA. There is also evidence of rapidly rising HIV epidemics among IDUs in a few MENA countries. Earlier evidence suffered from methodological limitations, but the quality of evidence has increased significantly in recent years. Regardless, all evidence consistently indicates that HIV has already established itself among a number of IDU populations in MENA, while it is still at low or nil prevalence in other populations. Levels of HIV prevalence among populations where the infection is already established are comparable to those observed in other regions.

The levels of risky behavior practices, such as the use of nonsterile injecting equipment, have been documented to be high, confirming the potential for further HIV spread among IDUs. The levels of HCV prevalence among IDUs have also been documented in the intermediate to high range, confirming the potential for further HIV spread. IDUs are sexually active and report high levels of risky sexual behavior, indicating substantial overlap of risks among the three key priority groups: IDUs, men who have sex with men (MSM), and FSWs. Levels of comprehensive HIV knowledge vary across the region, with both high and low levels documented in different settings.

The IDU risk context suggests the possibility of further concentrated HIV epidemics among IDUs in MENA over the next decade. The low or nil HIV prevalence in a number of IDU populations could be due to HIV not yet being introduced into these populations; HIV having been only recently introduced; or the nature of the injecting network structure among IDUs. There is an urgent need for HIV research to better understand transmission dynamics, risky behavior practices, and risk group sizes, and to be able to use this information to plan and implement more effective prevention and care services for IDUs.

Considering the above data, there are opportunities to prevent IDU epidemics in the region through needle exchange programs, access to frequent testing, prevention of heroin uptake, safe sex messages, and condom distribution.

BIBLIOGRAPHY

Aaraj, E. Unknown. "Report on the Situation Analysis on Vulnerable Groups in Beirut, Lebanon."

Aceijas, C., S. R. Friedman, H. L. Cooper, L. Wiessing, G. V. Stimson, and M. Hickman. 2006. "Estimates of Injecting Drug Users at the National and Local Level in Developing and Transitional Countries, and Gender and Age Distribution." *Sex Transm Infect* 82 Suppl 3: iii10–17.

Aceijas, C., G. V. Stimson, M. Hickman, and T. Rhodes. 2004. "Global Overview of Injecting Drug Use and HIV Infection among Injecting Drug Users." *AIDS* 18: 2295–303.

Aceijas, C., and T. Rhodes. 2007. "Global Estimates of Prevalence of HCV Infection among Injecting Drug Users." *Int J Drug Policy* 18: 352–58.

Achakzai, M., M. Kassi, and P. M. Kasi. 2007. "Seroprevalences and Co-Infections of HIV, Hepatitis C Virus and Hepatitis B Virus in Injecting Drug Users in Quetta, Pakistan." *Trop Doct* 37: 43–45.

Action Aid Afghanistan. 2006. "HIV AIDS in Afghanistan: A Study on Knowledge, Attitude, Behavior, and Practice in High Risk and Vulnerable Groups in Afghanistan."

Agha, A., S. Parviz, M. Younus, and Z. Fatmi. 2003. "Socio-Economic and Demographic Factors Associated with Injecting Drug Use among Drug Users in Karachi, Pakistan." *J Pak Med Assoc* 53: 511–16.

Ahmadi, J., N. Maharlooy, and M. Alishahi. 2004. "Substance Abuse: Prevalence in a Sample of Nursing Students." *J Clin Nurs* 13: 60–64.

Ahmed, M. A., T. Zafar, H. Brahmbhatt, G. Imam, S. Ul Hassan, J. C. Bareta, and S. A. Strathdee. 2003. "HIV/AIDS Risk Behaviors and Correlates of Injection Drug Use among Drug Users in Pakistan." *J Urban Health* 80: 321–29.

Alami, K. 2009. "Tendances récentes de l'épidémie à VIH/SIDA en Afrique du nord." Presentation, Research and AIDS Workshop in North Africa, Marrakech, Morocco.

Algeria MOH (Ministry of Health). Unknown. *Rapport de l'enquête nationale de séro-surveillance sentinelle du VIH et de la syphilis en Algérie 2004–2005.*

Al-Haddad, M. K., B. Z. Baig, and R. A. Ebrahim. 1997. "Epidemiology of HIV and AIDS in Bahrain." *J Commun Dis* 29: 321–28.

Al-Haddad, M. K., A. S. Khashaba, B. Z. Baig, and S. Khalfan. 1994. "HIV Antibodies among Intravenous Drug Users in Bahrain." *J Commun Dis* 26: 127–32.

Alizadeh, A. H., S. M. Alavian, K. Jafari, and N. Yazdi. 2005. "Prevalence of Hepatitis C Virus Infection and Its Related Risk Factors in Drug Abuser Prisoners in Hamedan—Iran." *World J Gastroenterol* 11: 4085–89.

Altaf, A., A. Memon, N. Rehman, and S. Shah. 2004. "Harm Reduction among Injection Drug Users in Karachi, Pakistan." International AIDS Conference 2004, Bangkok. Abstract WePeC5992.

Altaf, A., N. Saleem, S. Abbas, and R. Muzaffar. 2009. "High Prevalence of HIV Infection among Injection Drug Users (IDUs) in Hyderabad and Sukkur, Pakistan." *J Pak Med Assoc* 59: 136–40.

Altaf, A., S. A. Shah, N. A. Zaidi, A. Memon, R. Nadeem ur, and N. Wray. 2007. "High Risk Behaviors of Injection Drug Users Registered with Harm Reduction Programme in Karachi, Pakistan." *Harm Reduct J* 4: 7.

Asouab, F. 2005. "Risques VIH/SIDA chez UDI et plan d'action 2006–2010." Ministry of Health, Morocco.

Baqi, S. 1995. "HIV Seroprevalence and Risk Factors in Drug Abusers in Karachi." Second National Symposium, Aga Khan University.

Baqi, S., N. Nabi, S. N. Hasan, A. J. Khan, O. Pasha, N. Kayani, R. A. Haque, I. U. Haq, M. Khurshid, S. Fisher-Hoch, S. P. Luby, and J. B. McCormick. 1998. "HIV Antibody Seroprevalence and Associated Risk Factors in Sex Workers, Drug Users, and Prisoners in Sindh, Pakistan." *J Acquir Immune Defic Syndr Hum Retrovirol* 18: 73–79.

Beyrer, C. 2002. "Human Immunodeficiency Virus (HIV) Infection Rates and Drug Trafficking: Fearful Symmetries." *Bull Narcotics* 54.

Beyrer, C., M. H. Razak, K. Lisam, J. Chen, W. Lui, and X. F. Yu. 2000. "Overland Heroin Trafficking Routes and HIV-1 Spread in South and South-East Asia." *AIDS* 14: 75–83.

Bokhari, A., N. M. Nizamani, D. J. Jackson, N. E. Rehan, M. Rahman, R. Muzaffar, S. Mansoor, H. Raza, K. Qayum, P. Girault, E. Pisani, and I. Thaver. 2007. "HIV Risk in Karachi and Lahore, Pakistan: An Emerging Epidemic in Injecting and Commercial Sex Networks." *Int J STD AIDS* 18: 486–92.

Bolhari, J., M. Alvandi, P. Afshar, A. Bayanzadeh, M. Rezaii, and A. Rahimi Movaghar. 2002. "Assessment of Drug Abuse in Iranian Prisons." United National Drug Control Programme (UNDCP).

Day, C., B. Nassirimanesh, A. Shakeshaft, and K. Dolan. 2006. "Patterns of Drug Use among a Sample of Drug Users and Injecting Drug Users Attending a General Practice in Iran." *Harm Reduct J* 3: 2.

Eftekhar, M., M.-M. Gouya, A. Feizzadeh, N. Moshtagh, H. Setayesh, K. Azadmanesh, and A.-R. Vassigh. 2008. "Bio-Behavioural Survey on HIV and Its Risk Factors among Homeless Men Who Have Sex with Men in Tehran, 2006–07."

Egypt MOH (Ministry of Health), and Population National AIDS Program. 2006. *HIV/AIDS Biological and Behavioral Surveillance Survey.* Summary report.

El-Ghazzawi, E., G. Hunsmann, and J. Schneider. 1987. "Low Prevalence of Antibodies to HIV-1 and HTLV-I in Alexandria, Egypt." *AIDS Forsch* 2: 639.

El-Ghazzawi, E., L. Drew, L. Hamdy, E. El-Sherbini, Sel D. Sadek, and E. Saleh. 1995. "Intravenous Drug Addicts: A High Risk Group for Infection with Human Immunodeficiency Virus, Hepatitis Viruses, Cytomegalo Virus and Bacterial Infections in Alexandria Egypt." *J Egypt Public Health Assoc* 70: 127–50.

El-Sayed, N., M. Abdallah, A. Abdel Mobdy, A. Abdel Sattar, E. Aoun, F. Beths, G. Dallabetta, M. Rakha, C. Soliman, and N. Wasef. 2002. "Evaluation of Selected Reproductive Health Infections in Various Egyptian Population Groups in Greater Cairo." MOHP, IMPACT/FHI/USAID.

Elshimi, T., M. Warner-Smith, and M. Aon. 2004. "Blood-Borne Virus Risks of Problematic Drug Users in Greater Cairo." UNAIDS and UNODC, Geneva.

Emmanuel, F., S. Akhtar, A. Attarad, and C. Kamran. 2004. "HIV Risk Behavior and Practices among Heroin Addicts in Lahore, Pakistan." *Southeast Asian J Trop Med Public Health* 35: 940–48.

Emmanuel, F., and M. Fatima. 2008. "Coverage to Curb the Emerging HIV Epidemic among Injecting Drug Users in Pakistan: Delivering Prevention Services Where Most Needed." *Int J Drug Policy* 19 Suppl 1: S59–64.

Farhoudi, B., A. Montevalian, M. Motamedi, M. M. Khameneh, M. Mohraz, M. Rassolinejad, S. Jafari, P. Afshar, I. Esmaili, and L. Mohseni. 2003. "Human Immunodeficiency Virus and HIV-Associated Tuberculosis Infection and Their Risk Factors in Injecting Drug Users in Prison in Iran."

Gerberding, J. L. 1995. "Management of Occupational Exposures to Blood-Borne Viruses." *N Engl J Med* 332: 444–51.

Gheiratmand, R., R. Navipour, M. R. Mohebbi, and A. K. Mallik. 2005. "Uncertainty on the Number of

HIV/AIDS Patients: Our Experience in Iran." *Sex Transm Infect* 81: 279–80.

Ghys, P. D., W. Bazant, M. G. Monteiro, S. Calvani, and S. Lazzari. 2001. "The Epidemics of Injecting Drug Use and HIV in Asia." *AIDS* 15 Suppl 5: S91–99.

Goldmann, D. A. 2002. "Blood-Borne Pathogens and Nosocomial Infections." *J Allergy Clin Immunol* 110: S21–26.

Groterah, A. 2002. "Drug Abuse and HIV/AIDS in the Middle East and North Africa: A Situation Assessment." UNODC, internal document.

Hafeiz, H. B. 1995. "Socio-Demographic Correlates and Pattern of Drug Abuse in Eastern Saudi Arabia." *Drug Alcohol Depend* 38: 255–59.

Haque, N., T. Zafar, H. Brahmbhatt, G. Imam, S. ul Hassan, and S. A. Strathdee. 2004. "High-Risk Sexual Behaviours among Drug Users in Pakistan: Implications for Prevention of STDs and HIV/AIDS." *Int J STD AIDS* 15: 601–7.

Hermez, J. Unknown. "HIV/AIDS Prevention through Outreach to Vulnerable Populations in Beirut, Lebanon." Final report. Lebanon National AIDS Program, Lebanon.

Hermez, J., E. Aaraj, O. Dewachi, and N. Chemaly. Unknown. "HIV/AIDS Prevention among Vulnerable Groups in Beirut, Lebanon." Lebanon National AIDS Program, PowerPoint presentation.

Imani, R., A. Karimi, R. Rouzbahani, and A. Rouzbahani. 2008. "Seroprevalence of HBV, HCV and HIV Infection among Intravenous Drug Users in Shahr-e-Kord, Islamic Republic of Iran." *East Mediterr Health J* 14: 1136–41.

Ingold, R. 1994. "Rapid Assessment on Illicit Drug Use in Great Beirut." UNDCP.

Iqbal, J., and N. Rehan. 1996. "Sero-Prevalence of HIV: Six Years' Experience at Shaikh Zayed Hospital, Lahore." *J Pak Med Assoc* 46: 255–58.

Iqbal, N. 2000. "Substance Dependence: A Hospital Based Survey." *Saudi Med J* 21: 51–57.

Iran Center for Disease Management. 2005. "AIDS/HIV Surveillance Report." Ministry of Health.

———. 2006. "Treatment and Medical Education." Islamic Republic of Iran HIV/AIDS situation and response analysis.

Jahani, M. R., P. Kheirandish, M. Hosseini, H. Shirzad, S. A. Seyedalinaghi, N. Karami, P. Valiollahi, M. Mohraz, and W. McFarland. 2009. "HIV Seroconversion among Injection Drug Users in Detention, Tehran, Iran." *AIDS* 23: 538–40.

Jenkins, C. 2006. "Report on Sex Worker Consultation in Iran." Sponsored by UNAIDS and UNFPA, Dec 2–18, 2006.

Jenkins, C., and D. A. Robalino. 2003. *HIV in the Middle East and North Africa: The Cost of Inaction.* Orientations in Development Series, World Bank.

Khani, M., and M. M. Vakili. 2003. "Prevalence and Risk Factors of HIV, Hepatitis B Virus, and Hepatitis C Virus Infections in Drug Addicts among Zanjan Prisoners." *Arch Iranian Med* 6: 1–4.

Khawaja, Z. A., L. Gibney, A. J. Ahmed, and S. H. Vermund. 1997. "HIV/AIDS and Its Risk Factors in Pakistan." *AIDS* 11: 843–48.

Kheirandish, P., S. SeyedAlinaghi, M. Hosseini, M. Jahani, H. Shirzad, M. Foroughi, M. Seyed Ahmadian, H. Jabbari, M. Mohraz, and W. McFarland. 2009. "Prevalence and Correlates of HIV Infection among Male Injection Drug Users in Detention, Tehran, Iran." Unpublished.

Kilani, B., L. Ammari, C. Marrakchi, A. Letaief, M. Chakroun, M. Ben Jemaa, H. T. Ben Aissa, F. Kanoun, and T. Ben Chaabene. 2007. "Seroepidemiology of HCV-HIV Coinfection in Tunisia." *Tunis Med* 85: 121–23.

Kuo, I., S. ul-Hasan, N. Galai, D. L. Thomas, T. Zafar, M. A. Ahmed, and S. A. Strathdee. 2006. "High HCV Seroprevalence and HIV Drug Use Risk Behaviors among Injection Drug Users in Pakistan." *Harm Reduct J* 3: 26.

Lau, J. T., J. Thomas, and C. K. Lin. 2002. "HIV-Related Behaviours among Voluntary Blood Donors in Hong Kong." *AIDS Care* 14: 481–92.

Mathers, B. M., L. Degenhardt, B. Phillips, L. Wiessing, M. Hickman, S. A. Strathdee, A. Wodak, S. Panda, M. Tyndall, A. Toufik, and R. P. Mattick. 2008. "Global Epidemiology of Injecting Drug Use and HIV among People Who Inject Drugs: A Systematic Review." *Lancet* 372: 1733–45.

Mayhew, S., M. Collumbien, A. Qureshi, L. Platt, N. Rafiq, A. Faisel, N. Lalji, and S. Hawkes. 2009. "Protecting the Unprotected: Mixed-Method Research on Drug Use, Sex Work and Rights in Pakistan's Fight against HIV/AIDS." *Sex Transm Infect* 85 Suppl 2: ii31–36.

Mimouni, B., and N. Remaoun. 2006. "Etude du Lien Potentiel entre l'Usage Problématique de Drogues et le VIH/SIDA en Algérie 2004–2005." Ministry of Higher Education, Algeria.

Ministry of Health and Medical Education of Iran. 2004. *AIDS/HIV Surveillance Report,* Fourth Quarter. Tehran.

Mishwar. 2008. "An Integrated Bio-Behavioral Surveillance Study among Four Vulnerable Groups in Lebanon: Men Who Have Sex with Men; Prisoners; Commercial Sex Workers and Intravenous Drug Users." Internal document, final report, American University of Beirut and World Bank, Beirut, Lebanon.

Mohammad Alizadeh, A. H., S. M. Alavian, K. Jafari, and N. Yazdi. 2003. "Prevalence of Hbs Ag, Hc Ab & Hiv Ab in the Addict Prisoners of Hammadan Prison (Iran, 1998)." *Journal of Research in Medical Sciences* 7: 311–13.

Mojtahedzadeh, V., N. Razani, M. Malekinejad, M. Vazirian, S. Shoaee, M. B. Saberi Zafarghandi, A. L. Hernandez, and J. S. Mandel. 2008. "Injection Drug Use in Rural Iran: Integrating HIV Prevention into Iran's Rural Primary Health Care System." *AIDS Behav* 12: S7–12.

Morocco MOH (Ministry of Health). 2007. *Surveillance sentinelle du VIH, résultats 2006 et tendances de la séro-prévalence du VIH.*

———. Unknown. "Situation épidémiologique actuelle du VIH/SIDA au Maroc."

Mostashari, G., UNODC (United Nations Office on Drugs and Crime), and M. Darabi. 2006. "Summary of the Iranian Situation on HIV Epidemic." NSP Situation Analysis.

Narenjiha, H., H. Rafiey, A. Baghestani, et al. 2005. "Rapid Situation Assessment of Drug Abuse and Drug Dependence in Iran." DARIUS Institute (draft version, in Persian).

Nassirimanesh, B. 2002. "Proceedings of the Abstract for the Fourth National Harm Reduction Conference." Harm Reduction Coalition, Seattle, USA.

Neaigus, A. 1998. "The Network Approach and Interventions to Prevent HIV among Injection Drug Users." *Public Health Rep* 113 Suppl 1: 140–50.

Neaigus, A., S. R. Friedman, R. Curtis, D. C. Des Jarlais, R. T. Furst, B. Jose, P. Mota, B. Stepherson, M. Sufian, T. Ward, et al. 1994. "The Relevance of Drug Injectors' Social and Risk Networks for Understanding and Preventing HIV Infection." *Soc Sci Med* 38: 67–78.

Neaigus, A., M. Miller, S. R. Friedman, D. L. Hagen, S. J. Sifaneck, G. Ildefonso, and D. C. des Jarlais. 2001. "Potential Risk Factors for the Transition to Injecting among Non-Injecting Heroin Users: A Comparison of Former Injectors and Never Injectors." *Addiction* 96: 847–60.

Njoh, J., and S. Zimmo. 1997a. "Prevalence of Antibodies to Hepatitis C Virus in Drug-Dependent Patients in Jeddah, Saudi Arabia. *East Afr Med J* 74: 89–91.

Njoh, J., and S. Zimmo. 1997b. "The Prevalence of Human Immunodeficiency Virus among Drug-Dependent Patients in Jeddah, Saudi Arabia." *J Subst Abuse Treat* 14: 487–88.

Oman MOH (Ministry of Health). 2006. "HIV Risk among Heroin and Injecting Drug Users in Muscat, Oman." Quantitative survey, preliminary data.

Othman, B. M., and F. S. Monem. 2002. "Prevalence of Hepatitis C Virus Antibodies among Intravenous Drug Abusers and Prostitutes in Damascus, Syria." *Saudi Med J* 23: 393–95.

Pakistan National AIDS Control Program. 2005a. *HIV Second Generation Surveillance in Pakistan.* National Report Round 1. Ministry of Health, Pakistan, and Canada-Pakistan HIV/AIDS Surveillance Project.

———. 2005b. "Pilot Study in Karachi & Rawalpindi." Ministry of Health Canada-Pakistan HIV/AIDS Surveillance Project, Integrated Biological & Behavioral Surveillance 2004–5.

———. 2005c. *National Study of Reproductive Tract and Sexually Transmitted Infections: Survey of High Risk Groups in Lahore and Karachi.* Ministry of Health, Pakistan.

———. 2006-7. *HIV Second Generation Surveillance in Pakistan.* National Report Round II. Ministry of Health, Pakistan, and Canada-Pakistan HIV/AIDS Surveillance Project.

———. 2008. *HIV Second Generation Surveillance in Pakistan.* National Report Round III. Ministry of Health, Pakistan, Canada-Pakistan HIV/AIDS Surveillance Project.

Parviz, S., Z. Fatmi, A. Altaf, J. B. McCormick, S. Fischer-Hoch, M. Rahbar, and S. Luby. 2006. "Background Demographics and Risk Behaviors of Injecting Drug Users in Karachi, Pakistan." *Int J Infect Dis* 10: 364–71.

Platt, L, P. Vickerman, M. Collumbien, S. Hasan, N. Lalji, S. Mayhew, R. Muzaffar, A. Andreasen, and S. Hawkes. 2009. "Prevalence of HIV, HCV and Sexually Transmitted Infections among Injecting Drug Users in Rawalpindi and Abbottabad, Pakistan: Evidence for an Emerging Injection-Related HIV Epidemic." *Sex Transm Infect* 85 Suppl 2: ii17–22.

Rahbar, A. R., S. Rooholamini, and K. Khoshnood. 2004. "Prevalence of HIV Infection and Other Blood-Borne Infections in Incarcerated and Non-Incarcerated Injection Drug Users (IDUs) in Mashhad, Iran." *International Journal of Drug Policy* 15: 151–55.

Rai, M. A., H. J. Warraich, S. H. Ali, and V. R. Nerurkar. 2007. "HIV/AIDS in Pakistan: The Battle Begins." *Retrovirology* 4: 22.

Ramia, S., J. Mokhbat, A. Sibai, S. Klayme, and R. Naman. 2004. "Exposure Rates to Hepatitis C and G Virus Infections among HIV-Infected Patients: Evidence of Efficient Transmission of HGV by the Sexual Route." *Int J STD AIDS* 15: 463–66.

Ray Kim, W. 2002. "Global Epidemiology and Burden of Hepatitis C." *Microbes Infect* 4: 1219–25.

Razzaghi, E. M., A. R. Movaghar, T. C. Green, and K. Khoshnood. 2006. "Profiles of Risk: A Qualitative Study of Injecting Drug Users in Tehran, Iran." *Harm Reduct J* 3: 12.

Razzaghi, E., B. Nassirimanesh, P. Afshar, K. Ohiri, M. Claeson, and R. Power. 2006. "HIV/AIDS Harm Reduction in Iran." *Lancet* 368: 434–35.

Razzaghi, E., A. Rahimi, and M. Hosseini. 1999. *Rapid Situation Assessment (RSA) of Drug Abuse in Iran*. Tehran: Prevention Department, State Welfare Organization, Ministry of Health, I.R. of Iran and United Nations International Drug Control Program.

Reid, G., and G. Costigan. 2002. "Revisiting the Hidden Epidemic: A Situation Assessment of Drug Use in Asia in the Context of HIV/AIDS." Centre for Harm Reduction, the Burnet Institute, Melbourne.

Rhodes, T., C. Lowndes, A. Judd, L. A. Mikhailova, A. Sarang, A. Rylkov, M. Tichonov, K. Lewis, N. Ulyanova, T. Alpatova, V. Karavashkin, M. Khutorskoy, M. Hickman, J. V. Parry, and A. Renton. 2002. "Explosive Spread and High Prevalence of HIV Infection among Injecting Drug Users in Togliatti City, Russia." *AIDS* 16: F25–31.

Ryan, S. 2006. "Travel Report Summary." UNAIDS, Kabul, Afghanistan, February 27–March 7, 2006.

Salama, I. I., N. K. Kotb, S. A. Hemeda, and F. Zaki. 1998. "HIV/AIDS Knowledge and Attitudes among Alcohol and Drug Abusers in Egypt." *J Egypt Public Health Assoc* 73: 479–500.

Saleem, N. H., A. Adrien, and A. Razaque. 2008. "Risky Sexual Behavior, Knowledge of Sexually Transmitted Infections and Treatment Utilization among a Vulnerable Population in Rawalpindi, Pakistan." *Southeast Asian J Trop Med Public Health* 39: 642–48.

Saleh, E., W. McFarland, G. Rutherford, J. Mandel, M. El-Shazaly, and T. Coates. 2000. "Sentinel Surveillance for HIV and Markers for High Risk Behaviors among STD Clinic Attendees in Alexandria, Egypt." XIII International AIDS Conference, Durban, South Africa, Poster MoPeC2398.

Sanders-Buell, E., M. D. Saad, A. M. Abed, M. Bose, C. S. Todd, S. A. Strathdee, B. A. Botros, N. Safi, K. C. Earhart, P. T. Scott, N. Michael, and F. E. McCutchan. 2007. "A Nascent HIV Type 1 Epidemic among Injecting Drug Users in Kabul, Afghanistan Is Dominated by Complex AD Recombinant Strain, CRF35_AD." *AIDS Res Hum Retroviruses* 23: 834–39.

Sarkar, K., S. Panda, N. Das, and S. Sarkar. 1997. "Relationship of National Highway with Injecting Drug Abuse and HIV in Rural Manipur, India." *Indian J Public Health* 41: 49–51.

Schmitt, A., and J. Sofer. 1992. *Sexuality and Eroticism among Males in Moslem Countries*. New York: Harrington Park Press.

Shah, S. A., and A. Altaf. 2004. "Prevention and Control of HIV/AIDS among Injection Drug Users in Pakistan: A Great Challenge." *J Pak Med Assoc* 54: 290–91.

Shah, S. A., A. Altaf, S. A. Mujeeb, and A. Memon. 2004. "An Outbreak of HIV Infection among Injection Drug Users in a Small Town in Pakistan: Potential for National Implications." *Int J STD AIDS* 15: 209.

Shakeshaft, A., B. Nassirimanesh, C. Day, and K. A. Dolan. 2005. "Perceptions of Substance Use, Treatment Options and Training Needs among Iranian Primary Care Physicians." *Int J Equity Health* 4: 7.

Shareef, A., A. J. Burqan, A. Abed, E. Kalloub, and A. Alaiwi. 2006. "Drug Abuse Situation and ANGA Needs Study." PowerPoint presentation.

Shareef, A., I. Abu AlAjeen, A. Ailaiwi, Z. Mezeh, M. Shaheen, A. Helles, and A. Abed. 2006. "Assessment Study of the Drug Demand and Supply Status in Palestine, and the Urgent Needs of the Anti-Narcotic General Administration (ANGA)." Palestine Authority, Ministry of Interior, Police Headquarter Anti-Narcotic General Administration. UNODC PAL-06 Project supporting Palestinian ANGA.

Sindh AIDS Control Program. 2004. Surveillance data, government of Sindh, Pakistan.

Strathdee, S. A., T. Zafar, H. Brahmbhatt, A. Baksh, and S. ul Hassan. 2003. "Rise in Needle Sharing among Injection Drug Users in Pakistan during the Afghanistan War." *Drug Alcohol Depend* 71: 17–24.

Sy, T., and M. M. Jamal. 2006. "Epidemiology of Hepatitis C Virus (HCV) Infection." *Int J Med Sci* 3: 41–46.

Syria Mental Health Directorate. 2008. "Assessment of HIV Risk and Sero-Prevalence among Drug Users in Greater Damascus." Programme SNA, Syrian Ministry of Health, UNODC, UNAIDS.

Talaie, H., S. H. Shadnia, A. Okazi, A. Pajouhmand, H. Hasanian, and H. Arianpoor. 2007. "The Prevalence of Hepatitis B, Hepatitis C and HIV Infections in Non-IV Drug Opioid Poisoned Patients in Tehran, Iran." *Pak J Biol Sci* 10: 220–24.

Tawilah, J., and O. Tawil. 2001. "Visit to Sultane of Oman." Travel Report Summary, National AIDS Programme at the Ministry of Health in Muscat and Salalah, WHO Representative Office, WHO/EMRO.

Tehrani, F. R., and H. Malek-Afzalip. 2008. "Knowledge, Attitudes and Practices concerning HIV/AIDS among Iranian At-Risk Sub-Populations." *Eastern Mediterranean Health Journal* 14.

Todd, C. S., A. M. Abed, S. A. Strathdee, P. T. Scott, B. A. Botros, N. Safi, and K. C. Earhart. 2007. "HIV, Hepatitis C, and Hepatitis B Infections and Associated Risk Behavior in Injection Drug Users, Kabul, Afghanistan." *Emerg Infect Dis* 13: 1327–31.

Todd, C. S., N. Safi, and S. A. Strathdee. 2005. "Drug Use and Harm Reduction in Afghanistan." *Harm Reduct J* 2: 13.

UNAIDS. 2008. "Notes on AIDS in the Middle East and North Africa." RST, MENA.

UNAIDS and WHO. 2001. *AIDS Epidemic Update 2001*. Geneva.

———. 2002a. *AIDS Epidemic Update 2002*. Geneva.

———. 2002b. "Epidemiological Fact Sheet on HIV/AIDS and Sexually Transmitted Infections, 2002 Update." Libya. Geneva.

———. 2003. *AIDS Epidemic Update 2003*. Geneva.

———. 2005. *AIDS Epidemic Update 2005*. Geneva.

———. 2007. *AIDS Epidemic Update 2007*. Geneva.

United Nations Drug Control Programme. 2002. "Drug Abuse in Pakistan." Results from the Year 2000 National Assessment. Global Assessment Programme on Drug Abuse, Narcotics Control Division A-NFGoP.

UNODC (United Nations Office for Drugs and Crime). 2003. *Afghanistan: Opium Survey 2003*. UNODC-Crop Monitoring.

———. 2004. *World Drug Report*.

———. 2005a. *World Drug Report 2005, Volume I: Analysis*.

———. 2005b. *World Drug Report, Volume II: Statistics*.

———. 2007. *World Drug Report 2007*.

UNODCP (United Nations Office for Drug Control and Crime Prevention) and UNAIDS. 1999. "Baseline Study of the Relationship between Injecting Drug Use, HIV and Hepatitis C among Male Injecting Drug Users in Lahore." UNDCP and UNAIDS, Islamabad.

———. 2002. "Global Illicit Drug Trends." New York.

Ur Rehman, N., F. Emmanuel, and S. Akhtar. 2007. "HIV Transmission among Drug Users in Larkana, Pakistan." *Trop Doct* 37: 58–59.

Watts, D. M., N. T. Constantine, M. F. Sheba, M. Kamal, J. D. Callahan, and M. E. Kilpatrick. 1993. "Prevalence of HIV Infection and AIDS in Egypt over Four Years of Surveillance (1986–1990)." *J Trop Med Hyg* 96: 113–17.

Westermeyer, J. 1976. "The Pro-Heroin Effects of Anti-Opium Laws in Asia." *Arch Gen Psychiatry* 33: 1135–39.

Wodak, A. 1997. "Report to WHO/EMRO regarding Control of HIV among and from Injecting Drug Users in the Islamic Republic of Iran." Unpublished.

World Bank. 2006. *HIV/AIDS in Afghanistan*. World Bank, South Asia Region (SAR).

———. 2008. "Mapping and Situation Assessment of Key Populations at High Risk of HIV in Three Cities of Afghanistan." Human Development Sector, SAR AIDS Team, World Bank.

Xiao, Y., S. Kristensen, J. Sun, L. Lu, and S. H. Vermund. 2007. "Expansion of HIV/AIDS in China: Lessons from Yunnan Province." *Soc Sci Med* 64: 665–75.

Zafar, T., H. Brahmbhatt, G. Imam, S. ul Hassan, and S. A. Strathdee. 2003. "HIV Knowledge and Risk Behaviors among Pakistani and Afghani Drug Users in Quetta, Pakistan." *J Acquir Immune Defic Syndr* 32: 394–98.

Zali, M. R., R. Aghazadeh, A. Nowroozi, and H. Amir-Rasouly. 2001. "Anti-HCV Antibody among Iranian IV Drug Users: Is It a Serious Problem?" *Arch Iranian Med* 4: 115–19.

Zamani, S., S. Ichikawa, B. Nassirimanesh, M. Vazirian, K. Ichikawa, M. M. Gouya, P. Afshar, M. Ono-Kihara, S. M. Ravari, and M. Kihara. 2007. "Prevalence and Correlates of Hepatitis C Virus Infection among Injecting Drug Users in Tehran." *Int J Drug Policy* 18: 359–63.

Zamani, S., M. Kihara, M. M. Gouya, M. Vazirian, B. Nassirimanesh, M. Ono-Kihara, S. M. Ravari, A. Safaie, and S. Ichikawa. 2006. "High Prevalence of HIV Infection Associated with Incarceration among Community-Based Injecting Drug Users in Tehran, Iran." *J Acquir Immune Defic Syndr* 42: 342–46.

Zamani, S., M. Kihara, M. M. Gouya, M. Vazirian, M. Ono-Kihara, E. M. Razzaghi, and S. Ichikawa. 2005. "Prevalence of and Factors Associated with HIV-1 Infection among Drug Users Visiting Treatment Centers in Tehran, Iran." *AIDS* 19: 709–16.

Zamani, S., M. Vazirian, B. Nassirimanesh, E. M. Razzaghi, M. Ono-Kihara, S. Mortazavi Ravari, M. M. Gouya, and M. Kihara. 2008. "Needle and Syringe Sharing Practices among Injecting Drug Users in Tehran: A Comparison of Two Neighborhoods, One with and One without a Needle and Syringe Program." *AIDS Behav* DOI 10.1007/s10461-008-9404-2.

Chapter **3**

Men Who Have Sex with Men and HIV

This chapter focuses on the biological evidence for the extent of human immunodeficiency virus (HIV) spread among men who have sex with men (MSM), the behavioral evidence for sexual and injecting risk practices among this population group, and the context of homosexuality in the Middle East and North Africa (MENA).

HIV PREVALENCE AMONG MSM

HIV transmission between men who have sex with men has been reported in most MENA countries.[1] Table 3.1 describes the results of available point-prevalence surveys for MSM, including male sex workers (MSWs), *hijras*[2] (transgender individuals[3]), and *hijra* sex workers (HSWs). The available prevalence levels indicate a considerable HIV spread among MSM in MENA. Although some prevalence levels are low, this should not be interpreted as limited potential for future spread. HIV prevalence among *hijras* in one study in Pakistan was 0% in 1998, but syphilis prevalence was at 37%.[4] This suggests substantial levels of sexual risk behavior and potential for HIV infectious spread if HIV is introduced into sexual networks involving

this population. This has been confirmed because recent data have shown some rapidly rising epidemics among MSWs and *hijras* in Pakistan.[5] There is also a pattern of increasing HIV prevalence among MSM in other regions with a similar sociocultural background, such as in Indonesia in Southeast Asia.[6]

PREVALENCE OF HOMOSEXUALITY

Men who have sex with men form the most hidden and stigmatized risk group of all HIV risk groups in MENA. They are often subjected to harassment and even brutality.[7] Homosexual identities existed throughout Arab and Islamic history and are well described, including celebrated historical figures.[8] Arab and Islamic cultures treated homosexuals for much of history largely with indifference.[9] Despite homophobic inclinations at the individual level, there was no presence historically of an ideology of homophobia similar to that which existed in the West.[10] In

---

[1] WHO/EMRO Regional Database on HIV/AIDS; Jenkins and Robalino, "HIV in the Middle East and North Africa"; Schmitt and Sofer, *Sexuality and Eroticism*.
[2] Mainly in Pakistan and Afghanistan.
[3] Bokhari et al., "HIV Risk in Karachi and Lahore, Pakistan."
[4] Baqi et al., "Seroprevalence of HIV" (1999; 2006).

[5] Pakistan National AIDS Control Program, *HIV Second Generation Surveillance* (Rounds I, II, and III).
[6] Commission on AIDS in Asia, *Redefining AIDS in Asia*; Pisani et al., "HIV, Syphilis Infection, and Sexual Practices."
[7] Yuzgun, "Homosexuality and Police Terror in Turkey"; Symington, "Egypt"; Moszynski, "Egyptian Doctors."
[8] Al-Jahiz, *Letters of Al-Jahiz, Volume 2*; Abu-Nuwwas, *Poetry Collection of Abu-Nuwwas*; As-Siyuti, *History of the Caliphs*.
[9] Boswell, *Christianity, Social Tolerance, and Homosexuality*.
[10] Abukhalil, "Gender Boundaries and Sexual Categories in the Arab World."

Table 3.1 HIV Prevalence among MSM in MENA

Country	HIV prevalence among MSM
Egypt, Arab Republic of	1.4% (UNAIDS and WHO 2003; El-Rahman 2004; Family Health International 2007; El-Sayyed et al. 2008) 6.2% (Egypt MOH and Population National AIDS Program 2006)
Lebanon	3.6% (Mishwar 2008))
Morocco	4.4% (Alami 2009)
Pakistan	3.9% (MSWs; Bokhari et al. 2007) 0.0% (MSWs; Bokhari et al. 2007) 4.0% (MSWs; Bokhari et al. 2007) 0.4% (average of different cities with a range of 0–4.0; MSWs; Pakistan National AIDS Control Program 2005) 1.5% (average of different cities with a range of 0–7.5; MSWs; Pakistan National AIDS Control Program 2006–07) 0.9% (average of different cities with a range of 0–3.1; MSWs; Pakistan National AIDS Control Program 2008) 0.8% (average of different cities with a range of 0–1.6; HSWs; Pakistan National AIDS Control Program 2005) 1.8% (average of different cities with a range of 0–14.0; HSWs; Pakistan National AIDS Control Program 2006–07) 6.4% (average of different cities with a range of 0–27.6; HSWs; Pakistan National AIDS Control Program 2008) 1.5% (*hijras*; Bokhari et al. 2007) 0.5% (*hijras*; Bokhari et al. 2007) 0.0% (*hijras*; Baqi et al. 1999) 1.0% (*hijras*; Khan, A. A. et al. 2008) 0.5% (MSWs; *banthas*[a]; Hawkes et al. 2009) 0.0% (MSWs; *banthas*; Hawkes et al. 2009) 0.0% (MSWs; *khotkis*[b]; Rawalpindi; Hawkes et al. 2009) 0.0% (MSWs; *khotkis*; Abbottabad; Hawkes et al. 2009) 2.5% (MSWs; *khusras*[c]; Hawkes et al. 2009) 0.0% (MSWs; *khusras*; Hawkes et al. 2009)
Sudan	9.3% (Elrashied 2006)

a. Biological males with a male gender identity.
b. Biological males who dress as men but have "female soul" and feminized traits.
c. Transgenders who dress as women; they are often known as *hijras*.

medieval times, the regularity and apparent tolerance of male same-sex relations in the Arab and Islamic world were viewed in the West as a sign of moral decadence.[11]

There are no reliable estimates of the number of MSM in MENA. "Ever engaging" in anal sex is probably a poor definition for MSM in the context of this region. Male same-sex sexual behavior in MENA should not be understood in terms of the Western paradigm of rigid distinction between homosexuals and heterosexuals despite recent Westernization of lifestyles.[12] Sexual identities are more complex and intertwined and there is a full spectrum between these two distinctions.[13]

Drawing on the experience in India, gender segregation, delayed marriage, difficulty in accessing females for sex, and overcrowded living conditions can contribute to casual anal same-sex contacts.[14] It is possibly not uncommon for adolescent boys to have sex with each other,[15] for older men to pursue sex with boys,[16] and for married men to have extramarital

---

[11] Abukhalil, "Gender Boundaries and Sexual Categories in the Arab World."
[12] Ibid.

[13] Ibid.
[14] Pappas et al., "Males Who Have Sex with Males."
[15] Busulwa, "HIV/AIDS Situation Analysis Study."
[16] Khawaja et al., "HIV/AIDS and Its Risk Factors in Pakistan."

homosexual relationships.[17] Peer pressure at a young age and family instability were identified as reasons for engaging in same-sex anal sex and male sex work in Sudan.[18]

Male same-sex sexual behavior in MENA extends well beyond the concept of an active MSM population and takes multiple forms. In Pakistan, there is a complex tapestry of MSM activity including *hijras* or *khusras* (transvestites who dress as women and often practice male sex work), *khotkis* (biological males who dress as men but have "female soul" and feminized traits and who practice male sex work), *banthas* (biological males with a male gender identity who often practice male sex work), *zenanas* (she-males), *maalishias* (masseurs and mainly boys), and *chavas* (MSM who switch sex roles) among other forms.[19]

Various studies have documented same-sex anal sex among MENA populations. In the Arab Republic of Egypt, 77.4% of male street children reported ever having sex with males and 37.1% reported being forced to have sex with males.[20] In Lebanon, 8.4% of prisoners reported anal sex with a man in prison.[21] In the Islamic Republic of Iran, 29% of single, sexually active males in Tehran reported homosexual contacts with no definition provided for the kind of contacts.[22] In Pakistan, 11.3% of truck drivers reported ever having sex with an MSW, and 49.3% reported ever having sex with a man.[23] In another study, 21.9% of truck drivers had sex with a male or *hijra*.[24] Among truck drivers attending an STD (sexually transmitted disease) clinic, 53% reported anal sex with males.[25] Among prisoners, 26% reported sexual relations with other males prior to incarceration,[26] and among migrants, 1.7% reported ever having sex with a man.[27] History of urethritis and genital ulcer disease among male prisoners was associated with same-sex anal sex.[28]

In Sudan, 2% of males in mainly rural populations reported sex with males.[29] Among truck drivers, 0.2% reported having had sexual relations with both sexes, and 0.5% reported having had sex only with males.[30] Among prisoners, 2.2% reported having sex with males.[31] Taking advantage of boys and unemployed males for anal sex has also been reported in Sudan.[32] In the Republic of Yemen, it is estimated that there are 25,000 MSM, although there is no basis provided for this estimate.[33]

There are also few estimates of the prevalence of commercial sex among men. In Pakistan, there were an estimated average of 2.3 MSWs and 2.4 HSWs per 1,000 adult men across different cities.[34] The range of prevalence varied from 1 to 4.8 per 1,000 adult men for MSWs and 0.4 to 3.7 per 1,000 adult men for HSWs.[35]

These data on male same-sex sexual behavior suggest that the prevalence of homosexuality in MENA is comparable to global levels of a few percentage points of the male population engaging in anal sex with males.[36]

MEN WHO HAVE SEX WITH MEN AND RISK BEHAVIOR

This section discusses risk behaviors and practices in relation to HIV among MSM, including sexual behavior and partnership formation, commercial sex, condom use, heterosexual sex, and injecting drug use. A few studies have also documented substantial levels of sexually transmitted infections (STIs) among MSM, suggesting potential for future HIV epidemics (see chapter 10 on STIs).

[17] Khawaja et al., "HIV/AIDS and Its Risk Factors in Pakistan."

[18] Elrashied, "Generating Strategic Information."

[19] Hawkes et al., "HIV and Other Sexually Transmitted Infections"; Collumbien et al., "Understanding the Context"; Rajabali et al., "HIV and Homosexuality in Pakistan."

[20] Egypt MOH and Population National AIDS Program, *HIV/AIDS Biological and Behavioral Surveillance Survey.*

[21] Mishwar, "An Integrated Bio-Behavioral Surveillance Study."

[22] Ministry of Health and Medical Education of Iran, "Treatment and Medical Education."

[23] Agha, "Potential for HIV Transmission."

[24] Bokhari et al., "HIV Risk in Karachi and Lahore, Pakistan."

[25] Khawaja et al., "HIV/AIDS and Its Risk Factors in Pakistan."

[26] Baqi et al., "HIV Antibody Seroprevalence."

[27] Faisel and Cleland, "Study of the Sexual Behaviours."

[28] Akhtar and Luby, "Risk Behaviours."

[29] SNAP, UNICEF, and UNAIDS, "Baseline Study."

[30] Farah and Hussein, "HIV Prevalence."

[31] Assal, "HIV Prevalence."

[32] Ati, "HIV/AIDS/STIs Social and Geographical Mapping."

[33] Al-Serouri, "Assessment of Knowledge."

[34] Pakistan National AIDS Control Program, *HIV Second Generation Surveillance* (Round I).

[35] Ibid.

[36] McFarland and Caceres, "HIV Surveillance"; W. McFarland, personal communication (2008); UNAIDS, Epidemiological Software and Tools, http://www.unaids.org/en/KnowledgeCentre/HIVData/Epidemiology/ epi_software2007.asp.; Mercer et al., "Behaviourally Bisexual Men."

Sexual behavior and partnerships

Evidence on sexual partnership formation among MSM indicates substantial risk behavior. In Egypt, 90% of MSM reported more than one sexual partner,[37] with 82% of MSM being insertive and 51% being receptive.[38] In another study, 65.8% of MSM took both receptive and insertive sexual roles, 24.8% had only receptive roles, and 8.2% were exclusively insertive.[39] Sixty-seven percent of MSM reported having five concurrent sexual partners,[40] and 80.8% had ever had sex with multiple partners per act.[41] Being forced by their partners to practice anal sex in the last year was reported by 6.3% of MSM.[42]

In the Islamic Republic of Iran, 81.9% of MSM reported different kinds of sexual partnerships in the last six months including steady, casual, commercial, and female partnerships.[43] Forty-six percent reported six or more sexual partnerships in the last six months, and 9.93% reported only one kind of sexual partnership.[44] The partners were described as steady in 61.2% of the cases, sex workers in 53.8%, and casual in 82.2%.[45] Being victimized in coercive sex was reported by 47.8% of MSM.[46] Also among these MSM, 43% had ever tested for HIV, 82.3% reported being imprisoned at least once (mainly for drug use), and 64% reported a history of suicide attempts.[47]

In Lebanon, 74.3% of MSM reported having a regular sexual partner, 51.8% a casual partner, and 54.5% a commercial sex partner during the last month.[48] On average, MSM reported 9.47 partners in the past 12 months.[49] In Oman, MSM injecting drug users (IDUs) reported a mean number of two sexual partners.[50] In Sudan, 97.2% of MSM reported more than one concurrent partner,[51] and receptive MSM reported a mean of eight noncommercial partners in the last six months.[52] In addition to anal sex, 57.2% of MSM in Sudan reported engaging in oral sex, with virtually all doing so without condoms.[53] In Tunisia, 90.1% of MSM reported multiple anal sex partners in the last six months and 12% paid for sex with MSWs.[54] Among South Asian men from Bangladesh, India, and Pakistan, MSM aged 14–16, 17–20, 21–35, and 36–45 years averaged 2, 5, 42, and 35 sex partners per year, respectively.[55]

Male sex work

Sex work appears to be common among MSM in MENA who possibly use it to support their living in an environment of stigma and poor support networks.[56] Commercial sex among MSM was reported by various studies as 42%[57] and 20%[58] in Egypt, 36% in Lebanon,[59] and 67%[60] and 75.5%[61] in Sudan.

The practice of MSW in MENA reflects an environment of high risk and of considerable overlap with female commercial sex networks (see section on overlap below). In Afghanistan, male sex work is secretive and occurs in small networks in the homes of clients at a frequency of three clients per day.[62] In studies in Pakistan, MSWs reported an average of 2.3,[63] 2.1,[64] and 1.9[65] clients per working day, and an average of

[37] El-Sayed et al., "Evaluation of Selected Reproductive Health Infections."

[38] Egypt MOH and Population National AIDS Program, *HIV/AIDS Biological and Behavioral Surveillance Survey.*

[39] El-Sayyed, Kabbash, and El-Gueniedy, "Risk Behaviours."

[40] El-Sayed et al., "Knowledge, Attitude, and Practice."

[41] El-Sayyed, Kabbash, and El-Gueniedy, "Risk Behaviours."

[42] El-Sayed et al., "Knowledge, Attitude, and Practice."

[43] Eftekhar et al., "Bio-Behavioural Survey."

[44] Ibid.

[45] Ibid.

[46] Ibid.

[47] Ibid.

[48] Hermez et al., "HIV/AIDS Prevention among Vulnerable Groups"; Dewachi, "Men Who Have Sex with Other Men."

[49] Hermez et al., "HIV/AIDS Prevention among Vulnerable Groups."

[50] Oman MOH, "HIV Risk."

[51] Anonymous, "Improving HIV/AIDS Response."

[52] Elrashied, "Generating Strategic Information."

[53] Ibid.

[54] Hsairi and Ben Abdallah, "Analyse de la situation de vulnérabilité."

[55] Khan and Hyder, "HIV/AIDS among Men Who Have Sex with Men."

[56] International HIV/AIDS Alliance, "Spreading the Word."

[57] Egypt MOH and Population National AIDS Program, *HIV/AIDS Biological and Behavioral Surveillance Survey.*

[58] El-Sayed et al., "Knowledge, Attitude, and Practice."

[59] Mishwar, "An Integrated Bio-Behavioral Surveillance Study."

[60] Elrashied, "Prevalence, Knowledge and Related Risky Sexual Behaviours."

[61] Anonymous, "Improving HIV/AIDS Response."

[62] World Bank, "Mapping and Situation Assessment."

[63] Pakistan National AIDS Control Program, *HIV Second Generation Surveillance* (Round I).

[64] Pakistan National AIDS Control Program, *HIV Second Generation Surveillance* (Round II).

[65] Pakistan National AIDS Control Program, *HIV Second Generation Surveillance* (Round III).

31.1,[66] 25.8,[67] and 20.3[68] clients per month. In these same studies, HSWs reported an average of 2.5,[69] 2.5,[70] and 2.59[71] clients per working day, and an average of 36.3,[72] 32.0,[73] and 49.07[74] clients per month, respectively. In another study from Pakistan, different groups of MSWs reported a mean of 3.2 to 7.0 clients in the last week and a mean of 1.8 to 4.0 *new* clients in the last week.[75] The mean number of years in sex work was reported to be between 6.7 and 12.5 years.[76] *Hijras* constitute about one-quarter of all male sex workers in Pakistan.[77] Their clients are reported to be businessmen, drivers, students, police/military, rickshaw drivers, and the unemployed.[78]

Also from studies in Pakistan, 51% of *hijras* reported new clients in the past week with a median of one, and 68% reported regular clients with a median of three.[79] Payment to anyone for anal sex was reported in several studies by 20%,[80] 10%,[81] and 4.5%[82] of MSWs; 21.1%[83] of HSWs; and 15%[84] of *hijras*. Noncommercial partners in the last month were reported in studies by 37.7%,[85]

34.6%,[86] and 31.8%[87] of MSWs; 21.1%,[88] 32.9%,[89] and 44.0%[90] of HSWs; and 40%[91] of *hijras*. Close to half of the MSWs and HSWs used alcohol or drugs during sex in the last six months[92] or in the last month.[93] *Hijras* performed oral sex with 39% of their one-time clients and 42% of their regular clients.[94] Selling blood for money in the last six months was reported by 2.4% of MSWs and 1.6% of HSWs.[95]

In further evidence from Pakistan, MSWs reported four clients in the last week and 28% reported having sex with a nonpaying male in the last month.[96] Twenty-seven percent to 32% of different groups of MSWs also reported paying to have sex with other males or *hijras* in the last month.[97] *Hijras* reported four partners in the last week,[98] and 95% of HSWs have had sex with other *hijras*.[99] Seventeen percent to 19% of MSWs reported selling blood for profit.[100] Most *hijras* (84%) in one study were found to have engaged in sex work within the last month and 99% within the last year.[101] Increasingly among MSWs and HSWs in Pakistan, clients are found by roaming around in public places such as bus stops and markets, or through mobile phones and client referral, instead of through the traditional pimp or a *guru* (the leader or patron of a small group of *hijras*).[102]

[66] Pakistan National AIDS Control Program, *HIV Second Generation Surveillance* (Round I).

[67] Pakistan National AIDS Control Program, *HIV Second Generation Surveillance* (Round II).

[68] Pakistan National AIDS Control Program, *HIV Second Generation Surveillance* (Round III).

[69] Pakistan National AIDS Control Program, *HIV Second Generation Surveillance* (Round I).

[70] Pakistan National AIDS Control Program, *HIV Second Generation Surveillance* (Round II).

[71] Pakistan National AIDS Control Program, *HIV Second Generation Surveillance* (Round III).

[72] Pakistan National AIDS Control Program, *HIV Second Generation Surveillance* (Round I).

[73] Pakistan National AIDS Control Program, *HIV Second Generation Surveillance* (Round II).

[74] Pakistan National AIDS Control Program, *HIV Second Generation Surveillance* (Round III).

[75] Hawkes et al., "HIV and Other Sexually Transmitted Infections."

[76] Ibid.

[77] Pakistan National AIDS Control Program, *HIV Second Generation Surveillance* (Round I); Khan et al., "Correlates and Prevalence of HIV."

[78] Khan et al., "Correlates and Prevalence of HIV."

[79] Ibid.

[80] Pakistan National AIDS Control Program, *HIV Second Generation Surveillance* (Round I).

[81] Pakistan National AIDS Control Program, *HIV Second Generation Surveillance* (Round II).

[82] Pakistan National AIDS Control Program, *HIV Second Generation Surveillance* (Round III).

[83] Pakistan National AIDS Control Program, *HIV Second Generation Surveillance* (Round I).

[84] Khan et al., "Correlates and Prevalence of HIV."

[85] Pakistan National AIDS Control Program, *HIV Second Generation Surveillance* (Round I).

[86] Pakistan National AIDS Control Program, *HIV Second Generation Surveillance* (Round II).

[87] Pakistan National AIDS Control Program, *HIV Second Generation Surveillance* (Round III).

[88] Pakistan National AIDS Control Program, *HIV Second Generation Surveillance* (Round I).

[89] Pakistan National AIDS Control Program, *HIV Second Generation Surveillance* (Round II).

[90] Pakistan National AIDS Control Program, *HIV Second Generation Surveillance* (Round III).

[91] Khan et al., "Correlates and Prevalence of HIV."

[92] Pakistan National AIDS Control Program, *HIV Second Generation Surveillance* (Rounds I, II, and III).

[93] Hawkes et al., "HIV and Other Sexually Transmitted Infections."

[94] Khan et al., "Correlates and Prevalence of HIV."

[95] Pakistan National AIDS Control Program, *HIV Second Generation Surveillance* (Round III).

[96] Bokhari et al., "HIV Risk in Karachi and Lahore, Pakistan."

[97] Ibid.

[98] Ibid.

[99] Khan et al., "Correlates and Prevalence of HIV."

[100] Pakistan National AIDS Control Program, "Pilot Study in Karachi & Rawalpindi."

[101] Khan et al., "Correlates and Prevalence of HIV."

[102] Pakistan National AIDS Control Program, *HIV Second Generation Surveillance* (Rounds I, II, and III).

In Sudan, 63.7% of MSM reported being forced to have anal sex; that anal sex was necessary to secure employment, alcohol, or drugs; or that sex work was practiced for financial reasons.[103] About 25% of receptive MSM had at least 1 commercial sex partner per day with a mean of 10 insertive partners in the last six months.[104] Seventy-one percent of MSM reported a commercial sex partner in the last six months.[105] A study among female sex workers (FSWs) in Sudan reported that FSWs host young MSWs in their houses to offer both heterosexual and homosexual sex to clients who wish to engage in both activities.[106]

MSWs and HSWs report other sources of income. The majority of MSWs and HSWs in Pakistan reported working as laborers, factory workers, bus/van conductors, tailors, shopkeepers, beggars, dancers, and *malishi* (masseurs).[107] Close to half of MSWs and HSWs were illiterate.[108] High levels of sexual abuse were reported among *hijras* in Pakistan. Between 12% and 27% of different MSW and HSW groups reported being sexually violated by police in the last year, and between 24% and 39% reported providing free sex to police in the last year.[109] Between 10% and 18% of these MSWs and HSWs reported that their first sex was forced.[110]

Condom use

Reported condom use among MSM varies substantially, although overall it is more on the low side. In different studies in Egypt, 19% of MSM regularly used condoms[111]; 2%,[112] 19%,[113] and 19.2%[114] used condoms consistently; and 9.2% used condoms during last commercial sex.[115] Twenty-two percent of MSM in Egypt reported

difficulty in obtaining condoms and 38% reported difficulty using them,[116] but three quarters of MSM had heard of male condoms.[117] In studies in the Islamic Republic of Iran, 19.4%, 59.5%, and 59.9% of MSM used condoms during last anal sex with steady partners, commercial sex partners, and casual partners, respectively.[118] In Lebanon, two studies found that 47.1% and 54.5% of MSM always used condoms with regular partners and noncommercial casual partners, respectively.[119] In Oman, 68%–100% of different groups of MSM IDUs used condoms in the last year.[120]

In Pakistan, condom use during last anal sex with a client was reported by 24% of MSWs and 21% of HSWs.[121] Condom use during last oral sex with a client was reported by 13% of MSWs and 15% of HSWs.[122] Among MSWs, 34.7% reported condom use at last sex with a paying client and 32.5% with a nonpaying partner.[123] For HSWs, the percentages were 32.3 and 26, respectively.[124] Studies reported consistent condom use in the last month by 7.2%[125] and 8%[126] of MSWs, and 5.6%[127] and 7.5%[128] of HSWs. In further studies, 4% of *hijras* and 3.1% of MSWs used condoms consistently,[129] and 17% of MSWs used a condom with a nonpaying female in the last month.[130] Among the reasons cited for not using condoms among MSM in Pakistan are not liking them, partners' objection, lack of availability, and not thinking of them as necessary.[131]

---

[103] Elrashied, "Generating Strategic Information."
[104] Ibid.
[105] Ibid.
[106] Yousif, "Health Education Programme."
[107] Pakistan National AIDS Control Program, *HIV Second Generation Surveillance* (Rounds I, II, and III).
[108] Pakistan National AIDS Control Program, *HIV Second Generation Surveillance* (Rounds I and II).
[109] Hawkes et al., "HIV and Other Sexually Transmitted Infections."
[110] Ibid.
[111] El-Rahman, "Risky Behaviours for HIV/AIDS Infection."
[112] El-Sayed et al., "Knowledge, Attitude, and Practice."
[113] El-Sayed et al., "Evaluation of Selected Reproductive Health Infections."
[114] El-Sayyed, Kabbash, and El-Gueniedy, "Risk Behaviours."
[115] Egypt MOH and Population National AIDS Program, *HIV/AIDS Biological and Behavioral Surveillance Survey.*

[116] El-Sayed et al., "Evaluation of Selected Reproductive Health Infections."
[117] Egypt MOH and Population National AIDS Program, *HIV/AIDS Biological and Behavioral Surveillance Survey.*
[118] Eftekhar et al., "Bio-Behavioural Survey."
[119] Hermez et al., "HIV/AIDS Prevention among Vulnerable Groups"; Dewachi, "Men Who Have Sex with Other Men."
[120] Oman MOH, "HIV Risk."
[121] Pakistan National AIDS Control Program, *HIV Second Generation Surveillance* (Round I).
[122] Pakistan National AIDS Control Program, *HIV Second Generation Surveillance* (Round I).
[123] Pakistan National AIDS Control Program, *HIV Second Generation Surveillance* (Round III).
[124] Ibid.
[125] Pakistan National AIDS Control Program, *HIV Second Generation Surveillance* (Round I).
[126] Pakistan National AIDS Control Program, *HIV Second Generation Surveillance* (Round II).
[127] Pakistan National AIDS Control Program, *HIV Second Generation Surveillance* (Round I).
[128] Pakistan National AIDS Control Program, *HIV Second Generation Surveillance* (Round II).
[129] Saleem, Adrien, and Razaque, "Risky Sexual Behavior."
[130] Bokhari et al., "HIV Risk in Karachi and Lahore, Pakistan."
[131] Pakistan National AIDS Control Program, *HIV Second Generation Surveillance* (Round III).

In Sudan, 50.9% of MSM used condoms every time or almost every time, 58.5% used a condom during last sex with a commercial sex partner, 48.5% used a condom during last sex with a non-commercial partner, and 72.9% had ever used condoms. Among these MSM, 89.4% used condoms when they had sex with females during the last six months.[132] Over 50% of MSM in Sudan were not aware of the risk of HIV transmission in unprotected anal intercourse and 85.3% did not use condoms because they were not available.[133] In Tunisia, 46.4% of MSM used condoms during last nonpaid sex; 19.7% of MSM used condoms consistently during nonpaid sex[134]; 53.7% of MSM used condoms consistently during sex with females; 55.4% of MSM used condoms during last paid sex; and 4.3% used condoms consistently during paid anal sex.[135] Further data on condom use among MSM can be found in table 8.1.

The evidence summarized above suggests that the majority of anal same-sex acts in MENA are unprotected against HIV.

Engagement of MSM in heterosexual risk behavior

Several studies have documented a considerable overlap between homosexual sex and heterosexual sex in MENA, thereby allowing HIV to spread between homosexual and heterosexual risk networks. In Egypt, ever having sex with FSWs was reported by 73.3% of MSM older than 25 years[136] and 29.3% of younger MSM.[137] Forty-four percent of MSM were found to be bisexually active.[138] Also in Egypt, studies reported current marriage to a female partner by 5.6%[139] and 30%[140] of MSM, ever being married was reported by 13%,[141] and ever having sex with a female was reported by 56.2%.[142] In the Islamic Republic of Iran, 51.8% of

MSM reported ever being married, 87.7% reported having female partners in the last six months, and 14.5% reported living currently with a female partner.[143] In Lebanon, 52.2% of MSM reported ever having a female sex partner.[144]

In Pakistan, three studies reported, respectively, that 14.7%,[145] 12.4%,[146] and 10.5%[147] of MSWs, and 15.3%,[148] 17.4%,[149] and 12.2%[150] of HSWs were married. In another study, 8% of *hijras* were married and 20% have had sex with a woman.[151] Also in Pakistan, a study reported that 10%–19% of different groups of MSWs and HSWs were married.[152] Paying a female for sex in the last month was reported by 42.7% of MSWs in one study,[153] and 12%–39% of MSWs in another study.[154] Nine percent to 24% of MSWs had also had sex with a nonpaying female in the last month.[155] In studies in Sudan, 22.9% of MSM reported ever being married,[156] 17.3% reported currently being married,[157] and 61.2%[158] and 69.2%[159] reported ever having sex with a female.[160] In Tunisia, 31.1% of MSM reported having sex with females.[161]

Female sexual partners of MSM are vulnerable to HIV. The presence of heterosexual marriage among MSM, and generally sexual contacts with female partners, puts these partners at risk of HIV infection.[162]

[132] Elrashied, "Generating Strategic Information."

[133] Elrashied, "Prevalence, Knowledge and Related Risky Sexual Behaviours."

[134] Hsairi and Ben Abdallah, "Analyse de la situation de vulnérabilité."

[135] Ibid.

[136] El-Rahman, "Risky Behaviours for HIV/AIDS Infection"; El-Sayyed, Kabbash, and El-Gueniedy, "Risk Behaviours."

[137] El-Sayyed, Kabbash, and El-Gueniedy, "Risk Behaviours."

[138] El-Sayed et al., "Knowledge, Attitude, and Practice."

[139] Egypt MOH and Population National AIDS Program, *HIV/AIDS Biological and Behavioral Surveillance Survey.*

[140] El-Sayed et al., "Knowledge, Attitude, and Practice."

[141] Egypt MOH and Population National AIDS Program, *HIV/AIDS Biological and Behavioral Surveillance Survey.*

[142] Ibid.

[143] Eftekhar et al., "Bio-Behavioural Survey."

[144] Hermez et al., "HIV/AIDS Prevention among Vulnerable Groups."

[145] Pakistan National AIDS Control Program, *HIV Second Generation Surveillance* (Round I).

[146] Pakistan National AIDS Control Program, *HIV Second Generation Surveillance* (Round II).

[147] Pakistan National AIDS Control Program, *HIV Second Generation Surveillance* (Round III).

[148] Pakistan National AIDS Control Program, *HIV Second Generation Surveillance* (Round I).

[149] Pakistan National AIDS Control Program, *HIV Second Generation Surveillance* (Round II).

[150] Pakistan National AIDS Control Program, *HIV Second Generation Surveillance* (Round III).

[151] Khan et al., "Correlates and Prevalence of HIV."

[152] Hawkes et al., "HIV and Other Sexually Transmitted Infections."

[153] Pakistan National AIDS Control Program, *HIV Second Generation Surveillance* (Round III).

[154] Bokhari et al., "HIV Risk in Karachi and Lahore, Pakistan."

[155] Ibid.

[156] Elrashied, "Generating Strategic Information."

[157] Ibid.

[158] Ibid.

[159] Anonymous, "Improving HIV/AIDS Response."

[160] Elrashied, "Generating Strategic Information."

[161] Hsairi and Ben Abdallah, "Analyse de la situation de vulnérabilité."

[162] Jenkins, "Male Sexual Diversity and Culture"; Khilji, "Combating HIV/AIDS amongst Zenana Youth."

Engagement of MSM in injecting drug risk behavior

MSM report considerable levels of drug use, both in injecting and noninjecting forms. In Egypt, 10.9% of MSM injected drugs in the previous 12 months and 79.3% reported ever using noninjecting drugs.[163] In the Islamic Republic of Iran, 53% of MSM injected drugs in the last month and hepatitis C virus (HCV) prevalence was high at 48.8%, attesting to the overlap between MSM and IDU risk factors.[164] Studies in Pakistan reported that 4%–17%[165] and 1%–2%[166] of *hijras* and 7%–9%[167] and 4%[168] of MSWs injected drugs. Also in Pakistan, studies reported that 5%,[169] 5.2%,[170] and 4.2%[171] of MSWs and 5.3%,[172] 6.3%,[173] and 4.6%[174] of HSWs injected drugs in the last six months. Further reported by these studies, 10.1%,[175] 9.5%,[176] and 4.2%[177] of MSWs and 8.4%,[178] 6.4,[179] and 6.3%[180] of HSWs had sex with IDUs in the last six months. In yet another study in Pakistan, between 0% and 3% of different groups of MSWs reported IDU in the last year, between 19% and 25% reported IDU sex partners in the last year, and between 0% and 2% had a husband or lover who is an IDU.[181] In Sudan, 24.4% of MSM used drugs.[182] In Tunisia, 14.7% of MSM reported IDU within the last year.[183]

KNOWLEDGE OF HIV/AIDS

Levels of HIV knowledge among MSM in MENA appear to vary, probably reflecting the socioeconomic status of each MSM group. In Egypt, almost all MSM in one study have heard of HIV/AIDS and the majority were able to identify several transmission modes, but about one-quarter of MSM had misconceptions.[184] In the Islamic Republic of Iran, 82.4% of MSM were aware of HIV/AIDS and 50.6% knew of someone who was living with HIV.[185] Seventy-five percent also knew that they can protect themselves by using condoms, and 87.4% knew of the risk of infection from using nonsterile injecting equipment.[186] In Lebanon, almost all MSM were aware of HIV/AIDS, its transmission modes, the condom's role in prevention, and other prevention measures, but 43.3% perceived no chance of becoming infected with HIV.[187] Separate studies in Pakistan found that 72.1%,[188] 63.5%,[189] and 62.1%[190] of MSWs perceived no risk of HIV infection. Among HSWs, the percentages were 83.7,[191] 77.8,[192] and 59.2.[193] In Sudan, 98.3% of MSM have heard of HIV/AIDS,[194] but misconceptions were prevalent.[195] Some MSM harbored the belief that keeping to an insertive role

[163] Egypt MOH and Population National AIDS Program, *HIV/AIDS Biological and Behavioral Surveillance Survey.*

[164] Eftekhar et al., "Bio-Behavioural Survey."

[165] Pakistan National AIDS Control Program, "Pilot Study in Karachi & Rawalpindi."

[166] Bokhari et al., "HIV Risk in Karachi and Lahore, Pakistan."

[167] Pakistan National AIDS Control Program, "Pilot Study in Karachi & Rawalpindi."

[168] Bokhari et al., "HIV Risk in Karachi and Lahore, Pakistan."

[169] Pakistan National AIDS Control Program, *HIV Second Generation Surveillance* (Round I).

[170] Pakistan National AIDS Control Program, *HIV Second Generation Surveillance* (Round II).

[171] Pakistan National AIDS Control Program, *HIV Second Generation Surveillance* (Round III).

[172] Pakistan National AIDS Control Program, *HIV Second Generation Surveillance* (Round I).

[173] Pakistan National AIDS Control Program, *HIV Second Generation Surveillance* (Round II).

[174] Pakistan National AIDS Control Program, *HIV Second Generation Surveillance* (Round III).

[175] Pakistan National AIDS Control Program, *HIV Second Generation Surveillance* (Round I).

[176] Pakistan National AIDS Control Program, *HIV Second Generation Surveillance* (Round II).

[177] Pakistan National AIDS Control Program, *HIV Second Generation Surveillance* (Round III).

[178] Pakistan National AIDS Control Program, *HIV Second Generation Surveillance* (Round I).

[179] Pakistan National AIDS Control Program, *HIV Second Generation Surveillance* (Round II).

[180] Pakistan National AIDS Control Program, *HIV Second Generation Surveillance* (Round III).

[181] Hawkes et al., "HIV and Other Sexually Transmitted Infections."

[182] Elrashied, "Generating Strategic Information."

[183] Hsairi and Ben Abdallah, "Analyse de la situation de vulnérabilité."

[184] Egypt MOH and Population National AIDS Program, *HIV/AIDS Biological and Behavioral Surveillance Survey.*

[185] Eftekhar et al., "Bio-Behavioural Survey."

[186] Ibid.

[187] Hermez et al., "HIV/AIDS Prevention among Vulnerable Groups"; Dewachi, "Men Who Have Sex with Other Men."

[188] Pakistan National AIDS Control Program, *HIV Second Generation Surveillance* (Round I).

[189] Pakistan National AIDS Control Program, *HIV Second Generation Surveillance* (Round II).

[190] Pakistan National AIDS Control Program, *HIV Second Generation Surveillance* (Round III).

[191] Pakistan National AIDS Control Program, *HIV Second Generation Surveillance* (Round I).

[192] Pakistan National AIDS Control Program, *HIV Second Generation Surveillance* (Round II).

[193] Pakistan National AIDS Control Program, *HIV Second Generation Surveillance* (Round III).

[194] Anonymous, "Improving HIV/AIDS Response."

[195] Elrashied, "Generating Strategic Information."

protects fully from HIV infection and most MSM believed that the risk of contracting HIV through anal sex was smaller than that of vaginal sex.[196]

ANALYTICAL SUMMARY

Although evidence is still limited, there has been a considerable increase in knowledge relating to MSM and HIV in MENA in the last few years. MSM are the most hidden and stigmatized risk group of all HIV risk groups. Nevertheless, homosexuality exists in this region at levels comparable to those in other regions, with a small percentage of the male population engaging in anal sex with males.

HIV has already been documented to be spreading among MSM, with apparently a rapidly rising epidemic in at least one country (Pakistan). HIV prevalence among MSM is already at considerable levels in several other countries, but data are still too limited to document the trend. Data on risk behaviors indicate high levels of sexual risk behavior such as multiple sexual partnerships of different kinds, low condom use, and high prevalence of sex work among MSM. MSM risk behaviors overlap considerably with heterosexual sex and injecting drug risk behaviors. Levels of STIs prevalence are substantial, suggesting epidemic potential for HIV. Levels of comprehensive HIV knowledge vary across the region, with both high and low levels being documented in different settings.

The MSM risk context suggests the possibility of concentrated HIV epidemics among MSM as well as HIV infections among their female partners over the next decade. Indeed, there may already be concentrated HIV epidemics among MSM in several MENA countries, but definitive and conclusive data are lacking. There is an urgent need for HIV surveillance to better understand the transmission dynamics and to plan and implement more effective prevention and care services among MSM in MENA.

The key to preventing a considerable HIV epidemic among MSM is expanding prevention and treatment efforts, such as condom distribution, counseling, HIV testing, and social and medical services.

---

[196] Elrashied, "Generating Strategic Information."

BIBLIOGRAPHY

Abukhalil, A. 1997. "Gender Boundaries and Sexual Categories in the Arab World." *Fem Issues* 15: 91–104.

Abu-Nuwwas, Al-Hasan. 1962. *Diwan Abu Nuwwas (Poetry Collection of Abu-Nuwwas)*. Dar Sadir, Beirut.

Agha, S. 2000. "Potential for HIV Transmission among Truck Drivers in Pakistan." *AIDS* 14: 2404–6.

Akhtar, S., and S. P. Luby. 2002. "Risk Behaviours Associated with Urethritis and Genital Ulcer Disease in Prison Inmates, Sindh, Pakistan." *East Mediterr Health J* 8: 776–86.

Alami, K. 2009. "Tendances récentes de l'épidémie à VIH/SIDA en Afrique du nord." Presentation, Research and AIDS Workshop in North Africa, Marrakech, Morocco.

Al-Jahiz. 1965. "Kitab Mufakharat Al-Jawari wa-l-Ghilman." In *Harun, Abd-us-Salam Muhammad*, ed., *Rasa'il Al-Jahiz (Letters of Al-Jahiz)*, Vol. 2. Maktabat Al-Khanj, Cairo, Egypt.

Al-Serouri, A. W. 2005. "Assessment of Knowledge, Attitudes and Beliefs about HIV/AIDS among Young People Residing in High Risk Communities in Aden Governatore, Republic of Yemen." Society for the Development of Women & Children (SOUL), Education, Health, Welfare; United Nations Children's Fund, Yemen Country Office, HIV/AIDS Project.

Anonymous. 2007. "Improving HIV/AIDS Response among Most at Risk Population in Sudan." Orientation Workshop, April 16.

Assal, M. 2006. "HIV Prevalence, Knowledge, Attitude, Practices, and Risk Factors among Prisoners in Khartoum State, Sudan."

As-Siyuti. *Tarikh Al-Khulafa' (History of the Caliphs)*. Ahmad Al-Babi al-Halabi, 1305 A.H., Cairo.

Ati, H. A. 2005. "HIV/AIDS/STIs Social and Geographical Mapping of Prisoners, Tea Sellers and Commercial Sex Workers in Port Sudan Town, Red Sea State." Draft 2, Ockenden International, Sudan.

Baqi, S., N. Nabi, S. N. Hasan, A. J. Khan, O. Pasha, N. Kayani, R. A. Haque, I. U. Haq, M. Khurshid, S. Fisher-Hoch, S. P. Luby, and J. B. McCormick. 1998. "HIV Antibody Seroprevalence and Associated Risk Factors in Sex Workers, Drug Users, and Prisoners in Sindh, Pakistan." *J Acquir Immune Defic Syndr Hum Retrovirol* 18: 73–79.

Baqi, S., S. A. Shah, M. A. Baig, S. A. Mujeeb, and A. Memon. 1999. "Seroprevalence of HIV, HBV, and Syphilis and Associated Risk Behaviours in Male Transvestites (Hijras) in Karachi, Pakistan." *Int J STD AIDS* 10: 300–04.

———. 2006. "Seroprevalence of HIV, HBV and Syphilis and Associated Risk Behaviours in Male Transvestites (Hijras) in Karachi, Pakistan." *J Pak Med Assoc* 56: S17–21.

Bokhari, A., N. M. Nizamani, D. J. Jackson, N. E. Rehan, M. Rahman, R. Muzaffar, S. Mansoor, H. Raza, K. Qayum, P. Girault, E. Pisani, and I. Thaver. 2007. "HIV Risk in Karachi and Lahore, Pakistan: An Emerging Epidemic in Injecting and Commercial Sex Networks." *Int J STD AIDS* 18: 486–92.

Boswell, J. 1980. *Christianity, Social Tolerance, and Homosexuality*. University of Chicago Press.

Busulwa, R. 2003. "HIV/AIDS Situation Analysis Study." Conducted in Hodeidah, Taiz and Hadhramut, Republic of Yemen.

Collumbien, M., A. A. Qureshi, S. H. Mayhew, N. Rizvi, A. Rabbani, B. Rolfe, R. K. Verma, H. Rehman, and R. Naveed i. 2009. "Understanding the Context of Male and Transgender Sex Work Using Peer Ethnography." *Sex Transm Infect* 85 Suppl 2: ii3–7.

Commission on AIDS in Asia. 2008. *Redefining AIDS in Asia: Crafting an Effective Response*. New Delhi, India: Oxford University Press. Presented to Ban Ki-moon, UN Secretary General, on March 26, 2008. Oxford University Press.

Dewachi, O. 2001. "Men Who Have Sex with Other Men and HIV AIDS: A Situation Analysis in Beirut, Lebanon; HIV/AIDS Prevention through Outreach to Vulnerable Populations." Final report, April 29.

Eftekhar, M., A. Feizzadeh, N. Moshtagh, H. Setayesh, K. Azadmanesh, and A.-R. Vassigh. 2009. "HIV and HCV Prevalence and Related Risk Factors among Street-Based Men Who Have Sex with Men."

Eftekhar, M., M.-M. Gouya, A. Feizzadeh, N. Moshtagh, H. Setayesh, K. Azadmanesh, and A.-R. Vassigh. 2008. "Bio-Behavioural Survey on HIV and Its Risk Factors among Homeless Men Who Have Sex with Men in Tehran, 2006–07."

Egypt MOH (Ministry of Health), and Population National AIDS Program. 2006. *HIV/AIDS Biological and Behavioral Surveillance Survey*. Summary report.

El-Rahman, A. 2004. "Risky Behaviours for HIV/AIDS Infection among a Sample of Homosexuals in Cairo City, Egypt." XV International AIDS Conference, Bangkok, July 11–16, Abstract WePeC6146.

Elrashied, S. M. 2006a. "Generating Strategic Information and Assessing HIV/AIDS Knowledge, Attitude and Behaviour and Practices as well as Prevalence of HIV1 among MSM in Khartoum State, 2005." A draft report submitted to Sudan National AIDS Control Programme. Together Against AIDS Organization (TAG). Khartoum, Sudan.

———. 2006b. "Prevalence, Knowledge and Related Risky Sexual Behaviours of HIV/AIDS among Receptive Men Who Have Sex with Men (MSM) in Khartoum State, Sudan, 2005." XVI International AIDS Conference, Toronto, August 13–18, Abstract TUPE0509.

El-Sayed, N., M. Abdallah, A. Abdel Mobdy, A. Abdel Sattar, E. Aoun, F. Beths, G. Dallabetta, M. Rakha, C. Soliman, and N. Wasef. 2002. "Evaluation of Selected Reproductive Health Infections in Various Egyptian Population Groups in Greater Cairo." MOHP, IMPACT/FHI/USAID.

El-Sayed, N., A. Darwish, M. El-Geneidy, and M. Mehrez. 1994. "Knowledge, Attitude, and Practice of Homosexuals Regarding HIV in Egypt." National AIDS Program, Ministry of Health and Population, Egypt.

El-Sayyed, N., I. A. Kabbash, and M. El-Gueniedy. 2008. "Risk Behaviours for HIV/AIDS Infection among Men Who Have Sex with Men in Cairo, Egypt." *East Mediterr Health J* 14: 905–15.

Faisel, A., and J. Cleland. 2006. "Study of the Sexual Behaviours and Prevalence of STIs among Migrant Men in Lahore, Pakistan." Arjumand and Associates, Centre for Population Studies, London School of Hygiene and Tropical Medicine.

Family Health International. 2007. "USAID's Implementing AIDS Prevention and Care (IMPACT) Project, Middle East and North Africa Region Final Report." March 2005–June 2007.

Farah, M. S., and S. Hussein. 2006. "HIV Prevalence, Knowledge, Attitude, Practices and Risk Factors among Truck Drivers in Khartoum State." Grey Report. Sudan National AIDS Program.

Hawkes, S., M. Collumbien, L. Platt, N. Lalji, N. Rizvi, A. Andreasen, J. Chow, R. Muzaffar, H. ur-Rehman, N. Siddiqui, S. Hasan, and A. Bokhari. 2009. "HIV and Other Sexually Transmitted Infections among Men, Transgenders and Women Selling Sex in Two Cities in Pakistan: A Cross-Sectional Prevalence Survey." *Sex Transm Infect* 85 Suppl 2: ii8–16.

Hermez, J., E. Aaraj, O. Dewachi, and N. Chemaly. "HIV/AIDS Prevention among Vulnerable Groups in Beirut, Lebanon." PowerPoint presentation, Lebanon National AIDS Program.

Hsairi, M., and S. Ben Abdallah. 2007. "Analyse de la situation de vulnérabilité vis-à-vis de l'infection à VIH des hommes ayant des relations sexuelles avec des hommes." For ATL MST sida NGO–Tunis Section, National AIDS Programme/DSSB, UNAIDS. Final report abridged version.

International HIV/AIDS Alliance. 2007. "Spreading the Word," http://www.aidsalliance.org/sw50794.asp, accessed on January 12.

Jenkins, C. 2004. "Male Sexual Diversity and Culture: Implications for HIV Prevention and Care." Prepared for UNAIDS.

Jenkins, C., and D. A. Robalino. 2003. *HIV in the Middle East and North Africa: The Cost of Inaction*. Orientations in Development Series. Washington, D.C.: World Bank.

Khan, A. A., N. Rehan, K. Qayyum, and A. Khan. 2008. "Correlates and Prevalence of HIV and Sexually Transmitted Infections among Hijras (Male Transgenders) in Pakistan." *Int J STD AIDS* 19: 817–20.

Khan, O. A., and A. A. Hyder. 1998. "HIV/AIDS among Men Who Have Sex with Men in Pakistan." *Sex Health Exch* 12–13, 15.

Khan, S., and T. Khilji. 2002. "Pakistan Enhanced HIV/AIDS Program: Social Assessment and Mapping of Men Who Have Sex with Men (MSM) in Lahore, Pakistan." Naz Foundation International, Luknow.

Khawaja, Z. A., L. Gibney, A. J. Ahmed, and S. H. Vermund. 1997. "HIV/AIDS and Its Risk Factors in Pakistan." *AIDS* 11: 843–48.

Khilji, N. K. 2004. "Combating HIV/AIDS amongst Zenana Youth in Lahore Pakistan." XV International AIDS Conference, Bangkok, Thailand, July 11. *Int Conf AIDS* 15, Abstract WePeD6350.

McFarland, W., and C. F. Caceres. 2001. "HIV Surveillance among Men Who Have Sex with Men." *AIDS* 15 Suppl 3: S23–32.

Mercer, C. H., G. J. Hart, A. M. Johnson, and J. A. Cassell. 2009. "Behaviourally Bisexual Men as a Bridge Population for HIV and Sexually Transmitted Infections? Evidence from a National Probability Survey." *Int J STD AIDS* 20: 87–94.

Ministry of Health and Medical Education of Iran. 2006. "Treatment and Medical Education." Islamic Republic of Iran HIV/AIDS situation and response analysis.

Mishwar. 2008. "An Integrated Bio-Behavioral Surveillance Study among Four Vulnerable Groups in Lebanon: Men Who Have Sex with Men; Prisoners; Commercial Sex Workers and Intravenous Drug Users." Internal report, American University of Beirut and World Bank, Beirut, Lebanon.

Mostashari, G., UNODC (United Nations Office on Drugs and Crime), and M. Darabi. 2006. "Summary of the Iranian Situation on HIV Epidemic." NSP Situation Analysis.

Moszynski, P. 2008. "Egyptian Doctors Who Took Part in Forced HIV Testing 'Violated Medical Ethics.'" *BMJ* 336: 855.

Oman MOH (Ministry of Health). 2006. "HIV Risk among Heroin and Injecting Drug Users in Muscat, Oman." Quantitative survey, preliminary data.

Pakistan National AIDS Control Program. 2004. "Pilot Study in Karachi & Rawalpindi, Integrated Behavioral and Biological Surveillance." Ministry of Health, Pakistan, and Canada-Pakistan HIV/AIDS Surveillance Project.

———. 2005. *HIV Second Generation Surveillance in Pakistan*. National Report Round 1. Ministry of Health, Pakistan, and Canada-Pakistan HIV/AIDS Surveillance Project.

———. 2006–7. *HIV Second Generation Surveillance in Pakistan*. National Report Round II. Ministry of Health, Pakistan, and Canada-Pakistan HIV/AIDS Surveillance Project.

———. 2008. *HIV Second Generation Surveillance in Pakistan*. National Report Round III. Ministry of Health, Pakistan, Canada-Pakistan HIV/AIDS Surveillance Project.

Pappas, G., O. Khan, J. Wright, S. Khan, and J. O'Neill. 2001. "Males Who Have Sex with Males (MSM) and HIV/AIDS in India: The Hidden Epidemic." *AIDS Public Policy Journal* 16: 4–17.

Pisani, E., P. Girault, M. Gultom, N. Sukartini, J. Kumalawati, S. Jazan, and E. Donegan. 2004. "HIV, Syphilis Infection, and Sexual Practices among Transgenders, Male Sex Workers, and Other Men Who Have Sex with Men in Jakarta, Indonesia." *Sex Transm Infect* 80: 536–40.

Rajabali, A., S. Khan, H. J. Warraich, M. R. Khanani, and S. H. Ali. 2008. "HIV and Homosexuality in Pakistan." *Lancet Infect Dis* 8: 511–15.

Saleem, N. H., A. Adrien, and A. Razaque. 2008. "Risky Sexual Behavior, Knowledge of Sexually Transmitted Infections and Treatment Utilization among a Vulnerable Population in Rawalpindi, Pakistan." *Southeast Asian J Trop Med Public Health* 39: 642–48.

Schmitt, A., and J. Sofer. 1992. *Sexuality and Eroticism among Males in Moslem Countries*. New York: Harrington Park Press.

SNAP (Sudan National AIDS Program), UNICEF (United Nations Children's Fund), and UNAIDS (United Nations Joint Programme on HIV/AIDS). 2005. "Baseline Study on Knowledge, Attitudes, and Practices on Sexual Behaviors and HIV/AIDS Prevention amongst Young People in Selected States in Sudan." HIV/AIDS KAPB Report. Projects and Research Department (AFROCENTER Group).

Symington, A. 2008. "Egypt: Court Convicts Men for 'Debauchery.'" *HIV AIDS Policy Law Rev* 13: 63–64.

UNAIDS (United Nations Joint Programme on HIV/ AIDS), and WHO (World Health Organization). 2003. *AIDS Epidemic Update 2003*. Geneva.

World Bank. 2008. "Mapping and Situation Assessment of Key Populations at High Risk of HIV in Three Cities of Afghanistan." Human Development Sector, South Asia Region (SAR) AIDS Team, World Bank, Washington, D.C.

Yousif, M. E. A. 2006. "Health Education Programme among Female Sex Workers in Wad Medani Town-Gezira State." Grey Report, final.

Yuzgun, A. 1993. "Homosexuality and Police Terror in Turkey." *J Homosex* 24: 159–69.

Chapter 4

Commercial Sex and HIV

This chapter focuses on the biological evidence for the extent of human immunodeficiency virus (HIV) spread among female sex workers (FSWs), the behavioral evidence for sexual and injecting risk practices among this population group, and the context of commercial sex in the Middle East and North Africa (MENA).[1]

HIV PREVALENCE AMONG FSWs

There is documented evidence of some HIV spread among FSWs in MENA. Table 4.1 contains the results of the available point-prevalence surveys conducted among FSWs. Generally speaking, HIV prevalence continues to be at low levels among FSWs in most countries, though at levels much higher than those in the general population (chapter 6). HIV does not appear to be well established among many commercial sex networks in MENA. In three countries, Djibouti, Somalia, and Sudan, HIV prevalence for FSWs has reached high levels in at least parts of these countries, but still at lower levels than those found in hyperendemic HIV epidemics in sub-Saharan Africa.[2]

Repeatedly in MENA, there are reports of men becoming infected from FSWs. Among reported cases in Saudi Arabia, about 90% of the men who were infected with HIV heterosexually received the infection from FSWs, with the remaining 10% becoming infected from their wives.[3] HIV prevalence in Southern Sudan

was 14% among men who reported sexual contacts with an FSW, but was 0% among men who denied such contacts.[4]

CONTEXT OF COMMERCIAL SEX IN MENA

This section highlights key social, economic, and political factors that force women to engage in sex work in MENA. This profession should not be seen as either strictly voluntary or forced,[5] and it must be understood in terms of livelihood and gender perspective.[6] Lack of marketable skills, low educational level, inability to engage in meaningful economic activity, lack of viable alternatives, and higher income through sex work are key factors in preventing FSWs from seeking other alternative professions and are contributing to their marginalization.[7] Social and economic stresses, including drug use, divorce, legal and social restrictions on women's work, family troubles leading to runaway girls, domestic violence, history of being abused, survival while husband is in jail and unemployment, are increasingly forcing women to engage in sex work in MENA.[8]

---

[1] Male sex workers (MSWs) are included among MSM.

[2] Morison et al., "Commercial Sex and the Spread of HIV."

[3] Alrajhi, Halim, and Al-Abdely, "Mode of Transmission of HIV-1."

[4] McCarthy, Khalid, and El Tigani, "HIV-1 Infection in Juba, Southern Sudan."

[5] ACORD, "Socio Economic Research."

[6] ACORD, "Qualitative Socio Economic Research."

[7] Ati, "HIV/AIDS/STIs Social and Geographical Mapping"; ACORD, "Qualitative Socio Economic Research."

[8] Pakistan National AIDS Control Program, *HIV Second Generation Surveillance in Pakistan* (Rounds I and II); Razzaghi et al., "Profiles of Risk"; Jenkins, "Report on Sex Worker Consultation in Iran"; Saleem, Adrien, and Razaque, "Risky Sexual Behavior"; Štulhofer and Božicevic, "HIV Bio-Behavioural Survey"; Sepehrad,"The Role of Women "; Dareini, "Rise in Iranian Prostitution"; Daher and Zayat, "A Matter of Life."

Table 4.1 HIV Prevalence among FSWs in MENA

Country	HIV prevalence among FSWs
Afghanistan	0.0% (World Bank 2008)
Algeria	1.7% (Fares et al. 2004; Institut de Formation Paramédicale de Parnet 2004) 2.0% (Fares et al. 2004) 9.0% (Fares et al. 2004) 10.0% (Unknown, "Statut de la réponse nationale") 3.0% (Algeria MOH [unknown]) 4.0% (Algeria MOH [unknown]) 2.8% (Alami 2009) 3.7% (Alami 2009) 3.9% (Alami 2009) 6.9% (Alami 2009) 10.7% (Alami 2009) 10.0% (Alami 2009)
Djibouti	3.9% (street-based; Etchepare 2001) 9.0% (street-based; Etchepare 2001) 41.4% (street-based; Etchepare 2001) 39.5% (street-based; Etchepare 2001) 51.3% (street-based; Etchepare 2001) 55.8% (street-based; Etchepare 2001) >50.0% (street-based; Etchepare 2001) 2.0% (Fox et al. 1989) 4.6% (street-based; Rodier et al. 1993) 41.7% (street-based; Rodier et al. 1993) 41.0% (street-based; Rodier et al. 1993) 36.0% (street-based; Rodier et al. 1993) 70.0% (street-based; Marcelin et al. 2001; Marcelin et al. 2002) 1.4% (bar-based; Etchepare 2001) 2.7% (bar-based; Etchepare 2001) 5.0% (bar-based; Etchepare 2001) 7.0% (bar-based; Marcelin et al. 2001; Marcelin et al. 2002) 14.2% (bar-based; Etchepare 2001) 15.3% (bar-based; Rodier et al. 1993) 21.7% (bar-based; Etchepare 2001) 25.6% (bar-based; Etchepare 2001) ≈50% (Philippon et al. 1997)
Egypt, Arab Republic of	0.8% (Egypt MOH and Population National AIDS Program 2006) 0.0% (Watts et al. 1993)
Iran, Islamic Republic of	0.0% (Jahani et al. 2005) 0.0% (Tassie [unknown]) 2.67% (WHO/EMRO Regional Database on HIV/AIDS)
Lebanon	0.0% (Mishwar 2008)
Morocco	1.4% (WHO/EMRO Regional Database on HIV/AIDS) 2.3% (Morocco MOH 2003–04, 2005; Khattabi and Alami 2005) 3.14% (Khattabi and Alami 2005) 2.03% (Khattabi and Alami 2005) 2.95% (Khattabi and Alami 2005) 2.52% (Khattabi and Alami 2005) 2.36% (Khattabi and Alami 2005) 0.9% (female prisoners imprisoned for sex work; Khattabi and Alami 2005) 0.0% (female prisoners imprisoned for sex work; Morocco MOH 2007) 4.41% (Khattabi and Alami 2005) 0.0% (Khattabi and Alami 2005) 1.95% (Khattabi and Alami 2005) 2.1% (Alami 2009) 0.33% (Morocco MOH 2007) 0.0% (Morocco MOH 2007)

Table 4.1 (*Continued*)

Country	HIV prevalence among FSWs
Pakistan	0.0% (Iqbal and Rehan 1996) 0.0% (Baqi et al. 1998) 0.0% (Bokhari et al. 2007) 0.5% (Bokhari et al. 2007) 0.2% (Pakistan National AIDS Control Program 2005) 0.02% (Pakistan National AIDS Control Program 2006–07) 0.2% (UNFPA 2009) 0.0% (Rawalpindi; Hawkes et al. 2009) 0.0% (Abbottabad; Hawkes et al. 2009)
Somalia	0.0% (Jama et al. 1987) 0.0% (Burans et al. 1990) 2.1% (Watts et al. 1994) 2.4% (Corwin et al. 1991) 8.3% (Corwin et al. 1991) 0.0% (Corwin et al. 1991) 0.6% (Ahmed et al. 1991) 5.2% (Testa and Kriitmaa 2009)
Sudan	0.0% (Burans et al. 1990) 16.0% (Southern Sudan; McCarthy, Khalid, and El Tigani 1995) 4.4% (Ahmed 2004d) 1.55% (FSWs and tea sellers; Basha 2006) 1.7% (Anonymous 2007)
Tunisia	2.3% (UNAIDS 2008)
Turkey	0.0% (Orak, Dalkilic, and Ozbal 1991) 0.0% (Gul et al. 2008) 0.0% (Tiras et al. 1998)
Yemen, Republic of	4.5% (Al-Serouri 2005; WHO, UNICEF, and UNAIDS 2006) 2.7% (Al-Serouri 2005; WHO, UNICEF, and UNAIDS 2006) 7.0% (Al-Serouri 2005; WHO, UNICEF, and UNAIDS 2006; Al-Qadhi 2001) 1.3% (Štulhofer and Božicevic 2008)

Economic pressures, acute poverty, and mere survival are repeatedly cited as the main immediate factors leading women to engage in sex work.[9] Sex work is the only source of income for a large fraction of sex workers,[10] and FSWs often carry the burden of supporting several children, husbands, parents, and other relatives, in addition to supporting themselves.[11] The payment for sex work is sometimes made not by cash, but rather by consumable commodities such as food and clothes, highlighting the survival nature of some of the sex work in MENA.[12]

Family disruption leading to economic pressure is often cited as a key cause of sex work. Failure in marriage, punishing husband or family out of grievances, and being forced by a husband or other male relatives to do sex work are commonly reported.[13] FSWs often report being lured into this profession by people close to them.[14] Male pimps are often the father, husband, or boyfriend of the FSW.[15]

---

[9] Busulwa, "HIV/AIDS Situation Analysis Study"; Ati, "HIV/AIDS/STIs Social and Geographical Mapping"; ACORD, "Socio Economic Research"; ACORD, "Qualitative Socio Economic Research"; Zargooshi, "Characteristics of Gonorrhoea."

[10] Anonymous, "Improving HIV/AIDS Response"; ACORD, "Socio Economic Research"; Syria National AIDS Programme, "HIV/AIDS Female Sex Workers."

[11] Ati, "HIV/AIDS/STIs Social and Geographical Mapping"; ACORD, "Socio Economic Research"; ACORD, "Qualitative Socio Economic Research."

[12] ACORD, "Socio Economic Research"; ACORD, "Qualitative Socio Economic Research."

[13] Busulwa, "HIV/AIDS Situation Analysis Study"; ACORD, "Socio Economic Research"; ACORD, "Qualitative Socio Economic Research"; Daher and Zayat, "A Matter of Life"; Syria National AIDS Programme, "HIV/AIDS Female Sex Workers."

[14] Yousif, "Health Education Programme"; Syria National AIDS Programme, "HIV/AIDS Female Sex Workers."

[15] Soins Infirmiers et Developpement Communautaire, "Mapping for FSW and IDU Report."

FSWs in MENA often report high levels of sexual violence and abuse.[16] The abuse takes different forms including verbal, physical, sexual, or being pimped against their will.[17] The perpetrators of the abuse are often clients, husbands, lovers, and neighbors as well as the police and other state actors.[18] Eight percent of FSWs in Pakistan in one study reported being sexually violated by police in the last year and 35% reported providing free sex to police in the last year.[19] Five percent of these FSWs reported that their first sex was forced.[20]

Political conflicts and social and economic inequalities also fuel sexual exploitation and trafficking of women across national boundaries.[21] Several countries in MENA are source or transit countries for women and children trafficked for the purpose of sexual exploitation at destination countries within MENA.[22] The occupation of Iraq in 2003 has led to abductions of women and girls to be sold for prostitution, or being violently forced to engage in sex work for survival or because of economic necessity, both inside Iraq and in neighboring countries.[23]

Though the vast majority of sex work in MENA is driven by economic necessity, there is evidence of "means-to-an-end" or lifestyle sex work involving middle class young women who use commercial sex to pay for education fees while attending universities, or to attain social prestige by purchasing luxury goods to maintain a higher lifestyle.[24] The recent rapid increase in the age at marriage among women creates a window of vulnerability where women may succumb to sex work with the lure of incentives and presents.[25] Young women sometimes find themselves trapped or tricked into sex work by friends and colleagues already involved in sex work, either as a cover-up of their activities or as a silencing tactic.[26]

FORMS OF COMMERCIAL SEX

Sex work is prevalent all over MENA and its forms are changing rapidly due to the changes in the socioeconomic conditions and the use of modern communications, such as mobile phones. Commercial sex, long an invisible trade in this part of the world, is now becoming visible in large cities, even in once very conservative and traditional societies.[27] It is taking place at different venues including homes, hotels, nightclubs, streets, brothels, Kothikhana ("grand houses"),[28] client homes,[29] massage parlors, "pimp"-run or individually run permanent houses,[30] "red flats,"[31] beaches,[32] rental houses near army bases and market places,[33] truck stops,[34] and in bazaars.[35]

As in other regions, commercial sex has a complex tapestry and it is difficult to provide a clear-cut definition of this practice as it involves contacts with sex workers, other forms of transactional sex, and other nonregular sexual contacts.[36] It takes a variety of forms, including that of street children and runaway adolescents controlled by older adults[37]; high-class mobile FSWs[38]; mobile-phone networks[39]; "call girls"[40];

---

[16] Pakistan National AIDS Control Program, *HIV Second Generation Surveillance* (Round I and II); Mayhew et al., "Protecting the Unprotected"; Štulhofer and Božicevic, "HIV Bio-Behavioural Survey"; Syria National AIDS Programme, "HIV/AIDS Female Sex Workers."

[17] Mayhew et al., "Protecting the Unprotected."

[18] Ibid.

[19] Hawkes et al., "HIV and Other Sexually Transmitted."

[20] Ibid.

[21] Huda, "Sex Trafficking in South Asia."

[22] Ibid.

[23] Al-Ali, "Reconstructing Gender"; Al-Ali, "Iraqi Women: Untold Stories"; Hassan, "Iraqi Women under Occupation."

[24] Busulwa, "HIV/AIDS Situation Analysis Study"; Algeria MOH, *Rapport de l'enquête nationale de séro-surveillance*; Jenkins, "Report on Sex Worker Consultation in Iran"; Ati, "HIV/AIDS/STIs Social and Geographical Mapping."

[25] Ati, "HIV/AIDS/STIs Social and Geographical Mapping."

[26] Ibid.

[27] Busulwa, "HIV/AIDS Situation Analysis Study"; Jenkins, "Report on Sex Worker Consultation in Iran."

[28] Kothikhana are generally small premises that are rented by a madam and/or broker where a small number of FSWs engage in sex work (Pakistan National AIDS Control Program, *HIV Second Generation Surveillance* [Rounds I, II, and III]); Blanchard, Khan, and Bokhari, "Variations in the Population Size."

[29] ACORD, "Socio Economic Research."

[30] Ati, "HIV/AIDS/STIs Social and Geographical Mapping."

[31] El-Gawhary, *Sex Tourism in Cairo*.

[32] Štulhofer and Božicevic, "HIV Bio-Behavioural Survey."

[33] ACORD, "Socio Economic Research"; ACORD, "Qualitative Socio Economic Research."

[34] Štulhofer and Božicevic, "HIV Bio-Behavioural Survey."

[35] World Bank, "Mapping and Situation Assessment."

[36] Morison et al., "Commercial Sex"; Carael et al., "Clients of Sex Workers"; Lowndes et al., "Role of Core and Bridging Groups"; Aral and St. Lawrence, "The Ecology of Sex Work and Drug Use"; Aral et al., "The Social Organization of Commercial Sex."

[37] Ati, "HIV/AIDS/STIs Social and Geographical Mapping."

[38] Ibid.

[39] Busulwa, "HIV/AIDS Situation Analysis Study."

[40] Pakistan National AIDS Control Program, *HIV Second Generation Surveillance* (Round II).

sex work covered under other professions[41]; arrangement for clients through pimps/aunty[42]; reliance on older clients[43]; solicitation of sex at truck stops[44]; FSWs accompanying truck drivers for a whole trip[45]; and arranging for clients through taxis. In the more conservative parts of MENA, sex work is often based at homes with interaction with clients through phones, such as in Afghanistan.[46] Increasingly mobile phones are used to facilitate sex work, such as through female brokers in the Arab Republic of Egypt,[47] or simply by direct phone contacts with clients such as in Pakistan.[48] This is leading to a larger dispersion of the FSW population into the community.[49]

PREVALENCE OF COMMERCIAL SEX

Knowledge of the sizes of commercial sex networks, including group size estimations of FSWs and the proportion of men who sexually contact FSWs, is needed to assess the HIV epidemic potential and to estimate the resources needed for HIV prevention in this priority group.

FSWs risk group size estimation

There are no reliable estimates of the number of FSWs in MENA. Globally speaking, sex work varies widely across regions and can be as high as 7% of the female population.[50] Sex workers are never a negligible part of the total population of a community.[51]

It is estimated that there are 30,000 to 60,000 FSWs in the Islamic Republic of Iran.[52] It is also estimated that there are 5,000 FSWs in the Republic of Yemen,[53] and 1,500 street-based FSWs in Djibouti.[54] In the three cities of Kabul, Jalalabad, and Mazar-i-Sharif in Afghanistan, there are an estimated 1,160 FSWs, including 898 in Kabul alone.[55]

Few estimates are available on the prevalence of sex work among women in MENA. In three cities in Afghanistan, there were on average 1.9 FSWs per 1,000 women, with the highest concentration in Mazar-i-Sharif at 2.8 FSWs per 1,000 women.[56] In a study among hospital attendees in Morocco, 0.5% reported engaging in sex work.[57] In Pakistan, mapping has found that there are between 4.5 and 12.6 FSWs per 1,000 adult women, or between 4.2 and 11.4 FSWs per 1,000 adult men.[58] In Sudan, 1.4% of females in a mainly rural population reported engaging in commercial sex.[59] Also in Sudan, exchanging sex for money was reported by 0.5% of antenatal clinic (ANC) women attendees[60] and 1% of tea sellers.[61]

The above estimates suggest that the ratio of women in MENA who engage in sex work may range from about 1 to 10 FSWs per 1,000 adult women (0.1% up to 1%). This estimate is consistent with the prevalence of FSWs in Indonesia and Malaysia, two predominantly Muslim nations, at 0.4%[62] and 0.9%,[63] respectively. It is also consistent with the global range of the percentage of women who engage in sex work, but it is on the low side of this range.[64]

Clients of FSWs

Clients of sex workers come from all sectors of society and often include military personnel, police and other members of security forces,

[41] Ati, "HIV/AIDS/STIs Social and Geographical Mapping."

[42] Pakistan National AIDS Control Program, "Pilot Study in Karachi & Rawalpindi."

[43] Ibid.

[44] Farah and Hussein, "HIV Prevalence."

[45] Ibid.

[46] World Bank, "Mapping and Situation Assessment."

[47] Jenkins and Robalino, "HIV in the Middle East and North Africa."

[48] Pakistan National AIDS Control Program, *HIV Second Generation Surveillance* (Round II); Hawkes et al., "HIV and Other Sexually Transmitted Infections."

[49] Pakistan National AIDS Control Program, *HIV Second Generation Surveillance* (Round II).

[50] Vandepitte et al., "Estimates of the Number of Female Sex Workers."

[51] Ibid.

[52] Ministry of Health and Medical Education of Iran, "Treatment and Medical Education"; Mostashari, UNODC, and Darabi, "Summary of the Iranian Situation on HIV Epidemic."

[53] Al-Serouri, "Assessment of Knowledge"; Lambert, "HIV and Development Challenges."

[54] Rodier et al., "Trends of Human Immunodeficiency Virus."

[55] World Bank, "Mapping and Situation Assessment."

[56] Ibid.

[57] Chaouki et al., "The Viral Origin of Cervical Cancer."

[58] Pakistan National AIDS Control Program, *HIV Second Generation Surveillance* (Round I); Blanchard, Khan, and Bokhari, "Variations in the Population Size."

[59] SNAP, UNICEF, and UNAIDS, "Baseline Study."

[60] Ahmed, *Antenatal.*

[61] Ahmed, *Tea Sellers.*

[62] Indonesia MOH, *National Estimates of Adult HIV Infection, Indonesia.*

[63] WHO, *Consensus Report.*

[64] Blanchard, Khan, and Bokhari, "Variations in the Population Size"; Vandepitte et al., "Estimates of the Number of Female Sex Workers"; Blanchard et al., "Variability in the Sexual Structure."

public officials, youth, truck drivers, sailors, migrant workers, traders, rich business people, single men with well-paying jobs, men with frequent travel, and Persian Gulf country tourists.[65] Several studies assessed the prevalence of sexual contacts with sex workers. Broadly speaking, levels of contacts appear comparable to those in other regions, but on the low side.[66] In Afghanistan, 39% of truck drivers reported having access to FSWs and 7% have had sex with FSWs in the last 12 months.[67] In Jordan, most voluntary counseling and testing (VCT) attendees reported contacts with sex workers as the reason for attending VCT services (Jordan National AIDS Program, personal communication). In Pakistan, 34% of truck drivers[68] and 34.7% of migrant workers[69] reported contacts with FSWs.[70]

In Somalia, 48% of a group of healthy men reported contacts with FSWs.[71] Also in Somalia, a group of predominantly soldiers attending sexually transmitted disease (STD) clinics reported contacts with sex workers at a frequency of 1.51 contacts per week.[72] In Sudan, 3.1% of mainly rural populations in six states,[73] 7.6% of prisoners,[74] 71% of a group of truck drivers and prisoners,[75] and 57% of a group of soldiers, truck drivers, outpatients, and Ethiopian refugees reported contacts with FSWs.[76] Also in Sudan, 11.7% of military personnel,[77] 8.1% of truck drivers,[78] and 8.6% of prisoners[79] reported paying for sex. Among STD clinic attendees, 49.3% acquired their STD from sex workers.[80] Among mostly Sudanese refugees in Ethiopia, 46% of males reported having ever had sex with an FSW,

and 31% reported a sexual contact with an FSW within the last three months.[81]

The number of clients of sex workers is much bigger than that of the number of FSWs. In Pakistan, for example, the average number of clients per sex worker per month was 33.7.[82] Therefore, the size of commercial sex networks is substantially bigger than that of IDUs and MSM risk networks, implying a substantially larger potential bridging population. The number of clients of sex workers in one study in Pakistan was found to be much larger than that of spouses of IDUs.[83]

COMMERCIAL SEX AND RISK BEHAVIOR

This section reviews evidence on different aspects of sexual risk behavior among FSWs, including frequency of contacts with clients, nature of commercial sex networks, condom use, STI (sexually transmitted infection) transmission, anal and oral sex, and engagement of FSWs in injecting drug risk behavior.

Frequency of contacts with clients

The higher the frequency of sexual contacts with clients, the larger the potential for HIV to spread in commercial sex networks. Data suggest that FSWs in MENA have an average of about one client or less per *calendar* day, but a higher number per work day, broadly consistent with, but on the low side of, global trends.[84] In Afghanistan, FSWs reported an average of 13.1 clients per month in one study,[85] and in another study, 84% of them reported having one or two clients per working day, with 14% reporting three clients daily.[86] In the Islamic Republic of Iran, it is estimated that FSWs have five to nine customers per week,[87]

[65] Busulwa, "HIV/AIDS Situation Analysis Study"; Action Aid Afghanistan, "HIV AIDS in Afghanistan"; Ati, "HIV/AIDS/STIs Social and Geographical Mapping"; ACORD, "Socio Economic Research."
[66] Carael et al., "Clients of Sex Workers."
[67] Action Aid Afghanistan, "HIV AIDS in Afghanistan."
[68] Agha, "Potential for HIV Transmission."
[69] Faisel and Cleland, "Study of the Sexual Behaviours."
[70] Agha, "Potential for HIV Transmission."
[71] Ismail et al., "Sexually Transmitted Diseases in Men."
[72] Burans et al., "HIV Infection Surveillance in Mogadishu, Somalia."
[73] SNAP, UNICEF, and UNAIDS, "Baseline Study."
[74] Assal, "HIV Prevalence."
[75] Burans et al., "Serosurvey of Prevalence."
[76] McCarthy et al., "Hepatitis B and HIV in Sudan."
[77] Ahmed, *Military.*
[78] Ahmed, *Truck Drivers.*
[79] Ahmed, *Prisoners.*
[80] Taha et al., "Study of STDs."

[81] Holt et al., "Planning STI/HIV Prevention."
[82] Blanchard, Khan, and Bokhari, "Variations in the Population Size."
[83] Ibid.
[84] Morison et al., "Commercial Sex"; Lau et al., "A Study on Female Sex Workers"; Strathdee et al., "Characteristics of Female Sex Workers"; Elmore-Meegan, Conroy, and Agala, "Sex Workers in Kenya"; Wilson et al., "Sex Worker."
[85] World Bank, "Mapping and Situation Assessment."
[86] Action Aid Afghanistan, "HIV AIDS in Afghanistan."
[87] Mostashari, UNODC, and Darabi, "Summary of the Iranian Situation on HIV Epidemic."

with another report indicating an average of nine customers per week.[88] In Lebanon, FSWs reported an average of 3.1 nonregular partners and 2.1 regular partners per week, with a monthly average of 11.7 sexual partners.[89] Almost all FSWs (97%) in another study had more than five clients within the last month.[90] Also in Lebanon, most FSWs reported three to seven clients each week.[91]

In Pakistan, 7%–48% of FSWs in different settings reported more than 20 clients last month, and more than 80% of the FSWs reported less than one paid client per day.[92] The median number of clients per week in another study was three one-time clients and four regular clients.[93] In further studies from Pakistan, FSWs reported 4.5,[94] 4.6,[95] and 2.6[96] clients per workday and 31.6,[97] 36,[98] 33.1,[99] and 23[100] clients per month. Young FSWs were found to have the highest client volume.[101] Another study from Pakistan reported a mean of 5.5 clients in the past week, with a mean of 1.7 new clients in the past week.[102] This suggests that the number of new clients is relatively low, with many FSWs servicing a few regular clients.[103] The mean number of years in sex work was reported to be 13.9 years.[104]

In Sudan, more than half of FSWs reported more than two clients per day in Khartoum State,[105] and an average of four clients per week was reported in the Red Sea State.[106] The demand for sex work was found to rise during holidays, festivals, and at the end of the month.[107] In Southern Sudan, FSWs reported about two clients per day.[108] In the Syrian Arab Republic, 86.8% of FSWs reported one to three clients per day.[109] FSWs often report sexual activity with other sexual partners beyond sex work such as 53.8%[110] and 43.2%[111] in two studies of FSWs in Pakistan, and 57%[112] in a study in Syria.

Alcohol consumption is associated with higher sexual risk behavior and HIV infection,[113] and there is some evidence in MENA of alcohol and drug use in the context of commercial sex. In Pakistan, for example, in two studies, 27.4%[114] and 28.2%[115] of FSWs reported taking alcohol or drugs in the context of sex work in the last six months.

Structure of commercial sex networks

The data on the nature of commercial sex networks are limited. In parts of MENA, such as in Egypt, FSWs do not appear to form strong networks and do not have close ties.[116] This pattern appears to hold true in Lebanon as well, where FSWs have limited interaction among themselves due to intense competition.[117] In Southern Sudan, 92.8% of FSWs were working individually and not through mediators or organized sex work.[118] Understanding the network structure of sex workers and their clients is important in understanding the transmission patterns of HIV

[88] Ministry of Health and Medical Education of Iran, "Treatment and Medical Education."
[89] Hermez et al., "HIV/AIDS Prevention among Vulnerable Groups."
[90] Mishwar, "An Integrated Bio-Behavioral Surveillance Study."
[91] Rady, "Knowledge, Attitudes and Prevalence of Condom Use."
[92] Pakistan National AIDS Control Program, "Pilot Study in Karachi & Rawalpindi."
[93] Bokhari et al., "HIV Risk in Karachi and Lahore, Pakistan."
[94] Pakistan National AIDS Control Program, *HIV Second Generation Surveillance* (Round I).
[95] Blanchard, Khan, and Bokhari, "Variations in the Population Size."
[96] Pakistan National AIDS Control Program, *HIV Second Generation Surveillance* (Round II).
[97] Pakistan National AIDS Control Program, *HIV Second Generation Surveillance* (Round I).
[98] Blanchard, Khan, and Bokhari, "Variations in the Population Size."
[99] Pakistan National AIDS Control Program, *HIV Second Generation Surveillance* (Round II).
[100] Saleem, Adrien, and Razaque, "Risky Sexual Behavior."
[101] Pakistan National AIDS Control Program, *HIV Second Generation Surveillance* (Round I).
[102] Hawkes et al., "HIV and Other Sexually Transmitted Infections."
[103] Ibid.
[104] Ibid.
[105] ACORD, "Qualitative Socio Economic Research."

[106] Ati, "HIV/AIDS/STIs Social and Geographical Mapping."
[107] Ibid.
[108] ACORD, "Socio Economic Research."
[109] Syria National AIDS Programme, "HIV/AIDS Female Sex Workers."
[110] Pakistan National AIDS Control Program, *HIV Second Generation Surveillance* (Round I).
[111] Pakistan National AIDS Control Program, *HIV Second Generation Surveillance* (Round II).
[112] Syria National AIDS Programme, "HIV/AIDS Female Sex Workers."
[113] Mbulaiteye et al., "Alcohol and HIV"; Kaljee et al., "Alcohol Use"; Fisher, Bang, and Kapiga, "The Association between HIV Infection and Alcohol Use."
[114] Pakistan National AIDS Control Program, *HIV Second Generation Surveillance* (Round I).
[115] Pakistan National AIDS Control Program, *HIV Second Generation Surveillance* (Round II).
[116] Family Health International, "Implementing AIDS Prevention and Care (IMPACT) Project."
[117] Mishwar, "An Integrated Bio-Behavioral Surveillance Study."
[118] ACORD, "Socio Economic Research."

and other STIs in commercial sex networks.[119] Clustering of commercial sex networks into smaller subnetworks can reduce the overall STI prevalence among FSWs.[120] Given the limitations of the data, it is not possible to infer the connectivity of commercial sex networks in MENA.

Condom use

Reported condom use among FSWs varies substantially in MENA, although it appears to have been increasing in recent years. And while condom use is already at intermediate to high levels in several settings in MENA, it is still overall at low levels, particularly in the parts of MENA that are experiencing concentrated HIV epidemics among commercial sex workers, such as in Southern Sudan. This suggests that the majority of at-risk commercial sex acts in MENA are unprotected against HIV.

A number of studies documented condom use among FSWs in MENA. In Afghanistan, 36% of FSWs had ever used condoms.[121] In Egypt, 6% of FSWs always used condoms,[122] 56% had ever used condoms,[123] and 6.8% used condoms with noncommercial partners during last sex.[124] In the Islamic Republic of Iran, 24% and 83.2% of two FSW groups used condoms with the most recent client.[125] In studies in Lebanon, 28.1%, 34.8%, and 11.9% of FSWs reported that they always used condoms with nonregular clients, regular clients, and regular partners, respectively.[126] Almost 21% of these FSWs have never used condoms.[127] In a more recent study, 98%, 94%, and 43% of FSWs used condoms during last sex with a nonregular partner, a regular partner, and a regular client, respectively.[128]

In Pakistan, 17%–18% of FSWs in different settings always used condoms and 19%–26% did not use condoms during the last month.[129] In another study, 29%–49% of FSWs used a condom with a one-time client during last sex, 26%–47% used a condom with a regular client during last sex, and 21% used a condom with a nonpaying male during last sex.[130] Condom use during anal or oral sex was found to be more limited than its use in vaginal sex; only 7.9% of FSWs used a condom during last anal sex and 32.4% during last oral sex.[131] Also in Pakistan, 10% of migrant workers who had sex with FSWs used condoms.[132]

In Sudan, 13% of FSWs used condoms regularly,[133] and as reported in different studies, 10.3%,[134] 24.6%,[135] 57.8%,[136] and 23%[137] had ever used condoms. In yet another study, only 2% of clients of FSWs used condoms during last sex.[138] According to studies in Syria, 13.2%, 20.6%, 51%, and 15.2% always used condoms, often used condoms, sometimes used condoms, and never used condoms, respectively.[139] In Tunisia, only 37% of FSWs always used condoms, and 65% had ever used condoms, even though these FSWs are legal sex workers with free access to primary care centers.[140] In the Republic of Yemen, 57.1% of FSWs used a condom during last paid sex, 28.8% used a condom during last nonpaid sex, 50% used condoms consistently with nonregular clients, and 58% used condoms consistently with regular clients.[141] Further data on condom use among FSWs can be found in table 8.2.

Knowledge of condoms for HIV prevention, or as a birth control measure, appears to be rather high among FSWs, but still low in some

[119] Ghani and Aral, "Patterns of Sex Worker-Client Contacts."
[120] Ibid.
[121] World Bank, "Mapping and Situation Assessment."
[122] El-Sayed et al., "Evaluation of Selected Reproductive Health Infections."
[123] Ibid.
[124] Egypt MOH and Population National AIDS Program, HIV/AIDS Biological and Behavioral Surveillance Survey.
[125] Jahani et al., "Distribution and Risk Factors."; Ardalan et al., "Sex for Survival."
[126] Hermez et al., "HIV/AIDS Prevention among Vulnerable Groups."
[127] Hermez, "HIV/AIDS Prevention through Outreach."
[128] Mishwar, "An Integrated Bio-Behavioral Surveillance Study."

[129] Pakistan National AIDS Control Program, "Pilot Study in Karachi & Rawalpindi."
[130] Bokhari et al., "HIV Risk in Karachi and Lahore, Pakistan."
[131] Pakistan National AIDS Control Program, HIV Second Generation Surveillance (Round II).
[132] Faisel and Cleland, "Study of the Sexual Behaviours"; Faisel and Cleland, "Migrant Men."
[133] Ati, "HIV/AIDS/STIs Social and Geographical Mapping."
[134] Ahmed, Sex Sellers.
[135] ACORD, "Qualitative Socio Economic Research."
[136] Ati, "HIV/AIDS/STIs Social and Geographical Mapping."
[137] Anonymous, "Improving HIV/AIDS Response."
[138] SNAP, UNICEF, and UNAIDS, "Baseline Study."
[139] Syria National AIDS Programme, "HIV/AIDS Female Sex Workers."
[140] Hassen et al., "Cervical Human Papillomavirus Infection."
[141] Štulhofer and Božicevic, "HIV Bio-Behavioural Survey."

MENA settings. Only 41%[142] in Afghanistan and 17.2%,[143] 28%,[144] 45%,[145] and 45.1%[146] in studies in Sudan were aware of condoms. Condoms are often not seen as an HIV prevention measure, but as a contraceptive measure.[147] Between 37% and 77% of FSWs in Pakistan knew that condoms can prevent HIV.[148] The dominant mode of HIV prevention reported by FSWs in Sudan was minimizing the number of sexual partners.[149]

Knowledge of condoms does not necessarily translate into actual use. A fraction of FSWs do not perceive condom use as necessary, such as 29.1% of FSWs in Syria.[150] Only a quarter of FSWs in Southern Sudan negotiate condom use with their clients.[151] FSWs may not have the power to negotiate condom use,[152] and fear insistence on condom use would upset customers and result in clients leaving them for other FSWs or offering a lower price.[153] Dire financial need undermines the ability of FSWs to negotiate condom use,[154] and partner refusal and low desirability are two other barriers to condom use. In Syria, 45.2% of FSWs reported partner refusal as the reason for not using condoms and 25.9% reported that they do not like using them.[155] Some FSWs are also willing not to use condoms in exchange for a higher price such as in Lebanon,[156] Sudan,[157] and the Republic of Yemen.[158]

Access to condoms appears to be variable even within each MENA country. In the Republic of Yemen, FSWs in Aden reported easy access to condoms while other FSWs in other parts of the country reported difficulty in obtaining them.[159]

In Egypt, 44% of FSWs reported difficulty in getting condoms and 89% reported difficulty in using them.[160] One-third to two-thirds of FSWs in different settings in Pakistan reported that condoms were readily available.[161]

Commercial sex and STI transmission

A number of studies have documented substantial levels of STIs among FSWs (chapter 10 on STIs). Furthermore, a number of studies have documented STI transmission during contacts with FSWs, confirming the presence of active commercial sex networks all over MENA and indicating the heightened risk of exposure to HIV and other STIs in these networks. In the Islamic Republic of Iran, 64% of gonorrhea patients reported acquiring their infection through contacts with street-based FSWs.[162] In Kuwait, 77% of STD clinic attendees reported acquiring their infection from FSWs.[163] A similar outcome was found in another study in Kuwait where the common source of STIs was contact with FSWs.[164] The contacts occurred both in (50%) and outside (48%) of Kuwait.[165]

In Lebanon, a large fraction of the HIV infections acquired abroad were through contacts with FSWs.[166] In Pakistan, a history of urethritis or genital ulcer disease among male prisoners was associated with sex with FSWs.[167] The majority of Pakistanis who acquired HIV while working in the Persian Gulf region reported contacts with FSWs as the source of their infection.[168] Among truck drivers attending STD clinics in Pakistan, 40% reported contact with FSWs.[169] Also in Pakistan, 78% of STD clinic attendees who acquired STIs heterosexually reported that the source of infection was a sex

[142] World Bank, "Mapping and Situation Assessment."
[143] ACORD, "Qualitative Socio Economic Research."
[144] Ati, "HIV/AIDS/STIs Social and Geographical Mapping."
[145] Ahmed, Sex Sellers.
[146] Anonymous, "Improving HIV/AIDS Response."
[147] ACORD, "Socio Economic Research"; Ahmed, Sex Sellers.
[148] Bokhari et al., "HIV Risk in Karachi and Lahore, Pakistan."
[149] ACORD, "Qualitative Socio Economic Research."
[150] Syria National AIDS Programme, "HIV/AIDS Female Sex Workers."
[151] ACORD, "Socio Economic Research."
[152] ACORD, "Socio Economic Research"; ACORD, "Qualitative Socio Economic Research."
[153] Ati, "HIV/AIDS/STIs Social and Geographical Mapping"; ACORD, "Qualitative Socio Economic Research."
[154] ACORD, "Socio Economic Research."
[155] Syria National AIDS Programme, "HIV/AIDS Female Sex Workers."
[156] Hermez et al., "HIV/AIDS Prevention among Vulnerable Groups."
[157] Ati, "HIV/AIDS/STIs Social and Geographical Mapping."
[158] Štulhofer and Božicevic, "HIV Bio-Behavioural Survey."
[159] Busulwa, "HIV/AIDS Situation Analysis Study."

[160] El-Sayed et al., "Evaluation of Selected Reproductive Health Infections."
[161] Pakistan National AIDS Control Program, "Pilot Study in Karachi & Rawalpindi."
[162] Zargooshi, "Characteristics of Gonorrhoea."
[163] Al-Mutairi et al., "Clinical Patterns."
[164] Al-Fouzan and Al-Mutairi, "Overview."
[165] Al-Owaish et al., "HIV/AIDS Prevalence."
[166] Pieniazek et al., "Introduction of HIV-2."
[167] Akhtar and Luby, "Risk Behaviours."
[168] Shah et al., "HIV-Infected Workers Deported"; Baqi, Kayani, and Khan, "Epidemiology and Clinical Profile of HIV/AIDS "; Khan et al., "HIV-1 Subtype A Infection."
[169] Khawaja et al., "HIV/AIDS and Its Risk Factors in Pakistan."

worker.[170] In Saudi Arabia, 90% of men who were infected with HIV heterosexually acquired it from FSWs.[171] In Somalia, two studies reported that 40%[172] and 54%[173] of STD clinic attendees reported contacts with FSWs. In Sudan, 49.3% of STD patients reported acquiring their infection from FSWs.[174] HIV prevalence in Southern Sudan was 14% among men who reported contacts with FSWs, but 0% among men who denied such contacts.[175]

Anal sex, oral sex, and STIs as cofactors

Several studies have documented anal and oral sex practices in MENA. In Pakistan, FSWs in different cities reported having anal sex with a range of 0.6–4.1 clients last month.[176] In Sudan, about 55% of FSWs reported engaging in anal sex and 40% did so regularly.[177] Most often this was demanded or imposed by clients, but on occasion FSWs opted for anal sex to avoid pregnancy or to avoid having vaginal sex during menstruation.[178] The HIV transmission probability per coital act in unprotected receptive anal intercourse (0.0082)[179] is much higher than that of vaginal intercourse (0.0015).[180]

Oral sex appears to be common and was reported by 40% of FSWs in a study in Sudan.[181] In Pakistan, FSWs in different cities reported oral sex with a range of 0.6–3.8 clients last month.[182]

Only 3% of FSWs in a study in Sudan reported refraining from sex while suffering from a reproductive tract infection, a practice of concern considering the biological association of HIV transmission and STI coinfections.[183]

Engagement of FSWs in injecting drug risk behavior

FSWs report considerable levels of drug use both in injecting and noninjecting forms, and also report having sex with IDUs. These facts highlight the ease by which HIV can move between IDUs and FSWs. In particular, FSWs who inject drugs, or female IDUs who exchange sex for money or drugs, form subgroups at a heightened risk of HIV exposure, as has been seen in Asia.[184] These FSWs are highly marginalized and in urgent need of prevention and care programs.

Several studies have documented drug use among FSWs and sexual contacts with IDUs, but the data on female IDUs exchanging sex for money are limited. In Egypt, 9.3% of FSWs injected drugs and 78.8% used drugs.[185] In the Islamic Republic of Iran, 2% of a group of mainly FSWs injected drugs and 15.3% reported noninjecting drug use.[186] In another study, 2.5% of FSWs injected drugs and 60% used drugs.[187] In Pakistan, 20% of FSWs reported that they had clients whom they knew to inject drugs and 1%–2% of FSWs reported injecting drugs.[188] Also, in two studies in Pakistan, 3.3%[189] and 2.3%[190] of FSWs reported injecting drugs in the last six months and 13.5%[191] and 9.9%[192] had sex with IDUs. In yet more studies from Pakistan, 3% of FSWs reported injecting drugs in the last year,[193] 36% reported having sex with an IDU in the last year,[194] 20.3% reported IDUs as clients,[195] 22.4% reported lovers who inject drugs,[196] and 26% reported having a husband who injects drugs.[197]

[170] Rehan, "Profile of Men."

[171] Alrajhi, Halim, and Al-Abdely, "Mode of Transmission of HIV-1."

[172] Burans et al., "HIV Infection Surveillance in Mogadishu, Somalia."

[173] Ismail et al., "Sexually Transmitted Diseases in Men."

[174] Omer et al., "Sexually Transmitted Diseases in Sudanese Males."

[175] McCarthy, Khalid, and El Tigani, "HIV-1 Infection in Juba, Southern Sudan."

[176] Pakistan National AIDS Control Program, HIV Second Generation Surveillance (Round I).

[177] Ati, "HIV/AIDS/STIs Social and Geographical Mapping."

[178] Ibid.

[179] Vittinghoff et al., "Per-Contact Risk."

[180] Wawer et al., "Rates of HIV-1 Transmission."

[181] Ati, "HIV/AIDS/STIs Social and Geographical Mapping."

[182] Pakistan National AIDS Control Program, HIV Second Generation Surveillance (Round I).

[183] Korenromp et al., "Estimating the Magnitude."

[184] Commission on AIDS in Asia, Redefining AIDS in Asia.

[185] Egypt MOH and Population National AIDS Program, HIV/AIDS Biological and Behavioral Surveillance Survey.

[186] Jahani et al., "Distribution and Risk Factors."

[187] Tehrani and Malek-Afzalip, "Knowledge, Attitudes and Practices."

[188] Bokhari et al., "HIV Risk in Karachi and Lahore, Pakistan."

[189] Pakistan National AIDS Control Program, HIV Second Generation Surveillance (Round I).

[190] Pakistan National AIDS Control Program, HIV Second Generation Surveillance (Round II).

[191] Pakistan National AIDS Control Program, HIV Second Generation Surveillance (Round I).

[192] Pakistan National AIDS Control Program, HIV Second Generation Surveillance (Round II).

[193] Mayhew et al., "Protecting the Unprotected"; Hawkes et al., "HIV and Other Sexually Transmitted Infections."

[194] Hawkes et al., "HIV and Other Sexually Transmitted Infections."

[195] Mayhew et al., "Protecting the Unprotected."

[196] Ibid.

[197] Hawkes et al., "HIV and Other Sexually Transmitted Infections."

In Sudan, 4.8% of FSWs used drugs and 14.5% reported substance abuse among their clients.[198] In Syria and the Republic of Yemen, 10%[199] and 2%[200] of FSWs injected drugs, respectively.

KNOWLEDGE OF HIV/AIDS

Levels of HIV knowledge among sex workers appear to vary substantially in MENA. In Afghanistan, only 4% of FSWs in one study had heard of HIV/AIDS,[201] but in another study most FSWs reported knowing of HIV/AIDS, though very few ever tested for it.[202] In Egypt, all FSWs were aware of HIV and some of its transmission modes, but still had misconceptions about its transmission.[203] In the Islamic Republic of Iran, FSWs were found to be significantly less knowledgeable about HIV/AIDS than both youth and truck drivers.[204]

In Lebanon, almost all FSWs were aware of HIV/AIDS, its transmission modes, the condom's role in prevention, and other prevention measures.[205] However, 21.5% of these FSWs perceived no chance of becoming infected with HIV, possibly because of condom use.[206] In two studies in Pakistan, 60%[207] and 68%–98%[208] of FSWs reported ever hearing of HIV/AIDS, but only 15%–39% of FSWs felt at risk of HIV infection.[209] In Somalia, both men and women not engaged in sex work were found to know more than FSWs about HIV/AIDS.[210] In Sudan, 75.5% of FSWs were aware of HIV and its symptoms, and 54.9% were aware of some of its transmission modes.[211] In the Republic of Yemen, 85.9% of FSWs perceived no high risk of HIV infection.[212]

FSWs seek treatment for STIs through self-treatment or through friends rather than through knowledgeable health personnel.[213] They continue to suffer from unavailability of medical and support services,[214] and continue to fear pursuing such services due to social stigmatization, marginalization, and law enforcement.[215] All of the above factors contribute to the precarious and vulnerable position that FSWs endure in MENA.

ANALYTICAL SUMMARY

Commercial sex is prevalent all over MENA, although at lower levels compared to other regions. Economic pressure, family disruption or dysfunction, and political conflicts are major pressures for commercial sex in MENA. Roughly 0.1% to 1% of women appear to exchange sex for money or other commodities, and a few percentage points of men report sexual contacts with FSWs. Accordingly, commercial sex networks are the largest of the three key priority group networks in MENA.

There is considerable evidence on HIV prevalence and risk behavior practices among FSWs in MENA. Earlier evidence suffered from methodological limitations, but the quality of evidence has improved significantly in recent years. Regardless, all evidence suggests that HIV prevalence continues to be at low levels among FSWs in most countries, though at levels much higher than those in the general population. HIV does not appear to be well established in many commercial sex networks in MENA. In three countries, however (Djibouti, Somalia, and Sudan), HIV prevalence has reached high levels, indicating concentrated HIV epidemics in at least parts of these countries. Nevertheless, HIV prevalence in these countries is at lower levels than those found in hyperendemic HIV epidemics in sub-Saharan Africa.

FSWs report considerable levels of sexual risk behavior including roughly one client per calendar day; low levels of condom use, particularly in areas of concentrated HIV epidemics among

[198] Ati, "HIV/AIDS/STIs Social and Geographical Mapping."

[199] UNAIDS, "Notes on AIDS in the Middle East and North Africa"; Syria National AIDS Programme, "HIV/AIDS Female Sex Workers."

[200] Štulhofer and Božicevic, "HIV Bio-Behavioural Survey."

[201] Action Aid Afghanistan, "HIV AIDS in Afghanistan."

[202] World Bank, "Mapping and Situation Assessment."

[203] Egypt MOH and Population National AIDS Program, *HIV/AIDS Biological and Behavioral Surveillance Survey.*

[204] Tehrani and Malek-Afzalip, "Knowledge, Attitudes and Practices."

[205] Hermez et al., "HIV/AIDS Prevention among Vulnerable Groups."

[206] Ibid.

[207] Ali and Khanani, *Interventions Aimed at Behavior Modification.*

[208] Bokhari et al., "HIV Risk in Karachi and Lahore, Pakistan."

[209] Ibid.

[210] Corwin et al., "HIV-1 in Somalia."

[211] Anonymous, "Improving HIV/AIDS Response."

[212] Štulhofer and Božicevic, "HIV Bio-Behavioural Survey."

[213] Tehrani and Malek-Afzalip, "Knowledge, Attitudes and Practices."

[214] Mohebbi, "Female Sex Workers and Fear of Stigmatisation."

[215] Zargooshi, "Characteristics of Gonorrhoea."

FSWs; anal and oral sex in addition to vaginal sex; having clients or sexual partners who inject drugs; and injecting drugs themselves. Considerable levels of STI prevalence other than HIV are found among FSWs. STD clinic attendees repeatedly report acquiring STDs through paid sex. Levels of comprehensive HIV knowledge among FSWs vary across the region, with both high and low levels being documented in different settings.

The above factors suggest a potential for further HIV spread among FSWs, but probably not at high levels in most countries, except for Djibouti, Somalia, and Sudan. Near universal male circumcision, with its efficacy against HIV acquisition (chapter 6), and the lower risk behavior compared to other regions may prevent massive or even concentrated HIV epidemics among FSWs from materializing in most countries in MENA for at least a decade, if ever. Furthermore, the dynamics of HIV infection among FSWs are different from those for MSM and IDUs. FSWs are infected by their clients who are at lower risk behavior than themselves, as opposed to MSM and IDUs who are infected by members of their own risk group.

Yet HIV prevalence among FSWs will be at levels much higher than those among the general population. Subgroups within FSWs may be particularly at high risk of HIV, such as those who inject drugs, those who have clients who inject drugs, and female IDUs who exchange sex for money or drugs, as well as FSWs with low socioeconomic status who have poor HIV knowledge or are not able to afford or negotiate condom use. These subgroups are highly marginalized and in dire need of prevention and care programs. Furthermore, all FSWs are in need of prevention and care services not only because of HIV, but also because of the considerable levels of other STIs in this population. Dedicated STI services for FSWs need to be established, and in settings where they are already established, they need to be expanded.

BIBLIOGRAPHY

ACORD (Agency for Co-operation and Research in Development). 2005. "Socio Economic Research on HIV/AIDS Prevention among Informal Sex Workers." Federal Ministry of Health, Sudan National AIDS Control Program, and the World Health Organization.

———. 2006. "Qualitative Socio Economic Research on Female Sex Workers and Their Vulnerability to HIV/ AIDS in Khartoum State."

Action Aid Afghanistan. 2006. "HIV AIDS in Afghanistan: A Study on Knowledge, Attitude, Behavior, and Practice in High Risk and Vulnerable Groups in Afghanistan."

Agha, S. 2000. "Potential for HIV Transmission among Truck Drivers in Pakistan." *AIDS* 14: 2404–6.

Ahmed, S. M. 2004a. *Antenatal: Situation Analysis-Behavioral Survey Results & Discussions*. Report. Sudan National AIDS Control Program.

———. 2004b. *Military: Situation Analysis-Behavioral Survey Results & Discussions*. Report. Sudan National AIDS Control Program.

———. 2004c. *Prisoners: Situation Analysis-Behavioral Survey Results & Discussions*. Report. Sudan National AIDS Control Program.

———. 2004d. *Sex Sellers: Situation Analysis-Behavioral Survey Results & Discussions*. Report. Sudan National AIDS Control Program.

———. 2004e. *Tea Sellers: Situation Analysis-Behavioral Survey Results & Discussions*. Report. Sudan National AIDS Control Program.

———. 2004f. *Truck Drivers: Situation Analysis-Behavioral Survey Results & Discussions*. Report. Sudan National AIDS Control Program.

Ahmed, H. J., K. Omar, S. Y. Adan, A. M. Guled, L. Grillner, and S. Bygdeman. 1991. "Syphilis and Human Immunodeficiency Virus Seroconversion during a 6-Month Follow-Up of Female Prostitutes in Mogadishu, Somalia." *Int J STD AIDS* 2: 119–23.

Akhtar, S., and S. P. Luby. 2002. "Risk Behaviours Associated with Urethritis and Genital Ulcer Disease in Prison Inmates, Sindh, Pakistan." *East Mediterr Health J* 8: 776–86.

Al-Ali, N. 2005. "Reconstructing Gender: Iraqi Women between Dictatorship, War, Sanctions and Occupation." *Third World Quarterly* 26: 739–58.

———. 2007. "Iraqi Women: Untold Stories from 1948 to the Present."

Alami, K. 2009. "Tendances récentes de l'épidémie à VIH/SIDA en Afrique du nord." Presentation, Research and AIDS Workshop in North Africa, Marrakech, Morocco.

Al-Fouzan, A., and N. Al-Mutairi. 2004. "Overview of Incidence of Sexually Transmitted Diseases in Kuwait." *Clin Dermatol* 22: 509–12.

Algeria MOH (Ministry of Health). Unknown. *Rapport de l'enquête nationale de séro-surveillance*.

Ali, S., and R. Khanani. 1996. *Interventions Aimed at Behavior Modification of Commercial Sex Workers in Pakistan*. Karachi: Pakistan AIDS Prevention Society.

Al-Mutairi, N., A. Joshi, O. Nour-Eldin, A. K. Sharma, I. El-Adawy, and M. Rijhwani. 2007. "Clinical Patterns of Sexually Transmitted Diseases, Associated Sociodemographic Characteristics, and Sexual Practices in the Farwaniya Region of Kuwait." *Int J Dermatol* 46: 594–99.

Al-Owaish, R. A., S. Anwar, P. Sharma, and S. F. Shah. 2000. "HIV/AIDS Prevalence among Male Patients in Kuwait." *Saudi Med J* 21: 852–59.

Al-Qadhi, H. 2001. "A Silent Threat in Yemen: Confronting HIV/AIDS Choices." United Nations Development Programme.

Alrajhi, A. A., M. A. Halim, and H. M. Al-Abdely. 2004. "Mode of Transmission of HIV-1 in Saudi Arabia." *AIDS* 18: 1478–80.

Al-Serouri, A. W. 2005. "Assessment of Knowledge, Attitudes and Beliefs about HIV/AIDS among Young People Residing in High Risk Communities in Aden Governorate, Republic of Yemen." Society for the Development of Women & Children (SOUL), Education, Health, Welfare, United Nations Children's Fund, Yemen Country Office, HIV/AIDS Project.

Anonymous. 2007. "Improving HIV/AIDS Response among Most at Risk Population in Sudan." Orientation Workshop, April 16.

Aral, S. O., and J. S. St. Lawrence. 2002. "The Ecology of Sex Work and Drug Use in Saratov Oblast, Russia." *Sex Transm Dis* 29: 798–805.

Aral, S. O., J. S. St Lawrence, L. Tikhonova, E. Safarova, K. A. Parker, A. Shakarishvili, and C. A. Ryan. 2003. "The Social Organization of Commercial Sex Work in Moscow, Russia." *Sex Transm Dis* 30: 39–45.

Ardalan, A., K. H. Na'ini, A. M. Tabrizi, and A. Jazayeri. 2002. "Sex for Survival: The Future of Runaway Girls." *Social Welfare Research Quarterly* 2: 187–219.

Assal, M. 2006. "HIV Prevalence, Knowledge, Attitude, Practices, and Risk Factors among Prisoners in Khartoum State, Sudan." Grey Report.

Ati, H. A. 2005. "HIV/AIDS/STIs Social and Geographical Mapping of Prisoners, Tea Sellers and Commercial Sex Workers in Port Sudan Town, Red Sea State." Ockenden International, Sudan. Draft 2.

Baqi, S., N. Kayani, and J. A. Khan. 1999. "Epidemiology and Clinical Profile of HIV/AIDS in Pakistan." *Trop Doct* 29: 144–48.

Baqi, S., N. Nabi, S. N. Hasan, A. J. Khan, O. Pasha, N. Kayani, R. A. Haque, I. U. Haq, M. Khurshid, S. Fisher-Hoch, S. P. Luby, and J. B. McCormick. 1998. "HIV Antibody Seroprevalence and Associated Risk Factors in Sex Workers, Drug Users, and Prisoners in Sindh, Pakistan." *J Acquir Immune Defic Syndr Hum Retrovirol* 18: 73–79.

Basha, H. M. 2006. "Vulnerable Population Research in Darfur." Grey Report.

Blanchard, J. F., S. Halli, B. M. Ramesh, P. Bhattacharjee, R. G. Washington, J. O'Neil, and S. Moses. 2007. "Variability in the Sexual Structure in a Rural Indian Setting: Implications for HIV Prevention Strategies." *Sex Transm Infect* 83 Suppl 1: i30–36.

Blanchard, J. F., A. Khan, and A. Bokhari. 2008. "Variations in the Population Size, Distribution and Client Volume among Female Sex Workers in Seven Cities of Pakistan." *Sex Transm Infect* 84 Suppl 2: ii24–27.

Bokhari, A., N. M. Nizamani, D. J. Jackson, N. E. Rehan, M. Rahman, R. Muzaffar, S. Mansoor, H. Raza, K. Qayum, P. Girault, E. Pisani, and I. Thaver. 2007. "HIV Risk in Karachi and Lahore, Pakistan: An Emerging Epidemic in Injecting and Commercial Sex Networks." *Int J STD AIDS* 18: 486–92.

Burans, J. P., E. Fox, M. A. Omar, A. H. Farah, S. Abbass, S. Yusef, A. Guled, M. Mansour, R. Abu-Elyazeed, and J. N. Woody. 1990. "HIV Infection Surveillance in Mogadishu, Somalia." *East Afr Med J* 67: 466–72.

Burans, J. P., M. McCarthy, S. M. el Tayeb, A. el Tigani, J. George, R. Abu-Elyazeed, and J. N. Woody. 1990. "Serosurvey of Prevalence of Human Immunodeficiency Virus amongst High Risk Groups in Port Sudan, Sudan." *East Afr Med J* 67: 650–55.

Busulwa, R. 2003. "HIV/AIDS Situation Analysis Study." Conducted in Hodeidah, Taiz and Hadhramut, Republic of Yemen. Grey Report.

Carael, M., E. Slaymaker, R. Lyerla, and S. Sarkar. 2006. "Clients of Sex Workers in Different Regions of the World: Hard to Count." *Sex Transm Infect* 82 Suppl 3: iii26–33.

Chaouki, N., F. X. Bosch, N. Munoz, C. J. Meijer, B. El Gueddari, A. El Ghazi, J. Deacon, X. Castellsague, and J. M. Walboomers. 1998. "The Viral Origin of Cervical Cancer in Rabat, Morocco." *Int J Cancer* 75: 546–54.

Commission on AIDS in Asia. 2008. *Redefining AIDS in Asia: Crafting an Effective Response*. New Delhi, India: Oxford University Press. Presented to Ban Ki-moon, UN Secretary General, on March 26, 2008. Oxford University Press.

Corwin, A. L., J. G. Olson, M. A. Omar, A. Razaki, and D. M. Watts. 1991. "HIV-1 in Somalia: Prevalence and Knowledge among Prostitutes." *AIDS* 5: 902–4.

Daher, C., and D. Zayat. 2007. "A Matter of Life: Views, Perceptions, and Practices of Commercial Sex Workers and Intravenous Drug Users regarding HIV/AIDS Risk Behaviors." Grey Report.

Dareini, A. 2002. "Rise in Iranian Prostitution Blamed on Strict Sex Rules, Economy." Associated Press September 15.

Dewachi, O. 2001. "Men Who Have Sex with Other Men and HIV AIDS: A Situation Analysis in Beirut, Lebanon; HIV/AIDS Prevention through Outreach to Vulnarable Populations." Grey Report, April 29.

Egypt MOH (Ministry of Health), and Population National AIDS Program. 2006. *HIV/AIDS Biological and Behavioral Surveillance Survey*. Summary report.

El-Gawhary, K. 1995. *Sex Tourism in Cairo*. Middle East Report (September–October). Middle East Research and Information Project.

Elmore-Meegan, M., R. M. Conroy, and C. B. Agala. 2004. "Sex Workers in Kenya, Numbers of Clients and Associated Risks: An Exploratory Survey." *Reprod Health Matters* 12: 50–57.

El-Sayed, N., M. Abdallah, A. Abdel Mobdy, A. Abdel Sattar, E. Aoun, F. Beths, G. Dallabetta, M. Rakha, C. Soliman, and N. Wasef. 2002. "Evaluation of Selected Reproductive Health Infections in Various Egyptian Population Groups in Greater Cairo." MOHP, IMPACT/FHI/USAID.

Etchepare, M. 2001. "Programme National de Lutte contre le SIDA et les MST." Draft report, World Bank Mission for Health Project Strategy Development, Djibouti.

Faisel, A., and J. Cleland. 2006a. "Migrant Men: A Priority for HIV Control in Pakistan?" *Sex Transm Infect* 82: 307–10.

———. 2006b. "Study of the Sexual Behaviours and Prevalence of STIs among Migrant Men in Lahore, Pakistan." Arjumand and Associates, Centre for Population Studies, London School of Hygiene and Tropical Medicine.

Family Health International. 2007. "Implementing AIDS Prevention and Care (IMPACT) Project." USAID, Egypt Final Report, April 1999–September 2007.

Farah, M. S., and S. Hussein. 2006. "HIV Prevalence, Knowledge, Attitude, Practices and Risk Factors among Truck Drivers in Khartoum State." Grey Report. Sudan National AIDS Program.

Fares, G., et al. 2004. *Rapport sur l'enquête nationale de sero-surveillance sentinelle du VIH et de la syphilis en Algérie en 2004.* Ministère de la Santé de la population et de la reforme hospitalière, Alger, Décembre.

Fisher, J. C., H. Bang, and S. H. Kapiga. 2007. "The Association between HIV Infection and Alcohol Use: A Systematic Review and Meta-Analysis of African Studies." *Sex Transm Dis* 34: 856–63.

Fox, E., R. L. Haberberger, E. A. Abbatte, S. Said, D. Polycarpe, and N. T. Constantine. 1989. "Observations on Sexually Transmitted Diseases in Promiscuous Males in Djibouti." *J Egypt Public Health Assoc* 64: 561–69.

Ghani, A. C., and S. O. Aral. 2005. "Patterns of Sex Worker-Client Contacts and Their Implications for the Persistence of Sexually Transmitted Infections." *J Infect Dis* 191 Suppl 1: S34–41.

Gul, U., A. Kilic, B. Sakizligil, S. Aksaray, S. Bilgili, O. Demirel, and C. Erinckan. 2008. "Magnitude of Sexually Transmitted Infections among Female Sex Workers in Turkey." *J Eur Acad Dermatol Venereol* 22: 1123–24.

Hassan, G. 2005. "Iraqi Women under Occupation." *Brussells Tribunal* (www.brusselstribunal.org), May.

Hassen, E., A. Chaieb, M. Letaief, H. Khairi, A. Zakhama, S. Remadi, and L. Chouchane. 2003. "Cervical Human Papillomavirus Infection in Tunisian Women." *Infection* 31: 143–48.

Hawkes, S., M. Collumbien, L. Platt, N. Lalji, N. Rizvi, A. Andreasen, J. Chow, R. Muzaffar, H. ur-Rehman, N. Siddiqui, S. Hasan, and A. Bokhari. 2009. "HIV and Other Sexually Transmitted Infections among Men, Transgenders and Women Selling Sex in Two Cities in Pakistan: A Cross-Sectional Prevalence Survey." *Sex Transm Infect* 85 Suppl 2: ii8–16.

Hermez, J. Unknown. "HIV/AIDS Prevention through Outreach to Vulnerable Populations in Beirut, Lebanon." Grey Report, Beirut, Lebanon.

Hermez, J., E. Aaraj, O. Dewachi, and N. Chemaly. Unknown. "HIV/AIDS Prevention among Vulnerable Groups in Beirut, Lebanon." PowerPoint presentation, Lebanon National AIDS Program, Beirut.

Holt, B. Y., P. Effler, W. Brady, J. Friday, E. Belay, K. Parker, and M. Toole. 2003. "Planning STI/HIV Prevention among Refugees and Mobile Populations: Situation Assessment of Sudanese Refugees." *Disasters* 27: 1–15.

Huda, S. 2006. "Sex Trafficking in South Asia." *Int J Gynaecol Obstet* 94: 374–81.

Indonesia MOH (Ministry of Health). 2002. *National Estimates of Adult HIV Infection, Indonesia.* Workshop report.

Institut de Formation Paramédicale de Parnet. 2004. *Rapport de la réunion d'évaluation a mis-parcours de l'enquête de sero-surveillance du VIH.* Juin.

Iqbal, J., and N. Rehan. 1996. "Sero-Prevalence of HIV: Six Years' Experience at Shaikh Zayed Hospital, Lahore." *J Pak Med Assoc* 46: 255–58.

Ismail, S. O., H. J. Ahmed, L. Grillner, B. Hederstedt, A. Issa, and S. M. Bygdeman. 1990. "Sexually Transmitted Diseases in Men in Mogadishu, Somalia." *Int J STD AIDS* 1: 102–6.

Jahani, M. R., S. M. Alavian, H. Shirzad, A. Kabir, and B. Hajarizadeh. 2005. "Distribution and Risk Factors of Hepatitis B, Hepatitis C, and HIV Infection in a Female Population with 'Illegal Social Behaviour.'" *Sex Transm Infect* 81: 185.

Jama, H., L. Grillner, G. Biberfeld, S. Osman, A. Isse, M. Abdirahman, and S. Bygdeman. 1987. "Sexually Transmitted Viral Infections in Various Population Groups in Mogadishu, Somalia." *Genitourin Med* 63: 329–32.

Jenkins, C., and D. A. Robalino. 2003. "HIV in the Middle East and North Africa: The Cost of Inaction." Orientations in Development Series. Washington, DC: World Bank.

Kaljee, L. M., B. L. Genberg, T. T. Minh, L. H. Tho, L. T. Thoa, and B. Stanton. 2005. "Alcohol Use and HIV Risk Behaviors among Rural Adolescents in Khanh Hoa Province Viet Nam." *Health Educ Res* 20: 71–80.

Khan, S., M. A. Rai, M. R. Khanani, M. N. Khan, and S. H. Ali. 2006. "HIV-1 Subtype A Infection in a Community of Intravenous Drug Users in Pakistan." *BMC Infect Dis* 6: 164.

Khattabi, H., and K. Alami. 2005. "Surveillance sentinelle du VIH, Résultats 2004 et tendance de la séroprévalence du VIH." Morocco Ministry of Health, UNAIDS.

Khawaja, Z. A., L. Gibney, A. J. Ahmed, and S. H. Vermund. 1997. "HIV/AIDS and Its Risk Factors in Pakistan." *AIDS* 11: 843–48.

Korenromp, E. L., S. J. de Vlass, N. J. Nagelkerke, and J. D. Habbema. 2001. "Estimating the Magnitude of STD Cofactor Effects on HIV Transmission: How Well Can It Be Done?" *Sex Transm Dis* 28: 613–21.

Lambert, L. 2007. "HIV and Development Challenges in Yemen: Which Grows Fastest?" *Health Policy and Planning* 22: 60.

Lau, J. T., H. Y. Tsui, P. C. Siah, and K. L. Zhang. 2002. "A Study on Female Sex Workers in Southern China (Shenzhen): HIV-Related Knowledge, Condom Use and STD History." *AIDS Care* 14: 219–33.

Lowndes, C. M., M. Alary, H. Meda, C. A. Gnintoungbe, L. Mukenge-Tshibaka, C. Adjovi, A. Buve, L. Morison, M. Laourou, L. Kanhonou, and S. Anagonou. 2002. "Role of Core and Bridging Groups in the Transmission Dynamics of HIV and STIs in Cotonou, Benin, West Africa." *Sex Transm Infect* 78 Suppl 1: i69–77.

Marcelin, A. G., M. Grandadam, P. Flandre, J. L. Koeck, M. Philippon, E. Nicand, R. Teyssou, H. Agut, J. M. Huraux, and N. Dupin. 2001. "Comparative Study of Heterosexual Transmission of HIV-1, HSV-2 and KSHV in Djibouti." *8th Retrovir Oppor Infect* (abstract no. 585).

Marcelin, A. G., M. Grandadam, P. Flandre, E. Nicand, C. Milliancourt, J. L. Koeck, M. Philippon, R. Teyssou, H. Agut, N. Dupin, and V. Calvez. 2002. "Kaposi's Sarcoma Herpesvirus and HIV-1 Seroprevalences in Prostitutes in Djibouti." *J Med Virol* 68: 164–67.

Mayhew, S., M. Collumbien, A. Qureshi, L. Platt, N. Rafiq, A. Faisel, N. Lalji, and S. Hawkes. 2009. "Protecting the Unprotected: Mixed-Method Research on Drug Use, Sex Work and Rights in Pakistan's Fight against HIV/AIDS." *Sex Transm Infect* 85 Suppl 2: ii31–36.

Mbulaiteye, S. M., A. Ruberantwari, J. S. Nakiyingi, L. M. Carpenter, A. Kamali, and J. A. Whitworth. 2000. "Alcohol and HIV: A Study among Sexually Active Adults in Rural Southwest Uganda." *Int J Epidemiol* 29: 911–15.

McCarthy, M. C., J. P. Burans, N. T. Constantine, A. A. el-Hag, M. E. el-Tayeb, M. A. el-Dabi, J. G. Fahkry, J. N. Woody, and K. C. Hyams. 1989. "Hepatitis B and HIV in Sudan: A Serosurvey for Hepatitis B and Human Immunodeficiency Virus Antibodies among Sexually Active Heterosexuals." *Am J Trop Med Hyg* 41: 726–31.

McCarthy, M. C., I. O. Khalid, and A. El Tigani. 1995. "HIV-1 Infection in Juba, Southern Sudan." *J Med Virol* 46: 18–20.

Ministry of Health and Medical Education of Iran. 2006. "Treatment and Medical Education." Islamic Republic of Iran HIV/AIDS situation and response analysis.

Mishwar. 2008. "An Integrated Bio-Behavioral Surveillance Study among Four Vulnerable Groups in Lebanon: Men Who Have Sex with Men; Prisoners; Commercial Sex Workers and Intravenous Drug Users." Mid-term Report, American University of Beirut and World Bank.

Mohebbi, M. R. 2005. "Female Sex Workers and Fear of Stigmatisation." *Sex Transm Infect* 81: 180–81.

Morison, L., H. A. Weiss, A. Buve, M. Carael, S. C. Abega, F. Kaona, L. Kanhonou, J. Chege, and R. J. Hayes. 2001. "Commercial Sex and the Spread of HIV in Four Cities in Sub-Saharan Africa." *AIDS* 15 Suppl 4: S61–69.

Morocco MOH (Ministry of Health, Ministère de la Santé). 2003–4. *Bulletin épidemiologique de surveillance du VIH/SIDA et des infections sexuellement transmissibles.* Rabat, Ministère de la Santé Maroc.

———. 2005. *Bulletin épidemiologique de surveillance du VIH/SIDA et des infections sexuellement transmissibles.* Rabat, Ministère de la Santé Maroc.

———. 2007. *Surveillance sentinelle du VIH, résultats 2006 et tendances de la séroprévalence du VIH.*

Mostashari, G., UNODC (United Nations Office on Drugs and Crime), and M. Darabi. 2006. "Summary of the Iranian Situation on HIV Epidemic." NSP Situation Analysis.

Omer, E. E., M. H. Ali, O. M. Taha, M. A. Ahmed, and S. A. Abbaro. 1982. "Sexually Transmitted Diseases in Sudanese Males." *Trop Doct* 12: 208–10.

Orak, S., A. E. Dalkilic, and Y. Ozbal. 1991. "Serological Investigation of HIV Infections, HBsAg and Syphilis in Prostitutes in Elazig." *Mikrobiyol Bul* 25: 51–56.

Pakistan National AIDS Control Program. 2005a. *HIV Second Generation Surveillance in Pakistan.* National Report Round 1. Ministry of Health, Pakistan, and Canada-Pakistan HIV/AIDS Surveillance Project.

———. 2005b. "Pilot Study in Karachi & Rawalpindi." Ministry of Health Canada-Pakistan HIV/AIDS Surveillance Project, Integrated Biological & Behavioral Surveillance 2004–5.

———. 2006–7. *HIV Second Generation Surveillance in Pakistan.* National Report Round II. Ministry of Health, Pakistan, and Canada-Pakistan HIV/AIDS Surveillance Project.

———. 2008. *HIV Second Generation Surveillance in Pakistan.* National Report Round III. Ministry of Health, Pakistan, Canada-Pakistan HIV/AIDS Surveillance Project.

Philippon, M., M. Saada, M. A. Kamil, and H. M. Houmed. 1997. "Attendance at a Health Center by Clandestine Prostitutes in Djibouti." *Sante* 7: 5–10.

Pieniazek, D., J. Baggs, D. J. Hu, G. M. Matar, A. M. Abdelnoor, J. E. Mokhbat, M. Uwaydah, A. R. Bizri, A. Ramos, L. M. Janini, A. Tanuri, C. Fridlund, C. Schable, L. Heyndrickx, M. A. Rayfield, and W. Heneine. 1998. "Introduction of HIV-2 and Multiple HIV-1 Subtypes to Lebanon." *Emerg Infect Dis* 4: 649–56.

Rady, A. 2005. "Knowledge, Attitudes and Prevalence of Condom Use among Female Sex Workers in Lebanon: Behavioral Surveillance Study." UNFPA.

Razzaghi, E. M., A. R. Movaghar, T. C. Green, and K. Khoshnood. 2006. "Profiles of Risk: A Qualitative Study of Injecting Drug Users in Tehran, Iran." *Harm Reduct J* 3: 12.

Rehan, N. 2006. "Profile of Men Suffering from Sexually Transmitted Infections in Pakistan." *J Pak Med Assoc* 56: S60–65.

Rodier, G. R., B. Couzineau, G. C. Gray, C. S. Omar, E. Fox, J. Bouloumie, and D. Watts. 1993. "Trends of Human Immunodeficiency Virus Type-1 Infection in Female Prostitutes and Males Diagnosed with a Sexually Transmitted Disease in Djibouti, East Africa." *Am J Trop Med Hyg* 48: 682–86.

Saleem, N. H., A. Adrien, and A. Razaque. 2008. "Risky Sexual Behavior, Knowledge of Sexually Transmitted Infections and Treatment Utilization among a Vulnerable Population in Rawalpindi, Pakistan." *Southeast Asian J Trop Med Public Health* 39: 642–48.

Sepehrad, R. 2002. "The Role of Women in Iran's New Popular Revolution." *Brown J World Aff* 9: 217.

Shah, S. A., O. A. Khan, S. Kristensen, and S. H. Vermund. 1999. "HIV-Infected Workers Deported from the Gulf States: Impact on Southern Pakistan." *Int J STD AIDS* 10: 812–14.

SNAP (Sudan National AIDS Program), UNICEF (United Nations Children's Fund), and UNAIDS (United Nations Joint Programme on HIV/AIDS). 2005. "Baseline Study on Knowledge, Attitudes, and Practices on Sexual Behaviors and HIV/AIDS Prevention amongst Young People in Selected States in Sudan." HIV/AIDS KAPB Report. Projects and Research Department (AFROCENTER Group).

Soins Infirmiers et Developpement Communautaire. 2008. "Mapping for FSW and IDU Report." Grey Report.

Strathdee, S. A., R. Lozada, S. J. Semple, P. Orozovich, M. Pu, H. Staines-Orozco, M. Fraga-Vallejo, H. Amaro, A. Delatorre, C. Magis-Rodriguez, and T. L. Patterson. 2008. "Characteristics of Female Sex Workers with U.S. Clients in Two Mexico-U.S. Border Cities." *Sex Transm Dis* 35: 263–68.

Štulhofer, A., and I. Božicevic. 2008. "HIV Bio-Behavioural Survey among FSWs in Aden, Yemen." Grey Report.

Syria National AIDS Programme. 2004. "HIV/AIDS Female Sex Workers KABP Survey in Syria." Grey Report.

Taha, O. M., M. H. Ali, E. E. Omer, M. A. Ahmed, and S. A. Abbaro. 1979. "Study of STDs in Patients Attending Venereal Disease Clinics in Khartoum, Sudan." *Br J Vener Dis* 55: 313–15.

Tassie, J.-M. Unknown. "Assignment Report HIV/AIDS/STD Surveillance in I.R. of Iran." UNAIDS, Mission Internal Report.

Tehrani, F. R., and H. Malek-Afzalip. 2008. "Knowledge, Attitudes and Practices concerning HIV/AIDS among Iranian At-Risk Sub-Populations." *Eastern Mediterranean Health Journal* 14.

Testa, A. C., and K. Kriitmaa. 2009. "HIV and Syphilis Bio-Behavioural Surveillance Survey (BSS+) among Female Transactional Sex Workers in Hargeisa, Somaliland." International Organization for Migration, World Health Organization.

Tiras, M. B., O. Karabacak, Ö. Himmetoglu, and S. Yüksel. 1998. "Seroprevalence of Hepatitis B and HIV Infection in High-Risk Turkish Population." *Turkiye Klinikleri J Gynecol Obst* 8: 157–58.

UNAIDS (United Nations Joint Programme on HIV/AIDS). 2008. "Notes on AIDS in the Middle East and North Africa." RST, MENA.

UNFPA (United Nations Population Fund). 2009. "UNFPA, Local NGO Partner for HIV Education Efforts Aimed at Pakistani Sex Workers." *Kaisernetwork Daily News* January 7.

Unknown. "Statut de la réponse nationale: Caractéristiques de l'épidémie des IST/VIH/SIDA." Algeria.

Vandepitte, J., R. Lyerla, G. Dallabetta, F. Crabbe, M. Alary, and A. Buve. 2006. "Estimates of the Number of Female Sex Workers in Different Regions of the World." *Sex Transm Infect* 82 Suppl 3: iii18–25.

Vittinghoff, E., J. Douglas, F. Judson, D. McKirnan, K. MacQueen, and S. P. Buchbinder. 1999. "Per-Contact Risk of Human Immunodeficiency Virus Transmission between Male Sexual Partners." *Am J Epidemiol* 150: 306–11.

Watts, D. M., N. T. Constantine, M. F. Sheba, M. Kamal, J. D. Callahan, and M. E. Kilpatrick. 1993. "Prevalence of HIV Infection and AIDS in Egypt over Four Years of Surveillance (1986–1990)." *J Trop Med Hyg* 96: 113–17.

Watts, D. M., A. L. Corwin, M. A. Omar, and K. C. Hyams. 1994. "Low Risk of Sexual Transmission of Hepatitis C Virus in Somalia." *Trans R Soc Trop Med Hyg* 88: 55–56.

Wawer, M. J., R. H. Gray, N. K. Sewankambo, D. Serwadda, X. Li, O. Laeyendecker, N. Kiwanuka, G. Kigozi, M. Kiddugavu, T. Lutalo, F. Nalugoda, F. Wabwire-Mangen, M. P. Meehan, and T. C. Quinn. 2005. "Rates of HIV-1 Transmission per Coital Act, by Stage of HIV-1 Infection, in Rakai, Uganda." *J Infect Dis* 191: 1403–9.

WHO (World Health Organization). 1999. *Consensus Report on STI, HIV, and AIDS Epidemiology, Malaysia.* Regional Office for the Western Pacific.

WHO, UNICEF (United Nations Children's Fund), and UNAIDS (United Nations Joint Programme on HIV/AIDS). 2006. "Yemen, Epidemiological Facts Sheets on HIV/AIDS and Sexually Transmitted Infections."

Wilson, D., P. Chiroro, S. Lavelle, and C. Mutero. 1989. "Sex Worker, Client Sex Behaviour and Condom Use in Harare, Zimbabwe." *AIDS Care* 1: 269–80.

World Bank. 2008. "Mapping and Situation Assessment of Key Populations at High Risk of HIV in Three Cities of Afghanistan." Human Development Sector, South Asia Region (SAR) AIDS Team, World Bank.

Yousif, M. E. A. 2006. "Health Education Programme among Female Sex Workers in Wad Medani Town-Gezira State." Final Report.

Zargooshi, J. 2002. "Characteristics of Gonorrhoea in Kermanshah, Iran." *Sex Transm Infect* 78: 460–61.

Chapter 5

Potential Bridging Populations and HIV

This chapter focuses on the biological evidence for the extent of human immunodeficiency virus (HIV) spread among potential bridging populations, the behavioral evidence for sexual and injecting risk practices among these population groups, and the context of bridging the infection to the general population in the Middle East and North Africa (MENA).

CONTEXT OF BRIDGING POPULATIONS IN MENA

Bridging populations are defined as the populations that bridge HIV infections from the high-risk priority groups to the low-risk general population. These conventionally include groups such as clients of female sex workers (FSWs), truck drivers, taxi drivers, military personnel, fishermen, sailors, migrant labor, and the sexual partners of injecting drug users (IDUs), FSWs, and men who have sex with men (MSM). A sizable segment of the MENA population belongs to these groups. Djibouti has a major trade corridor with Ethiopia and large military installations of foreign troops that facilitated a strong demand for an active and complex sex trade that caters to truck drivers, foreign military personnel, and the local population.[1] It is estimated that there are 2,000 international truck drivers

and 60,000 domestic drivers in Afghanistan,[2] and 1 million truck drivers in Pakistan.[3] Migrant males constitute 15%–20% of all adult men in Pakistan.[4]

Given the limited HIV prevalence found in MENA, one must be cautious in labeling any population group in the region as a bridging population. The evidence on the role of conventionally defined bridging populations in the HIV epidemics in MENA needs to be well established. Based on current evidence as discussed below, one cannot conclude that there is a clear contribution of such populations in the HIV epidemic. Therefore bridging populations have been labeled here as *potential bridging populations* to highlight the specific nature of their context in MENA.

HIV PREVALENCE IN POTENTIAL BRIDGING POPULATIONS

HIV point-prevalence surveys of potential bridging populations are still limited in MENA. Table 5.1 lists available data. The low HIV prevalence found in these surveys, along with the context of HIV spread in the rest of risk groups, suggests that HIV spread may be still limited in

---

[1] El-Saharty and Ali, "An Effective Well-Coordinated Response to HIV in Djibouti."

[2] Ryan, "Travel Report Summary."

[3] Agha, "Potential for HIV Transmission."

[4] Faisel and Cleland, "Study of the Sexual Behaviours"; Faisel and Cleland, "Migrant Men."

Table 5.1 HIV Prevalence in Potential Bridging Populations in MENA

Country	HIV prevalence in potential bridging populations
Jordan	0.0% (military personnel; Jordan National AIDS Program, personal communication)
Iran, Islamic Republic of	0.0% (truck drivers; S. Seyed Alinaghi, personal communication [2009])
Morocco	1.0% (truck drivers; Bennani and Alami 2006) 0.0% (truck drivers; Morocco MOH 2007) 0.0% (sailors; Khattabi and Alami 2005) 0.28% (sailors; Bennani and Alami 2006) 0.62% (sailors; Morocco MOH 2007)
Pakistan	0.0% (truck drivers; Ahmed et al. 1995) 0.0% (truck drivers; Bokhari et al. 2007) 1.0% (truck drivers; Bokhari et al. 2007) 0.6% (seafarers; Mujeeb and Hafeez 1993)
Sudan	0.0% (truck drivers; Burans et al. 1990) 0.5% (truck drivers; Farah and Hussein 2006) 1.1% (truck drivers; Ahmed 2004b) 1.7% (military personnel; McCarthy et al. 1989) 0.5% (military personnel; Ahmed 2004a) 2.9% (military personnel; Yei town, Southern Sudan; SNAP, NSNAC, and UNAIDS 2006) 0.8% (military personnel; Rumbek town, Southern Sudan; SNAP, NSNAC, and UNAIDS 2006) 14% (clients of FSWs; Southern Sudan; McCarthy, Khalid, and El Tigani 1995)
Other	1.54% (truck drivers[a]; Botros et al. 2007)

[a] A complex network of truck drivers serving Europe, the Russian Federation, Caucasus, Central Asia, China, and the Middle East.

bridging populations in MENA, apart from Djibouti, Somalia, and Sudan.

POTENTIAL BRIDGING POPULATIONS AND RISK BEHAVIOR

Several studies have documented risk behaviors among potential bridging populations in MENA. In Afghanistan, 39% of truck drivers reported access to FSWs and 7% paid for sex in the last 12 months.[5] In Djibouti, 22.7% of dockers had two or three wives and of those who had one wife, 53.2% of their wives were living away in Ethiopia.[6] Among truck drivers, 14% were in polygamous unions, 24.8% had more than one sex partner, 18.4% had a nonregular sex partner, and 17.5% had contacted FSWs in the previous year.[7] In the Islamic Republic of Iran, 38.3% of truck drivers reported premarital or extramarital sex and 35.2% had never used condoms.[8]

In Pakistan, 40% of truck drivers attending a sexually transmitted disease (STD) clinic reported contact with FSWs and 53% reported male same-sex contacts.[9] Most truck drivers in one study were married, but they were away from their wives for up to two months at a time.[10] Among them, 34% had sex with an FSW, 11.3% had sex with a male sex worker (MSW), and 49.3% had sex with a man. Most truckers had limited knowledge of HIV and were not aware that condoms can protect against HIV. Only 3%–6% of them used condoms during last sex with a nonspousal partner. In another study, 32.3% of truck drivers paid for sex with a female, 1.7% used a condom during last sex with an FSW, 21.9% had sex with a male or *hijra*, and 0% used condoms during last sex with a male or *hijra*.[11] Truck drivers in Pakistan are reported to have male helpers or "cleaners" who accompany them during their travel and who may be expected to have sex with the driver.[12] Syphilis

[5] Action Aid Afghanistan, "HIV AIDS in Afghanistan."
[6] O' Grady, *WFP Consultant Visit to Djibouti Report.*
[7] Ibid.
[8] Tehrani and Malek-Afzalip, "Knowledge, Attitudes and Practices."

[9] Khawaja et al., "HIV/AIDS and Its Risk Factors in Pakistan."
[10] Agha, "Potential for HIV Transmission."
[11] Bokhari et al., "HIV Risk in Karachi and Lahore, Pakistan."
[12] Khawaja et al., "HIV/AIDS and Its Risk Factors in Pakistan."

prevalence has been reported as 9.4% among truck drivers, indicating considerable prevalence of risk behaviors.[13]

Among urban migrant males in Pakistan, 63.5% had sex with one or more nonmarital partners, 34.7% had sex with an FSW, and 1.7% had sex with a man.[14] About half of the nonmarital partners over the last year were FSWs and the other half were identified as female "friends." Three-quarters of those who reported having sex with a female friend also reported having sex with an FSW. Most of the high-risk behaviors were concentrated, but not confined to, between puberty and marriage.

In Somalia, 30.3% of traveling merchants and drivers had more than one sexual partner in the previous year,[15] and the majority of truck drivers reported contacts with FSWs.[16] In Sudan, 2.4% of truck drivers had ever used condoms, 29.6% had premarital or extramarital sex, 12.9% had premarital sex, and 8.1% had paid for sex.[17] In another study, 55% of truck drivers reported no current sexual partners, 13.4% reported one partner, 7.4% reported two partners, 10.8% reported three partners, and 13.4% reported more than three partners.[18] Among them, 3.4% had sex before marriage, 0.2% had sex with males and females, 0.5% had sex only with males, and 72.1% had heard of condoms but only 8.9% ever used them.[19] Among military personnel, 2.7% had ever used condoms, 42.5% had premarital or extramarital sex, 5.2% had premarital sex, and 11.7% had paid for sex.[20] In another study, 39.6% of sexually active military personnel had one sexual partner, 13.4% had two partners, 12.5% had three partners, and 31.2% had more than three partners.[21]

A study among truck drivers serving a complex network from Europe, the Russian Federation, Caucasus, Central Asia, China, and the Middle East found that 1.9% of the drivers

were IDUs.[22] The study also reported prevalence of sexual contacts with FSWs and other males and that these contacts were associated with HIV prevalence.

Existing evidence suggests considerable levels of sexual risk behavior among potential bridging populations including sexual contacts with FSWs and other nonmarital females as well as other males. There is hardly any evidence on injecting drug practices among these population groups.

VULNERABILITY OF SEXUAL PARTNERS OF PRIORITY POPULATIONS

A key highlight of HIV epidemiology in MENA is the vulnerability of sexual partners of both priority populations and FSW clients to HIV infection, and their limited role in transmitting HIV to the general population. Women are especially vulnerable because most risk behaviors in MENA are practiced by men. The majority of women living with HIV in MENA were infected through their husbands or partners, who were mostly not aware of their infections.[23] Ninety-seven percent of women living with HIV in Saudi Arabia were infected by their husbands.[24] Seventy-six percent of women living with HIV in the Islamic Republic of Iran were also infected by their husbands, who were predominantly IDUs.[25] HIV infections are repeatedly found among pregnant women with no identifiable risk behaviors, suggesting that the risk factor is heterosexual sex with the spouse.[26] The average age at HIV infection among women in the West Bank and Gaza is close to a decade younger than that of men, and most women were infected by their husbands.[27]

Given the low levels of risk behavior in the general population (chapters 6 and 10), sexual partners of priority populations appear to rarely engage in risky behavior (beyond sexual contacts with their partners who engage in risk

[13] WHO/EMRO, "Prevention and Control."

[14] Faisel and Cleland, "Study of the Sexual Behaviours"; Faisel and Cleland, "Migrant Men."

[15] WHO/EMRO, "Presentation of WHO Somalia's Experience."

[16] Burans et al., "HIV Infection Surveillance in Mogadishu, Somalia."

[17] Ahmed, Truck Drivers.

[18] Farah and Hussein, "HIV Prevalence."

[19] Ibid.

[20] Ahmed, Military.

[21] Sudan National HIV/AIDS Control Program, HIV/AIDS/STIs Prevalence.

[22] Botros et al., "HIV Prevalence and Risk Behaviours."

[23] McGirk, "Religious Leaders Key."

[24] Alrajhi, Halim, and Al-Abdely, "Mode of Transmission of HIV-1."

[25] Ramezani, Mohraz, and Gachkar, "Epidemiologic Situation"; Burrows, Wodak, and WHO, Harm Reduction in Iran.

[26] Aidaoui, Bouzbid, and Laouar, "Seroprevalence of HIV Infection."

[27] UNAIDS, "Key Findings."

behaviors), and probably rarely spread the infection further. In this sense, they are not a bridging population that would pass the infection into the general population. This aspect of HIV epidemiology in MENA could be one of the factors behind the consistently very low HIV prevalence found in the general population (chapter 6).

ANALYTICAL SUMMARY

A sizable fraction of the MENA population belongs to what can be labeled as *potential bridging populations*. Evidence on HIV prevalence, other STIs' prevalence, sexual risk behavior measures, and drug injecting practices among potential bridging populations remains rather limited. Existing evidence suggests considerable levels of sexual risk behavior among potential bridging populations, but limited HIV prevalence, except possibly for Djibouti, Somalia, and Sudan.

The limited HIV prevalence among potential bridging populations is probably a consequence of the low HIV prevalence among FSWs and the high coverage of male circumcision among men. In this sense, these populations are not key contributors to the dynamics of HIV infectious spread in MENA and are not effectively bridging populations capable of spreading the infection further to the general population.

Indeed, a key characteristic of sexual partners of priority populations in this region is their vulnerability to HIV, rather than their role in HIV spread. Sexual partners of priority groups are enduring a sizable proportion of the HIV disease burden, though they rarely transmit the infection further, except to their own children. Women are especially vulnerable because most risk behaviors are practiced by men. HIV prevention efforts in MENA should address this key vulnerability.

BIBLIOGRAPHY

Action Aid Afghanistan. 2006. "HIV AIDS in Afghanistan: A Study on Knowledge, Attitude, Behavior, and Practice in High Risk and Vulnerable Groups in Afghanistan."

Agha, S. 2000. "Potential for HIV Transmission among Truck Drivers in Pakistan." *AIDS* 14: 2404–6.

Ahmed, A. J., N. Hassan, O. Pasha, S. Fisher-Hoch, J. B. McCormick, and S. P. Luby. 1995. "Prevalence of STDs among Long-Distance Truck Drivers in Pakistan." Proceedings of the Conference on HIV Surveillance, Karachi, Pakistan.

Ahmed, S. M. 2004a. *Military: Situation Analysis-Behavioral Survey Results & Discussions.* Report. Sudan National AIDS Control Program.

———. 2004b. *Truck Drivers: Situation Analysis-Behavioral Survey Results & Discussions.* Report. Sudan National AIDS Control Program.

Aidaoui, M., S. Bouzbid, and M. Laouar. 2008. "Seroprevalence of HIV Infection in Pregnant Women in the Annaba Region (Algeria)." *Rev Epidemiol Sante Publique* 56: 261–66.

Alrajhi, A. A., M. A. Halim, and H. M. Al-Abdely. 2004. "Mode of Transmission of HIV-1 in Saudi Arabia." *AIDS* 18: 1478–80.

Bennani, A., and K. Alami. 2006. "Surveillance sentinelle VIH, résultats 2005 et tendances de la séroprévalence du VIH." Morocco Ministry of Health, UNAIDS.

Bokhari, A., N. M. Nizamani, D. J. Jackson, N. E. Rehan, M. Rahman, R. Muzaffar, S. Mansoor, H. Raza, K. Qayum, P. Girault, E. Pisani, and I. Thaver. 2007. "HIV Risk in Karachi and Lahore, Pakistan: An Emerging Epidemic in Injecting and Commercial Sex Networks." *Int J STD AIDS* 18: 486–92.

Botros, B. A., Q. Aliyev, M. Saad, M. Monteville, A. Michael, Z. Nasibov, H. Mustafaev, P. Scott, J. Sanchez, J. Carr, and K. Earhart. 2007. "HIV Prevalence and Risk Behaviours among International Truck Drivers in Azerbaijan." 17th European Congress of Clinical Microbiology and Infectious Diseases (ECCMID) and 25th International Congress of Chemotherapy (ICC), Munich, Germany.

Burans, J. P., E. Fox, M. A. Omar, A. H. Farah, S. Abbass, S. Yusef, A. Guled, M. Mansour, R. Abu-Elyazeed, and J. N. Woody. 1990. "HIV Infection Surveillance in Mogadishu, Somalia." *East Afr Med J* 67: 466–72.

Burrows, D., A. Wodak, and WHO (World Health Organization). 2005. *Harm Reduction in Iran: Issues in National Scale-Up.* Report for WHO.

El-Saharty, S., and O. Ali. 2006. "An Effective Well-Coordinated Response to HIV in Djibouti." World Bank Global HIV/AIDS Program.

Faisel, A., and J. Cleland. 2006a. "Migrant Men: A Priority for HIV Control in Pakistan?" *Sex Transm Infect* 82: 307–10.

———. 2006b. "Study of the Sexual Behaviours and Prevalence of STIs among Migrant Men in Lahore, Pakistan." Arjumand and Associates, Centre for Population Studies, London School of Hygiene and Tropical Medicine.

Farah, M. S., and S. Hussein. 2006. "HIV Prevalence, Knowledge, Attitude, Practices and Risk Factors among Truck Drivers in Khartoum State." Grey Report. Sudan National AIDS Program.

Khattabi, H., and K. Alami. 2005. "Surveillance sentinelle du VIH, Résultats 2004 et tendance de la séroprévalence du VIH." Morocco Ministry of Health, UNAIDS.

Khawaja, Z. A., L. Gibney, A. J. Ahmed, and S. H. Vermund. 1997. "HIV/AIDS and Its Risk Factors in Pakistan." *AIDS* 11: 843–48.

McCarthy, M. C., K. C. Hyams, A. el-Tigani el-Hag, M. A. el-Dabi, M. el-Sadig el-Tayeb, I. O. Khalid, J. F. George, N. T. Constantine, and J. N. Woody. 1989. "HIV-1 and Hepatitis B Transmission in Sudan." *AIDS* 3: 725–29.

McCarthy, M. C., I. O. Khalid, and A. El Tigani. 1995. "HIV-1 Infection in Juba, Southern Sudan." *J Med Virol* 46: 18–20.

McGirk, J. 2008. "Religious Leaders Key in the Middle East's HIV/AIDS Fight." *Lancet* 372: 279–80.

Morocco MOH (Ministry of Health). 2007. *Surveillance sentinelle du VIH, résultats 2006 et tendances de la séro-prévalence du VIH.*

Mujeeb, S. A., and A. Hafeez. 1993. "Prevalence and Pattern of HIV Infection in Karachi." *J Pak Med Assoc* 43: 2–4.

O'Grady, M. 2004. *WFP Consultant Visit to Djibouti Report.* United Nations World Food Programme, July 30.

Ramezani, A., M. Mohraz, and L. Gachkar. 2006. "Epidemiologic Situation of Human Immuno-deficiency Virus (HIV/AIDS Patients) in a Private Clinic in Tehran, Iran." *Arch Iran Med* 9: 315–18.

Ryan, S. 2006. "Travel Report Summary." Kabul, Afghanistan. UNAIDS, February 27–March 7, 2006.

SNAP (Sudan National AIDS Program), NSNAC (New Sudan National AIDS Council), and UNAIDS (United Nations Joint Programme on HIV/AIDS). 2006. "Scaling-up HIV/AIDS Response in Sudan." National Consultation on the Road towards Universal Access to Prevention, Treatment, Care, and Support.

Sudan National HIV/AIDS Control Program. 2004. *HIV/AIDS/STIs Prevalence, Knowledge, Attitude, Practices and Risk Factors among University Students and Military Personnel.* Federal Ministry of Health, Khartoum.

Tehrani, F. R., and H. Malek-Afzalip. 2008. "Knowledge, Attitudes and Practices concerning HIV/AIDS among Iranian At-Risk Sub-Populations." *Eastern Mediterranean Health Journal* 14.

UNAIDS (United Nations Joint Programme on HIV/AIDS). 2007. "Key Findings on HIV Status in the West Bank and Gaza." Working document, UNAIDS Regional Support Team for the Middle East and North Africa.

WHO/EMRO (World Health Organization, Eastern Mediterranean Region). 2000. "Presentation of WHO Somalia's Experience in Supporting the National Response." Somalia. Regional Consultation towards Improving HIV/AIDS & STD Surveillance in the Countries of EMRO, Beirut, Lebanon, Oct 30–Nov 2.

———. 2007. "Prevention and Control of Sexually Transmitted Infections in the WHO Eastern Mediterranean Region." Intercountry meeting, PowerPoint presentation.

Chapter 6

General Population and HIV

This chapter focuses on the biological evidence for the extent of human immunodeficiency virus (HIV) spread among the general population, the behavioral evidence for sexual risk practices among this population group, and the context of the general population in the Middle East and North Africa (MENA).

HIV PREVALENCE IN THE GENERAL POPULATION

HIV prevalence has been measured in a number of general population groups in MENA. Prevalence levels are very low in all countries with the exception Djibouti, Somalia, and Sudan. Tables 6.1–6.3 and C.1 (appendix c) list the results of available point-prevalence surveys in population-based and national surveys; among antenatal clinic (ANC) attendees and other pregnant women; blood donors; and other different subpopulation groups in MENA.

The data below indicate that there is no evidence of a substantial HIV epidemic in the general population in any of the MENA countries. There appears to be very limited HIV transmission within the general population in MENA, apart from Djibouti, Somalia, and Sudan. In these nations, HIV is already generalized in parts

Table 6.1 HIV Prevalence in Population-Based Surveys in MENA

Country	HIV prevalence
Djibouti	2.9% (national; Djibouti, Ministère de La Santé, and Association Internationale de Développement 2002) 3.4% (in Djibouti-ville; UNAIDS 2008) 1.1% (out of Djibouti-ville; UNAIDS 2008) 2.0% (Maslin et al. 2005) 2.2% (Maslin et al. 2005)
Iran, Islamic Republic of	0.0% (Hamadan province; Amini et al. 1993) 0.01% (Massarrat and Tahaghoghi-Mehrizi 2002)
Libya	0.13% (Libya National Center for the Prevention of and Control of Infectious Diseases 2005) 0.67% (Alkoufra; El-Gadi, Abudher, and Sammud 2008) 0.4% (Tripoli; El-Gadi, Abudher, and Sammud 2008)
Sudan	2.6% (national; SNAP 2005a) 2.0% (national; UNAIDS and WHO 2003) 1.6% (national; Sudan MOH 2006) 1.4% (national; SNAP 2008) 0.4% (Rumbek town, Southern Sudan; Kaiser et al. 2006) 4.4% (Yei town, Southern Sudan; Kaiser et al. 2006) 2.7% (in overall in Yei area; Southern Sudan; SNAP, NSNAC, and UNAIDS 2006)

Table 6.2 HIV Prevalence among ANC Attendees and Other Pregnant Women in MENA

Country	HIV prevalence
Afghanistan	0.0% (Todd et al. 2007; Todd et al. 2008)
Algeria	1.0% (Institut de Formation Paramédicale de Parnet 2004) 0.53% (Aidaoui, Bouzbid, and Laouar 2008) 0.7% (Algeria MOH [unknown]) 0.9% (Algeria MOH [unknown]) 0.2% (Alami 2009) 0.14% (Alami 2009) 0.09 (Alami 2009) 0.5% (Alami 2009) 0.23% (Alami 2009)
Djibouti	2.5% (Unknown 2002)
Iran, Islamic Republic of	0.02% (Ministry of Health and Medical Education of Iran 2006) ≈0.1% (WHO/EMRO 2007a) 0.5% (SeyedAlinaghi 2009) 0.05% (Sharifi-Mood and Keikha 2008)
Mauritania	0.4% (WHO 2002)
Morocco	0.03% (Khattabi and Alami 2005) 0.0025% (Khattabi and Alami 2005) 0.014% (Khattabi and Alami 2005) 0.0% (WHO/EMRO Regional Database on HIV/AIDS) 0.12% (Khattabi and Alami 2005; Morocco MOH 2006) 0.13% (UNAIDS/WHO 2005; Morocco MOH 2006) 0.04% (Elharti et al. 2002) 0.02% (Elharti et al. 2002) 0.01% (Elharti et al. 2002) 0.07% (Elharti et al. 2002) 0.15% (Khattabi and Alami 2005) 0.10% (Khattabi and Alami 2005) 0.08% (Alami 2009) 0.06% (Bennani and Alami 2006)
Somalia	0.0% (Jama et al. 1987) 0.9% (WHO 2004c) 0.9% (Somaliland; WHO 2004c) 1.4% (Somaliland; WHO 2004c) 1.3% (Somaliland; WHO 2004c; Somaliland Ministry of Health and Labour 2007) 0.7% (Somaliland Ministry of Health and Labour 2007) 1.6% (Somaliland Ministry of Health and Labour 2007) 0.0% (Somaliland Ministry of Health and Labour 2007) 2.3% (Somaliland Ministry of Health and Labour 2007) 0.6% (Somaliland Ministry of Health and Labour 2007) 1.1% (Somaliland Ministry of Health and Labour 2007) 1.6% (Somaliland Ministry of Health and Labour 2007) 2.7% (Somaliland Ministry of Health and Labour 2007) 0.0% (Somaliland Ministry of Health and Labour 2007) 1.3% (Somaliland Ministry of Health and Labour 2007) 2.2% (Somaliland Ministry of Health and Labour 2007) 0.8% (Somaliland Ministry of Health and Labour 2007) 1.0% (Puntland; WHO 2004b) 0.6% (central Somalia; WHO 2004c) 0.7% (refugees; UNHCR 2003) 1.4% (refugees; UNHCR 2005) 1.0% (refugees; UNHCR 2006–07a) 1.5% (refugees; UNHCR 2006–07a) 1.6% (refugees; UNHCR 2006–07a) 1.2% (refugees; UNHCR 2006–07a)

Table 6.2 *(Continued)*

Country	HIV prevalence
	0.6% (refugees; UNHCR 2006–07a)
	0.7% (refugees; UNHCR 2006–07a)
	1.9% (refugees; UNHCR 2006–07a)
	0.1% (refugees; PMTCT attendees; UNHCR 2006–07a)
Sudan	1.0% (national; Sudan National AIDS/STIs Program 2008; Sudan National HIV/AIDS Control Program 2005b)
	1.0% (Ahmed 2004b)
	0.58% (national; Sudan National AIDS/STIs Program 2008)
	0.5% (Gutbi and Eldin 2006)
	1.57% (IDPs; SNAP and UNAIDS 2006)
	0.26% (refugees; Sudan National AIDS/STIs Program 2008)
	0.27% (IDPs; Sudan National AIDS/STIs Program 2008)
	6–8% (Southern Sudan; UNAIDS and WHO 2003)
	3.4% (Southern Sudan; Southern Sudan AIDS Commission 2007)
	2.3% (Southern Sudan; NSNAC and UNAIDS 2006)
	0–11.1% (various locations; Southern Sudan; Southern Sudan AIDS Commission 2007)
	3.0% (Juba, Southern Sudan; Basha 2006)
	4.0% (Juba, Southern Sudan; Basha 2006)
	2.3% (Yei town; Southern Sudan; SNAP, NSNAC, and UNAIDS 2006; Kaiser et al. 2006)
	2.3% (Rumbek town; Southern Sudan; SNAP, NSNAC, and UNAIDS 2006; Kaiser et al. 2006)
	1.6% (Tambura; Southern Sudan; NSNAC and UNAIDS 2006)
	2.0% (Ezo; Southern Sudan; NSNAC and UNAIDS 2006)
	7.2% (Yambio; Southern Sudan; NSNAC and UNAIDS 2006)
	8.7% (Yambio; villages near main road; Southern Sudan; NSNAC and UNAIDS 2006)
	3.0% (Yambio; villages away from main road; Southern Sudan; NSNAC and UNAIDS 2006)
	0.19% (North Sudan; Sudan National AIDS/STIs Program 2008)
	0.66% (PMTCT attendees; North Sudan; SNAP 2008; NSNAC and UNAIDS 2006)
	0.14% (urban; North Sudan; Sudan National AIDS/STIs Program 2008)
	0.33% (rural; North Sudan; Sudan National AIDS/STIs Program 2008)
	2.0% (West Nile; North Sudan; Sudan MOH 2006)
	1.5% (Red Sea; North Sudan; Sudan National HIV/AIDS Control Program 2005b)
	0.0% (Algadarif; North Sudan; Sudan National HIV/AIDS Control Program 2005b)
	0.0% (Kassala; North Sudan; Sudan National HIV/AIDS Control Program 2005b)
	0.0% (Upper Nile; North Sudan; Sudan National HIV/AIDS Control Program 2005b)
	0.98% (Algazira; North Sudan; Sudan National HIV/AIDS Control Program 2005b)
	0.0% (Algazira; North Sudan; SNAP and UNAIDS 2006)
	0.0% (Blue Nile; North Sudan; SNAP and UNAIDS 2006)
	0.0% (West Kurdufan; North Sudan; SNAP and UNAIDS 2006)
	0.0% (North Darfur; North Sudan; SNAP and UNAIDS 2006)
	2.2% (White Nile; North Sudan; Sudan National HIV/AIDS Control Program 2005b; SNAP and UNAIDS 2006)
	0.0% (Upper Nile; North Sudan; SNAP and UNAIDS 2006)
	1–5% (Khartoum; North Sudan; UNAIDS 2000)
	0.25% (Khartoum; North Sudan; Gutbi and Eldin 2006)
	0.5% (Khartoum 1; North Sudan; Sudan National HIV/AIDS Control Program 2005b; Gutbi and Eldin 2006)
	0.25% (Khartoum 2; North Sudan; Sudan National HIV/AIDS Control Program 2005b; Gutbi and Eldin 2006)
	0.25% (Khartoum 3; North Sudan; Sudan National AIDS Control Program 2005b; Gutbi and Eldin 2006)
	0.8% (Khartoum; North Sudan; Ahmed 2004b)
	1.38% (Khartoum; North Sudan; Gassmelseed et al. 2006)
	5.0% (refugees; IRC 2002)
	1.2% (refugees; UNHCR 2006–07b)
	0.8% (PMTCT attendees; UNHCR 2006–07b)

Note: IDP = internally displaced person; PMTCT = prevention of mother-to-child transmission.

Table 6.3 HIV Prevalence among Blood Donors in MENA

Country	HIV prevalence
Afghanistan	0.0% (Dupire et al. 1999) 0.0006% (Afghanistan Central Blood Bank 2006)
Algeria	0.01% (Unknown 2002) 0.02% (Unknown 2002) 0.08% (Unknown 2002) 0.01% (Unknown 2002)
Djibouti	0.0% (Marcelin et al. 2001) 1.9% (Dray et al. 2005) 3.4% (Massenet and Bouh 1997)
Egypt, Arab Republic of	0.0% (Constantine et al. 1990) 0.0% (El-Ghazzawi, Hunsmann, and Schneider 1987) 0.0% (Kandela 1993) 0.02% (Watts et al. 1993) 0.0% (Quinti et al. 1995)
Iran, Islamic Republic of	0.0018% (Rezvan, Abolghassemi, and Kafiabad 2007) 0.009% (Rezvan, Abolghassemi, and Kafiabad 2007) 0.005% (Rezvan, Abolghassemi, and Kafiabad 2007) 0.005% (Rezvan, Abolghassemi, and Kafiabad 2007) 0.0% (Pourshams et al. 2005) 0.003% (Khedmat et al. 2007)
Jordan	0.004% (Al Katheeb, Tarawneh, and Awidi 1988) 0.0% (Jordan National AIDS Program, personal communication)
Kuwait	0.01% (Kuwaitis; Ameen et al. 2005) 0.00% (non-Kuwaiti Arabs; Ameen et al. 2005)
Mauritania	0.6% (WHO 2002) 0.8% (WHO 2002)
Morocco	0.02% (Elmir et al. 2002; Elharti 2002)
Pakistan	0.15% (Abdul Mujeeb and Hashmi 1988) 0.0% (Mujeeb et al. 1991) 0.003% (Kayani et al. 1994) 0.052% (Pakistan National Institute of Health 1992) 0.064% (Pakistan National Institute of Health 1995) 0.02% (Kakepoto et al. 1996) 0.0% (Iqbal and Rehan 1996) 0–0.06% (Sultan, Mehmood, and Mahmood 2007) 0.0% (college students; Mujeeb, Aamir, and Mehmood 2006; Abdul Mujeeb, Aamir, and Mehmood 2000)
Qatar	0.03% (Qatar 2008)
Saudi Arabia	0.02% (Al Rasheed et al. 1988) 0.0% (El-Hazmi 2004) 0.0% (Alamawi et al. 2003)
Somalia	1.0% (Kulane et al. 2000) 0.8% (WHO 2003)
Sudan	0–11% (various locations; Southern Sudan; NSNAC and UNAIDS 2006) 7.0% (Labone; Southern Sudan; NSNAC and UNAIDS 2006) 13.5% (Chukudum; Southern Sudan; NSNAC and UNAIDS 2006) 12.7% (Yei; Southern Sudan; NSNAC and UNAIDS 2006) 0.05% (Hashim et al. 1997) 0.9% (Winsbury 1996) 0.8–1.8% (WHO/EMRO 2007a) 1.25% (SNAP 2008)

Table 6.3 *(Continued)*

Country	HIV prevalence
Turkey	0.005% (Afsar et al. 2008) 0.0% (Afsar et al. 2008) 0.0% (Afsar et al. 2008) 0.015% (Coskun et al. 2008) 0–0.66% (Arabaci et al. 2003)
West Bank and Gaza	0.006% (Maayan et al. 1994) 0.0% (Yassin et al. 2001)
Yemen, Republic of	0.1–0.3% (WHO/EMRO 2007a) 0.04% (Yemen National AIDS Control Programme 1998) 0.29% (Yemen National AIDS Control Programme 2001) 0.02% (WHO/EMRO Regional Database on HIV/AIDS)

of these countries, as defined technically by prevalence larger than 1% among pregnant women.[1]

Southern Sudan is of particular concern and could already be in a state of general population HIV epidemic, but conclusive evidence is still lacking. Technically speaking, the HIV epidemics in Djibouti and parts of Somalia are already generalized, but the context of HIV infection and risk groups in these countries suggest that HIV dynamics are mainly focused around concentrated epidemics in the commercial sex networks. The generalization of the epidemic, being larger than 1% among pregnant women, mainly reflects the large commercial sex networks in these countries in the context of major trade corridors, large foreign military installations, and political conflict. HIV prevalence in these countries is also much lower than HIV prevalence in countries in sub-Saharan Africa that truly have a general population HIV epidemic.[2]

GENERAL POPULATION AND RISK BEHAVIOR

Data on sexual behavior among the general population continue to be rather limited. In particular, it does not appear that any nationwide sexual behavior survey has ever been conducted in MENA. Several studies, however, collected a reasonable amount of data in a few countries and these data provide a partial profile of sexual behavior in the general population. Below is a review of evidence on different aspects of risky behavior among the general population, including the nature of sexual behavior, nonconventional marriage forms and polygamy, and the overall nature and trends of risky behavior. Further data on sexual risk behavior among key vulnerable subgroups in the general population, such as prisoners, youth, and mobile populations, can be found in chapter 9. Further data on condom use and HIV knowledge and attitudes in the general population can be found in chapter 8. Levels of sexually transmitted infections (STIs) in the general population can be found in chapter 10.

Nature of sexual behavior

Two case-control studies in Algeria and Morocco examining the epidemiology of human papillomavirus (HPV) infection, an STI that causes cervical cancer, provided valuable data on the sexual behavior of general population women who were in the control arm of this study. In the Algeria study, almost 30% of women reported more than one lifetime sexual partner, with 5% reporting three or more partners.[3] Twenty-six percent of the women reported that their husbands had extramarital affairs with other women and 25% were unsure about their husbands' extramarital affairs. Thirty-four percent reported that their husbands had sex with female sex workers (FSWs) and 10% were unsure about their husbands' contacts with FSWs. Women in polygamous marriages (6% of women) were at higher risk of cervical cancer, suggesting that polygamy implies a higher level of sexual risk

---

[1] Pisani et al., "HIV Surveillance."

[2] UNAIDS/WHO, *AIDS Epidemic Update 2007.*

[3] Hammouda et al., "Cervical Carcinoma in Algiers."

behavior than monogamy. Widowed and divorced women were also at higher risk of cervical cancer, also suggesting higher levels of sexual risk behavior. The pattern of apparently higher levels of risky behavior among widowed or divorced women was also seen in Djibouti, where single, divorced, separated, or widowed women were found to have significantly higher HIV prevalence (8.2%) compared to married women (2.3%).[4]

In the Morocco study, almost 20% of women reported more than one lifetime sexual partner, with 2% reporting more than three partners.[5] Six percent reported having more than one partner before reaching 20 years of age, and 2% reported having nonspousal sexual partnerships. One woman out of 203 women reported engaging in sex work. The study also reported a mean of 1.3 lifetime sexual partners, a median of 1, and a range of 1–4, and that the median age at first sex was 18 years. Condom use was limited with only 16% of women having ever used condoms. Polygamous unions were reported by 12% of women and polygamy was associated with cervical cancer, although not with statistical significance as in the Algeria study.[6]

A behavioral surveillance study among the general population in Juba, Southern Sudan, also provided valuable data.[7] Thirty-one percent of unmarried men 15–24 years of age and 62% of unmarried men 25–49 years of age had ever had sex.[8] Among women, the corresponding percentages were 8 and also 8, respectively.[9] Casual sex in the last year was reported by 11.7% of men and 1.5% of women.[10] The mean number of casual partners in the last year among those who had casual sex was two for both men and women.[11] Casual sex was found to be much more common among unmarried men (19%) than married men (4%).[12] In the last year, 1.7% of men[13] reported paying for sex and 0.2% of

women reported exchanging sex for money.[14] Three percent of women, but no men, reported ever being forced to have sex.[15]

Other studies have provided further data on sexual behavior. In Afghanistan, studies found that 0.2% and 0.7% of spouses reported that their husbands engaged in extramarital sexual contacts with men or boys, and other women, respectively.[16] In the Islamic Republic of Iran, among runaways and other women seeking safe haven, 40% of those sexually active reported that their first sexual contact was with someone other than their husband, and 6% reported a history of rape.[17] In another study, 38% of clients of FSWs were married, suggesting that marriage does not preclude contact with FSWs.[18]

In Lebanon, 62.8% of the general population in one study had their first sexual intercourse prior to age 20, 32.1% had multiple sexual partners, 22.4% had casual sex, and 36% had paid for sex.[19] In another study, 52% of men were sexually active before age 20, and 22% of unmarried men had sexual relations with nonregular partners.[20] In a third study, 30.8% of the general population was sexually active but unmarried, and 13% of them had nonspousal regular partners.[21] Of those who reported nonspousal regular partners, almost 20% had more than one partner. Of the respondents, 33.3% had their sexual debut between the ages of 15 and 20 years, and 42.9% were sexually active by age 25.[22] Among the sexually active population, 16.8% had nonregular sexual partners and 31.4% paid money or gifts for sex.[23]

In Pakistan, 6% of general population respondents had extramarital affairs and only 5% had ever used condoms.[24] In another study, the average frequency of coital acts, whether marital or extramarital, was 3.5 per week.[25] In

[4] Unknown, "Surveillance des infections à VIH."
[5] Chaouki et al., "The Viral Origin of Cervical Cancer."
[6] Hammouda et al., "Cervical Carcinoma in Algiers."
[7] UNHCR, "HIV Behavioural Surveillance Survey."
[8] Ibid.
[9] Ibid.
[10] Ibid.
[11] Ibid.
[12] Ibid.
[13] Ibid.

[14] Ibid.
[15] Ibid.
[16] Todd et al., "Seroprevalence and Correlates of HIV" (2008).
[17] Hajiabdolbaghi et al., "Insights from a Survey."
[18] Zargooshi, "Characteristics of Gonorrhoea."
[19] Lebanon National AIDS Control Program, "General Population Evaluation Survey."
[20] WHO/EMRO, "Prevention and Control of Sexually Transmitted Infections."
[21] Jurjus et al., "Knowledge, Attitudes, Beliefs, and Practices."
[22] Ibid.
[23] Ibid.
[24] Raza et al., "Knowledge, Attitude and Behaviour."
[25] Naim and Bhutto, "Sexuality during Pregnancy."

Oman, 13% of male members of social clubs reported extramarital relations in the last year.[26] In Somalia, 34% of general population men and 22.5% of general population women had more than one sexual partner in the previous year.[27] The average age at first sex was 17 years for males and 15 years for females.[28] Also in Somalia, 32% of women attending STD (sexually transmitted disease) clinics were unmarried,[29] and 4% of pregnant women attending ANC centers were also unmarried.[30] Among Somali refugees in Kenya, HIV prevalence was associated with polygamy, although not with statistical significance.[31]

In Sudan, 14.9% of males and 5.7% of females of mainly rural populations in six states reported extramarital sex at the present time, but only 2.2% of males and 1.2% of females used condoms during last sex.[32] Sexual contacts between males were reported by 2% of the males, and commercial sex was reported by 3.1% of males and 1.4% of females.[33] In further studies from Sudan, 12% of adults reported a nonregular sexual partner in the last year,[34] and premarital or extramarital sex was reported by 14.4% of university students,[35] 5.4% of ANC women attendees,[36] 10.3% of tea sellers,[37] and 15.3% of tuberculosis (TB) patients.[38] Furthermore, premarital sex was reported by 1.2% of ANC women attendees,[39] 0.5% of tea sellers,[40] and 1% of TB patients.[41] In Southern Sudan, 44% of sexually active men and 4% of women reported that they have had sex with another person apart from their spouse or regular sexual partner.[42] Median age at first sex was

13.8 for males and 18 for females.[43] Recent extramarital sex was reported by 4.5% of males and 1.7% of females.[44]

Nonconventional marriage forms and polygamy

Anecdotal evidence suggests an increasing prevalence of nonconventional forms of marriage in MENA.[45] One of these forms is *zawaj al-muta'a* or *sigheh* (temporary marriage), sanctioned among Shiites, but not among Sunnis, and common in the Islamic Republic of Iran and Lebanon.[46] This form of marriage is legally permitted in the Islamic Republic of Iran and consists of a marriage contract between a man and a woman agreeing, often privately and verbally, to marry each other for a fixed term that can range from 1 hour to 99 years.[47] *Sigheh* appears to be common in the Islamic Republic of Iran, such as among divorced women with limited financial resources.[48] It was also encouraged by political leaders following the Islamic Revolution and is seen as an alternative to premarital or extramarital sex.[49] Over a quarter of the youth (27.1%) in the Islamic Republic of Iran and almost half of the truck drivers (43.3%) found *sigheh* more acceptable than extramarital sex.[50] Institutionalizing temporary marriages through the construction of "chastity houses," where women would be paid for sex according to some established rules, was suggested by some scholars in the Islamic Republic of Iran, but this was never enacted.[51]

Another form of nonconventional marriage is *'urfi* marriage (clandestine marriage).[52] This form is religiously sanctioned among Sunnis and Shiites, but has no legal bearings. It is most common in the Arab Republic of Egypt and there is anecdotal evidence suggesting that it is increasing in prevalence in this country.[53] While there are no reliable estimates of the number of

[26] Jenkins and Robalino, "HIV in the Middle East and North Africa."

[27] WHO/EMRO, "Presentation of WHO Somalia's Experience."

[28] WHO, *2004 First National Second Generation HIV/AIDS/STI Sentinel Surveillance Survey (Somalia)*.

[29] Somaliland Ministry of Health and Labour, *Somaliland 2007*.

[30] WHO, *2004 First National Second Generation HIV/AIDS/STI Sentinel Surveillance Survey (Somalia)*.

[31] UNHCR, *HIV Sentinel Surveillance among Antenatal Clients*.

[32] SNAP, UNICEF, and UNAIDS, "Baseline Study on Knowledge."

[33] Ibid.

[34] SNAP, *Situation Analysis*.

[35] Ahmed, *University Students*.

[36] Ahmed, *Antenatal*.

[37] Ahmed, *Tea Sellers*.

[38] Ahmed, *TB Patients*.

[39] Ahmed, *Antenatal*.

[40] Ahmed, *Tea Sellers*.

[41] Ahmed, *TB Patients*.

[42] NSNAC and UNAIDS, *HIV/AIDS Integrated Report South Sudan*.

[43] Ibid.

[44] Ibid.

[45] Rashad and Osman, "Nuptiality in Arab Countries."

[46] Roudi-Fahimi and Ashford, "Sexual & Reproductive Health."

[47] Mohammad et al., "Sexual Risk-Taking Behaviors among Boys"; Haeri, "Temporary Marriage."

[48] Aghajanian, *Family and Family Change in Iran*.

[49] Haeri, "Temporary Marriage."

[50] Tehrani and Malek-Afzalip, "Knowledge, Attitudes and Practices."

[51] Sepehrad, "The Role of Women "; Recknagel and Gorgin, "Iran."

[52] Roudi-Fahimi and Ashford, "Sexual & Reproductive Health"; DeJong et al., "The Sexual and Reproductive Health of Young People."

[53] Beamish, "Adolescent Reproductive Health in Egypt."

'urfi marriages, there were nearly 10,000 cases of contested paternity due to 'urfi marriages in Egyptian courts in 1998.[54]

A third type of nonconventional marriage is "travelers' marriage," including "summer marriages" and *jawaz* (or *nikah*) *al misyar*. Summer marriages typically occur between wealthy tourists from rich MENA countries and poor women or girls from poor MENA countries, and last only for the duration of the summer, after which the marriage is often dissolved.[55] *Jawaz al misyar* is common mainly in the Persian Gulf region and is an arrangement by which a man marries without the housing and financial responsibilities that are expected from him in a conventional marriage.[56] The couples continue to live separately from each other and see each other when they please. *Jawaz al misyar* is generally sanctioned among Sunnis, but is forbidden among Shiites.

There is very limited evidence on the levels of sexual risk behavior implied by these kinds of marriages and whether they are effectively a "legitimization" of premarital and extramarital sex. One study in the Islamic Republic of Iran reported that temporary marriages appear to be associated with exposure to STIs. Twenty-four percent of male gonorrhea patients reported acquiring the infection from temporary wives.[57]

Although polygamy is common in MENA, it appears to be in decline.[58] The percentage of women in polygamous unions is estimated (not necessarily from representative populations) at 6% in Algeria,[59] 6.8% in Jordan,[60] 12.5% in Kuwait,[61] 3% in Lebanon,[62] 12% in Morocco,[63] 5% in the Syrian Arab Republic,[64] and 26% in the United Arab Emirates.[65] Among Somali refugees in Kenya, 18.7% of married women were in polygamous unions.[66] In Sudan, the percentage of people of different population groups who reported having more than one husband/

wife was 0% among university students,[67] 7% among military personnel,[68] 24.2% among married military personnel,[69] 14.5% among prisoners,[70] 12.6% among truck drivers,[71] 13% among internally displaced persons,[72] 14.2% among tea sellers,[73] 1.8% among street children,[74] 11.8% among ANC women attendees,[75] 14.1% among FSWs,[76] 13.3% among TB patients,[77] 15.7% among STD clinic attendees,[78] and 15.7% among suspected AIDS patients.[79] There was no definition given to distinguish whether these percentages represent sequential or polygamous marriages or whether these marriages include spousal relationships not necessarily sanctioned by religion or state. These measures, however, suggest the prevalence of multiple marriages in Sudan.

Concurrency of sexual partnerships and heterogeneity in sexual risk behavior are conducive to the spread of HIV in the population.[80] Polygamy has been associated with higher risk of exposure to STIs in sub-Saharan Africa.[81] The permissive attitudes toward polygamy have been suggested as an explanation of higher HIV rates among a minority of Muslim communities in sub-Saharan Africa.[82] Polygamy was found to be associated with cervical cancer in two studies in Algeria[83] and Morocco.[84] Nevertheless, lower STI prevalence was reported among women in polygamous marriages compared to women in nonpolygamous marriages in the United Arab Emirates.[85] The association between polygamy

[54] Rashad et al., "Marriage in the Arab World."

[55] DeJong et al., "The Sexual and Reproductive Health of Young People."

[56] Rashad et al., "Marriage in the Arab World."

[57] Zargooshi, "Characteristics of Gonorrhoea."

[58] Foster, "Young Women's Sexuality in Tunisia."

[59] Hammouda et al., "Cervical Carcinoma in Algiers."

[60] Naffa, "Jordanian Women: Past and Present."

[61] Chaleby, "Women of Polygamous Marriages."

[62] Jurjus et al., "Knowledge, Attitudes, Beliefs, and Practices."

[63] Chaouki et al., "The Viral Origin of Cervical Cancer."

[64] Roudi-Fahimi and Ashford, "Sexual & Reproductive Health."

[65] Ghazal-Aswad et al., "Prevalence of Chlamydia Trachomatis Infection."

[66] UNHCR, *HIV Sentinel Surveillance among Antenatal Clients.*

[67] Ahmed, *University Students.*

[68] Ahmed, *Military.*

[69] Sudan National HIV/AIDS Control Program, *HIV/AIDS/STIs Prevalence.*

[70] Ahmed, *Prisoners.*

[71] Ahmed, *Truck Drivers.*

[72] Ahmed, *Internally Displaced People.*

[73] Ahmed, *Tea Sellers.*

[74] Ahmed, *Street Children.*

[75] Ahmed, *Antenatal.*

[76] Ahmed, *Sex Sellers.*

[77] Ahmed, *TB Patients.*

[78] Ahmed, *STDs.*

[79] Ahmed, *AIDS Patients.*

[80] Kretzschmar and Morris, "Measures of Concurrency in Networks"; Morris, "Sexual Networks and HIV"; Watts and May, "The Influence of Concurrent Partnerships"; May and Anderson, "The Transmission Dynamics."

[81] Obasi et al., "Antibody to Herpes Simplex Virus Type 2."

[82] Kapiga, "Determinants of Multiple Sexual Partners"; Kapiga and Lugalla, "Sexual Behaviour Patterns."

[83] Hammouda et al., "Cervical Carcinoma in Algiers."

[84] Chaouki et al., "The Viral Origin of Cervical Cancer."

[85] Ghazal-Aswad et al., "Prevalence of Chlamydia Trachomatis Infection."

and STI risk of exposure is complex in MENA, because polygamy tends to be associated with closed sexual networks rather than open and intertwined networks.[86] However, the above evidence does give credence to the possibility that polygamy could be associated with higher risk of exposure to STIs within the context of this region.

Overall nature and trends of sexual risk behavior

The above evidence suggests that the levels of sexual risk behavior among the general population in MENA appear to be rather low in comparison to other regions.[87] The MENA population views sex outside of marriage very negatively, particularly for women.[88] Premarital sex is one of the leading causes of suicide among young women. In Algeria, 30% of women who commit suicide are pregnant but unmarried.[89] In Turkey, hymen examination is the most frequent cause of suicide among young Turkish women.[90]

Most of the sexual risk behavior appears to be practiced by men rather than women. Nevertheless, women endure a large share of the STD burden through exposures to infected husbands. Sex with an infected partner was found to be a significant predictor of women's exposure to STDs in Egypt.[91] Infection with STDs in Morocco was more associated with male rather than female sexual behavior.[92]

Most of the sexual risk behavior appears to be concentrated in, but not confined to, youth and before marriage. Eighty-one percent of STD clinic attendees in Kuwait were either single or married patients living alone.[93] Most of them were in the 21–30 years age group. Nonetheless, sexual risk exists for all age groups, its form varying depending on the age group.

There appears to be a substantial gap in age in sexual partnerships between men and women, with women marrying older men.

Intergenerational sex puts women at higher risk of exposure to STIs.[94] Among women who had cervical cancer and reported first marriage/intercourse before age 15 in Morocco, 57% married a husband in the 20–30 years age range and 19% married a husband older than 30 years of age.[95] Intergenerational sex has been implicated as the main reason behind the large gap in HIV prevalence between men and women in sub-Saharan Africa.[96] Though age at marriage has increased rapidly over the last three decades,[97] a substantial fraction of women still marry at an early age. Early age at marriage was found to be associated with higher risk of exposure to STIs in two studies of women in MENA.[98]

While the overall levels of sexual risk behaviors appear to be rather low, there are indications that they are increasing in MENA. Behavioral surveys in Lebanon and Turkey suggest increased risky behavior among youth.[99] Anecdotal evidence points to increases in sexual activity, sexual risk behavior, and STIs among boys and girls.[100]

MALE CIRCUMCISION

Male circumcision is nearly universal in MENA,[101] and there is extensive scientific evidence for its protective effects against HIV, including a measured efficacy of 60% against HIV infection established in three randomized clinical trials.[102] Southern Sudan is the only part of MENA where universal male circumcision is not the norm. A study in Juba, Southern Sudan, found that only 44% of men were circumcised (90% of Muslim men and 39% of non-Muslim men).[103] The prevalence of male circumcision is

[86] Huff, "Male Circumcision: Cutting the Risk?"

[87] Wellings et al., "Sexual Behaviour in Context"; Durex, "Global Sex Survey 2005."

[88] Sakalli-Ugurlu and Glick, "Ambivalent Sexism."

[89] International Planned Parenthood Federation, "Unsafe Abortion."

[90] Gursoy and Vural, "Nurses' and Midwives' Views."

[91] Mostafa and Roshdy, "Risk Profiles."

[92] Ryan et al., "Reproductive Tract Infections."

[93] Al-Mutairi et al., "Clinical Patterns."

[94] Chaouki et al., "The Viral Origin of Cervical Cancer"; Burchell et al., "Chapter 6."

[95] Chaouki et al., "The Viral Origin of Cervical Cancer."

[96] Hallett et al., "Behaviour Change"; Gregson et al., "Sexual Mixing Patterns."

[97] Rashad, "Demographic Transition."

[98] Chaouki et al., "The Viral Origin of Cervical Cancer"; Hassen et al., "Cervical Human Papillomavirus Infection."

[99] Kassak et al., "Final Working Protocol"; Yamazhan et al., "Attitudes towards HIV/AIDS."

[100] Busulwa, "HIV/AIDS Situation Analysis Study."

[101] Weiss et al., "Male Circumcision."

[102] Auvert et al., "Randomized, Controlled Intervention Trial"; Bailey et al., "Male Circumcision"; Gray et al., "Male Circumcision."

[103] UNHCR, "HIV Behavioural Surveillance Survey."

probably lower in the rural areas in Southern Sudan, out of Juba. Male circumcision should be considered as a prevention intervention for HIV in Southern Sudan. It must be stressed, however, that male circumcision is only partially protective and does not fully prevent HIV infection.

Female "circumcision," more appropriately labeled as female genital mutilation, is also prevalent in several MENA countries and is not associated with any protective effects against HIV.[104] The prevalence of female genital mutilation is estimated at 98% in Djibouti,[105] 97.3% in Egypt,[106] 94% in southern Somalia,[107] 89% in Sudan,[108] and 22.6% in the Republic of Yemen.[109] Although three-quarters of girls in Egypt undergo this procedure by medically trained personnel,[110] this may not be the case in other countries. Female genital mutilation is associated with infections and other health complications that may potentially put females, biologically speaking, at higher risk of HIV infection.[111]

ANALYTICAL SUMMARY

There is considerable evidence on the levels of HIV prevalence among the general population in MENA. HIV prevalence is very low in all countries, except Djibouti, Somalia, and Sudan. There is no evidence for a substantial HIV epidemic in the general population in any of the MENA countries.

Apart from Djibouti, Somalia, and Sudan, there appears to be very limited HIV transmission within the general population. Southern Sudan is of particular concern and could be already in a state of general population HIV epidemic, but conclusive evidence is still lacking. Though the HIV epidemic in Djibouti and parts

of Somalia is technically already generalized, the epidemiology of HIV infection in these nations suggests that there is no sustainable general population epidemic. The dynamics of HIV infection in these nations are focused mainly around concentrated epidemics in commercial sex networks in the context of special circumstances of risk and vulnerability largely not present in the rest of the MENA countries. HIV prevalence in these countries is still at levels much lower than those found in the hyperendemic HIV epidemics in sub-Saharan Africa.

Sexual behavior data in the general population in MENA remain rather limited. Existing evidence suggests that sexual risk behaviors in the general population are present, but at rather low levels in comparison to other regions. Spousal sexual partnerships in MENA seem to be in a state of change with nonconventional forms of marriage increasing in prevalence. Levels of sexual risk behavior appear to be increasing, particularly among youth, though probably not to a level that can support an HIV epidemic in the general population. Available sexual risk behavior measures suggest limited potential for a sustainable HIV epidemic in the general population in at least the foreseeable future, if ever.

STI prevalence data, including herpes simplex virus type 2 (HSV-2), HPV, syphilis, gonorrhea, and chlamydia, indicate low prevalence of these infections among the general population in MENA in comparison to other regions (chapter 10). Unsafe abortions are also at low levels in MENA compared to other regions (chapter 10). These proxy measures of sexual risk behavior imply low levels of risky behavior in MENA. This further indicates limited potential for a sustainable HIV epidemic in the general population.

Male circumcision is almost universal in MENA,[112] and is associated with a biological efficacy against HIV infection.[113] Male circumcision is associated with lower HIV prevalence at the population level,[114] and its role in HIV dynamics appears to be "quarantining" HIV sustainable transmission to within higher risk groups with

[104] DeJong et al., "The Sexual and Reproductive Health of Young People."

[105] Roudi-Fahimi and Ashford, "Sexual & Reproductive Health."

[106] El-Zanaty and Way, *Egypt Demographic and Health Survey.*

[107] Scott et al., "Low Prevalence of Human Immunodeficiency Virus-1."

[108] Sudan Department of Statistics, *Sudan Demographic and Health Survey 1989/1990.*

[109] Roudi-Fahimi and Ashford, "Sexual & Reproductive Health"; Yemen Central Statistical Organization, *Yemen Demographic, Maternal and Child Health Survey 1997.*

[110] Roudi-Fahimi and Ashford, "Sexual & Reproductive Health."

[111] Obermeyer, "The Consequences of Female Circumcision"; Obermeyer, "The Health Consequences of Female Circumcision"; Bailey, Neema, and Othieno, "Sexual Behaviors."

[112] Weiss et al., "Male Circumcision."

[113] Auvert et al., "Randomized, Controlled Intervention Trial"; Bailey et al., "Male Circumcision"; Gray et al., "Male Circumcision."

[114] Weiss et al., "Male Circumcision"; Drain et al., "Male Circumcision."

limited inroads into the general population.[115] This further indicates limited potential for a sustainable HIV epidemic in the general population.

At a global level, there is no evidence for a sustainable general population HIV epidemic apart from specific parts of sub-Saharan Africa.[116] It is inconceivable that MENA will be the exception to this pattern after consistently very low HIV prevalence in the general population over the two decades since the virus's introduction into the MENA population in the 1980s.

All of the above considerations affirm that it is unlikely that the MENA region will experience a sustainable or substantial HIV epidemic in the general population in at least the foreseeable future, if ever. Nevertheless, prevention resources in MENA continue to be focused among the general population, as opposed to priority groups, despite its lowest risk of HIV exposure of all HIV risk groups. HIV programs focused on the general population in MENA should stress stigma reduction, rather than personal risk reduction, and prevention efforts should be focused on priority populations.

BIBLIOGRAPHY

Abdul Mujeeb, S., K. Aamir, and K. Mehmood. 2000. "Seroprevalence of HBV, HCV and HIV Infections among College Going First Time Voluntary Blood Donors." *J Pak Med Assoc* 50: 269–70.

Abdul Mujeeb, S., and M. R. Hashmi. 1988. "A Study of HIV-Antibody in Sera of Blood Donors and People at Risk." *J Pak Med Assoc* 38: 221–22.

Afghanistan Central Blood Bank. 2006. *Report of Testing of Blood Donors from March–December, 2006.* Ministry of Public Health, Kabul, Afghanistan.

Afsar, I., S. Gungor, A. G. Sener, and S. G. Yurtsever. 2008. "The Prevalence of HBV, HCV and HIV Infections among Blood Donors in Izmir, Turkey." *Indian J Med Microbiol* 26: 288–89.

Aghajanian, A. 2001. *Family and Family Change in Iran.* Fayetteville: Fayetteville State University.

Ahmed, S. M. 2004a. *AIDS Patients: Situation Analysis-Behavioral Survey Results & Discussions.* Report. Sudan National AIDS Control Program.

———. 2004b. *Antenatal: Situation Analysis-Behavioral Survey Results & Discussions.* Report. Sudan National AIDS Control Program.

———. 2004c. *Internally Displaced People: Situation Analysis-Behavioral Survey Results & Discussions.* Report. Sudan National AIDS Control Program.

———. 2004d. *Military: Situation Analysis-Behavioral Survey Results & Discussions.* Report. Sudan National AIDS Control Program.

———. 2004e. *Prisoners: Situation Analysis-Behavioral Survey Results & Discussions.* Report. Sudan National AIDS Control Program.

———. 2004f. *Sex Sellers: Situation Analysis-Behavioral Survey Results & Discussions.* Report. Sudan National AIDS Control Program.

———. 2004g. *STDs: Situation Analysis-Behavioral Survey Results & Discussions.* Report. Sudan National AIDS Control Program.

———. 2004h. *Street Children: Situation Analysis-Behavioral Survey Results & Discussions.* Report. Sudan National AIDS Control Program.

———. 2004i. *TB Patients: Situation Analysis-Behavioral Survey Results & Discussions.* Report. Sudan National AIDS Control Program.

———. 2004j. *Tea Sellers: Situation Analysis-Behavioral Survey Results & Discussions.* Report. Sudan National AIDS Control Program.

———. 2004k. *Truck Drivers: Situation Analysis-Behavioral Survey Results & Discussions.* Report. Sudan National AIDS Control Program.

———. 2004l. *University Students: Situation Analysis-Behavioral Survey, Results & Discussions.* Report. Sudan National AIDS Control Program.

Aidaoui, M., S. Bouzbid, and M. Laouar. 2008. "Seroprevalence of HIV Infection in Pregnant Women in the Annaba Region (Algeria)." *Rev Epidemiol Sante Publique* 56: 261–66.

Al Katheeb, M. S., M. S. Tarawneh, and A. S. Awidi. 1988. "Antibodies to HIV in Jordanian Blood Donors and Patients with Congenital Bleeding Disorders." IV International Conference on AIDS, Stockholm, abstract 5003.

Al Rasheed, A. M., D. Fairclough, Abu Al Sand, and A. O. Osoba. 1988. "Screening for HIV Antibodies among Blood Donors at Riadh Armed Forces Hospital." IV International Conference on AIDS, Stockholm, abstract 5001.

Alamawi, S., A. Abutaleb, L. Qasem, S. Masoud, Z. Memish, K. Al Khairy, O. Kheir, S. Bernvil, and A. H. Hajeer. 2003. "HIV-1 p24 Antigen Testing in Blood Banks: Results from Saudi Arabia." *Br J Biomed Sci* 60: 102–4.

Alami, K. 2009. "Tendances récentes de l'épidémie à VIH/SIDA en Afrique du nord." Presentation, Research and AIDS Workshop in North Africa, Marrakech, Morocco.

Algeria MOH (Ministry of Health). "Rapport de l'enquête nationale de séro-surveillance sentinelle du VIH et de la syphilis en Algérie 2004–2005."

Al-Mutairi, N., A. Joshi, O. Nour-Eldin, A. K. Sharma, I. El-Adawy, and M. Rijhwani. 2007. "Clinical Patterns of Sexually Transmitted Diseases, Associated Sociodemographic Characteristics, and Sexual

Practices in the Farwaniya Region of Kuwait." *Int J Dermatol* 46: 594–99.

Alsallaq, R. A., B. Cash, H. A. Weiss, I. M. Longini, S. B. Omer, M. J. Wawer, R. H. Gray, and L. J. Abu-Raddad. Forthcoming. "Quantitative Assessment of the Role of Male Circumcision in HIV Epidemiology at the Population Level." *Epidemics.*

Ameen, R., N. Sanad, S. Al-Shemmari, I. Siddique, R. I. Chowdhury, S. Al-Hamdan, and A. Al-Bashir. 2005. "Prevalence of Viral Markers among First-Time Arab Blood Donors in Kuwait." *Transfusion* 45: 1973–80.

Amini, S., M. F. Mahmoodi, S. Andalibi, and A. A. Solati. 1993. "Seroepidemiology of Hepatitis B, Delta and Human Immunodeficiency Virus Infections in Hamadan Province, Iran: A Population Based Study." *J Trop Med Hyg* 96: 277–87.

Arabaci, F., H. A. Sahin, I. Sahin, and S. Kartal. 2003. "Kan donörlerinde HBV, HCV, HIV ve VDRL seropozitifligi." *Klimik Derg* 16: 18–20.

Auvert, B., D. Taljaard, E. Lagarde, J. Sobngwi-Tambekou, R. Sitta, and A. Puren. 2005. "Randomized, Controlled Intervention Trial of Male Circumcision for Reduction of HIV Infection Risk: The ANRS 1265 Trial." *PLoS Med* 2: e298.

Bailey, R. C., S. Moses, C. B. Parker, K. Agot, I. Maclean, J. N. Krieger, C. F. M. Williams, R. T. Campbell, and J. O. Ndinya-Achola. 2007. "Male Circumcision for HIV Prevention in Young Men in Kisumu, Kenya: A Randomised Controlled Trial." *Lancet* 369: 643–56.

Bailey, R. C., S. Neema, and R. Othieno. 1999. "Sexual Behaviors and Other HIV Risk Factors in Circumcised and Uncircumcised Men in Uganda." *J Acquir Immune Defic Syndr* 22: 294–301.

Basha, H. M. 2006. "Vulnerable Population Research in Darfur."

Beamish, J. 2003. "Adolescent Reproductive Health in Egypt: Status, Policies, Programs, and Issues Policy Project." Unpublished memo.

Bennani, A., and K. Alami. 2006. "Surveillance sentinelle VIH, résultats 2005 et tendances de la séro-prévalence du VIH." Morocco Ministry of Health, UNAIDS.

Burchell, A. N., R. L. Winer, S. de Sanjose, and E. L. Franco. 2006. "Chapter 6: Epidemiology and Transmission Dynamics of Genital HPV Infection." *Vaccine* 24 Suppl 3: S52–61.

Busulwa, R. 2003. "HIV/AIDS Situation Analysis Study." Conducted in Hodeidah, Taiz and Hadhramut, Republic of Yemen.

Chaleby, K. 1985. "Women of Polygamous Marriages in an Inpatient Psychiatric Service in Kuwait." *J Nerv Ment Dis* 173: 56–58.

Chaouki, N., F. X. Bosch, N. Munoz, C. J. Meijer, B. El Gueddari, A. El Ghazi, J. Deacon, X. Castellsague, and J. M. Walboomers. 1998. "The Viral Origin of Cervical Cancer in Rabat, Morocco." *Int J Cancer* 75: 546–54.

Chemtob, D., and S. F. Srour. 2005. "Epidemiology of HIV Infection among Israeli Arabs." *Public Health* 119: 138–43.

Constantine, N. T., M. F. Sheba, D. M. Watts, Z. Farid, and M. Kamal. 1990. "HIV Infection in Egypt: A Two and a Half Year Surveillance." *J Trop Med Hyg* 93: 146–50.

Coskun, O., C. Gul, H. Erdem, O. Bedir, and C. P. Eyigun. 2008. "Prevalence of HIV and Syphilis among Turkish Blood Donors." *Ann Saudi Med* 28: 470.

DeJong, J., R. Jawad, and I. Mortagy, and B. Shepard. 2005. "The Sexual and Reproductive Health of Young People in the Arab Countries and Iran." *Reprod Health Matters* 13: 49–59.

Djibouti (Ministère de La Santé) and Association Internationale de Développement. 2002. *Epidémie a VIH/SIDA/IST en République de Djibouti; Tome I: Analyse de la Situation et Analyse de la Réponse Nationale.* Décembre.

Drain, P. K., D. T. Halperin, J. P. Hughes, J. D. Klausner, and R. C. Bailey. 2006. "Male Circumcision, Religion, and Infectious Diseases: An Ecologic Analysis of 118 Developing Countries." *BMC Infect Dis* 6: 172.

Dray, X., R. Dray-Spira, J. A. Bronstein, and D. Mattera. 2005. "Prevalences of HIV, Hepatitis B and Hepatitis C in Blood Donors in the Republic of Djibouti." *Med Trop (Mars)* 65: 39–42.

Dupire, B., A. K. Abawi, C. Ganteaume, T. Lam, P. Truze, and G. Martet. 1999. "Establishment of a Blood Transfusion Center at Kabul (Afghanistan)." *Sante* 9: 18–22.

Durex. 2005. "Durex Global Sex Survey 2005."

El-Gadi, S., A. Abudher, and M. Sammud. 2008. "HIV-Related Knowledge and Stigma among High School Students in Libya." *Int J STD AIDS* 19: 178–83.

El-Ghazzawi, E., G. Hunsmann, and J. Schneider. 1987. "Low Prevalence of Antibodies to HIV-1 and HTLV-I in Alexandria, Egypt." *AIDS Forsch* 2: 639.

Elharti, E., A. Zidouh, R. Mengad, O. Bennani, and R. Elaouad. 2002. "Monitoring HIV through Sentinel Surveillance in Morocco." *East Mediterr Health J* 8: 141–49.

El-Hazmi, M. M. 2004. "Prevalence of HBV, HCV, HIV-1, 2 and HTLV-I/II Infections among Blood Donors in a Teaching Hospital in the Central Region of Saudi Arabia." *Saudi Med J* 25: 26–33.

Elmir, E., S. Nadia, B. Ouafae, M. Rajae, S. Amina, and A. Rajae el. 2002. "HIV Epidemiology in Morocco: A Nine-Year Survey (1991–1999)." *Int J STD AIDS* 13: 839–42.

El-Zanaty, F., and A. Way. 2001. *Egypt Demographic and Health Survey.* Calverton, MD: Ministry of Health and Population Egypt, National Population Council and ORC Macro.

Foster, A. 2002. "Young Women's Sexuality in Tunisia: The Health Consequences of Misinformation among University Students." In *Everyday Life in the Muslim Middle East*, ed. D. L. Bowen and E. A. Early, 98–110. Bloomington: Indiana University Press.

Gassmelseed, D. E., A. M. Nasr, S. M. Homeida, M. A. Elsheikh, and I. Adam. 2006. "Prevalence of HIV Infection among Pregnant Women of the Central Sudan." *J Med Virol* 78: 1269–70.

Ghazal-Aswad, S., P. Badrinath, N. Osman, S. Abdul-Khaliq, S. Mc Ilvenny, and I. Sidky. 2004. "Prevalence of Chlamydia Trachomatis Infection among Women in a Middle Eastern Community." *BMC Womens Health* 4: 3.

Gray, R. H., G. Kigozi, D. Serwadda, F. Makumbi, S. Watya, F. Nalugoda, N. Kiwanuka, L. H. Moulton, M. A. Chaudhary, M. Z. Chen, N. K. Sewankambo, F. Wabwire-Mangen, M. C. Bacon, C. F. M. Williams, P. Opendi, S. J. Reynolds, O. Laeyendecker, T. C. Quinn, and M. J. Wawer. 2007. "Male Circumcision for HIV Prevention in Men in Rakai, Uganda: A Randomised Trial." *Lancet* 369: 657–66.

Gregson, S., C. A. Nyamukapa, G. P. Garnett, P. R. Mason, T. Zhuwau, M. Caraël, S. K. Chandiwana, and R. M. Anderson. 2002. "Sexual Mixing Patterns and Sex-Differentials in Teenage Exposure to HIV Infection in Rural Zimbabwe." *Lancet* 359: 1896–1903.

Gursoy, E., and G. Vural. 2003. "Nurses' and Midwives' Views on Approaches to Hymen Examination." *Nurs Ethics* 10: 485–96.

Gutbi, O. S.-A., and A. M. G. Eldin. 2006. "Women Tea-Sellers in Khartoum and HIV/AIDS: Surviving Against the Odds." Grey Report, Khartoum, Sudan.

Haeri, S. 1994. "Temporary Marriage: An Islamic Discourse on Female Sexuality in Iran." In *The Eye of the Storm: Women in Post-Revolutionary Iran*, ed. M. Afkhami and E. Friedl, 98–114. New York, NY: Tauris Publishers.

Hajiabdolbaghi, M., N. Razani, N. Karami, P. Kheirandish, M. Mohraz, M. Rasoolinejad, K. Arefnia, Z. Kourorian, G. Rutherford, and W. McFarland. 2007. "Insights from a Survey of Sexual Behavior among a Group of At-Risk Women in Tehran, Iran, 2006." *AIDS Educ Prev* 19: 519–30.

Hallett, T. B., S. Gregson, J. J. Lewis, B. A. Lopman, and G. P. Garnett. 2007. "Behaviour Change in Generalised HIV Epidemics: Impact of Reducing Cross-Generational Sex and Delaying Age at Sexual Debut." *Sex Transm Infect* 83 Suppl 1: i50–54.

Hammouda, D., N. Munoz, R. Herrero, A. Arslan, A. Bouhadef, M. Oublil, B. Djedeat, B. Fontaniere, P. Snijders, C. Meijer, and S. Franceschi. 2005. "Cervical Carcinoma in Algiers, Algeria: Human Papillomavirus and Lifestyle Risk Factors." *Int J Cancer* 113: 483–89.

Hashim, M. S., M. A. Salih, A. A. el Hag, Z. A. Karrar, E. M. Osman, F. S. el-Shiekh, I. A. el Tilib, and N. E. Attala. 1997. "AIDS and HIV Infection in Sudanese Children: A Clinical and Epidemiological Study." *AIDS Patient Care STDS* 11: 331–37.

Hassen, E., A. Chaieb, M. Letaief, H. Khairi, A. Zakhama, S. Remadi, and L. Chouchane. 2003. "Cervical Human Papillomavirus Infection in Tunisian Women." *Infection* 31: 143–48.

Huff, B. 2000. "Male Circumcision: Cutting the Risk?" American Foundation for AIDS Research, August.

Institut de Formation Paramédicale de Parnet. 2004. *Rapport de la réunion d'évaluation a mis-parcours de l'enquête de sero-surveillance du VIH.* Juin.

International Planned Parenthood Federation. 1992. "Unsafe Abortion and Sexual Health in the Arab World: The Damascus Conference." Proceedings of the Damascus Conference, Arab World Region.

Iqbal, J., and N. Rehan. 1996. "Sero-Prevalence of HIV: Six Years' Experience at Shaikh Zayed Hospital, Lahore." *J Pak Med Assoc* 46: 255–58.

IRC (International Rescue Committee). 2002. *CDC. Kakuma Refugee Camp Sentinel Surveillance Report.* Nairobi.

Jama, H., L. Grillner, G. Biberfeld, S. Osman, A. Isse, M. Abdirahman, and S. Bygdeman. 1987. "Sexually Transmitted Viral Infections in Various Population Groups in Mogadishu, Somalia." *Genitourin Med* 63: 329–32.

Jenkins, C., and D. A. Robalino. 2003. "HIV in the Middle East and North Africa: The Cost of Inaction." Orientations in Development Series, World Bank.

Jurjus, A. R., J. Kahhaleh, National AIDS Program, and WHO/EMRO (World Health Organization/Eastern Mediterranean Regional Office). 2004. "Knowledge, Attitudes, Beliefs, and Practices of the Lebanese concerning HIV/AIDS." Grey Report, Beirut, Lebanon.

Kaiser, R., T. Kedamo, J. Lane, G. Kessia, R. Downing, T. Handzel, E. Marum, P. Salama, J. Mermin, W. Brady, and P. Spiegel. 2006. "HIV, Syphilis, Herpes Simplex Virus 2, and Behavioral Surveillance among Conflict-Affected Populations in Yei and Rumbek, Southern Sudan." *AIDS* 20: 942–44.

Kakepoto, G. N., H. S. Bhally, G. Khaliq, N. Kayani, I. A. Burney, T. Siddiqui, and M. Khurshid. 1996. "Epidemiology of Blood-Borne Viruses: A Study of Healthy Blood Donors in Southern Pakistan." *Southeast Asian J Trop Med Public Health* 27: 703–6.

Kandela, P. 1993. "Arab Nations: Attitudes to AIDS." *Lancet* 341: 884–85.

Kapiga, S. H. 1996. "Determinants of Multiple Sexual Partners and Condom Use among Sexually Active Tanzanians." *East Afr Med J* 73: 435–42.

Kapiga, S. H., and J. L. Lugalla. 2002. "Sexual Behaviour Patterns and Condom Use in Tanzania: Results from the 1996 Demographic and Health Survey." *AIDS Care* 14: 455–69.

Kassak, K., J. DeJong, Z. Mahfoud, R. Afifi, S. Abdurahim, M. L. Sami Ramia, F. El-Barbir, M. Ghanem, S. Shamra, K. Kreidiyyeh, and D. El-Khoury. 2008. "Final Working Protocol for an Integrated Bio-Behavioral Surveillance Study among Four Vulnerable Groups in Lebanon: Men Who Have Sex with Men; Prisoners; Commercial Sex Workers; and Intravenous Drug Users." Grey Report.

Kayani, N., A. Sheikh, A. Khan, C. Mithani, and M. Khurshid. 1994. "A View of HIV-I Infection in Karachi." *J Pak Med Assoc* 44: 8–11.

Khattabi, H., and K. Alami. 2005. "Surveillance senti-nelle du VIH, Résultats 2004 et tendance de la séro-prévalence du VIH." Morocco Ministry of Health, UNAIDS.

Khedmat, H., F. Fallahian, H. Abolghasemi, S. M. Alavian, B. Hajibeigi, S. M. Miri, and A. M. Jafari. 2007. "Seroepidemiologic Study of Hepatitis B Virus, Hepatitis C Virus, Human Immunodeficiency Virus and Syphilis Infections in Iranian Blood Donors." *Pak J Biol Sci* 10: 4461–66.

Kretzschmar, M., and M. Morris. 1996. "Measures of Concurrency in Networks and the Spread of Infectious Disease." *Mathematical Biosciences* 133: 165–95.

Kulane, A., A. A. Hilowle, A. A. Hassan, and R. Thorstensson. 2000. "Prevalence of HIV, HTLV I/II and HBV Infections during Long Lasting Civil Conflicts in Somalia." *Int Conf AIDS*: 13.

Lebanon National AIDS Control Program. 1996. "General Population Evaluation Survey Assessing Knowledge, Attitudes, Beliefs and Practices Related to HIV/AIDS in Lebanon." Ministry of Public Health.

Libya National Center for the Prevention of and Control of Infectious Diseases. 2005. "Results of the National Seroprevalence Survey." Summary document.

Maayan, S., E. Shinar, M. Aefani, M. Soughayer, R. Alkhoudary, S. Barshany, and N. Manny. 1994. "HIV-1 Prevalence among Israeli and Palestinian Blood Donors." *AIDS* 8: 133–34.

Marcelin, A. G., M. Grandadam, P. Flandre, J. L. Koeck, M. Philippon, E. Nicand, R. Teyssou, H. Agut, J. M. Huraux, and N. Dupin. 2001. "Comparative Study of Heterosexual Transmission of HIV-1, HSV-2 and KSHV in Djibouti." *8th Retrovir Oppor Infect* (abstract no. 585).

Maslin, J., C. Rogier, F. Berger, M. A. Khamil, D. Mattera, M. Grandadam, M. Caron, and E. Nicand. 2005. "Epidemiology and Genetic Characterization of HIV-1 Isolates in the General Population of Djibouti (Horn of Africa)." *J Acquir Immune Defic Syndr* 39: 129–32.

Massarrat, M. S., and S. Tahaghoghi-Mehrizi. 2002. "Iranian National Health Survey: A Brief Report." *Archives of Iranian Medicine* 2: 73–79.

Massenet, D., and A. Bouh. 1997. "Aspects of Blood Transfusion in Djibouti." *Med Trop (Mars)* 57: 202–5.

May, R. M., and R. M. Anderson. 1988. "The Transmission Dynamics of Human Immunodeficiency Virus (HIV)." *Philosophical Transactions of the Royal Society of London Series B-Biological Sciences* 321: 565–607.

Ministry of Health and Medical Education of Iran. 2006. "Treatment and Medical Education." Islamic Republic of Iran HIV/AIDS situation and response analysis.

Mohammad, K., F. K. Farahani, M. R. Mohammadi, S. Alikhani, M. Zare, F. R. Tehrani, A. Ramezankhani, A. Hasanzadeh, and H. Ghanbari. 2007. "Sexual Risk-Taking Behaviors among Boys Aged 15–18 Years in Tehran." *J Adolesc Health* 41: 407–14.

Morocco MOH (Ministry of Health). 2006. *Implementation of the Declaration of Commitment on HIV/AIDS*. 2006 National Report, Kingdom of Morocco.

Morris, M. 1997. "Sexual Networks and HIV." *AIDS* 11: S209–16.

Mostafa, S. R., and O. H. Roshdy. 1999. "Risk Profiles for Sexually Transmitted Diseases among Patients Attending the Venereal Disease Clinic at Alexandria Main University Hospital." *East Mediterr Health J* 5: 740–54.

Mujeeb, S. A., K. Aamir, and K. Mehmood. 2006. "Seroprevalence of HBV, HCV and HIV Infections among College Going First Time Voluntary Blood Donors." *J Pak Med Assoc* 56: S24–25.

Mujeeb, S. A., M. R. Khanani, T. Khursheed, and A. Siddiqui. 1991. "Prevalence of HIV-Infection among Blood Donors." *J Pak Med Assoc* 41: 253–54.

Naffa, S. 2004. "Jordanian Women: Past and Present." Grey Report.

Naim, M., and E. Bhutto. 2000. "Sexuality during Pregnancy in Pakistani Women." *J Pak Med Assoc* 50: 38–44.

NSNAC (New Sudan National AIDS Council), and UNAIDS (United Nations Joint Programme on HIV/AIDS). 2006. *HIV/AIDS Integrated Report South Sudan, 2004–2005*. With United Nations General Assembly Special Session on HIV/AIDS Declaration of Commitment.

Obasi, A., F. Mosha, M. Quigley, Z. Sekirassa, T. Gibbs, K. Munguti, J. Todd, H. Grosskurth, P. Mayaud, J. Changalucha, D. Brown, D. Mabey, and R. Hayes. 1999. "Antibody to Herpes Simplex Virus Type 2 as a Marker of Sexual Risk Behavior in Rural Tanzania." *J Infect Dis* 179: 16–24.

Obermeyer, C. M. 2003. "The Health Consequences of Female Circumcision: Science, Advocacy, and Standards of Evidence." *Med Anthropol Q* 17: 394–412.

———. 2005. "The Consequences of Female Circumcision for Health and Sexuality: An Update on the Evidence." *Cult Health Sex* 7: 443–61.

Pakistan National Institute of Health. 1992. *National AIDS Control Program Report*. Islamabad: Government of Pakistan.

———. 1995. *National AIDS Control Program Report*. Islamabad: Government of Pakistan.

Pisani, E., S. Lazzari, N. Walker, and B. Schwartlander. 2003. "HIV Surveillance: A Global Perspective." *J Acquir Immune Defic Syndr* 32 Suppl 1: S3–11.

Pourshams, A., R. Malekzadeh, A. Monavvari, M. R. Akbari, A. Mohamadkhani, S. Yarahmadi, N. Seddighi, M. Mohamadnejad, M. Sotoudeh, and A. Madjlessi. 2005. "Prevalence and Etiology of Persistently Elevated Alanine Aminotransferase Levels in Healthy Iranian Blood Donors." *Journal of Gastroenterology and Hepatology* 20: 229–33.

Qatar, state of. 2008. *Report on the Country Progress Indicators towards Implementing the Declaration of Commitment on HIV*. National Health Authority.

Quinti, I., E. Renganathan, E. El Ghazzawi, M. Divizia, G. Sawaf, S. Awad, A. Pana, and G. Rocchi. 1995. "Seroprevalence of HIV and HCV Infections in Alexandria, Egypt." *Zentralbl Bakteriol* 283: 239–44.

Rashad, H. 2000. "Demographic Transition in Arab Countries: A New Perspective." *Journal of Population Research* 17: 83–101.

Rashad, H., and M. Osman. 2003. "Nuptiality in Arab Countries: Changes and Implications." In *The New Arab Family, Cairo Papers in Social Science, Vol. 24, Nos. 1–2*, ed. N. Hopkins, 20–50. Cairo: American University in Cairo Press.

Rashad, H., M. I. Osman, F. Roudi-Fahimi, and Population Reference Bureau. 2005. "Marriage in the Arab World." Population Reference Bureau.

Raza, M. I., A. Afifi, A. J. Choudhry, and H. I. Khan. 1998. "Knowledge, Attitude and Behaviour towards AIDS among Educated Youth in Lahore, Pakistan." *J Pak Med Assoc* 48: 179–82.

Recknagel, C., and A. Gorgin. 2002. "Iran: Proposal Debated for Solving Prostitution with 'Chastity Houses.'" Prague, 7 August (RFE/RL).

Rezvan, H., H. Abolghassemi, and S. A. Kafiabad. 2007. "Transfusion-Transmitted Infections among Multitransfused Patients in Iran: A Review." *Transfus Med* 17: 425–33.

Roudi-Fahimi, F., and L. Ashford. 2008. "Sexual & Reproductive Health in the Middle East and North Africa. A Guide for Reporters." Population Reference Bureau.

Ryan, C. A., A. Zidouh, L. E. Manhart, R. Selka, M. Xia, M. Moloney-Kitts, J. Mahjour, M. Krone, B. N. Courtois, G. Dallabetta, and K. K. Holmes. 1998. "Reproductive Tract Infections in Primary Healthcare, Family Planning, and Dermatovenereology Clinics: Evaluation of Syndromic Management in Morocco." *Sex Transm Infect* 74 Suppl 1: S95–105.

Sakalli-Ugurlu, N., and P. Glick. 2003. "Ambivalent Sexism and Attitudes toward Women Who Engage in Premarital Sex in Turkey." *J Sex Res* 40: 296–302.

Scott, D. A., A. L. Corwin, N. T. Constantine, M. A. Omar, A. Guled, M. Yusef, C. R. Roberts, and D. M. Watts. 1991. "Low Prevalence of Human Immunodeficiency Virus-1 (HIV-1), HIV-2, and Human T Cell Lymphotropic Virus-1 Infection in Somalia." *American Journal of Tropical Medicine and Hygiene* 45: 653.

Sepehrad, R. 2002. "The Role of Women in Iran's New Popular Revolution." *Brown J World Aff* 9: 217.

SeyedAlinaghi, S. 2009. "Seroprevalence of HIV Infection among Pregnant Women in Tehran, Iran, by Rapid HIV Test." Personal communication.

Sharifi-Mood, B., and F. Keikha. 2008. "Seroprevalence of Human Immunodeficiency Virus (HIV) in Pregnant Women in Zahedan, Southeastern Iran." *Journal of Research in Medical Sciences* 13: 186–88.

SNAP (Sudan National AIDS Program). 2002. *Situation Analysis: Behavioral & Epidemiological Surveys & Response Analysis*. HIV/AIDS Strategic Planning Process Report, Federal Ministry of Health, Khartoum.

———. 2004. *HIV/AIDS/STIs Prevalence, Knowledge, Attitude, Practices and Risk Factors among University Students and Military Personnel*. Federal Ministry of Health, Khartoum.

———. 2005a. *National Policy on HIV/AIDS*. SNAP.

———. 2005b. *Sentinel Sero-Surveillance—2005 Data*. Annual newsletter, SNAP.

———. 2008. "Update on the HIV Situation in Sudan." PowerPoint presentation, SNAP.

SNAP (Sudan National AIDS Program), NSNAC (New Sudan National AIDS Council), and UNAIDS (United Nations Joint Programme on HIV/AIDS). 2006. "Scaling-up HIV/AIDS Response in Sudan." National Consultation on the Road towards Universal Access to Prevention, Treatment, Care and Support.

SNAP, and UNAIDS. 2006. "HIV/AIDS Integrated Report North Sudan, 2004–2005 (Draft)." With United Nations General Assembly Special Session on HIV/AIDS Declaration of Commitment.

SNAP, UNICEF (United Nations Childrens Fund), and UNAIDS. 2005. "Baseline Study on Knowledge, Attitudes, and Practices on Sexual Behaviors and HIV/AIDS Prevention amongst Young People in Selected States in Sudan." HIV/AIDS KAPB Report, Projects and Research Department (AFROCENTER Group).

Somaliland Ministry of Health and Labour. 2007. *Somaliland 2007 HIV/Syphilis Seroprevalence Survey, A Technical Report*. Ministry of Health and Labour in collaboration with the WHO, UNAIDS, UNICEF/GFATM, and SOLNAC.

Southern Sudan AIDS Commission. 2007. Southern Sudan ANC Sentinel Surveillance Data. U.S. Centers for Disease Control and Prevention (CDC), Sudan, and Southern Sudan AIDS Commission. Database.

Sudan Department of Statistics. 1991. *Sudan Demographic and Health Survey 1989/1990*. Ministry of Economic and National Planning Sudan, Macro International. Columbia MD: Department of Statistics and Macro International.

Sudan MOH (Ministry of Health). 2006. *2005 ANC Sentinel Sites Results*. Khartoum.

Sudan National AIDS/STIs Program. 2008. *2007 ANC HIV Sentinel Sero-survey, Technical Report*. Federal Ministry of Health, Preventive Medicine Directorate, Draft.

Sultan, F., T. Mehmood, and M. T. Mahmood. 2007. "Infectious Pathogens in Volunteer and Replacement Blood Donors in Pakistan: A Ten-Year Experience." *Int J Infect Dis* 11: 407–12.

Tehrani, F. R., and H. Malek-Afzalip. 2008. "Knowledge, Attitudes and Practices concerning HIV/AIDS among Iranian At-Risk Sub-Populations." *Eastern Mediterranean Health Journal* 14.

Todd, C. S., M. Ahmadzai, F. Atiqzai, S. Miller, J. M. Smith, S. A. Ghazanfar, and S. A. Strathdee. 2008. "Seroprevalence and Correlates of HIV, Syphilis, and Hepatitis B and C Virus among Intrapartum Patients in Kabul, Afghanistan." *BMC Infect Dis* 8: 119.

Todd, C. S., M. Ahmadzai, F. Atiqzai, H. Siddiqui, P. Azfar, S. Miller, J. M. Smith, S. A. S. Ghazanfar, and S. A. Strathdee. 2007. "Seroprevalence and Correlates of HIV, Syphilis, and Hepatitis B and C Infection among Antenatal Patients and Testing Practices and Knowledge among Obstetric Care Providers in Kabul." PowerPoint presentation.

UNAIDS (United Nations Joint Programme on HIV/AIDS). 2000. Epidemiological Country Fact Sheet, Sudan.

———. 2008. "Notes on AIDS in the Middle East and North Africa." RST, MENA.

UNAIDS, and WHO (World Health Organization). 2003. *AIDS Epidemic Update 2003*. Geneva.

———. 2005. *AIDS Epidemic Update 2005*. Geneva.

———. 2007. *AIDS Epidemic Update 2007*. Geneva.

UNHCR (United Nations High Commissioner for Refugees). 2003. *National AIDS and Sexually Transmitted*

Control Programme. HIV sentinel surveillance, Dadaab Refugee Camps, Nairobi, Kenya.

———. 2005. *National AIDS and Sexually Transmitted Control Programme.* Sentinel surveillance report, Dadaab Refugee Camps, Nairobi, Kenya, January–May 2005.

———. 2006–7a. *HIV Sentinel Surveillance among Antenatal Clients and STI Patients.* Dadaab Refugee Camps, Kenya.

———. 2006–7b. *HIV Sentinel Surveillance among Conflict Affected Populations.* Kakuma Refugee Camp—Refugees and Host Nationals, Great Lakes Initiative on HIV/AIDS.

———. 2007. "HIV Behavioural Surveillance Survey Juba Municipality, South Sudan." United Nations High Commissioner for Refugees.

Unknown. Unknown. "Statut de la réponse nationale: Caractéristiques de l'épidémie des IST/VIH/SIDA." Algeria, Grey Report.

Unknown. 2002. "Surveillance des infections à VIH et de la syphilis chez les femmes enceintes vues dans 8 centres de consultations prénatales dans le district de Djibouti." Grey Report.

Watts, C. H., and R. M. May. 1992. "The Influence of Concurrent Partnerships on the Dynamics of HIV/AIDS." *Math Biosci* 108: 89–104.

Watts, D. M., N. T. Constantine, M. F. Sheba, M. Kamal, J. D. Callahan, and M. E. Kilpatrick. 1993. "Prevalence of HIV Infection and AIDS in Egypt over Four Years of Surveillance (1986–1990)." *J Trop Med Hyg* 96: 113–17.

Weiss, H. A., D. Halperin, R. C. Bailey, R. J. Hayes, G. Schmid, and C. A. Hankins. 2008. "Male Circumcision for HIV Prevention: From Evidence to Action?" *AIDS* 22: 567–74.

Wellings, K., M. Collumbien, E. Slaymaker, S. Singh, Z. Hodges, D. Patel, and N. Bajos. 2006. "Sexual Behaviour in Context: A Global Perspective." *Lancet* 368: 1706–28.

WHO (World Health Organization). 2002. "HIV/AIDS Epidemiological Surveillance Report for the WHO African Region 2002 Update."

———. 2003. *WHO Somalia Statistic Report 2003.*

———. 2004a. *The 2004 First National Second Generation HIV/AIDS/STI Sentinel Surveillance Survey, Central South, Somalia, A Technical Report.*

———. 2004b. *The 2004 First National Second Generation HIV/AIDS/STI Sentinel Surveillance Survey, Puntland, Somalia, A Technical Report.*

———. 2004c. *The 2004 First National Second Generation HIV/AIDS/STI Sentinel Surveillance Survey, Somalia, A Technical Report.*

WHO/EMRO (World Health Organization, Eastern Mediterranean Region). 2000. "Presentation of WHO Somalia's Experience in Supporting the National Response." Regional Consultation towards Improving HIV/AIDS & STD Surveillance in the Countries of EMRO, Beirut, Lebanon, October 30–November 2.

———. 2007a. "HIV/AIDS Surveillance in Low Level and Concentrated HIV Epidemics. A Technical Guide for Countries in the WHO Eastern Mediterranean Region." Grey Report.

———. 2007b. "Prevention and Control of Sexually Transmitted Infections in the WHO Eastern Mediterranean Region." Intercountry meeting, PowerPoint presentation.

Winsbury, R. 1996. "Aiding Refugees in the Aftermath of Civil War." *AIDS Anal* Afr 6 (5): 3.

Yamazhan, T., D. Gokengin, E. Ertem, R. Sertoz, S. Atalay, and D. Serter. 2007. "Attitudes towards HIV/AIDS and Other Sexually Transmitted Diseases in Secondary School Students in Izmir, Turkey: Changes in Time." *Trop Doct* 37: 10–12.

Yassin, K., R. Awad, A. J. Tebi, A. Queder, and U. Laaser. 2001. "A Zero Prevalence of Anti-HIV in Blood Donors in Gaza: How Can It Be Sustained?" *AIDS* 15: 936–37.

Yemen Central Statistical Organization. 1998. *Yemen Demographic, Maternal and Child Health Survey 1997.* Macro International. Calverton, MD: Central Statistical Organization and Macro International.

Yemen National AIDS Control Programme. 1998. *AIDS/HIV Surveillance Report, Fourth Quarter 1998.* Ministry of Public Health.

———. 2001. *AIDS/HIV Surveillance Report, Fourth Quarter 2001.* Ministry of Public Health.

Zargooshi, J. 2002. "Characteristics of Gonorrhoea in Kermanshah, Iran." *Sex Transm Infect* 78: 460–61.

Chapter 7

Further Evidence Related to HIV Epidemiology in MENA

This chapter covers other relevant aspects of human immunodeficiency virus (HIV) epidemiology in the Middle East and North Africa (MENA) gleaned from various sources and available data.

HIV AND SEXUALLY TRANSMITTED DISEASE CLINIC ATTENDEES, VOLUNTARY COUNSELING AND TESTING ATTENDEES, AND SUSPECTED AIDS PATIENTS

HIV prevalence among sexually transmitted disease (STD) clinic attendees, voluntary counseling and testing (VCT) attendees, and suspected AIDS (acquired immune deficiency syndrome) patients has been reported for several MENA countries. Table D.1 (appendix D) lists the results of available point-prevalence surveys among these populations. Since STD clinic and VCT attendees are more likely to represent people who visited these centers because of perceived risks, the level of HIV prevalence among these populations hints at the risk of HIV exposure in a part of the population with specific identifiable risk behaviors.

There are also few measures of risky behavior among these population groups. A study on STD clinic attendees in Pakistan found that 55% acquired the STD heterosexually, 11.6% homosexually, and 18.4% bisexually.[1] Among STD clinic attendees[2] and suspected AIDS patients[3] in Sudan, 5.4% and 0% reported ever using a condom, 13.2% and 17.4% reported premarital and extramarital sex, 0.8% and 8.7% reported premarital sex, and 3.9% and 4.3% paid for sex, respectively. Consistently in MENA, studies report that the main source of the STD infection is sexual contact with female sex workers (FSWs), such as in the Islamic Republic of Iran,[4] Kuwait,[5] Pakistan,[6] Somalia,[7] and Sudan.[8]

Analytical summary

These results suggest that apart from Djibouti, Somalia, and Sudan, HIV prevalence among STD clinic and VCT attendees is generally low. HIV has clearly made inroads into the heterosexual high-risk networks in Djibouti, Somalia, and Sudan. The limited prevalence in the rest of the countries is likely a consequence of the low levels of HIV prevalence in the priority groups, FSWs in particular, since the main reason for attending an STD clinic in the region is sexual contact with FSWs.

---

[1] Rehan, "Profile of Men."

[2] Ahmed, *STDs*.

[3] Ahmed, *AIDS Patients*.

[4] Zargooshi, "Characteristics of Gonorrhoea."

[5] Al-Mutairi et al., "Clinical Patterns"; Al-Fouzan and Al-Mutairi, "Overview."

[6] Rehan, "Profile of Men."

[7] Burans et al., "HIV Infection Surveillance in Mogadishu, Somalia"; Ismail et al., "Sexually Transmitted Diseases in Men."

[8] Omer et al., "Sexually Transmitted Diseases in Sudanese Males."

Available data illustrate that the passive facility-based surveillance at STD clinics and VCT centers is to a large extent not capturing the dynamics of HIV transmission in MENA. An active surveillance among priority populations incorporating an integrated biobehavioral surveillance methodology would be a much more effective approach in generating interpretable data on HIV epidemiology in MENA.

HIV/AIDS AMONG TUBERCULOSIS PATIENTS

HIV/AIDS among tuberculosis (TB) patients is a useful indicator of the maturity of the HIV epidemic in a given setting because it reflects the presence of advanced HIV or AIDS cases in the population. Table D.2 (appendix D) summarizes the results of available point-prevalence surveys among TB patients.

Analytical summary

Available prevalence surveys among TB patients suggest that apart from Djibouti, Somalia, and Sudan, HIV prevalence among TB patients is generally low. HIV has clearly been making inroads into a subset of the populations in Djibouti, Somalia, and Sudan for at least a decade. The limited prevalence among TB patients in the rest of MENA countries is probably a consequence of either the recent introduction of HIV into high-risk networks or the very low levels of HIV prevalence in the whole population, except possibly for small pockets of high-risk priority groups.

FURTHER POINT-PREVALENCE SURVEYS

Table D.3 (appendix D) lists a summary of point-prevalence surveys extracted from the United Nations Joint Programme on HIV/AIDS (UNAIDS) epidemiological facts sheets on each MENA country over the years. Some of the data reported here are gleaned from country-based case notification surveillance reports[9] or are provided through national-level agencies. These surveys may not be conducted using sound methodology or internationally accepted guide-

lines for HIV surveillance. There is also very limited information on the populations on which these measurements were made. Given theses limitations, the prevalence levels may not be representative of the populations that they are supposed to represent. However, despite these limitations, these measures are useful to corroborate the rest of the point-prevalence surveys discussed in the previous chapters and, indeed, convey the same picture of HIV epidemiology in MENA.

Analytical summary

The further point-prevalence surveys in table D.3 are generally consistent with those reported in the previous chapters and follow similar patterns. Injecting drug users (IDUs) and men who have sex with men (MSM) are the key priority groups for HIV infectious spread in MENA, followed by FSWs, but mainly in Djibouti, Somalia, and Sudan. There is very limited HIV prevalence in the general population.

The fluctuations among some of these data may suggest a lack of representation. To maximize the explanatory power of point-prevalence data, MENA countries need to conduct point-prevalence measurements using consistent and standard methodology and internationally accepted guidelines for HIV surveillance.

HIV-POSITIVE RESULTS EXTRACTED FROM HIV/AIDS CASE NOTIFICATION SURVEILLANCE REPORTS

Many countries in MENA routinely test different population groups for HIV. These groups include blood tissue and organ donors, blood recipients, pregnant women, marriage applicants, university students, public sector employees, out-migrants (for visa to work abroad), in-migrants (for residency or visa renewal), prisoners, TB patients, suspected AIDS cases, VCT attendees, STD clinic attendees, sexual contacts of people living with HIV (PLHIV), "bar girls," FSWs, MSM, drug users, and IDUs.

The results of 53 million HIV tests reported to the World Health Organization (WHO), as part of the HIV/AIDS case notification surveillance reports, show an overall prevalence of

---

[9] WHO/EMRO Regional Database on HIV/AIDS.

0.09%.[10] Figure 7.1 displays the percentage of these tests that were positive among different population groups.[11] Figure 7.2 shows the distribution of HIV tests by population group. Not all countries report these tests and among those that do, they may not do so consistently. Therefore, these point-prevalence measurements may be subject to different kinds of selection bias, such as reflecting measurements from a few countries as opposed to others. There is also substantial intercountry and inter-population variability in HIV prevalence across these measures, suggesting the lack of representation.

The pattern emerging in these testing reports is that of consistently very low HIV prevalence in the general population in the majority of countries. HIV prevalence is nearly nil among blood donors, pregnant women, marriage applicants, kidney donors, and migrants. In over 3 million HIV tests conducted in the Syrian Arab Republic over eight years up to 2003, less than 300 HIV cases were identified.[12] Most HIV infections are found among priority and vulnerable populations, their sexual partners, or in populations with suspected infection or identifiable risks. Even in these populations, the majority of testing reports show relatively low HIV prevalence.

It is evident in figure 7.2 that the vast majority of HIV tests in MENA are conducted on populations at low risk of HIV infection. This suggests that resources may not be prioritized for testing the priority groups at high risk of infection. HIV testing in MENA appears to be disconnected with the reality of HIV epidemiology in the region. The reported numbers of positive tests have also fluctuated substantially in several countries in recent years. These fluctuations confirm the nonsustained and sporadic nature of HIV testing and the lack of standard and effective methodological surveillance by MENA countries. The Islamic Republic of Iran, for example, observed two large blips in reported cases in 1996 and 2001, which turned out to be

Figure 7.1 Fraction of HIV Tests That Are Positive in Different Population Groups in MENA

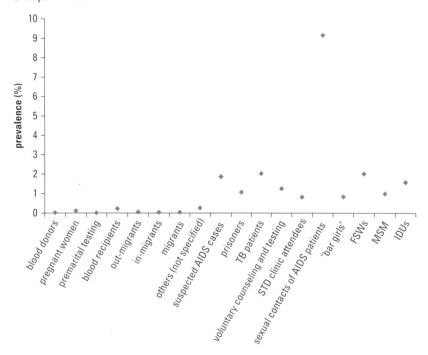

Source: WHO/EMRO Regional Database on HIV/AIDS.

Figure 7.2 Distribution of HIV Tests in MENA by Population Group

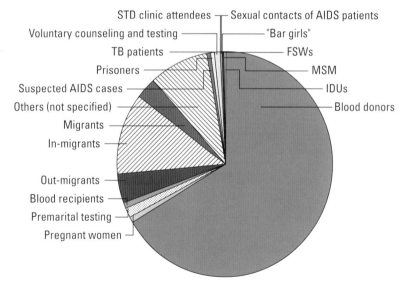

Source: WHO/EMRO Regional Database on HIV/AIDS.

<hr />

[10] Ibid.

[11] Ibid.

[12] Syria National AIDS Programme, "HIV/AIDS Female Sex Workers."

due to two testing campaigns in prisons in these respective years.[13]

Analytical summary

HIV prevalence in HIV testing surveys is generally consistent with the levels reported in the previous chapters and follows a similar pattern. There is very limited HIV prevalence in the general population. Most HIV infections are found among priority and vulnerable populations, their sexual partners, or in populations with suspected infection or identifiable risks.

Resources are not prioritized to testing high-risk priority groups. HIV testing appears to be disconnected with the reality of HIV epidemiology in MENA.

The fluctuations in the testing results suggest a lack of representation and nonsustained and sporadic HIV testing. There is no consistent, standard, and effective methodological surveillance in the countries of the region. Surveillance capacity needs to be enhanced and HIV testing procedures need to be standardized to generate interpretable data on HIV epidemiology. Tens of millions of HIV tests are routinely conducted every year in MENA, but these valuable data sources are not being utilized because of a lack of scientific capacity and methodological rigor.

DISTRIBUTION BY SEX OF REPORTED HIV CASES

Until recently, the vast majority of HIV infections in most countries in MENA were found among men. Men were 10, 4.4, 8.5, 1.6, 7, 3, and 2 times as likely as women to be infected in Bahrain,[14] Israel (Arab Israelis),[15] Lebanon,[16] Morocco,[17] Pakistan,[18] Saudi Arabia,[19] and

Sudan,[20] respectively. The percentages of HIV infections that are among men are 81% in the Arab Republic of Egypt,[21] 94% in the Islamic Republic of Iran,[22] 81.75% in Lebanon,[23] 70% in Oman,[24] 88.4% (up to 1997) in Pakistan,[25] and 79.4% in the West Bank and Gaza.[26] In Lebanon, the disease burden among men has even increased. The ratio of males versus females was 3.6 to 1 in the years 1984 to 1998,[27] but it increased to 8.5 to 1 by 2004.[28]

Nevertheless, the overall pattern in MENA appears to include an increasing proportion of females among HIV cases, such as in Algeria, Djibouti, Morocco, Pakistan, Sudan, and the Republic of Yemen.[29] In Algeria, the ratio of men to women decreased from 5.1 at the beginning of the epidemic to 1.1 in 2004.[30] The proportion of infections in women in Morocco has steadily increased to reach almost 50%, compared to 20% only five years earlier.[31] The ratio of men to women in the Republic of Yemen decreased from 4 to 1 in 1995, to 2 to 1 in 1999, and to 1 to 1 in 2000.[32] In Djibouti, the country with the highest HIV prevalence in MENA, women are already more affected by the disease than men. The prevalence is 3.6% among women and 3.1% among men in Djibouti-ville, and 1.7% among women and 0.3% among men in the rest of the country.[33]

Analytical summary

Most HIV infections in most MENA countries continue to be among men. This reflects the reality that most risk behaviors are practiced by

[13] Gheiratmand et al., "Uncertainty on the Number of HIV/AIDS Patients."

[14] Al-Haddad et al., "HIV Antibodies."

[15] Chemtob and Srour, "Epidemiology of HIV Infection."

[16] Jurjus et al., "Knowledge, Attitudes, Beliefs, and Practices."

[17] Elharti et al., "Some Characteristics of the HIV Epidemic in Morocco."

[18] Rajabali et al., "HIV and Homosexuality in Pakistan"; UNAIDS and WHO, AIDS Epidemic Update 2006.

[19] UNAIDS and WHO, AIDS Epidemic Update 2006.

[20] Sudan National HIV/AIDS Control Program, Annual Report.

[21] WHO/EMRO Regional Database on HIV/AIDS.

[22] Iran Center for Disease Management, AIDS/HIV Surveillance Report.

[23] Kassak et al., "Final Working Protocol."

[24] Tawilah and Tawil, Visit to Sultane of Oman.

[25] Khan and Hyder, "HIV/AIDS among Men."

[26] UNAIDS, "Key Findings."

[27] Kalaajieh, "Epidemiology of Human Immunodeficiency Virus."

[28] Jurjus et al., "Knowledge, Attitudes, Beliefs, and Practices."

[29] UNAIDS, "Notes on AIDS in the Middle East and North Africa"; Iqbal and Rehan, "Sero-Prevalence of HIV"; Kayani et al., "A View of HIV-I Infection in Karachi."

[30] Algeria MOH, "Rapport de l'enquête nationale de séro-surveillance."

[31] UNAIDS, "Notes on AIDS in the Middle East and North Africa"; Morocco MOH, "Situation épidémiologique"; Elharti et al., "Some Characteristics of the HIV Epidemic in Morocco."

[32] Lambert, "HIV and Development Challenges"; Al-Serouri, HIV/AIDS Situation and Response Analysis Report.

[33] WHO, "Summary Country Profile."

men rather than women. However, the proportion of females among PLHIV appears to be increasing. This pattern may suggest a maturation of the second wave of infection spread from men with identifiable risk behaviors to their wives, who are vulnerable to the infection despite engaging in no risky behavior of their own. HIV infections are repeatedly found among women with no identifiable risk behaviors, suggesting that the risk factor is heterosexual sex with the spouse.[34]

TRANSMISSION MODES

All transmission modes reported globally have been documented in MENA. There is considerable variability in which transmission mode is most common across MENA countries (table 7.1). Of the total number of reported HIV infections in the WHO/EMRO database of HIV/AIDS case notification surveillance reports,[35] the main transmission mode is unprotected vaginal and anal sex, followed by drug injection.[36] In a substantial percentage of HIV infections, the transmission mode continues to be characterized as unknown, such as in Saudi Arabia, where 26% of HIV infections appear to be with no reported identifiable risk factors.[37] Table 7.1 lists the transmission modes for a number of MENA countries.

Analytical summary

The MENA region is experiencing the same HIV transmission modes that exist in the rest of the regions. There is variability in the dominant transmission modes across MENA countries, reflecting the status of HIV dynamics in these countries. In countries with apparently no significant endemic transmission of HIV, the dominant mode is that of heterosexual sex, apparently reflecting mainly exogenous HIV infections related to exposures abroad among the nationals of these countries, or HIV transmissions to their sexual partners upon their

return. In the rest of the countries with endogenous HIV epidemics, the dominant transmission mode reflects the nature of the epidemics in these countries. For example, the dominant transmission mode in the Islamic Republic of Iran is injecting drug use, while the dominant mode in Sudan is heterosexual sex, echoing the nature of the epidemics in these two countries.

PATTERN OF EXOGENOUS HIV EXPOSURES IN MENA

HIV epidemiology in MENA exhibits one key aspect not captured in the conceptual framework used to understand HIV epidemiology (chapter 1). In a few MENA countries, there appears to be very limited endemic transmission of HIV in all of the population groups within the country, including priority populations. The number of newly diagnosed HIV infections continues to be rather stable, at low frequency with the majority reflecting sexual and injecting exposures abroad among the nationals of these countries, or HIV transmissions to their sexual partners upon their return.[38] The high mobility and migration levels are the drivers of this pattern, which has been persistent since the discovery of the epidemic, and continues to be seen even among recent HIV infections. In Jordan, in 450 out of 501 notified HIV/AIDS cases by 2006, HIV infections were acquired abroad.[39] In Lebanon, 45.36% of notified HIV/AIDS cases up to 2004 were linked to travel abroad.[40] Half of reported AIDS cases in the Republic of Yemen were linked to a travel history abroad.[41] It bears notice that some of these exposures, though exogenous to the country of the national, may still reflect exposures in another MENA country.

Analytical summary

HIV epidemiology in a few MENA countries appears to be dominated by the pattern of exogenous HIV exposures among the nationals

[34] Aidaoui, Bouzbid, and Laouar, "Seroprevalence of HIV Infection."
[35] WHO/EMRO Regional Database on HIV/AIDS.
[36] UNAIDS, "Notes on AIDS in the Middle East and North Africa."
[37] UNAIDS and WHO, AIDS Epidemic Update 2006.

[38] WHO/EMRO Regional Database on HIV/AIDS; L. J. Abu-Raddad, personal discussions with members of National AIDS Programs in MENA during 2006–9.
[39] Jordan National AIDS Program, personal communication.
[40] Jurjus et al., "Knowledge, Attitudes, Beliefs, and Practices."
[41] WHO, UNICEF, and UNAIDS, "Yemen, Epidemiological Facts Sheets."

Table 7.1 HIV Transmission Modes for a Number of MENA Countries

Country	Heterosexual transmission	Homosexual transmission	Injecting drug transmission	Blood or blood products transmission	Mother-to-child transmission
Algeria	45.71% Algeria MOH [unknown])				
Egypt, Arab Republic of	50.0% (UNAIDS and WHO 2005)	20.0% (UNAIDS and WHO 2005)			
Iran, Islamic Republic of			87.0% (Iran Center for Disease Management 2004) 82.0% (Gouya 2006) 78.0% (Hamadan province; Ghannad et al. 2009)	1.8% (Ministry of Health and Medical Education of Iran 2006) 0.35% (Hamadan province; Ghannad et al. 2009)	0.5% (Ministry of Health and Medical Education of Iran 2006) 1.0% (Hamadan province; Ghannad et al. 2009)
Jordan	52.0% (Jordan National AIDS Program, personal communication)		4.3% (Anonymous 2006)	31.0% (Jordan National AIDS Program, personal communication) 19.0% (UNAIDS 2006b)	1.7% (Anonymous 2006)
Kuwait	48.0% (Al-Fouzan and Al-Mutairi 2004)				
Lebanon	53.0% (Lebanon National AIDS Control Program 2008) 53.9% (up to 1998; Kalaajieh 2000) 56.0% (Kassak et al. 2008)	16.0% (Lebanon National AIDS Control Program 2008) 15.68% (Jurjus et al. 2004)	6.0% (Lebanon National AIDS Control Program 2008)	7.0% (Lebanon National AIDS Control Program 2008) 8.5% (up to 1998; Kalaajieh 2000)	3.0% (Lebanon National AIDS Control Program 2008) 4.3% (Kalaajieh 2000)
Morocco	77.0% (Elharti et al. 2002) 72.0% (Elharti et al. 2002) 80.0% (Alami 2009) 83.0% (Morocco MOH [unknown])	7.0% (Elharti et al. 2002) 4.0% (Alami 2009)	11.0% (Elharti et al. 2002) 4.0% (Alami 2009)	0.62% (Elharti et al. 2002) 1.0% (Alami 2009)	4.63% (Elharti et al. 2002) 3.0% (Alami 2009)
Pakistan		3.2% (Khan and Hyder 1998) 7.0% (Rajabali et al. 2008; UNAIDS and WHO 2006)			
Qatar	Main transmission mode (Qatar 2008)				

Table 7.1 *(Continued)*

Country	Heterosexual transmission	Homosexual transmission	Injecting drug transmission	Blood or blood products transmission	Mother-to-child transmission
Saudi Arabia	37.9% (Al-Mazrou et al. 2005)	2.5% (Al-Mazrou et al. 2005)	1.3% (Al-Mazrou et al. 2005)	25.0% (Al-Mazrou et al. 2005)	6.5% (Al-Mazrou et al. 2005)
	46.0% (Alrajhi, Halim, and Al-Abdely 2004)	5.0% (Alrajhi, Halim, and Al-Abdely 2004)	2.0% (Alrajhi, Halim, and Al-Abdely 2004)	26.0% (Alrajhi, Halim, and Al-Abdely 2004)	12.0% (Alrajhi, Halim, and Al-Abdely 2004)
Sudan	97.0% (UNAIDS and WHO 2007; SNAP, UNICEF, and UNAIDS 2005; Farah and Hussein 2006)				
Syrian Arab Republic	70.0% (Syria National AIDS Programme 2004)	8.0% (Syria National AIDS Programme 2004)	4.0% (Syria National AIDS Programme 2004)	12.0% (Syria National AIDS Programme 2004)	3.0% (Syria National AIDS Programme 2004)
Tunisia	56.3% (Kilani et al. 2007)	6.5% (men; Hsairi and Ben Abdallah 2007)	37.1% (Hsairi and Ben Abdallah 2007)		
	75.0% (women; Zouiten et al. 2002)				
	67.2% (women; Hsairi and Ben Abdallah 2007)				
	25.7% (men; Hsairi and Ben Abdallah 2007)				
West Bank and Gaza	52.0% (UNAIDS 2007)	1.0% (UNAIDS 2007)	4.7% (UNAIDS 2007)	17.6% (UNAIDS 2007)	
Yemen, Republic of	77.3% (Lambert 2007)	16.0% (Lambert 2007)		6.8% (Lambert 2007)	

of these countries, or HIV transmissions to their sexual partners upon their return. The weak surveillance systems of priority populations prevent us from definitively concluding whether this is indeed the dominant epidemiologic pattern in these countries. HIV could be still spreading among some of the priority groups, or within pockets of these populations, without awareness of this endemic spread. However, there is no evidence to date that such considerable endemic transmission exists in these countries.

Effective and repeated surveillance of priority populations (IDUs, MSM, and FSWs) is key for these countries to conclusively confirm that HIV spread is indeed limited in priority populations. This could also facilitate the detection of emerging epidemics and would offer a window of opportunity for targeted prevention at an early phase of an epidemic. Pakistan is a relevant example; after nearly two decades of an epidemiologic pattern of exogenous HIV exposures, HIV found its way to priority populations and has spread rapidly among IDUs and, to some extent, MSM.[42] Monitoring recent infections and examining the nature of exposures could also be useful in detecting emerging endemic transmission chains in these countries.

---

[42] Pakistan National AIDS Control Program, *HIV Second Generation Surveillance* (Rounds I, II, and III).

PARENTERAL HIV TRANSMISSIONS OTHER THAN INJECTING DRUG USE

Transmission of blood-borne pathogens occurs routinely in resource-limited settings and is considered a major public health problem in the developing world.[43] MENA is no exception to this rule, and there appears to be a lack of sufficient resources for screening blood and sterilizing medical equipment in several countries, including Afghanistan, Pakistan, Somalia, and the Republic of Yemen.[44] MENA as a whole suffers from high prevalence of unnecessary medical injections and transfusions, reuse of needles and syringes, needlestick injuries among health care workers (HCWs), and scarifications.[45] Public health systems are overstretched, leading to some careless attitudes toward safety measures.[46]

Standard precautions are not routinely implemented in public health care, and even less so in private practices such as among dentists[47] and in hemodialysis centers.[48] Injections are the preferred mode of therapy even when alternative modes are equally effective,[49] and some health practitioners see this as an opportunity for charging additional fees.[50] Injections by nonmedical providers are rampant,[51] such as in Afghanistan, where they were reported by 38%

of the participants of a study.[52] Financial limitations contribute to the reuse of syringes.[53]

Blood transfusions are performed even when not medically indicated[54]; a considerable share of the population reported such procedures. From 6.7% to 14.2% of diverse population groups in Sudan reported receiving a blood transfusion at least once in their lifetime.[55] Reuse of nonsterile blades and needles is not uncommon. Five percent of university students in Afghanistan used the nonsterile injecting needles of others and 20.8% used the nonsterile shaving sets of another person.[56] Thirty-one percent of university students and 19.4% of military personnel in Sudan used the nonsterile blades of others, and 4.8% and 8.6% used nonsterile needles with others, respectively.[57]

Occupational injuries among HCWs are common, such as in Morocco where they were found to be at high frequency, although they were rarely declared.[58] Forty-nine percent of HCWs in Egypt,[59] 58.9% in Morocco,[60] and 45% in Pakistan[61] reported a needlestick injury in the previous year.[62] Percutaneous injuries among HCWs in MENA are caused by needle recapping, handling of trash bags or linens, collision with sharps, concealed sharps, restless patients, handling and passing of devices, and invasive interventions such as surgery.[63]

The incidence of occupational exposures to infected blood and other fluids in the Islamic Republic of Iran, including exposures to fluids infected with HIV, hepatitis C virus (HCV), and hepatitis B virus (HBV), was documented at a rate of 53% exposures per person per year.[64] The

[43] Kane et al., "Transmission of Hepatitis"; Simonsen et al., "Unsafe Injections."

[44] Khawaja et al., "HIV/AIDS and Its Risk Factors in Pakistan"; World Bank Group, "World Bank Update 2005"; World Bank, *HIV/AIDS in Afghanistan*; WHO/EMRO, "Progress Report on HIV/AIDS and '3 by 5'"; UNAIDS, "Country Alignment and Harmonisation Support"; WHO/EMRO, *Progress towards Universal Access to HIV Prevention*; Luby et al., "Evaluation of Blood Bank Practices."

[45] Khawaja et al., "HIV/AIDS and Its Risk Factors in Pakistan"; World Bank Group, "World Bank Update 2005"; Yerly et al., "Nosocomial Outbreak"; Khattab et al., "Report on a Study of Women Living with HIV"; Burans et al., "Serosurvey of Prevalence"; Zafar et al., "Knowledge, Attitudes and Practices"; Hossini et al., "Knowledge and Attitudes"; Yemen MOH, *National Strategic Framework*; Kennedy, O'Reilly, and Mah, "The Use of a Quality-Improvement Approach."

[46] Zafar et al., "Knowledge, Attitudes and Practices."

[47] Askarian, Mirzaei, and McLaws, "Attitudes, Beliefs, and Infection Control"; Askarian, Mirzaei, and Cookson, "Knowledge, Attitudes, and Practice."

[48] Kabbash et al., "Risk Perception and Precautions."

[49] Janjua et al., "Population Beliefs"; Altaf et al., "Determinants of Therapeutic Injection Overuse."

[50] Janjua, Akhtar, and Hutin, "Injection Use."

[51] Janjua, Akhtar, and Hutin, "Injection Use"; Janjua, "Injection Practices."

[52] Todd et al., "Prevalence of Human Immunodeficiency Virus Infection."

[53] Janjua, "Injection Practices."

[54] Abdul Mujeeb, "Blood Transfusion."

[55] Ahmed, *Sex Sellers*; Ahmed, *Antenatal*; Ahmed, *Tea Sellers*; Ahmed, *Military*; Ahmed, *Truck Drivers*; Ahmed, *University Students*; Ahmed, *TB Patients*; Ahmed, *Internally Displaced People*; Ahmed, *Street Children*.

[56] Mansoor et al., "Gender Differences in KAP."

[57] Sudan National HIV/AIDS Control Program, *HIV/AIDS/STIs Prevalence*; Ahmed, *STDs*; Ahmed, *AIDS Patients*.

[58] Hossini et al., "Knowledge and Attitudes"; Laraqui et al., "Assessing Knowledge, Attitude, and Practice."

[59] Kabbash et al., "Risk Perception and Precautions."

[60] Laraqui et al., "Assessing Knowledge."

[61] Zafar et al., "Knowledge, Attitudes and Practices."

[62] Ibid.

[63] Kuruuzum et al., "Risk of Infection"; Jahan, "Epidemiology of Needlestick Injuries."

[64] Hadadi et al., "Occupational Exposure."

incidence of needlestick injuries in Saudi Arabia was estimated at 11% per nurse per year and 6% per doctor per year.[65] There is not sufficient knowledge of risks of needlestick injuries even among HCWs.[66] Despite what appeared to be good knowledge, the performance of HCWs for universal blood precautions in public hemodialysis units in Egypt was poor, and performance was worse in private units.[67]

At 4.3 per year, MENA has the highest rate of injections per person per year of all regions.[68] In Egypt, 26.8% of women in the 2005 Demographic and Health Survey reported receiving an injection in the last six months, with an average number of two injections.[69] MENA also has the highest levels of all regions of incidences of HBV (58.3%) and HCV infections (81.7%) attributable to contaminated injections.[70] It is estimated that 7.2% of HIV infections in the region are due to contaminated injections.[71] Every year in MENA, contaminated injections appear to be the cause of 2.5 million HBV infections, 645,000 HCV infections, and 2,200 HIV infections.[72] Reuse of needles and syringes; major and minor surgery; hospitalization; a history of invasive procedures; a history of dental procedures; high levels of injections; medical abortion; and formal and informal health care were repeatedly linked to HCV infection in MENA.[73]

Egypt has witnessed the world's largest iatrogenic transmission of blood-borne pathogens during the era of parenteral antischistosomal therapy.[74] This led to a massive increase in HCV and HBV infections in the general population, and today Egypt has the world's highest HCV prevalence.[75] The largest documented nosocomial (contracted as a result of being hospitalized)

outbreak in HIV/AIDS history occurred in a children's hospital in Libya and involved 402 children, 19 mothers (through breastfeeding), and two nurses.[76] The first documented HIV outbreak in renal dialysis centers in the history of the HIV epidemic occurred in Egypt,[77] which had a second HIV outbreak in renal dialysis centers as well.[78] HCV incidence among hemodialysis patients in Morocco was very high at 9.41% per person per year,[79] and moderately high in the Islamic Republic of Iran at 1.8% per person per year,[80] suggesting elevated levels of nosocomial transmissions. Incidence of blood-borne diseases was found to be common in dialysis centers in Jordan.[81]

There is at least one documented HIV infection in MENA that resulted from *hijamah* (traditional medicine practice of phlebotomy by applying glass cupping and skin scarification).[82] A history of *hijamah* has been associated with HCV infection in two Iranian studies.[83]

Parenteral transmission of HIV has been documented in several MENA countries and HIV prevalence has been measured among a number of populations at risk of parenteral HIV infection. Table 7.2 lists these HIV prevalence measurements. The sizable prevalence in these studies reflects infections that occurred mostly before improvements in safety precautions were implemented. Meanwhile, the nil prevalence mainly reflects point-prevalence surveys after safety precautions were implemented.

The above factors pose a concern as to whether there is substantial parenteral HIV transmission in MENA beyond IDU, and whether such transmission accounts for some of the HIV infections where apparently there are no identifiable risk behaviors. To address this question, and given the limitations on HIV data, the authors conducted a review of HCV prevalence in MENA.

[65] Jahan, "Epidemiology of Needlestick Injuries."

[66] Moghimi et al., "Knowledge, Attitude, and Practice."

[67] Kabbash et al., "Risk Perception and Precautions."

[68] Hauri, Armstrong, and Hutin, "The Global Burden of Disease."

[69] Measure DHS, "Egypt: Demographic and Health Survey 2005."

[70] Hauri, Armstrong, and Hutin, "The Global Burden of Disease."

[71] Ibid.

[72] Ibid.

[73] Barut et al., "Analysis of Risk Factors"; Idrees and Riazuddin, "Frequency Distribution"; Stoszek et al., "Prevalence of and Risk Factors"; Khan et al., "Prevalence of Hepatitis 'B' and 'C'"; Gulcan et al., "Evaluation of Risk Factors"; Abbas et al., "Prevalence and Mode of Spread"; Younus, Siddiqi, and Akhtar, "Reassessment of Selected Healthcare"; Ben Alaya Bouafif et al., "A Case Control Study."

[74] Frank et al., "The Role of Parenteral Antischistosomal Therapy."

[75] Waked et al., "High Prevalence of Hepatitis C."

[76] Yerly et al., "Nosocomial Outbreak"; Visco-Comandini et al., "Monophyletic HIV Type 1"; de Oliveira et al., "Molecular Epidemiology."

[77] Hassan et al., "HIV Infection."

[78] El Sayed et al., "Epidemic Transmission."

[79] Sekkat et al., "Prevalence of Anti-HCV Antibodies."

[80] Nemati et al., "Hepatitis C Virus Infection."

[81] Al Hijazat and Ajlouni, "Hepatitis B Infection."

[82] Alrajhi, Halim, and Al-Abdely, "Mode of Transmission."

[83] Zali et al., "Anti-HCV Antibody"; Hosseini Asl, Avijgan, and Mohamadnejad, "High Prevalence."

Table 7.2 HIV Prevalence among Populations at Risk of Parenteral HIV Infection (excluding IDUs)

Country	HIV prevalence among populations at risk of parenteral HIV infection
Bahrain	1.6% (children with hereditary hemolytic anemias; Al-Mahroos and Ebrahim 1995)
Egypt, Arab Republic of	4.8% (blood or blood products recipients; Watts et al. 1993)
Iran, Islamic Republic of	0.0% (thalassemia patients; Mirmomen et al. 2006)
	0.0% (thalassemia patients; Ansar and Kooloobandi 2002)
	0.0% (thalassemia patients; Alavian, Gholami, and Masarrat 2002)
	0.0% (thalassemia patients; Javadzadeh, Attar, and Taher Yavari 2006)
	0.0% (thalassemia patients; Khamispoor and Tahmasebi 1999)
	0.0% (thalassemia patients; Basiratnia, HosseiniAsl, and Avijegan 1999)
	0.0% (thalassemia patients; Kadivar et al., 2001)
	0.0% (thalassemia patients; Nakhaie and Talachian 2003)
	0.0% (thalassemia patients; Rezvan, Abolghassemi, and Kafiabad 2007)
	0.0% (thalassemia patients; Marcelin et al. 2001)
	0.0% (multitransfused thalassaemic children; Karimi and Ghavanini 2001b)
	0.71% (multitransfused patients with hemophilia; Karimi and Ghavanini 2001a)
	2.3% (hemophiliacs; Alavian, Ardeshiri, and Hajarizadeh 2001)
	0.0% (hemophiliacs; Karimi, Yarmohammadi, and Ardeshiri 2002)
	0.9% (hemophiliacs; Torabi et al. 2006)
	1.4% (hemophiliacs; Javadzadeh, Attar, and Taher Yavari 2006)
	0.0% (hemophiliacs; Mansour-Ghanaei et al. 2002)
	0.0% (hemophiliacs; Khamispoor and Tahmasebi 1999)
Jordan	0.0% (multitransfused patients; Al-Sheyyab, Batieha, and El-Khateeb 2001)
Lebanon	6.0% (multitransfused patients; Mokhbat et al. 1989)
Morocco	0.0% (hemodialysis patients; Boulaajaj et al. 2005)
Pakistan	0.98% (multitransfused patients; Mujeeb and Hafeez 1993; hemodialysis patients; Khamispoor and Tahmasebi 1999)
Qatar	38.5% (children with thalassemia; Novelli et al. 1987)
Saudi Arabia	1.3% (multitransfused thalassemic and sickle cell disease patients; El-Hazmi and Ramia 1989)
	0.0% (children undergoing cancer therapy; Bakir et al. 1995)
Tunisia	0.0% (hemodialysis patients; Hmida et al. 1995)
	8.6% (hemophiliacs; Langar et al. 2005)

HCV is a major cause of chronic liver disease and hepatocellular carcinoma.[84] HCV prevalence is a powerful proxy of the potential spread of HIV through the parenteral transmission modes in different populations,[85] and HCV is the most prevalent transfusion-transmitted infection.[86] It is also a better proxy of parenteral transmissions than HBV, which has other major nonparenteral trans-

mission modes.[87] Table D.4 (appendix D) summarizes the review of HCV prevalence. Although overall the region has the second highest HCV prevalence after sub-Saharan Africa,[88] this is largely due to the contribution of the high prevalence found in Egypt[89] and Pakistan.[90] For the rest of the countries, intermediate prevalence levels are found in the general population. These levels are not

---

[84] Colombo, Rumi, and Ninno, "Treatment of Chronic Hepatitis C in Europe."

[85] Goldmann, "Blood-Borne Pathogens and Nosocomial Infections"; Walker et al., "Epidemiology: Sexual Transmission of HIV in Africa"; Schmid et al., "Transmission of HIV-1."

[86] Rezvan, Abolghassemi, and Kafiabad, "Transfusion-Transmitted Infections."

[87] Maayan et al., "Exposure to Hepatitis."

[88] WHO, Global Surveillance and Control of Hepatitis C; WHO, Weekly Epidemiological Record.

[89] Frank et al., "The Role of Parenteral Antischistosomal Therapy."

[90] Raja and Janjua, "Epidemiology of Hepatitis C Virus Infection in Pakistan"; Khokhar, Gill, and Malik, "General Seroprevalence of Hepatitis "; Aslam et al., "Association between Smallpox Vaccination and Hepatitis C."

dissimilar to those found in the Americas, Asia, and Europe.[91]

Table D.4 suggests the following regarding the parenteral transmission of blood-borne pathogens in MENA:

1. There is ongoing transmission of HCV in the general population, largely at intermediate levels.

2. There are specific population groups that are at high risk of infection, such as hemodialysis patients, multitransfused patients, and household contacts of HCV-infected patients.[92]

3. There is ongoing blood-borne transmission in health facilities as evidenced by the higher prevalence of HCV among HCWs and hospitalized patients.

4. HCV prevalence is high among prisoners, suggesting that IDU and the use of nonsterile injecting and noninjecting utensils are common in prisons.

5. There is not sufficient awareness about the dangers of reusing the nonsterile injection equipment of others, as suggested by the higher prevalence among diabetes patients, who likely use self-administered or relative-administered injections.

6. Persons in certain professional categories might be at higher risk of becoming infected, or transmitting the infection, due to exposures to bodily fluids, such as barbers, who appear to have about a fivefold higher HCV prevalence than the general population (5% in Morocco[93] and 2.8% in Turkey[94]). HCV infection at barber shops has also been suggested in Pakistan.[95] Studies of traditional barbers in Morocco and Pakistan have shown that the risk of blood-borne infectious diseases was not known to barbers nor to their customers and that the hygiene conditions were deficient.[96] This is also of concern because there is a tradition in MENA of barbers practicing medicine.[97]

HCV prevalence is a proxy for the cumulative risk of parenteral transmission over an extended period of time and may not be representative of recent trends. It is plausible that more stringent safety precautions have been implemented recently. Improvements in blood safety measures have reduced HIV infections due to contaminated blood in MENA from 12.1% in 1993 to 0.4% in 2003.[98] In Lebanon and the West Bank and Gaza, no new HIV cases through blood transfusion have been detected for several years.[99] In the Islamic Republic of Iran, HCV prevalence among thalassemia patients decreased from 22.8% to 2.6% following the implementation of blood donor screening.[100] Also in the Islamic Republic of Iran, HCV prevalence among hemodialysis patients decreased from 18% in 2001 to 12% in 2006 in one study,[101] and from 14.4% in 1999 to 4.5% in 2006 in another study.[102] Similar reductions were also achieved for HBV in both the Islamic Republic of Iran and Turkey.[103] In Egypt, 95% of women in the 2005 Demographic and Health Survey reported that the medical provider followed basic injection safety procedures.[104]

Nevertheless, improvements in safety measures may not have been uniform across MENA. A study in Pakistan observed an increase in HCV prevalence in recent years.[105] There is evidence of ongoing HCV incidence at the household and population levels in Egypt,[106] and intrafamilial and household clustering of HCV infection in Pakistan.[107]

---

[91] Sy and Jamal, "Epidemiology of Hepatitis C Virus (HCV) Infection."

[92] Ali et al., "Hepatitis B and Hepatitis C in Pakistan."

[93] Zahraoui-Mehadji et al., "Infectious Risks."

[94] Candan et al., "Prevalence of Hepatitis."

[95] Raja and Janjua, "Epidemiology of Hepatitis C Virus Infection in Pakistan"; Ali et al., "Hepatitis B and Hepatitis C in Pakistan"; Khattak et al. "Factors Influencing Hepatitis C."

[96] Zahraoui-Mehadji et al., "Infectious Risks"; Janjua and Nizamy, "Knowledge and Practices of Barbers."

[97] Zahraoui-Mehadji et al., "Infectious Risks."

[98] UNAIDS, "Notes on AIDS in the Middle East and North Africa."

[99] UNAIDS, "Key Findings"; Jurjus et al., "Knowledge, Attitudes, Beliefs, and Practices."

[100] Mirmomen et al., "Epidemiology of Hepatitis."

[101] Taziki and Espahbodi, "Prevalence of Hepatitis."

[102] Alavian et al., "Hepatitis B and C."

[103] Rezvan, Abolghassemi, and Kafiabad, "Transfusion-Transmitted Infections"; Alavian et al., "Hepatitis B and C"; Kocak et al., "Trends in Major Transfusion-Transmissible Infections."

[104] Measure DHS, "Egypt: Demographic and Health Survey 2005."

[105] Mujeeb and Pearce, "Temporal Trends in Hepatitis B and C."

[106] Mujeeb and Pearce, "Temporal Trends in Hepatitis B and C"; Saleh et al., "Incidence and Risk Factors"; Mohamed et al., "Transmission of Hepatitis C Virus between Parents and Children"; Magder et al., "Estimation of the Risk of Transmission."

[107] Abbas et al., "Prevalence and Mode of Spread of Hepatitis."

Analytical summary

There have been steady improvements in recent years in MENA in safety measures related to HIV parenteral transmission modes, but a few countries are still lagging in achieving acceptable standards. In line with this progress, HIV parenteral transmissions, other than IDU, have been in decline in most MENA countries and have reached very low levels. Despite this progress, isolated HIV outbreaks, particularly in health care facilities, could still occur as they have in the past.

Some HIV infectious spread may be present along the same pathways that HCV is using to spread in MENA. The parenteral transmission modes other than IDU, however, are unlikely to be large enough to sustain an HIV epidemic considering that HIV transmission probability per exposure is much lower than that of HCV.[108] Despite the presence of exposures to blood and bodily fluids, the low endemicity of HIV, as well as HCV and HBV, in most of the region limits the infection risk to these pathogens.[109] Earlier speculation that the sub-Saharan Africa HIV epidemic was driven by unsafe injections[110] proved to be incorrect.[111] Yet, more precautions, including educational programs,[112] need to be implemented to avoid the unnecessary spread of HIV and other blood-borne pathogens along the parenteral transmission modes.

HIV MOLECULAR EPIDEMIOLOGY

Molecular epidemiology research in MENA is still limited, though such research could be valuable in tracking the evolution of the epidemic among different risk groups, understanding sexual and injecting risk networks of priority groups, and identifying transmission pathways among the populations of the region.[113] Several studies in MENA have examined the nature of HIV subtypes present in the region and have suggested the transmission pathways in the population.

In Algeria, despite substantial HIV subtype diversity,[114] subtype B was found to be the dominant strain, particularly in the north of the country, accounting for 56% of the samples studied.[115] There is, however, a high diversity in the recombinant subtypes in the southern part of Algeria bordering sub-Saharan Africa, with origins found in the vicinity of Algeria, such as in Niger.[116]

In Djibouti, an analysis of 34 isolates found that 73% were of subtype C, 18% of recombinants forms including CRF02_AG, 6% of subtype D, and 3% of subtype A.[117] Another study in Djibouti found subtype C to be the most prevalent, with the presence of subtypes A and D along with recombinant types.[118] Among French military personnel who served in Djibouti, mostly subtype C infections were found, though subtypes A and B were also found.[119]

An analysis of viral sequences among IDUs in the Islamic Republic of Iran found confined variability, suggesting the epidemic in the Islamic Republic of Iran is recent.[120] The viral sequences were found to be strongly related and formed a single cluster within subtype A, related, though not necessarily directly, to Ugandan and Kenyan isolates.[121] Interestingly, there was a lack of strong phylogenetic correlation between the sequences from the Islamic Republic of Iran and other Middle Eastern countries.[122] The virus may have been introduced to Iranian IDUs by a pilgrim visiting Mashhad, the Islamic Republic of Iran's holiest city.[123] Meanwhile, the analyses indicated that all hemophiliacs infected with HIV in the Islamic Republic of Iran are infected with HIV subtype B.[124] This suggests that there have been two parallel epidemics in

[108] Goldmann, "Blood-Borne Pathogens and Nosocomial Infections"; Gerberding, "Management of Occupational Exposures to Blood-Borne Viruses."

[109] Kuruuzum et al., "Risk of Infection."

[110] Gisselquist et al., "Let It Be Sexual"; Gisselquist et al., "HIV Infections."

[111] Schmid et al., "Transmission of HIV-1."

[112] Mishal et al., "Risk of Transmission."

[113] Sanders-Buell et al., "A Nascent HIV Type 1 Epidemic"; Piyasirisilp et al., "A Recent Outbreak"; McCutchan et al., "HIV-1 and Drug Trafficking."

[114] Bouzeghoub et al., "First Observation."

[115] Bouzeghoub et al., "High Diversity of HIV Type 1 in Algeria."

[116] Ibid.

[117] Maslin et al., "Epidemiology and Genetic Characterization."

[118] Ibid.

[119] Lasky et al., "Presence of Multiple Non-B Subtypes."

[120] Tagliamonte et al., "HIV Type 1 Subtype A"; Naderi et al., "Molecular and Phylogenetic Analysis."

[121] Tagliamonte et al., "HIV Type 1 Subtype A."

[122] Tagliamonte et al., "HIV Type 1 Subtype A"; Naderi et al., "Molecular and Phylogenetic Analysis."

[123] Tagliamonte et al., "HIV Type 1 Subtype A."

[124] Sarrami-Forooshani et al., "Molecular Analysis."

different risk populations in the Islamic Republic of Iran. The HIV epidemic among IDUs in Kabul, Afghanistan, has also been linked through sequence analyses to the Iranian epidemic.[125] One other study from the Islamic Republic of Iran supports a close link between the virus subtypes circulating in the Islamic Republic of Iran and Afghanistan.[126]

In Lebanon, a complex HIV subtype distribution pattern was found representing the infection's travel history from its point of origination.[127] Even within a single subtype, high levels of genetic intrasubtype diversity were found, suggesting multiple introductions of the virus to Lebanon.[128]

A study of a nosocomial HIV outbreak in a children's hospital in Libya linked the virus to a strain originating in West Africa.[129] In Morocco, 93.5% of HIV infections were found to be of subtype B.[130] More recent data, however, suggest an increasing diversity of subtypes, with 34% of the cases carrying nonsubtype B viruses.[131] In the West Bank and Gaza, subtype B was also dominant and the phylogenetic tree analyses indicated multiple introductions of HIV into the population.[132] Subtype A was the only subtype observed among a group of IDUs in Pakistan.[133]

In Saudi Arabia, high strain diversity suggesting multiple introductions was found, with subtypes C, G, B, D, and A accounting for 39.3%, 25%, 17.9%, 3.6%, and 1.8% of the infections, respectively.[134] Two kinds of sequences (CRF25_cpx and CRF43_02G) were found to form distinct subclusters, suggesting a transmission network within Saudi Arabia.[135]

In Sudan, 50% of the strains from blood donors in Khartoum were of subtype D and 30% of subtype C, with limited frequencies of subtypes A, B, and recombinant forms.[136] Some of the D subtype strains clustered with those in

East Africa, while others clustered with those in West Africa. The majority of strains were similar to those in Uganda, Kenya, and Ethiopia.

In Tunisia, subtype B was by far the dominant subtype.[137] In a study of 19 strains in the Republic of Yemen, 47.3% were of subtype B, 31.6% of subtype C, 10.5% of subtype D, 5.3% of subtype A, and 5.3% were recombinant forms.[138] Of the two subtype D strains, one clustered with strains from Uganda and the other with strains from Cameroon. The one subtype A strain was similar to a Cameroon variant. Overall, the strains found in the study suggest multiple introductions of HIV to the Republic of Yemen from East and West Africa, Europe, and India.

Analytical summary

It is difficult to draw firm conclusions from just a few studies, including a small number of HIV isolates that may be reflecting transmission patterns from the past. More often than not though, sequence analyses indicate multiple distinct subtypes in the isolated strains.[139] This suggests multiple introductions rather than endemic existence of genetically diverse HIV subtypes in a number of MENA countries. The diversity found in Algeria, Lebanon, Saudi Arabia, the West Bank and Gaza, and the Republic of Yemen may suggest that HIV dynamics are mainly driven by exogenous exposures, generally among the nationals of these countries while abroad, or HIV transmissions to their sexual partners upon their return. Most endogenous HIV infections could be direct transmissions from index cases following multiple introductions. HIV dynamics are not dominated by a specific epidemic in one or multiple risk groups.

On the other hand, the dominance of specific subtypes with limited sequence variability in Djibouti, the Islamic Republic of Iran, and Sudan, in addition to possibly two subclusters in Saudi Arabia, suggests that HIV infections are occurring in transmission chains that have been propagating locally for at least several years. This suggests a local epidemic-type HIV transmission in one or multiple risk groups.

[125] Sanders-Buell et al., "A Nascent HIV Type 1 Epidemic."
[126] Soheilli et al., "Presence of HIV-1 CRF35_AD in Iran."
[127] Pieniazek et al., "Introduction of HIV-2."
[128] Ibid.
[129] de Oliveira et al., "Molecular Epidemiology."
[130] Elharti et al., "HIV-1 Diversity in Morocco."
[131] Morocco MOH, "Situation épidémiologique."
[132] Gehring et al., "Molecular Epidemiology of HIV in Israel."
[133] Khan et al., "HIV-1 Subtype A."
[134] Badreddine et al., "Identification and Characterization of HIV Type 1."
[135] Yamaguchi et al., "Identification of New CRF43_02G and CRF25_cpx."
[136] Hierholzer et al., "HIV Type 1 Strains."
[137] Ben Halima et al., "First Molecular Characterization."
[138] Saad et al., "HIV Type 1 Strains."
[139] Earhart, "The Molecular Epidemiology of HIV-1 in Central Asia."

Needless to say, the above data show that HIV has no borders and is entering the region from multiple sources through nationals of MENA countries.

BIBLIOGRAPHY

Abbas, Z., N. L. Jeswani, G. N. Kakepoto, M. Islam, K. Mehdi, and W. Jafri. 2008. "Prevalence and Mode of Spread of Hepatitis B and C in Rural Sindh, Pakistan." *Trop Gastroenterol* 29: 210–16.

Abdul Mujeeb, S. 1993. "Blood Transfusion—A Potential Source of HIV/AIDS Spread." *J Pakistan Med Assoc* 43: 1.

Ahmed, S. M. 2004a. *AIDS Patients: Situation Analysis-Behavioral Survey Results & Discussions*. Report. Sudan National AIDS Control Program.

———. 2004b. *Antenatal: Situation Analysis-Behavioral Survey Results & Discussions*. Report. Sudan National AIDS Control Program.

———. 2004c. *Internally Displaced People: Situation Analysis-Behavioral Survey Results & Discussions*. Report, Sudan National AIDS Control Program.

———. 2004d. *Military Situation: Analysis-Behavioral Survey Results & Discussions*. Report. Sudan National AIDS Control Program.

———. 2004e. *Sex Sellers: Situation Analysis-Behavioral Survey Results & Discussions*. Report. Sudan National AIDS Control Program.

———. 2004f. *STDs: Situation Analysis-Behavioral Survey Results & Discussions*. Report. Sudan National AIDS Control Program.

———. 2004g. *Street Children: Situation Analysis-Behavioral Survey Results & Discussions.* Report. Sudan National AIDS Control Program.

———. 2004h. *TB Patients: Situation Analysis-Behavioral Survey Results & Discussions*. Report, Sudan National AIDS Control Program.

———. 2004i. *Tea Sellers: Situation Analysis-Behavioral Survey Results & Discussions*. Report. Sudan National AIDS Control Program.

———. 2004j. *Truck Drivers: Situation: Analysis-Behavioral Survey Results & Discussions*. Report. Sudan National AIDS Control Program.

———. 2004k. *University Students: Situation Analysis-Behavioral Survey, Results & Discussions.* Report. Sudan National AIDS Control Program.

Aidaoui, M., S. Bouzbid, and M. Laouar. 2008. "Sero-prevalence of HIV Infection in Pregnant Women in the Annaba Region (Algeria)." *Rev Epidemiol Sante Publique* 56: 261–66.

Al Hijazat, M., and Y. M. Ajlouni. 2008. "Hepatitis B Infection among Patients Receiving Chronic Hemo-dialysis at the Royal Medical Services in Jordan." *Saudi J Kidney Dis Transpl* 19: 260–67.

Alami, K. 2009. "Tendances récentes de l'épidémie à VIH/SIDA en Afrique du nord." Presentation, Research and AIDS Workshop in North Africa, Marrakech, Morocco.

Alavian, S. M., A. Ardeshiri, and B. Hajarizadeh. 2001. "Prevalence of HCV, HBV and HIV Infections among Hemophiliacs." *Transfusion Today* 49: 4–5.

Alavian, S. M., K. Bagheri-Lankarani, M. Mahdavi-Mazdeh, and S. Nourozi. 2008. "Hepatitis B and C in Dialysis Units in Iran: Changing the Epidemiology." *Hemodial Int* 12: 378–82.

Alavian, S. M., B. Gholami, and S. Masarrat. 2002. "Hepatitis C Risk Factors in Iranian Volunteer Blood Donors: A Case-Control Study." *J Gastroenterol Hepatol* 17: 1092–97.

Al-Fouzan, A., and N. Al-Mutairi. 2004. "Overview of Incidence of Sexually Transmitted Diseases in Kuwait." *Clin Dermatol* 22: 509–12.

Algeria MOH (Ministry of Health). Unknown. "Rapport de l'enquête nationale de séro-surveillance sentinelle du VIH et de la syphilis en Algérie 2004–2005." Grey Report.

Al-Haddad, M. K., A. S. Khashaba, B. Z. Baig, and S. Khalfan. 1994. "HIV Antibodies among Intravenous Drug Users in Bahrain." *J Commun Dis* 26: 127–32.

Ali, S. A., R. M. Donahue, H. Qureshi, and S. H. Vermund. 2009. "Hepatitis B and Hepatitis C in Pakistan: Prevalence and Risk Factors." *Int J Infect Dis* 13: 9–19.

Al-Mahroos, F. T., and A. Ebrahim. 1995. "Prevalence of Hepatitis B, Hepatitis C and Human Immune Deficiency Virus Markers among Patients with Hereditary Haemolytic Anaemias." *Ann Trop Paediatr* 15: 121–28.

Al-Mazrou, Y. Y., M. H. Al-Jeffri, A. I. Fidail, N. Al-Huzaim, and S. E. El-Gizouli. 2005. "HIV/AIDS Epidemic Features and Trends in Saudi Arabia." *Ann Saudi Med* 25: 100–04.

Al-Mutairi, N., A. Joshi, O. Nour-Eldin, A. K. Sharma, I. El-Adawy, and M. Rijhwani. 2007. "Clinical Patterns of Sexually Transmitted Diseases, Associated Sociodemographic Characteristics, and Sexual Practices in the Farwaniya Region of Kuwait." *Int J Dermatol* 46: 594–99.

Alrajhi, A. A., M. A. Halim, and H. M. Al-Abdely. 2004. "Mode of Transmission of HIV-1 in Saudi Arabia." *AIDS* 18: 1478–80.

Al-Serouri, A. W. 2000. *HIV/AIDS Situation and Response Analysis Report*. National AIDS Program, Ministry of Health, Yemen Republic.

Al-Sheyyab, M., A. Batieha, and M. El-Khateeb. 2001. "The Prevalence of Hepatitis B, Hepatitis C and Human Immune Deficiency Virus Markers in Multi-Transfused Patients." *J Trop Pediatr* 47: 239–42.

Altaf, A., Z. Fatmi, A. Ajmal, T. Hussain, H. Qahir, and M. Agboatwalla. 2004. "Determinants of Therapeutic Injection Overuse among Communities in Sindh, Pakistan." *J Ayub Med Coll Abbottabad* 16: 35–38.

Anonymous. 2006. *Scaling Up the HIV Response toward Universal Access to Prevention, Treatment, Care and Support in Jordan*. Summary report of the national consultation.

Ansar, M. M., and A. Kooloobandi. 2002. "Prevalence of Hepatitis C Virus Infection in Thalassemia and Haemodialysis Patients in North Iran-Rasht." *J Viral Hepat* 9: 390–92.

Askarian, M., K. Mirzaei, and B. Cookson. 2007. "Knowledge, Attitudes, and Practice of Iranian

Dentists with Regard to HIV-Related Disease." *Infect Control Hosp Epidemiol* 28: 83–87.

Askarian, M., K. Mirzaei, and M. L. McLaws. 2006. "Attitudes, Beliefs, and Infection Control Practices of Iranian Dentists Associated with HIV-Positive Patients." *Am J Infect Control* 34: 530–33.

Aslam, M., J. Aslam, B. D. Mitchell, and K. M. Munir. 2005. "Association between Smallpox Vaccination and Hepatitis C Antibody Positive Serology in Pakistani Volunteers." *J Clin Gastroenterol* 39: 243–46.

Badreddine, S., K. Smith, H. van Zyl, P. Bodelle, J. Yamaguchi, P. Swanson, S. G. Devare, and C. A. Brennan. 2007. "Identification and Characterization of HIV Type 1 Subtypes Present in the Kingdom of Saudi Arabia: High Level of Genetic Diversity Found." *AIDS Res Hum Retroviruses* 23: 667–74.

Bakir, T. M. F., K. M. Kurbaan, I. A. Fawaz, and S. Ramia. 1995. "Infection with Hepatitis Viruses (B and C) and Human Retro Viruses (HTLV-1 and HIV) in Saudi Children Receiving Cycled Cancer Chemotherapy." *Journal of Tropical Pediatrics* 41: 206–9.

Barut, S., U. Erkorkmaz, S. Yuce, and U. Uyeturk. 2008. "Analysis of Risk Factors in Anti-HCV Positive Patients in Gaziosmanpasa University Hospital, Tokat, Turkey." *Mikrobiyol Bul* 42: 675–80.

Basiratnia, M., S. M. K. HosseiniAsl, and M. Avijegan. 1999. "Hepatitis C Prevalence in Thalassemia Patients in Sharkord, Iran (Farsi)." *Shahrkord University Medical Science Journal* 4: 13–18.

Ben Alaya Bouafif, N., H. Triki, S. Mejri, O. Bahri, S. Chlif, J. Bettaib, S. Hechmi, K. Dellagi, and A. Ben Salah. 2007. "A Case Control Study to Assess Risk Factors for Hepatitis C among a General Population in a Highly Endemic Area of Northwest Tunisia." *Arch Inst Pasteur Tunis* 84: 21–27.

Ben Halima, M., C. Pasquier, A. Slim, T. Ben Chaabane, Z. Arrouji, J. Puel, S. Ben Redjeb, and J. Izopet. 2001. "First Molecular Characterization of HIV-1 Tunisian Strains." *J Acquir Immune Defic Syndr* 28: 94–96.

Boulaajaj, K., Y. Elomari, B. Elmaliki, B. Madkouri, D. Zaid, and N. Benchemsi. 2005. "Prevalence of Hepatitis C, Hepatitis B and HIV Infection among Haemodialysis Patients in Ibn-Rochd University Hospital, Casablanca." *Nephrol Ther* 1: 274–84.

Bouzeghoub, S., V. Jauvin, P. Pinson, M. H. Schrive, A. C. Jeannot, A. Amrane, B. Masquelier, H. Belabbes el, and H. J. Fleury. 2008. "First Observation of HIV Type 1 Drug Resistance Mutations in Algeria." *AIDS Res Hum Retroviruses* 24: 1467–73.

Bouzeghoub, S., V. Jauvin, P. Recordon-Pinson, I. Garrigue, A. Amrane, H. Belabbes el, and H. J. Fleury. 2006. "High Diversity of HIV Type 1 in Algeria." *AIDS Res Hum Retroviruses* 22: 367–72.

Burans, J. P., E. Fox, M. A. Omar, A. H. Farah, S. Abbass, S. Yusef, A. Guled, M. Mansour, R. Abu-Elyazeed, and J. N. Woody. 1990. "HIV Infection Surveillance in Mogadishu, Somalia." *East Afr Med J* 67: 466–72.

Burans, J. P., M. McCarthy, S. M. el Tayeb, A. el Tigani, J. George, R. Abu-Elyazeed, and J. N. Woody. 1990. "Serosurvey of Prevalence of Human Immuno-deficiency Virus amongst High Risk Groups in Port Sudan, Sudan." *East Afr Med J* 67: 650–55.

Candan, F., H. Alagozlu, O. Poyraz, and H. Sumer. 2002. "Prevalence of Hepatitis B and C Virus Infection in Barbers in the Sivas Region of Turkey." *Occup Med (Lond)* 52: 31–34.

Chemtob, D., and S. F. Srour. 2005. "Epidemiology of HIV Infection among Israeli Arabs." *Public Health* 119: 138–43.

Colombo, M., M. G. Rumi, and E. D. Ninno. 2003. "Treatment of Chronic Hepatitis C in Europe." *J Hepatobiliary Pancreat Surg* 10: 168–71.

de Oliveira, T., O. G. Pybus, A. Rambaut, M. Salemi, S. Cassol, M. Ciccozzi, G. Rezza, G. C. Gattinara, R. D'Arrigo, M. Amicosante, L. Perrin, V. Colizzi, and C. F. Perno. 2006. "Molecular Epidemiology: HIV-1 and HCV Sequences from Libyan Outbreak." *Nature* 444: 836–37.

Earhart, K. 2004. "The Molecular Epidemiology of HIV-1 in Central Asia." PowerPoint presentation.

El Sayed, N. M., P. J. Gomatos, C. M. Beck-Sague, U. Dietrich, H. von Briesen, S. Osmanov, J. Esparza, R. R. Arthur, M. H. Wahdan, and W. R. Jarvis. 2000. "Epidemic Transmission of Human Immunodeficiency Virus in Renal Dialysis Centers in Egypt." *J Infect Dis* 181: 91–97.

Elharti, E., M. Alami, H. Khattabi, A. Bennani, A. Zidouh, A. Benjouad, and R. El Aouad. 2002. "Some Characteristics of the HIV Epidemic in Morocco." *East Mediterr Health J* 8: 819–25.

Elharti, E., R. Elaouad, S. Amzazi, H. Himmich, Z. Elhachimi, C. Apetrei, J. C. Gluckman, F. Simon, and A. Benjouad. 1997. "HIV-1 Diversity in Morocco." *AIDS* 11: 1781–83.

El-Hazmi, M. A., and S. Ramia. 1989. "Frequencies of Hepatitis B, Delta and Human Immune Deficiency Virus Markers in Multi-Transfused Saudi Patients with Thalassaemia and Sickle-Cell Disease." *J Trop Med Hyg* 92: 1–5.

Farah, M. S., and S. Hussein. 2006. "HIV Prevalence, Knowledge, Attitude, Practices and Risk Factors among Truck Drivers in Khartoum State." Sudan National AIDS Program.

Frank, C., M. K. Mohamed, G. T. Strickland, D. Lavanchy, R. R. Arthur, L. S. Magder, T. El Khoby, Y. Abdel-Wahab, E. S. Aly Ohn, W. Anwar, and I. Sallam. 2000. "The Role of Parenteral Antischistosomal Therapy in the Spread of Hepatitis C Virus in Egypt." *Lancet* 355: 887–91.

Gehring, S., S. Maayan, H. Ruppach, P. Balfe, J. Juraszczyk, I. Yust, N. Vardinon, A. Rimlawi, S. Polak, Z. Bentwich, H. Rubsamen-Waigmann, and U. Dietrich. 1997. "Molecular Epidemiology of HIV in Israel." *J Acquir Immune Defic Syndr Hum Retrovirol* 15: 296–303.

Gerberding, J. L. 1995. "Management of Occupational Exposures to Blood-Borne Viruses." *N Engl J Med* 332: 444–51.

Ghannad, M. S., S. M. Arab, M. Mirzaei, and A. Moinipur. 2009. "Epidemiologic Study of Human Immunodeficiency Virus (HIV) Infection in the Patients Referred to Health Centers in Hamadan Province, Iran." *AIDS Res Hum Retroviruses* 25: 277–83.

Gheiratmand, R., R. Navipour, M. R. Mohebbi, and A. K. Mallik. 2005. "Uncertainty on the Number of HIV/AIDS Patients: Our Experience in Iran." *Sex Transm Infect* 81: 279–80.

Gisselquist, D., J. J. Potterat, S. Brody, and F. Vachon. 2003. "Let It Be Sexual: How Health Care Transmission of AIDS in Africa Was Ignored." *Int J STD AIDS* 14: 148–61.

Gisselquist, D., R. Rothenberg, J. Potterat, and E. Drucker. 2002. "HIV Infections in Sub-Saharan Africa Not Explained by Sexual or Vertical Transmission." *Int J STD AIDS* 13: 657–66.

Goldmann, D. A. 2002. "Blood-Borne Pathogens and Nosocomial Infections." *J Allergy Clin Immunol* 110: S21–26.

Gouya, M. M. 2006. *National Report on HIV and AIDS Cases*. Disease Management Center, Ministry of Health and Medical Education. Tehran: Islamic Republic of Iran.

Gulcan, A., E. Gulcan, A. Toker, I. Bulut, and Y. Akcan. 2008. "Evaluation of Risk Factors and Seroprevalence of Hepatitis B and C in Diabetic Patients in Kutahya, Turkey." *J Investig Med* 56: 858–63.

Hadadi, A., S. Afhami, M. Karbakhsh, and N. Esmailpour. 2008. "Occupational Exposure to Body Fluids among Healthcare Workers: A Report from Iran." *Singapore Med J* 49: 492–96.

Hassan, N. F., N. M. el Ghorab, M. S. Abdel Rehim, M. S. el Sharkawy, N. M. el Sayed, K. Emara, Y. Soltant, M. Sanad, R. G. Hibbs, and R. R. Arthur. 1994. "HIV Infection in Renal Dialysis Patients in Egypt." *AIDS* 8: 853.

Hauri, A. M., G. L. Armstrong, and Y. J. Hutin. 2004. "The Global Burden of Disease Attributable to Contaminated Injections Given in Health Care Settings." *Int J STD AIDS* 15: 7–16.

Hierholzer, M., R. R. Graham, I. El Khidir, S. Tasker, M. Darwish, G. D. Chapman, A. H. Fagbami, A. Soliman, D. L. Birx, F. McCutchan, and J. K. Carr. 2002. "HIV Type 1 Strains from East and West Africa Are Intermixed in Sudan." *AIDS Res Hum Retroviruses* 18: 1163–66.

Hmida, S., N. Mojaat, E. Chaouchi, T. Mahjoub, B. Khlass, S. Abid, and K. Boukef. 1995. "HCV Antibodies in Hemodialyzed Patients in Tunisia." *Pathol Biol* (Paris) 43: 581–83.

Hosseini Asl, S. K., M. Avijgan, and M. Mohamadnejad. 2004. "High Prevalence of HBV, HCV, and HIV Infections: In Gypsy Population Residing in Shar-e-kord." *Arch Iranian Med* 7: 22–24.

Hossini, C. H., D. Tripodi, A. E. Rahhali, M. Bichara, D. Betito, J. P. Curtes, and C. Verger. 2000. "Knowledge and Attitudes of Health Care Professionals with Respect to AIDS and the Risk of Occupational Transmission of HIV in 2 Moroccan Hospitals." *Sante* 10: 315–21.

Hsairi, M., and S. Ben Abdallah. 2007. "Analyse de la situation de vulnérabilité vis-à-vis de l'infection à VIH des hommes ayant des relations sexuelles avec des hommes." For ATL MST sida NGO–Tunis Section, National AIDS Programme/DSSB, UNAIDS. Final report, abridged version.

Idrees, M., and S. Riazuddin. 2008. "Frequency Distribution of Hepatitis C Virus Genotypes in Different Geographical Regions of Pakistan and Their Possible Routes of Transmission." *BMC Infect Dis* 8: 69.

Iqbal, J., and N. Rehan. 1996. "Sero-Prevalence of HIV: Six Years' Experience at Shaikh Zayed Hospital, Lahore." *J Pak Med Assoc* 46: 255–58.

Iran Center for Disease Management. 2004. *AIDS/HIV Surveillance Report* (April). Tehran: Ministry of Health and Medical Education.

Ismail, S. O., H. J. Ahmed, L. Grillner, B. Hederstedt, A. Issa, and S. M. Bygdeman. 1990. "Sexually Transmitted Diseases in Men in Mogadishu, Somalia." *Int J STD AIDS* 1: 102–6.

Jahan, S. 2005. "Epidemiology of Needlestick Injuries among Health Care Workers in a Secondary Care Hospital in Saudi Arabia." *Ann Saudi Med* 25: 233–38.

Janjua, N. Z. 2003. "Injection Practices and Sharp Waste Disposal by General Practitioners of Murree, Pakistan." *J Pak Med Assoc* 53: 107–11.

Janjua, N. Z., S. Akhtar, and Y. J. Hutin. 2005. "Injection Use in Two Districts of Pakistan: Implications for Disease Prevention." *Int J Qual Health Care* 17: 401–8.

Janjua, N. Z., Y. J. Hutin, S. Akhtar, and K. Ahmad. 2006. "Population Beliefs about the Efficacy of Injections in Pakistan's Sindh Province." *Public Health* 120: 824–33.

Janjua, N. Z., and M. A. Nizamy. 2004. "Knowledge and Practices of Barbers about Hepatitis B and C Transmission in Rawalpindi and Islamabad." *J Pak Med Assoc* 54: 116–19.

Javadzadeh, H., M. Attar, and M. Taher Yavari. 2006. "Study of the Prevalence of HBV, HCV, and HIV Infection in Hemophilia and Thalassemia Population of Yazd (Farsi)." *Khoon (Blood)* 2: 315–22.

Jurjus, A. R., J. Kahhaleh, National AIDS Program, and WHO/EMRO (World Health Organization, Eastern Mediterranean Regional Office). 2004. "Knowledge, Attitudes, Beliefs, and Practices of the Lebanese concerning HIV/AIDS." Beirut, Lebanon.

Kabbash, I. A., N. M. El-Sayed, A. N. Al-Nawawy, S. Abou Salem Mel, B. El-Deek, and N. M. Hassan. 2007. "Risk Perception and Precautions Taken by Health Care Workers for HIV Infection in Haemodialysis Units in Egypt." *East Mediterr Health J* 13: 392–407.

Kadivar, M. R., A. R. Mirahmadizadeh, A. Karimi, and A. Hemmati. 2001. "The Prevalence of HCV and HIV in Thalassemia Patients in Shiraz, Iran." *Medical Journal of Iranian Hospital* 4: 18–20.

Kalaajieh, W. K. 2000. "Epidemiology of Human Immunodeficiency Virus and Acquired Immunodeficiency Syndrome in Lebanon from 1984 through 1998." *Int J Infect Dis* 4: 209–13.

Kane, A., J. Lloyd, M. Zaffran, L. Simonsen, and M. Kane. 1999. "Transmission of Hepatitis B, Hepatitis C and Human Immunodeficiency Viruses through Unsafe Injections in the Developing World: Model-Based Regional Estimates." *Bull World Health Organ* 77: 801–7.

Karimi, M., and A. A. Ghavanini. 2001a. "Seroprevalence of Hepatitis B, Hepatitis C and Human Immunodeficiency Virus Antibodies among Multitransfused Thalassaemic Children in Shiraz, Iran." *J Paediatr Child Health* 37: 564–66.

———. 2001b. "Seroprevalence of HBsAg, Anti-HCV, and Anti-HIV among Haemophiliac Patients in Shiraz, Iran." *Haematologia (Budap)* 31: 251–55.

Karimi, M., H. Yarmohammadi, and R. Ardeshiri. 2002. "Inherited Coagulation Disorders in Southern Iran." *Haemophilia* 8: 740–44.

Kassak, K., J. DeJong, Z. Mahfoud, R. Afifi, S. Abdurahim, M. L. Sami Ramia, F. El-Barbir, M. Ghanem, S. Shamra, K. Kreidiyyeh, and D. El-Khoury. 2008. "Final Working Protocol for an Integrated Bio-Behavioral Surveillance Study among Four Vulnerable Groups in Lebanon: Men Who Have Sex with Men; Prisoners; Commercial Sex Workers; and Intravenous Drug Users." Grey Report.

Kayani, N., A. Sheikh, A. Khan, C. Mithani, and M. Khurshid. 1994. "A View of HIV-I Infection in Karachi." *J Pak Med Assoc* 44: 8–11.

Kennedy, M., D. O'Reilly, and M. W. Mah. 1998. "The Use of a Quality-Improvement Approach to Reduce Needlestick Injuries in a Saudi Arabian Hospital." *Clin Perform Qual Health Care* 6: 79–83.

Khamispoor, G., and R. Tahmasebi. 1999. "Prevalence of HIV, HBV, HCV and Syphilis in High Risk Groups of Bushehr Province (Farsi)." *Iranian South Medical Journal* 1: 53–59.

Khan, M. S., M. Jamil, S. Jan, S. Zardad, S. Sultan, and A. S. Sahibzada. 2007. "Prevalence of Hepatitis 'B' and 'C' in Orthopaedics Patients at Ayub Teaching Hospital Abbottabad." *J Ayub Med Coll Abbottabad* 19: 82–84.

Khan, O. A., and A. A. Hyder. 1998. "HIV/AIDS among Men Who Have Sex with Men in Pakistan." *Sex Health Exch* 12–13, 15.

Khan, S., M. A. Rai, M. R. Khanani, M. N. Khan, and S. H. Ali. 2006. "HIV-1 Subtype A Infection in a Community of Intravenous Drug Users in Pakistan." *BMC Infect Dis* 6: 164.

Khattab, H. A. S., M. A. Gineidy, N. Shorbagui, and N. Elnahal. 2007. "Report on a Study of Women Living with HIV in Egypt." Egyptian Society for Population Studies and Reproductive Health.

Khattak, M. N., S. Akhtar, S. Mahmud, and T. M. Roshan. 2008. "Factors Influencing Hepatitis C Virus Sero-Prevalence among Blood Donors in North West Pakistan." *J Public Health Policy* 29: 207–25.

Khawaja, Z. A., L. Gibney, A. J. Ahmed, and S. H. Vermund. 1997. "HIV/AIDS and Its Risk Factors in Pakistan." *AIDS* 11: 843–48.

Khokhar, N., M. L. Gill, and G. J. Malik. 2004. "General Seroprevalence of Hepatitis C and Hepatitis B Virus Infections in Population." *J Coll Physicians Surg Pak* 14: 534–36.

Kilani, B., L. Ammari, C. Marrakchi, A. Letaief, M. Chakroun, M. Ben Jemaa, H. T. Ben Aissa, F. Kanoun, and T. Ben Chaabene. 2007. "Seroepidemiology of HCV-HIV Coinfection in Tunisia." *Tunis Med* 85: 121–23.

Kocak, N., S. Hepgul, S. Ozbayburtlu, H. Altunay, M. F. Ozsoy, E. Kosan, Y. Aksu, G. Yilmaz, and A. Pahsa. 2004. "Trends in Major Transfusion-Transmissible Infections among Blood Donors over 17 Years in Istanbul, Turkey." *J Int Med Res* 32: 671–75.

Kuruuzum, Z., N. Yapar, V. Avkan-Oguz, H. Aslan, O. A. Ozbek, N. Cakir, and A. Yuce. 2008. "Risk of Infection in Health Care Workers Following Occupational Exposure to a Noninfectious or Unknown Source." *Am J Infect Control* 36: e27–31.

Lambert, L. 2007. "HIV and Development Challenges in Yemen: Which Grows Fastest?" *Health Policy and Planning* 22: 60.

Langar, H., H. Triki, E. Gouider, O. Bahri, A. Djebbi, A. Sadraoui, A. Hafsia, and R. Hafsia. 2005. "Blood-Transmitted Viral Infections among Haemophiliacs in Tunisia." *Transfusion clinique et biologique* 12: 301–5.

Laraqui, O., S. Laraqui, D. Tripodi, M. Zahraoui, A. Caubet, C. Verger, and C. H. Laraqui. 2008. "Assessing Knowledge, Attitude, and Practice on Occupational Blood Exposure in Caregiving Facilities, in Morocco." *Med Mal Infect* 38: 658–66.

Lasky, M., J. L. Perret, M. Peeters, F. Bibollet-Ruche, F. Liegeois, D. Patrel, S. Molinier, C. Gras, and E. Delaporte. 1997. "Presence of Multiple Non-B Subtypes and Divergent Subtype B Strains of HIV-1 in Individuals Infected after Overseas Deployment." *AIDS* 11: 43–51.

Lebanon National AIDS Control Program. 2008. "A Case Study on Behavior Change among Female Sex Workers." Beirut, Lebanon.

Luby, S., R. Khanani, M. Zia, Z. Vellani, M. Ali, A. H. Qureshi, A. J. Khan, S. Abdul Mujeeb, S. A. Shah, and S. Fisher-Hoch. 2000. "Evaluation of Blood Bank Practices in Karachi, Pakistan, and the Government's Response." *Health Policy Plan* 15: 217–22.

Maayan, S., E. N. Shufman, D. Engelhard, and D. Shouval. 1994. "Exposure to Hepatitis B and C and to HTLV-1 and 2 among Israeli Drug Abusers in Jerusalem." *Addiction* 89: 869–74.

Magder, L. S., A. D. Fix, N. N. Mikhail, M. K. Mohamed, M. Abdel-Hamid, F. Abdel-Aziz, A. Medhat, and G. T. Strickland. 2005. "Estimation of the Risk of Transmission of Hepatitis C between Spouses in Egypt Based on Seroprevalence Data." *Int J Epidemiol* 34: 160–65.

Mansoor, A. B., W. Fungladda, J. Kaewkungwal, and W. Wongwit. 2008. "Gender Differences in KAP Related to HIV/AIDS among Freshmen in Afghan Universities." *Southeast Asian J Trop Med Public Health* 39: 404–18.

Mansour-Ghanaei, F., M. S. Fallah, A. Shafaghi, M. Yousefi-Mashhoor, N. Ramezani, F. Farzaneh, and R. Nassiri. 2002. "Prevalence of Hepatitis B and C Seromarkers and Abnormal Liver Function Tests among Hemophiliacs in Guilan (Northern Province of Iran)." *Med Sci Monit* 8: CR797–800.

Marcelin, A. G., M. Grandadam, P. Flandre, J. L. Koeck, M. Philippon, E. Nicand, R. Teyssou, H. Agut, J. M. Huraux, and N. Dupin. 2001. "Comparative Study of Heterosexual Transmission of HIV-1, HSV-2 and KSHV in Djibouti." *8th Retrovir Oppor Infect* (abstract no. 585).

Maslin, J., C. Rogier, F. Berger, M. A. Khamil, D. Mattera, M. Grandadam, M. Caron, and E. Nicand. 2005. "Epidemiology and Genetic Characterization of HIV-1 Isolates in the General Population of Djibouti (Horn of Africa)." *J Acquir Immune Defic Syndr* 39: 129–32.

McCutchan, F., J. Carr, S. Tovanabutra, X.-F. Yu, C. Beyrer, and D. Birx. 2002. "HIV-1 and Drug Trafficking: Viral Strains Illuminate Networks and Provide Focus for Interventions." NIDA-Sponsored Satellite Sessions, XIV International AIDS Conference, Barcelona, Spain.

Measure DHS. 2006. "Egypt: Demographic and Health Survey 2005." Grey Report.

Ministry of Health and Medical Education of Iran. 2006. "Treatment and Medical Education." Islamic Republic of Iran HIV/AIDS situation and response analysis.

Mirmomen, S., S. M. Alavian, B. Hajarizadeh, J. Kafaee, B. Yektaparast, M. J. Zahedi, A. A. Azami, M. M. Hosseini, A. R. Faridi, K. Davari, and B. Hajibeigi. 2006. "Epidemiology of Hepatitis B, Hepatitis C, and Human Immunodeficiency Virus Infections in Patients with Beta-Thalassemia in Iran: A Multicenter Study." *Arch Iran Med* 9: 319–23.

Mishal, Y., C. Yosefy, E. Hay, D. Catz, E. Ambon, and R. Schneider. 1998. "Risk of Transmission of Viral Disease by Needle Punctures and Cuts in Hospital Health Care Workers." *Harefuah* 135: 337–39, 408.

Moghimi, M., S. A. Marashi, A. Kabir, H. R. Taghipour, A. H. Faghihi-Kashani, I. Ghoddoosi, and S. M. Alavian. 2009. "Knowledge, Attitude, and Practice of Iranian Surgeons about Blood-Borne Diseases." *J Surg Res* 151: 80–84.

Mohamed, M. K., M. Abdel-Hamid, M. N. Mikhail, F. Abdel-Aziz, A. Medhat, L. S. Magder, A. D. Fix, and G. T. Strickland. 2005. "Intrafamilial Transmission of Hepatitis C in Egypt." *Hepatology* 42: 683–87.

Mohamed, M. K., L. S. Magder, M. Abdel-Hamid, M. El-Daly, N. N. Mikhail, F. Abdel-Aziz, A. Medhat, V. Thiers, and G. T. Strickland. 2006. "Transmission of Hepatitis C Virus between Parents and Children." *Am J Trop Med Hyg* 75: 16–20.

Mokhbat, J. E., R. E. Naman, F. S. Rahme, A. E. Farah, K. L. Zahar, and A. Maalouf. 1989. "Clinical and Serological Study of the Human Immunodeficiency Virus Infection in a Cohort of Multi-Transfused Persons." *J Med Liban* 38: 9–14.

Morocco MOH (Ministry of Health). Unknown. "Situation épidémiologique actuelle du VIH/SIDA au Maroc."

Mujeeb, S. A., and A. Hafeez. 1993. "Prevalence and Pattern of HIV Infection in Karachi." *J Pak Med Assoc* 43: 2–4.

Mujeeb, S. A., and M. S. Pearce. 2008. "Temporal Trends in Hepatitis B and C Infection in Family Blood Donors from Interior Sindh, Pakistan." *BMC Infect Dis* 8: 43.

Naderi, H. R., M. Tagliamonte, M. L. Tornesello, M. Ciccozzi, G. Rezza, R. Farid, F. M. Buonaguro, and L. Buonaguro. 2006. "Molecular and Phylogenetic Analysis of HIV-1 Variants Circulating among Injecting Drug Users in Mashhad-Iran." *Infect Agent Cancer* 1: 4.

Nakhaie, S., and E. Talachian. 2003. "Prevalence and Characteristic of Liver Involvement in Thalassemia Patients with HCV in Ali-Asghar Children Hospital, Tehran, Iran (Farsi)." *Journal of Iranian University Medical Science* 37: 799–806.

Nemati, E., S. M. Alavian, S. Taheri, M. Moradi, V. Pourfarziani, and B. Einollahi. 2009. "Hepatitis C Virus Infection among Patients on Hemodialysis: A Report from a Single Center in Iran." *Saudi J Kidney Dis Transpl* 20: 147–53.

Novelli, V. M., H. Mostafavipour, M. Abulaban, F. Ekteish, J. Milder, and B. Azadeh. 1987. "High Prevalence of Human Immunodeficiency Virus Infection in Children with Thalassemia Exposed to Blood Imported from the United States." *Pediatr Infect Dis J* 6: 765–66.

Omer, E. E., M. H. Ali, O. M. Taha, M. A. Ahmed, and S. A. Abbaro. 1982. "Sexually Transmitted Diseases in Sudanese Males." *Trop Doct* 12: 208–10.

Pakistan National AIDS Control Program. 2005. *HIV Second Generation Surveillance in Pakistan.* National Report Round 1. Ministry of Health, Pakistan, and Canada-Pakistan HIV/AIDS Surveillance Project.

———. 2006–7. *HIV Second Generation Surveillance in Pakistan.* National Report Round II. Ministry of Health, Pakistan, and Canada-Pakistan HIV/AIDS Surveillance Project.

———. 2008. *HIV Second Generation Surveillance in Pakistan.* National Report Round III. Ministry of Health, Pakistan, Canada-Pakistan HIV/AIDS Surveillance Project.

Pieniazek, D., J. Baggs, D. J. Hu, G. M. Matar, A. M. Abdelnoor, J. E. Mokhbat, M. Uwaydah, A. R. Bizri, A. Ramos, L. M. Janini, A. Tanuri, C. Fridlund, C. Schable, L. Heyndrickx, M. A. Rayfield, and W. Heneine. 1998. "Introduction of HIV-2 and Multiple HIV-1 Subtypes to Lebanon." *Emerg Infect Dis* 4: 649–56.

Piyasirisilp, S., F. E. McCutchan, J. K. Carr, E. Sanders-Buell, W. Liu, J. Chen, R. Wagner, H. Wolf, Y. Shao, S. Lai, C. Beyrer, and X. F. Yu. 2000. "A Recent Outbreak of Human Immunodeficiency Virus Type 1 Infection in Southern China Was Initiated by Two Highly Homogeneous, Geographically Separated Strains, Circulating Recombinant Form AE and a Novel BC Recombinant." *J Virol* 74: 11286–95.

Qatar, State of. 2008. *Report on the Country Progress Indicators towards Implementing the Declaration of Commitment on HIV.* National Health Authority.

Raja, N. S., and K. A. Janjua. 2008. "Epidemiology of Hepatitis C Virus Infection in Pakistan." *J Microbiol Immunol Infect* 41: 4–8.

Rajabali, A., S. Khan, H. J. Warraich, M. R. Khanani, and S. H. Ali. 2008. "HIV and Homosexuality in Pakistan." *Lancet Infect Dis* 8: 511–15.

Rehan, N. 2006. "Profile of Men Suffering from Sexually Transmitted Infections in Pakistan." *J Pak Med Assoc* 56: S60–65.

Rezvan, H., H. Abolghassemi, and S. A. Kafiabad. 2007. "Transfusion-Transmitted Infections among Multi-Transfused Patients in Iran: A Review." *Transfus Med* 17: 425–33.

Saad, M. D., A. Al-Jaufy, R. R. Grahan, Y. Nadai, K. C. Earhart, J. L. Sanchez, and J. K. Carr. 2005. "HIV Type 1 Strains Common in Europe, Africa, and Asia Cocirculate in Yemen." *AIDS Res Hum Retroviruses* 21: 644–48.

Saleh, D. A., F. Shebl, M. Abdel-Hamid, S. Narooz, N. Mikhail, M. El-Batanony, S. El-Kafrawy, M. El-Daly, S. Sharaf, M. Hashem, S. El-Kamary, L. S. Magder, S. K. Stoszek, and G. T. Strickland. 2008. "Incidence and Risk Factors for Hepatitis C Infection in a Cohort of Women in Rural Egypt." *Trans R Soc Trop Med Hyg* 102: 921–28.

Sanders-Buell, E., M. D. Saad, A. M. Abed, M. Bose, C. S. Todd, S. A. Strathdee, B. A. Botros, N. Safi, K. C. Earhart, P. T. Scott, N. Michael, and F. E. McCutchan. 2007. "A Nascent HIV Type 1 Epidemic among Injecting Drug Users in Kabul, Afghanistan is Dominated by Complex AD Recombinant Strain, CRF35_AD." *AIDS Res Hum Retroviruses* 23: 834–39.

Sarrami-Forooshani, R., S. R. Das, F. Sabahi, A. Adeli, R. Esmaeili, B. Wahren, M. Mohraz, M. Haji-Abdolbaghi, M. Rasoolinejad, S. Jameel, and F. Mahboudi. 2006. "Molecular Analysis and Phylogenetic Characterization of HIV in Iran." *J Med Virol* 78: 853–63.

Schmid, G. P., A. Buve, P. Mugyenyi, G. P. Garnett, R. J. Hayes, B. G. Williams, J. G. Calleja, K. M. De Cock, J. A. Whitworth, S. H. Kapiga, P. D. Ghys, C. Hankins, B. Zaba, R. Heimer, and J. T. Boerma. 2004. "Transmission of HIV-1 Infection in Sub-Saharan Africa and Effect of Elimination of Unsafe Injections." *Lancet* 363: 482–88.

Sekkat, S., N. Kamal, B. Benali, H. Fellah, K. Amazian, A. Bourquia, A. El Kholti, and A. Benslimane. 2008. "Prevalence of Anti-HCV Antibodies and Seroconversion Incidence in Five Haemodialysis Units in Morocco." *Nephrol Ther* 4: 105–10.

Simonsen, L., A. Kane, J. Lloyd, M. Zaffran, and M. Kane. 1999. "Unsafe Injections in the Developing World and Transmission of Bloodborne Pathogens: A Review." *Bull World Health Organ* 77: 789–800.

SNAP (Sudan National AIDS Program), UNICEF (United Nations Children's Fund), and UNAIDS (United Nations Joint Programme on HIV/AIDS). 2005. "Baseline Study on Knowledge, Attitudes, and Practices on Sexual Behaviors and HIV/AIDS Prevention amongst Young People in Selected States in Sudan." HIV/AIDS KAPB Report, Projects and Research Department (AFROCENTER Group).

Soheilli, Z. S., Z. Ataiee, S. Tootian, M. Zadsar, S. Amini, K. Abadi, V. Jauvin, P. Pinson, H. J. Fleury, and S. Samiei. 2009. "Presence of HIV-1 CRF35_AD in Iran." *AIDS Res Hum Retroviruses* 25: 123–24.

Stoszek, S. K., M. Abdel-Hamid, S. Narooz, M. El Daly, D. A. Saleh, N. Mikhail, E. Kassem, Y. Hawash, S. El Kafrawy, A. Said, M. El Batanony, F. M. Shebl, M. Sayed, S. Sharaf, A. D. Fix, and G. T. Strickland. 2006. "Prevalence of and Risk Factors for Hepatitis C in Rural Pregnant Egyptian Women." *Trans R Soc Trop Med Hyg* 100: 102–7.

Sudan National HIV/AIDS Control Program. 2004a. *Annual Report*. Federal Ministry of Health, Khartoum.

———. 2004b. *HIV/AIDS/STIs Prevalence, Knowledge, Attitude, Practices and Risk Factors among University Students and Military Personnel*. Federal Ministry of Health, Khartoum.

Sy, T., and M. M. Jamal. 2006. "Epidemiology of Hepatitis C Virus (HCV) Infection." *Int J Med Sci* 3: 41–46.

Syria National AIDS Programme. 2004. "HIV/AIDS Female Sex Workers KABP Survey in Syria."

Tagliamonte, M., H. R. Naderi, M. L. Tornesello, F. Farid, F. M. Buonaguro, and L. Buonaguro. 2007. "HIV Type 1 Subtype A Epidemic in Injecting Drug User (IDU) Communities in Iran." *AIDS Res Hum Retroviruses* 23: 1569–74.

Tawilah, J., and O. Tawil. 2001. *Visit to Sultane of Oman*. Travel Report Summary. National AIDS Programme at the Ministry of Health in Muscat and Salalah and WHO Representative Office. World Health Organization, Regional Office for the Eastern Mediterranean.

Taziki, O., and F. Espahbodi. 2008. "Prevalence of Hepatitis C Virus Infection in Hemodialysis Patients." *Saudi J Kidney Dis Transpl* 19: 475–78.

Todd, C. S., Y. Barbera-Lainez, S. C. Doocy, A. Ahmadzai, F. M. Delawar, and G. M. Burnham. 2007. "Prevalence of Human Immunodeficiency Virus Infection, Risk Behavior, and HIV Knowledge among Tuberculosis Patients in Afghanistan." *Sex Transm Dis* 34: 878–82.

Torabi, S. A., K. Abcd-Ashtiani, R. Dchkhoda, A. N. Moghadam, M. K. Bahram, R. Dolatkhah, J. Babaei, and N. Taheri. 2006. "Prevalence of Hepatitis B, C and HIV in Hemophiliac Patients of East Azarbaijan in 2004." *Blood* 2: 291–99.

UNAIDS (United Nations Joint Programme on HIV/AIDS). 2006a. "Country Alignment and Harmonisation Support to Scaling Up the HIV/AIDS Response: The Somali Experience."

———. 2006b. "Common Country Assessment: Key Challenges in Health; HIV Prevention in Jordan."

———. 2007. "Key Findings on HIV Status in the West Bank and Gaza." Working document, RST, MENA.

———. 2008. "Notes on AIDS in the Middle East and North Africa." RST, MENA.

UNAIDS, and WHO (World Health Organization). 2005. *AIDS Epidemic Update 2005*. Geneva.

———. 2006. *AIDS Epidemic Update 2006*. Geneva.

———. 2007. *AIDS Epidemic Update 2007*. Geneva.

Visco-Comandini, U., G. Cappiello, G. Liuzzi, V. Tozzi, G. Anzidei, I. Abbate, A. Amendola, L. Bordi, M. A. Budabbus, O. A. Eljhawi, M. I. Mehabresh, E. Girardi, A. Antinori, M. R. Capobianchi, A. Sonnerborg, and G. Ippolito. 2002. "Monophyletic HIV Type 1 CRF02-AG in a Nosocomial Outbreak in Benghazi, Libya." *AIDS Res Hum Retroviruses* 18: 727–32.

Waked, I. A., S. M. Saleh, M. S. Moustafa, A. A. Raouf, D. L. Thomas, and G. T. Strickland. 1995. "High Prevalence of Hepatitis C in Egyptian Patients with Chronic Liver Disease." *Gut* 37: 105–7.

Walker, P. R., M. Worobey, A. Rambaut, E. C. Holmes, and O. G. Pybus. 2003. "Epidemiology: Sexual Transmission of HIV in Africa." *Nature* 422: 679.

Watts, D. M., N. T. Constantine, M. F. Sheba, M. Kamal, J. D. Callahan, and M. E. Kilpatrick. 1993. "Prevalence of HIV Infection and AIDS in Egypt over Four Years of Surveillance (1986–1990)." *J Trop Med Hyg* 96: 113–17.

WHO (World Health Organization). 1999a. "Global Surveillance and Control of Hepatitis C." Report of a WHO consultation organized in collaboration with the Viral Hepatitis Prevention Board, Antwerp, Belgium. *J Viral Hepat* 6: 35–47.

———. 1999b. *Weekly Epidemiological Record*. No. 49.

———. 2005. "Summary Country Profile for HIV/AIDS Treatment Scale-Up." Djibouti.

WHO/EMRO (Eastern Mediterranean Regional Office). 2005. "Progress Report on HIV/AIDS and '3 by 5.'" July, Cairo.

———. 2006. *Progress towards Universal Access to HIV Prevention, Treatment and Care in the Health Sector*. Report on a baseline survey for the year 2005 in the WHO Eastern Mediterranean Region. Draft.

WHO, UNICEF (United Nations Children's Fund), and UNAIDS (United Nations Joint Programme on HIV/AIDS). 2006. "Yemen, Epidemiological Facts Sheets on HIV/AIDS and Sexually Transmitted Infections."

World Bank. 2006. *HIV/AIDS in Afghanistan*. South Asia Region, World Bank.

World Bank Group. 2005. "World Bank Update 2005: HIV/AIDS in Pakistan." Washington, DC.

Yamaguchi, J., S. Badreddine, P. Swanson, P. Bodelle, S. G. Devare, and C. A. Brennan. 2008. "Identification of New CRF43_02G and CRF25_cpx in Saudi Arabia Based on Full Genome Sequence Analysis of Six HIV Type 1 Isolates." *AIDS Res Hum Retroviruses* 24: 1327–35.

Yemen MOH (Ministry of Health). Unknown. *National Strategic Framework for the Control and Prevention of HIV/AIDS in the Republic of Yemen*. Grey Report.

Yerly, S., R. Quadri, F. Negro, K. P. Barbe, J. J. Cheseaux, P. Burgisser, C. A. Siegrist, and L. Perrin. 2001. "Nosocomial Outbreak of Multiple Bloodborne Viral Infections." *J Infect Dis* 184: 369–72.

Younus, M., A. E. Siddiqi, and S. Akhtar. 2009. "Reassessment of Selected Healthcare Associated Risk Factors for HBV and HCV Infections among Volunteer Blood Donors, Karachi, Pakistan." *Cent Eur J Public Health* 17: 31–35.

Zafar, A., N. Aslam, N. Nasir, R. Meraj, and V. Mehraj. 2008. "Knowledge, Attitudes and Practices of Health Care Workers regarding Needle Stick Injuries at a Tertiary Care Hospital in Pakistan." *J Pak Med Assoc* 58: 57–60.

Zahraoui-Mehadji, M., M. Z. Baakrim, S. Laraqui, O. Laraqui, Y. El Kabouss, C. Verger, A. Caubet, and C. H. Laraqui. 2004. "Infectious Risks Associated with Blood Exposure for Traditional Barbers and Their Customers in Morocco." *Sante* 14: 211–16.

Zali, M. R., R. Aghazadeh, A. Nowroozi, and H. Amir-Rasouly. 2001. "Anti-HCV Antibody among Iranian IV Drug Users: Is It a Serious Problem?" *Arch Iranian Med* 4: 115–19.

Zargooshi, J. 2002. "Characteristics of Gonorrhoea in Kermanshah, Iran." *Sex Transm Infect* 78: 460–61.

Zouiten, F., A. Ben Said, L. Ammari, A. Slim, F. Kanoun, and T. Ben Chaabane. 2002. "AIDS in Tunisian Women: Study of 92 Cases." *Tunis Med* 80: 402–6.

Chapter 8

Condom Knowledge and Use and HIV/AIDS Knowledge and Attitudes

This chapter discusses condom knowledge and its use in the Middle East and North Africa (MENA) populations, and then delineates the characteristics of HIV/AIDS (human immunodeficiency virus/acquired immune deficiency syndrome) knowledge and attitudes in this region.

KNOWLEDGE OF CONDOM AS A PREVENTION METHOD AND ITS USE

Levels of general condom knowledge, levels of condom knowledge as a means of HIV prevention, and levels of condom use have been documented in different populations in multiple studies in MENA. Tables 8.1 and 8.2 summarize these levels for a number of MENA countries. Condom knowledge varies substantially within MENA, and it is rather low in resource-limited settings.

Condom knowledge does not necessarily mean condom knowledge as *a means of HIV prevention*. Parts of the populations have heard of condoms as a birth control method, but are not aware of its use for HIV prevention. Among rural populations in Sudan, 31.6% had heard of condoms, but only 4% identified them as a means of HIV prevention.[1] Avoidance of nonsanctioned sex is often cited as a means of HIV prevention rather than safe sex. Only 0.4% of tourism and industrial workers in the Arab Republic of Egypt reported knowing condoms can be used for HIV prevention.[2]

Condom knowledge as a means of HIV prevention does not necessarily relate to actual condom use. Only a fraction of those who are aware of the efficacy of condoms against HIV actually use condoms,[3] and they may do so out of pregnancy concerns rather than for HIV prevention.[4] Of those who use condoms, only a small minority use them consistently. In a nutshell, consistent condom use for HIV prevention is limited in MENA and the majority of at-risk sexual acts are not protected against HIV infection. Condom use is low even among the priority populations (table 8.2).

Repeatedly, pharmacies are cited as the most accessible source for condoms.[5] Several priority populations have reported limitations in condom accessibility and difficulty in using them, such as in Egypt, where 44% of female sex workers (FSWs) and 22% of men who have sex with men (MSM) had trouble obtaining condoms, and 89% of FSWs and 38% of MSM had trouble using them.[6] The most cited reasons for not using condoms are high condom prices,[7]

---

[1] SNAP, UNICEF, and UNAIDS, "Baseline Study on Knowledge."

[2] El-Sayed, Kabbash, and El-Gueniedy, "Knowledge, Attitude and Practices."

[3] Hajiabdolbaghi et al., "Insights from a Survey"; Ministry of Health and Medical Education of Iran, *AIDS/HIV Surveillance Report*; Syria MOH, *HIV/AIDS Female Sex Workers.*

[4] Faisel and Cleland, "Study of the Sexual Behaviours."

[5] Mohammad et al., "Sexual Risk-Taking Behaviors"; Hermez et al., "HIV/AIDS Prevention"; Jurjus et al., "Knowledge, Attitudes, Beliefs, and Practices."

[6] El-Sayed et al., "Evaluation of Selected Reproductive Health Infections."

[7] Tehrani and Malek-Afzalip, "Knowledge, Attitudes and Practices"; Ministry of Health and Medical Education of Iran, *AIDS/HIV Surveillance Report.*

Table 8.1 General Knowledge of Condoms including HIV Prevention, in Different Populations Groups in MENA

Country	Knowledge of condoms	Knowledge of condom use for HIV prevention
Afghanistan	25.0% (TB patients; Todd et al. 2007) 41.0% (FSWs; World Bank 2008)	
Egypt, Arab Republic of	10.0% (adolescents; El-Tawila et al. 1999)	60.0% (general population; Kabbash et al. 2007) 49.3% (MSM; El-Sayyed, Kabbash, and El-Gueniedy 2008)
Iran, Islamic Republic of	Majority (adolescents; Mohammadi et al. 2006)	Majority (adolescents; Mohammadi et al. 2006) 53.0% (adolescents; Yazdi et al. 2006) 42.0% (adolescents; prevent STIs; Mohammadi et al. 2006) 49.0% (university students; Simbar, Tehrani, and Hashemi 2005) 62.0% (male university students; Simbar, Tehrani, and Hashemi 2005) 39.0% (female university students; Simbar, Tehrani, and Hashemi 2005) 10.0% (prisoners; Khawaja et al. 1997) Nearly all (FSWs; Ministry of Health and Medical Education of Iran 2004)
Jordan	84.4% (general population women; Measure DHS 1998)	33.0% (general population women; Measure DHS 2003)
Lebanon	84.1% (general population; Jurjus et al. 2004)	
Morocco	37.5% (general population women; Morocco MOH 2004) 53.8% (youth; Morocco MOH, with GTZ, 2007) 73.4% (FSWs; Morocco MOH 2007)	37.5% (general population women; Zidouh [unknown]) 53% (youth; Morocco MOH, with GTZ, 2007) 53% (FSWs; Morocco MOH 2007)
Pakistan	94.0% *hijras* (Khan et al. 2008)	58.7% (obstetrics and gynecology clinic attendees; Haider et al. 2009) 19.5% (ever-married women; Measure DHS 2007) Minority (truck drivers; Agha 2000) 37%–77% (FSWs; Bokhari et al. 2007) 60.4% (FSWs; Pakistan National AIDS Control Program 2005) 64.0% (FSWs; Pakistan National AIDS Control Program 2006–07) 46.6% (IDUs; Pakistan National AIDS Control Program 2005) 44.3% (IDUs; Pakistan National AIDS Control Program 2006–07) 44.0% (IDUs; Pakistan National AIDS Control Program 2008) 63.7% (MSWs; Pakistan National AIDS Control Program 2005) 54.0% (MSWs; Pakistan National AIDS Control Program 2006–07) 61.7% (MSWs; Pakistan National AIDS Control Program 2008) 57.0% (HSWs; Pakistan National AIDS Control Program 2005) 50.2% (HSWs; Pakistan National AIDS Control Program 2006–07) 66.5% (HSWs; Pakistan National AIDS Control Program 2008) 69.0% *hijras* (Khan et al. 2008)
Somalia	23.0% (women under age 24; Population Studies Research Institute 2000)	
Sudan	71.9% (university students; Sudan National HIV/AIDS Control Program 2004) One-third (general population; Ahmed 2004b) 21.1% (general population; Southern Sudan; NSNAC and UNAIDS 2006) 89.0% (general population; men; Southern Sudan; UNHCR 2007) 71.0% (general population; women; Southern Sudan; UNHCR 2007) 31.6% (rural populations; SNAP, UNICEF, and UNAIDS 2005) 72.1% (truck drivers; Farah and Hussein 2006) 63.9% (prisoners; Assal 2006) 65.2% (military personnel; Sudan National HIV/AIDS Control Program 2004) 45.0% (FSWs; Sudan National HIV/AIDS Control Program 2004) 60.9% (FSWs; Yousif 2006) 17.2% (FSWs; ACORD 2006) 28.0% (FSWs; Ati 2005)	18.5% (street children; Ahmed 2004h) 27.4% (university students; Ahmed 2004l) 4.0% (rural populations; SNAP, UNICEF, and UNAIDS 2005) 5.2% (ANC women attendees; Ahmed 2004b) 10.2% (general population; Southern Sudan; NSNAC and UNAIDS 2006) 78.0% (general population; men; Southern Sudan; UNHCR 2007) 58.0% (general population; women; Southern Sudan; UNHCR 2007) 5.0% (tea sellers; Ahmed 2004j) 11.3% (internally displaced persons; Ahmed 2004c) 2.0% (police officers; Abdelwahab 2006) 5.7% (military personnel; Ahmed 2004d) 9.1% (prisoners; Ahmed 2004e) 7.5% (truck drivers; Ahmed 2004k) 12.8% (TB patients; Ahmed 2004i) 8.5% (STD clinic attendees; Ahmed 2004g) 4.3% (suspected AIDS patients; Ahmed 2004a) 5.3% (truck drivers; Farah and Hussein 2006) 17.0% (FSWs; Sudan National HIV/AIDS Control Program 2004) 17.3% (FSWs; Ahmed 2004f)

Table 8.1 *(Continued)*

Country	Knowledge of condoms	Knowledge of condom use for HIV prevention
	45.0% (FSWs; Sudan National HIV/AIDS Control Program 2004) 45.1% (FSWs; Anonymous 2007)	
Syrian Arab Republic		38.0% (IDUs; Syria Mental Health Directorate 2008)
Tunisia	89.2% (MSM; Hsairi and Ben Abdallah 2007)	
West Bank and Gaza		67.0% (youth; PFPPA 2005)
Yemen, Republic of	48.3% (general population, marginalized minority, and returnees from extended work abroad; Busulwa 2003)	28.5% (youth; Al-Serouri 2005) 49.4% (high school students; Raja and Farhan 2005) 51.9% (high school students; Gharamah and Baktayan 2006) 20.7% (general population, marginalized minority, and returnees from extended work abroad; Busulwa 2003)

Note: ANC = antenatal clinic; HSW = *hijra* sex worker; IDU = injecting drug user; STD = sexually transmitted disease; TB = tuberculosis.

Table 8.2 Condom Use among Different Population Groups in MENA

Country	Condom use
Afghanistan	0.0% (ever use; IDUs; Sanders-Buell et al. 2007) 17.0% (ever use; commercial sex; IDUs; World Bank 2008) 36.0% (ever use; FSWs; World Bank 2008)
Djibouti	48.4% (ever use; sexually active high school students; Rodier et al. 1993) 24.2% (always; sexually active high school students; Rodier et al. 1993) Rare (STD clinic attendees; Wassef et al. 1989) Not common (unlicensed FSWs; Wassef et al. 1989) Common (bar hostesses; Wassef et al. 1989)
Egypt, Arab Republic of	90.0% (casual sex; tourism workers; El-Sayed et al. 1996) 23.9% (contraceptive method; general population; Kabbash et al. 2007) Low (regular use; university students; Refaat 2004) 34.1% (ever use; regular partners; IDUs; Egypt MOH and Population National AIDS Program 2006) 12.8% (ever use; nonregular noncommercial partners; IDUs; Egypt MOH and Population National AIDS Program 2006) 11.8% (ever use; with CSWs; IDUs; Egypt MOH and Population National AIDS Program 2006) 66.0% (ever use; IDUs; Elshimi, Warner-Smith, and Aon 2004) 20.0% (ever use; IDUs; El-Sayed et al. 2002) 9.0% (always; IDUs; El-Sayed et al. 2002) 44.0% (ever use; FSWs; El-Sayed et al. 2002) 6.8% (last sex act with a noncommercial partner; FSWs; Egypt MOH and Population National AIDS Program 2006) 6.0% (always; FSWs; El-Sayed et al. 2002) 56.0% (ever use; FSWs; El-Sayed et al. 2002) 6.8% (last sex; noncommercial partners; IDUs; Egypt MOH and Population National AIDS Program 2006) 47.0% (ever use; MSM; El-Sayed et al. 2002) 19.0% (regularly; MSM; El-Rahman 2004) 2.0% (consistent; MSM; El-Sayed 1994) 19.0% (consistent; MSM; El-Sayed et al. 2002) 19.2% (consistent; MSM; El-Sayyed, Kabbash, and El-Gueniedy 2008) 9.2% (last commercial sex; MSM; Egypt MOH and Population National AIDS Program 2006) 12.7% (last noncommercial sex; MSM; Egypt MOH and Population National AIDS Program 2006) 21.0% (ever use; MSM; El-Sayed 1994) 47.9% (ever use; MSM; El-Sayyed, Kabbash, and El-Gueniedy 2008)

(continued)

Table 8.2 *(Continued)*

Country	Condom use
Iran, Islamic Republic of	71.7% (ever use; youth; Mohammad et al. 2007)
	48.0% (ever use; university students; Simbar, Tehrani, and Hashemi 2005)
	64.8% (ever use; truck drivers; Tehrani and Malek-Afzalip 2008)
	89.0% (recent; clients of FSWs; Zargooshi 2002)
	53.0% (ever use; IDUs; Zamani et al. 2005)
	52.0% (ever use; IDUs; Narenjiha et al. 2005)
	37.0% (last sex; IDUs; Zamani et al. 2005)
	11.3%–12.4% (ever use; IDU prisoners; Farhoudi et al. 2003)
	52.0% (ever use; FSWs; Tehrani and Malek-Afzalip 2008)
	50.0% (ever use; FSWs; Ministry of Health and Medical Education of Iran 2004)
	24%–83.2% (last client; FSWs; Jahani et al. 2005; Ardalan et al. 2002)
	19.4% (last anal sex; steady partners; MSM; Eftekhar et al. 2008)
	59.5% (last anal sex; commercial sex partners; MSM; Eftekhar et al. 2008)
	59.9% (last anal sex; casual partners; MSM; Eftekhar et al. 2008)
Jordan	Moderately high (nonmarital sex; youth; UNAIDS and WHO 2005)
	4.0% (last sex; general population women; Measure DHS 2003)
Kuwait	1.5% (recent use; STD clinic attendees; Al-Mutairi et al. 2007)
Lebanon	7.0% (current use; married women; Kulczycki 2004)
	24.0% (current use; married women; Kulczycki 2004)
	32.0% (ever use; general population; Lebanon National AIDS Control Program 1996)
	25.0% (last sex regular partnerships; general population; Jurjus et al. 2004)
	71.7% (last sex nonregular partnerships; general population; Jurjus et al. 2004)
	15.3% (ever use; general population; Jurjus et al. 2004)
	23.4% (last sex while drunk; prisoners; Mishwar 2008)
	88.0% (ever use; IDUs; Aaraj [unknown])
	59.0% (ever use; IDUs; Ingold 1994)
	5.8% (last sex; regular; IDUs; Aaraj [unknown]; Hermez et al. [unknown])
	34.6% (last sex; casual sex; IDUs; Aaraj [unknown]; Hermez et al. [unknown])
	39.3% (last sex; commercial sex, IDUs; Aaraj [unknown]; Hermez et al. [unknown])
	28.1% (always; nonregular clients; FSWs; Hermez et al. [unknown])
	34.8% (always; regular clients; FSWs; Hermez et al. [unknown])
	11.9% (always; regular partners; FSWs; Hermez et al [unknown])
	79.0% (ever use; FSWs; Hermez [unknown])
	98.0% (last sex; FSWs; Mishwar 2008)
	94.0% (last sex; FSWs; Mishwar 2008)
	43.0% (last sex; FSWs; Mishwar 2008)
	80.0% (last sex; FSWs; Rady 2005)
	32.3% (consistent; regular client; FSWs; Lebanon National AIDS Control Program 2008)
	26.2% (consistent; nonclient; FSWs; Lebanon National AIDS Control Program 2008)
	35.1% (consistent; vaginal sex; FSWs; Lebanon National AIDS Control Program 2008)
	13.9% (consistent; oral sex; FSWs; Lebanon National AIDS Control Program 2008)
	36.1% (consistent; anal sex; FSWs; Lebanon National AIDS Control Program 2008)
	88.0% (ever use; MSM; Aaraj [unknown])
	47.1% (always; regular partners; MSM; Hermez et al.; Dewachi 2001)
	54.5% (always; noncommercial casual partner; MSM; Hermez et al. [unknown]; Dewachi 2001)
	47.0% (last anal sex; regular partner; MSM; Mishwar 2008)
	66.0% (last anal sex; noncommercial casual partner; MSM; Mishwar 2008)
Morocco	16.0% (ever use; general population women; Chaouki et al. 1998)
	9.0% (regular use; incarcerated women; El Ghrari et al. 2007)
	10.0% (always; males; mainly IDUs; Asouab 2005; Morocco MOH [unknown])
	8.1% (usually; males; mainly IDUs; Asouab 2005)
	38.4% (rarely; males; mainly IDUs; Asouab 2005)
	43.6% (never; males; mainly IDUs; Asouab 2005)
	22.0% (always; females; mainly IDUs; Asouab 2005; Morocco MOH [unknown])

Table 8.2 *(Continued)*

Country	Condom use
	4.9% (usually; females; mainly IDUs; Asouab 2005)
	29.3% (rarely; females; mainly IDUs; Asouab 2005)
	43.9% (never; females; mainly IDUs; Asouab 2005)
	59.0% (consistent; vaginal sex; FSWs; Alami 2009)
	9.7% (almost always; vaginal sex; FSWs; Alami 2009)
	22.2% (sometimes; vaginal sex; FSWs; Alami 2009)
	26.1% (consistent; anal sex; FSWs; Alami 2009)
	10.9% (almost always; anal sex; FSWs; Alami 2009)
	13.0% (sometimes; anal sex; FSWs; Alami 2009)
Oman	53%–69% (ever use; IDUs; Oman MOH 2006)
	12%–25% (always; IDUs; Oman MOH 2006)
	68%–100% (last year; MSM; IDUs; Oman MOH 2006)
Pakistan	7.0% (contraceptive method; general population; Measure DHS 2007)
	6.0% (ever use; general population; Raza et al. 1998)
	10.0% (commercial sex; migrant workers; Faisel and Cleland 2006)
	25.0% (sex with a female friend; migrant workers; Faisel and Cleland 2006)
	3%–6% (last sex with a nonspousal partner; truck drivers; Agha 2000)
	1.7% (last sex with FSW; truck drivers; Bokhari et al. 2007)
	0.0% (last sex with male or *hijra*; truck drivers; Bokhari et al. 2007)
	40.0% (ever use; IDUs; Emmanuel and Fatima 2008)
	37.5% (ever use; IDUs; Lahore; Kuo et al. 2006)
	14.2% (ever use; IDUs; Quetta; Kuo et al. 2006)
	7.0% (ever use; IDUs; Parviz et al. 2006)
	34.0% (ever use; IDUs; Altaf et al. 2007)
	10.0% (ever use; IDUs; Haque et al. 2004)
	17%–34% (last commercial sex; IDUs; Bokhari et al. 2007)
	10%–25% (last anal sex sold to a man; IDUs; Bokhari et al. 2007)
	22%–39% (last vaginal or anal sex sold to a woman; IDUs; Bokhari et al. 2007)
	7%–13% (last anal sex paid to a man or *hijra*; IDUs; Bokhari et al. 2007)
	46%–66% (not used last 6 months; nonpaid partners; IDUs; Pakistan National AIDS Control Program 2005)
	49%–86% (not used last 6 months; commercial sex; IDUs; Pakistan National AIDS Control Program 2005)
	45.0% (last sex; IDUs; Platt et al. 2009)
	32.0% (last sex; IDUs; Platt et al. 2009)
	17%–18% (always; FSWs; Pakistan National AIDS Control Program 2005)
	74%–81% (last month; FSWs; Pakistan National AIDS Control Program 2005)
	29%–49% (last sex; one-time client; FSWs; Bokhari et al. 2007)
	26%–47% (last sex; regular client; FSWs; Bokhari et al. 2007)
	21.0% (last sex; noncommercial partners; FSWs; Bokhari et al. 2007)
	17.0% (consistent last month; FSWs; Saleem, Adrien, and Razaque 2008)
	68.0% (ever use; FSWs; Pakistan National AIDS Control Program 2005)
	34.0% (last sex; noncommercial partners; FSWs; Pakistan National AIDS Control Program 2005)
	18.0% (consistent last month; FSWs; Pakistan National AIDS Control Program 2005)
	23.0% (consistent last month; FSWs; Pakistan National AIDS Control Program 2006–07)
	34.0% (last vaginal sex; FSWs; Blanchard, Khan, and Bokhari 2008)
	45.0% (last vaginal sex; FSWs; Pakistan National AIDS Control Program 2006–07)
	38.0% (last commercial vaginal sex; FSWs; Hawkes et al. 2009)
	12.0% (consistent last month during commercial vaginal sex; FSWs; Hawkes et al. 2009)
	61.0% (last commercial anal sex; FSWs; Hawkes et al. 2009)
	54.0% (last commercial oral sex; FSWs; Hawkes et al. 2009)
	46.0% (last sex with husband; FSWs; Hawkes et al. 2009)
	15.0% (consistent last month with husband; FSWs; Hawkes et al. 2009)
	7.9% (last anal sex; FSWs; Pakistan National AIDS Control Program 2006–07)
	32.4% (last oral sex; FSWs; Pakistan National AIDS Control Program 2006–07)
	3.1% (consistent; MSWs; Saleem, Adrien, and Razaque 2008)

(continued)

Table 8.2 *(Continued)*

Country	Condom use
	24.0% (last anal sex; MSWs; Pakistan National AIDS Control Program 2005)
	13.0% (last oral sex; MSWs; Pakistan National AIDS Control Program 2005)
	34.0% (last commercial sex; MSWs; Pakistan National AIDS Control Program 2008)
	32.5% (last sex; noncommercial partners; MSWs; Pakistan National AIDS Control Program 2008)
	7.1% (consistent last month; MSWs; Pakistan National AIDS Control Program 2005)
	8.0% (consistent last month; MSWs; Pakistan National AIDS Control Program 2006–07)
	24.0% (consistent last month; commercial sex; MSWs; Pakistan National AIDS Control Program 2008)
	22.2% (consistent last month; noncommercial partners; MSWs; Pakistan National AIDS Control Program 2008)
	21.0% (last anal sex; HSWs; Pakistan National AIDS Control Program 2005)
	15.0% (last oral sex; HSWs; Pakistan National AIDS Control Program 2005)
	32.3% (last commercial sex; HSWs; Pakistan National AIDS Control Program 2008)
	26.0% (last sex; noncommercial partners; HSWs; Pakistan National AIDS Control Program 2008)
	7.5% (consistent last month; HSWs; Pakistan National AIDS Control Program 2005)
	5.6% (consistent last month; HSWs; Pakistan National AIDS Control Program 2006–07)
	19.7% (consistent last month; commercial sex; HSWs; Pakistan National AIDS Control Program 2008)
	19.6% (consistent last month; noncommercial partners; HSWs; Pakistan National AIDS Control Program 2008)
	20%–52% (ever use; *hijras;* Pakistan National AIDS Control Program 2005)
	20.0% (ever use; *hijras;* Baqi et al. 1999)
	4.0% (consistent; *hijras;* Saleem, Adrien, and Razaque 2008)
	18.0% (last sex; one-time client; *hijras;* Khan et al. 2008)
	12.0% (last receptive anal sex; one-time client; *hijras;* Khan et al. 2008)
	15.0% (last sex; regular client; *hijras;* Khan et al. 2008)
	13.0% (last receptive anal sex; regular client; *hijras;* Khan et al. 2008)
	9.0% (last sex; MSWs; Bokhari et al. 2007)
	17.0% (last month; nonpaying female; MSWs; Bokhari et al. 2007)
	23.0% (last commercial anal sex; *banthas;* Hawkes et al. 2009)
	31.0% (last commercial anal sex; *khotkis;* Hawkes et al. 2009)
	25.0% (last commercial anal sex; *khusras;* Hawkes et al. 2009)
	10.0% (consistent last month during commercial anal sex; *banthas;* Hawkes et al. 2009)
	8.0% (consistent last month during commercial anal sex; *khotkis;* Hawkes et al. 2009)
	4.0% (consistent last month during commercial anal sex; *khusras;* Hawkes et al. 2009)
	10.0% (last commercial oral sex; *banthas;* Hawkes et al. 2009)
	8.0% (last commercial oral sex; *khotkis;* Hawkes et al. 2009)
	4.0% (last commercial oral sex; *khusras;* Hawkes et al. 2009)
	0.0% (last sex with *gyria; banthas;* Hawkes et al. 2009)
	27.0% (last sex with *gyria; khotkis;* Hawkes et al. 2009)
	7.0% (last sex with *gyria; khusras;* Hawkes et al. 2009)
	0.0% (consistent last month with *gyria; banthas;* Hawkes et al. 2009)
	8.0% (consistent last month with *gyria; khotkis;* Hawkes et al. 2009)
	7.0% (consistent last month with *gyria; khusras;* Hawkes et al. 2009)
Somalia	12.7% (ever use; general population men; WHO 2004)
	5.0% (ever use; general population women; WHO 2004)
	2.6% (recent use; general population; Scott et al. 1991)
	14.0% (last sex; general population women; WHO/EMRO 2000)
	15.2% (last sex; general population men; WHO/EMRO 2000)
	10.3% (last sex; merchants/drivers; WHO/EMRO 2000)
Sudan	5.8% (ever use; street children; Ahmed 2004h)
	6.2% (ever use; university students; Ahmed 2004I)
	37.6% (ever use; university students; Sudan National HIV/AIDS Control Program 2004)
	3.6% (consistent; university students; Sudan National HIV/AIDS Control Program 2004)
	1.2% (last sex; rural population females; SNAP, UNICEF, and UNAIDS 2005)
	2.2% (last sex; rural population males; SNAP, UNICEF, and UNAIDS 2005)
	3.0% (last year; general population; Southern Sudan; NSNAC and UNAIDS 2006)
	2.0% (last sex with casual partner; general population; Sudan National HIV/AIDS Control Program 2004)

Table 8.2 *(Continued)*

Country	Condom use
	2.7% (ever use; ANC women attendees; Ahmed 2004b)
	5.0% (last sex with spouse; men; Southern Sudan; UNHCR 2007)
	1.0% (last sex with spouse; women; Southern Sudan; UNHCR 2007)
	31.0% (last sex with spouse; refugees; men; Southern Sudan; UNHCR 2007)
	5.0% (last sex with spouse; refugees; women; Southern Sudan; UNHCR 2007)
	46.3% (last sex with casual partner; men; Southern Sudan; UNHCR 2007)
	0.0% (last sex with casual partner; women; Southern Sudan; UNHCR 2007)
	22.5% (consistent with casual partner; men; Southern Sudan; UNHCR 2007)
	0.0% (consistent with casual partner; women; Southern Sudan; UNHCR 2007)
	0.0% (last sex with commercial partner; men; Southern Sudan; UNHCR 2007)
	0.0% (last sex with commercial partner; women; Southern Sudan; UNHCR 2007)
	16.0% (ever use among sexually active; men; Southern Sudan; UNHCR 2007)
	3.0% (ever use among sexually active; women; Southern Sudan; UNHCR 2007)
	1.0% (ever use; tea sellers; Ahmed 2004j)
	3.0% (ever use; internally displaced persons; IGAD 2006)
	5.0% (ever use; internally displaced persons; Ahmed 2004c)
	0.0% (ever use; Sudanese women refugees; Holt et al. 2003)
	8.9% (ever use; truck drivers; Farah and Hussein 2006)
	2.4% (ever use; truck drivers; Ahmed 2004k)
	2.7% (ever use; military personnel; Ahmed 2004d)
	4.0% (ever use; prisoners; Ahmed 2004e)
	15.8% (ever use; prisoners; Assal 2006)
	1.7% (ever use; TB patients; Ahmed 2004i)
	5.4% (ever use; STD clinic attendees; Ahmed 2004g)
	0.0% (ever use; suspected AIDS patients; Ahmed 2004a)
	10.4% (ever used; military personnel; Sudan National HIV/AIDS Control Program 2004)
	1.7% (consistent; military personnel; Sudan National HIV/AIDS Control Program 2004)
	2.0% (last sex; clients of FSWs; SNAP, UNICEF, and UNAIDS 2005)
	2.1% (regularly; FSWs and tea sellers; Basha 2006)
	10.3% (ever use; FSWs; Ahmed 2004f)
	16.7% (ever use; FSWs; Yousif 2006)
	13.0% (regularly; FSWs; Ati 2005)
	24.6% (ever use; FSWs; ACORD 2006)
	57.8% (ever use; FSWs; Ati 2005)
	23.0% (ever use; FSWs; Anonymous 2007)
	86.2% (ever use; MSM; Elrashied 2006)
	50.9% (every time or almost every time; MSM; Elrashied 2006)
	58.5% (last commercial sex; MSM; Elrashied 2006)
	48.5% (last noncommercial sex; MSM; Elrashied 2006)
	72.9% (ever use; MSM; Elrashied 2006)
	89.4% (last six months; female partners; MSM; Elrashied 2006)
Syrian Arab Republic	13.2% (always; FSWs; Syria MOH 2004)
	20.6% (often; FSWs; Syria MOH 2004)
	51.0% (sometimes; FSWs; Syria MOH 2004)
	15.2% (never; FSWs; Syria MOH 2004)
	39.0% (less than half the time; Syria Mental Health Directorate 2008)
	21.0% (more than half the time; Syria Mental Health Directorate 2008)
	19.0% (consistent; Syria Mental Health Directorate 2008)
	27.0% (less than half the time; commercial sex; Syria Mental Health Directorate 2008)
	5.0% (more than half the time; commercial sex; Syria Mental Health Directorate 2008)
	17.0% (consistent; commercial sex; Syria Mental Health Directorate 2008)
Tunisia	65.0% (ever use; FSWs; Hassen et al. 2003)
	37.0% (always; FSWs; Hassen et al. 2003)
	27.0% (sometimes; FSWs; Hassen et al. 2003)
	46.4% (last nonpaid sex; MSM; Hsairi and Ben Abdallah 2007)

(continued)

Table 8.2 *(Continued)*

Country	Condom use
	19.7% (consistent during nonpaid sex; MSM; Hsairi and Ben Abdallah 2007)
	53.7% (last sex with females; MSM; Hsairi and Ben Abdallah 2007)
	55.4% (last paid sex; MSM; Hsairi and Ben Abdallah 2007)
Turkey	70.0% (always; FSWs; Gul et al. 2008)
Yemen, Republic of	57.1% (last paid sex; FSWs; Štulhofer and Božicevic 2008)
	28.8% (last nonpaid sex; FSWs; Štulhofer and Božicevic 2008)
	50.0% (consistent; nonregular clients; FSWs; Štulhofer and Božicevic 2008)
	58.0% (consistent; regular clients; FSWs; Štulhofer and Božicevic 2008)

Note: ANC = antenatal clinic; CSW = commercial sex worker; HSW = *hijra* sex worker; IDU = injecting drug user; STD = sexually transmitted disease; TB = tuberculosis.

partner refusal,[8] pharmacies are too far,[9] not thinking of them as necessary,[10] or fear of imprisonment if caught possessing them (such as for FSWs and MSM).[11] Condom accessibility varies by population group. In Pakistan, condom accessibility at any time varied between 5.9% among truck drivers and 67.5% among FSWs.[12]

Condom use as a contraception method also appears to be low in MENA. In Jordan, 84.4% of women knew about condoms, but only 2.4% reported using them for family planning.[13] Several factors have been cited for their limited use as a contraception method including reduced sexual pleasure, inconvenience, adverse experiences, gender-related issues, and social stigma attached to condoms as a birth control method.[14] Nevertheless, effective national family planning programs appear to have increased condom knowledge and its use for HIV prevention, such as in the Islamic Republic of Iran, where relatively higher levels of condom knowledge and use can be found.[15] The Islamic Republic of Iran also appears to be the only MENA country to possess a condom manufacturing facility, which produces 45 million condoms per year.[16]

There appears to be a gender gap in condom knowledge. In the Islamic Republic of Iran, male college students were almost twice as likely as females, 62% versus 39%, to know about condoms as a sexually transmitted infection (STI) prevention method.[17] Lack of culturally sensitive and gender-specific information appears to contribute to this gap, suggesting the need for targeted, gender-specific, and culturally sensitive information regarding condom use for HIV prevention.[18] Men in MENA also appear to have a negative attitude toward condom use.[19]

Analytical summary

Condom knowledge varies in MENA and tends to be low in resource-limited settings. Although a substantial fraction of the MENA population knows about condoms, people are not as aware about their use for HIV prevention. Condom knowledge as a means of HIV prevention does not translate into actual condom use. And even when condoms are used for HIV prevention, they are not used consistently. Condom use is low even among the priority populations that are at the highest risk of infection. Though condoms are accessible from pharmacies in many parts of MENA, they are less accessible in other parts, particularly in resource-limited settings. All of these factors indicate that the majority of at-risk sexual acts in MENA are not protected against HIV infection.

[8] Tehrani and Malek-Afzalip, "Knowledge, Attitudes and Practices."
[9] Hermez et al., "HIV/AIDS Prevention."
[10] Khan et al., "Correlates and Prevalence of HIV."
[11] Rajabali et al., "HIV and Homosexuality in Pakistan"; Lebanon National AIDS Control Program, "A Case Study."
[12] Bokhari et al., "HIV Risk in Karachi and Lahore, Pakistan."
[13] Measure DHS, "Jordan Demographic and Health Survey 1997."
[14] Kulczycki, "The Sociocultural Context."
[15] Hajiabdolbaghi et al., "Insights from a Survey"; Roudi, "Iran's Revolutionary Approach."
[16] Mehryar, Ahmad-Nia, and Kazemipour, "Reproductive Health in Iran."

[17] Simbar, Tehrani, and Hashemi, "Reproductive Health Knowledge."
[18] Lazarus et al., "HIV/AIDS Knowledge."
[19] Ibid.

Knowledge of condoms as a means of HIV prevention needs to be increased and their use for safe sex must be highlighted. This would be best achieved through culturally sensitive and gender-specific awareness programs.

HIV/AIDS KNOWLEDGE AND ATTITUDES

One of the few areas relevant to HIV/AIDS for which there has been ample research in MENA is that of the levels of HIV/AIDS knowledge and attitudes in different population groups. The evidence confirms the variability in the levels of knowledge and nature of attitudes across and within MENA countries, but there are still key features that characterize much of HIV/AIDS knowledge and attitudes in this region.

Levels of HIV/AIDS basic knowledge

In the majority of MENA populations, the level of HIV/AIDS basic knowledge is high. In Egypt, 84.4% of ever-married women reported knowing about HIV/AIDS.[20] In Pakistan, 86.8% of migrant workers had heard of HIV/AIDS.[21] This high basic knowledge level has been seen in the majority of studies (table E.1 in appendix E). In some settings in MENA, however, low levels of basic knowledge have also been documented. In Afghanistan, 50.8% of women were aware of HIV/AIDS in one study and only 20% knew that HIV is sexually transmitted.[22] This limited basic knowledge has been observed in a minority of studies (table E.1 in appendix E).

Levels of HIV/AIDS comprehensive knowledge

Despite widespread basic knowledge, the level of comprehensiveness of HIV/AIDS knowledge is inadequate.[23] In Egypt, only 6.1% of ever-married women had comprehensive knowledge of HIV/AIDS.[24] In Somalia, only 4% of young women had comprehensive knowledge of HIV/AIDS.[25]

Many people may have heard of HIV/AIDS, but are unaware of its different transmission modes and clinical manifestations of infection and disease.[26] Knowledge of transmission modes is biased by the sociocultural context, where some transmission modes, such as sharing of injections, can be widely known, but other transmission modes, such as sexual relations within marriage, are not thought of as a transmission mode.[27] This pattern of low comprehensive knowledge has been seen in many studies (table E.2 in appendix E).

A few studies, however, have identified fairly good levels of comprehensive knowledge in specific populations, including a general population group in the Islamic Republic of Iran[28] and prisoners, FSWs, MSM, and injecting drug users (IDUs) in Lebanon.[29] Comparing knowledge, attitudes, and practices (KAP) surveys in Sudan from 2002 and 2005 found a substantial improvement in HIV/AIDS knowledge.[30] The level of HIV/AIDS knowledge appears to be steadily improving.

Levels of HIV/AIDS misinformation

There is a high level of misinformation and many misconceptions about HIV/AIDS in MENA.[31] In the Islamic Republic of Iran, one-third of high school students believed that HIV can be transmitted by mosquitoes.[32] In Saudi Arabia, 49% of health care workers (HCWs) identified casual kissing as a transmission mode.[33] In Sudan, one-fifth of antenatal clinic (ANC) attendees believed they could acquire HIV by sharing a meal with an HIV-positive person.[34] This high level of misinformation has been seen in many other studies (table E.3 in appendix E).

Perception of risk of HIV infection

Most people in MENA do not consider themselves at risk of HIV infection. In Djibouti, 80%

[20] Measure DHS, "Egypt: Demographic and Health Survey 2005."
[21] Faisel and Cleland, "Study of the Sexual Behaviours."
[22] Todd et al., "Seroprevalence and Correlates of HIV."
[23] Abolfotouh, "The Impact of a Lecture"; Farghaly and Kamal, "Study of the Opinion and Level of Knowledge about AIDS."
[24] Measure DHS, "Egypt: Demographic and Health Survey 2005."
[25] Somaliland Ministry of Health and Labour, *Somaliland 2007 HIV/Syphilis Seroprevalence Survey.*
[26] Genc et al., "AIDS Awareness and Knowledge."
[27] UNAIDS, "Key Findings."
[28] Montazeri, "AIDS Knowledge and Attitudes."
[29] Mishwar, "An Integrated Bio-Behavioral Surveillance Study"; Rady, "Knowledge, Attitudes and Prevalence."
[30] SNAP, UNICEF, and UNAIDS, "Baseline Study on Knowledge."
[31] Abolfotouh, "The Impact of a Lecture"; Farghaly and Kamal, "Study of the Opinion and Level of Knowledge about AIDS."
[32] Tavoosi et al., "Knowledge and Attitude."
[33] Mahfouz et al., "Knowledge and Attitudes."
[34] Ahmed, *Antenatal.*

of high school students reported not being at risk of HIV infection.[35] In Jordan, 82% of general population women reported not being at risk for HIV at all.[36] In the Republic of Yemen, 95.1% of secondary school students believed that young people are not susceptible to HIV infection.[37]

Attitudes toward people living with HIV

Attitudes toward people living with HIV (PLHIV) vary within and between populations, though generally the norm is that of negative and discriminatory attitudes. Different studies have documented both tolerant and intolerant attitudes, often even within the same population. In Egypt, 99% of general population women did not accept all four positive attitudes toward PLHIV, including caring for patients with AIDS-related illness, buying from HIV-positive shopkeepers, allowing HIV-positive women to teach, and being willing to disclose the infection of a family member.[38] The stigma, discrimination, and phobia are most worrying among HCWs. There is an environment of risk exaggeration in dealing with PLHIV,[39] such as among nurses in both Egypt[40] and the Islamic Republic of Iran.[41] Over half of Kuwaiti physicians would avoid contact with PLHIV.[42] These negative attitudes have been seen in many other studies (table E.4 in appendix E).

There is an immense stigma and human rights issues surrounding HIV in MENA.[43] Fear of stigmatization and feelings of anxiety, hopelessness, and depression are frequently reported by PLHIV.[44] High profile violations of basic rights of PLHIV have been widely reported.[45] The rights to confidentiality and consent are repeatedly violated.[46] Several aspects of human sexuality are deemed unacceptable.[47] The attitudes toward PLHIV depend strongly on the social acceptability of the transmission mode by which people become infected.[48] Religiosity has been associated with both positive[49] and negative[50] attitudes toward PLHIV.

The negative attitudes may be due in part to the invisible nature of the epidemic.[51] As a consequence of low HIV prevalence, most people have never been in contact with a patient with an AIDS-related illness. In the Syrian Arab Republic, only 2.8% of FSWs reported knowing a relative or a friend who was HIV positive.[52] The lack of comprehensive and proper knowledge of HIV/AIDS is a major factor in discriminatory attitudes. In the Islamic Republic of Iran, positive attitudes were found to be directly correlated with higher knowledge of this disease.[53] The increasing visibility of HIV in MENA may lead to improved attitudes toward PLHIV.

Despite prevailing negative attitudes, several studies have documented positive attitudes in a few MENA populations. In the Islamic Republic of Iran, 84% of general population respondents supported the social rights of PLHIV to work and study,[54] and 95% said that patients with AIDS-related illness deserve respect as human beings.[55] In Libya, 91% of high school students supported providing free care to PLHIV.[56] In Morocco, 68% of general population women said they would take care of PLHIV.[57] Encouragingly, there appears to be a trend of decreasing discrimination and stigmatization toward PLHIV. In Jordan, the percentages of youth who believed that PLHIV have the right to keep their illness a secret has increased from 18% in 1994,[58] to 29% in 1999,[59] and to 34.3% in 2005.[60]

[35] Rodier et al., "HIV Infection."

[36] Measure DHS, "Jordan: Demographic and Health Survey 1997."

[37] Gharamah and Baktayan, "Exploring HIV/AIDS Knowledge."

[38] Measure DHS, "Egypt: Demographic and Health Survey 2005."

[39] Duyan, Agalar, and Sayek, "Surgeons' Attitudes toward HIV/AIDS in Turkey."

[40] Shouman and Fotouh, "The Impact of Health Education."

[41] Askarian et al., "Knowledge about HIV Infection."

[42] Fido and Al Kazemi, "Survey of HIV/AIDS Knowledge."

[43] DeJong et al., "The Sexual and Reproductive Health."

[44] Kabbash et al., "Needs Assessment."

[45] Moszynski, "Egyptian Doctors."

[46] Mobeireek et al., "Information Disclosure and Decision-Making."

[47] Mohammadi et al., "Reproductive Knowledge, Attitudes and Behavior."

[48] Badahdah, "Saudi Attitudes towards People Living with HIV/AIDS."

[49] Paruk et al., "Compassion or Condemnation?"

[50] Badahdah, "Saudi Attitudes towards People Living with HIV/AIDS."

[51] UNAIDS, "Key Findings."

[52] Syria MOH, "HIV/AIDS Female Sex Workers."

[53] Mazloomy and Baghianimoghadam, "Knowledge and Attitude"; Hedayati-Moghaddam, "Knowledge of and Attitudes."

[54] Montazeri, "AIDS Knowledge and Attitudes in Iran."

[55] IRIB, "Poll of Teheran Public on AIDS (2006)."

[56] El-Gadi, Abudher, and Sammud, "HIV-Related Knowledge and Stigma."

[57] Zidouh, "VIH/SIDA et Infections sexuellement transmissibles."

[58] Jordan National AIDS Control Programme, *Report on the National KABP Survey* (1994).

[59] Jordan National AIDS Control Programme, *Report on the National KABP Survey* (1999).

[60] Jordan National AIDS Control Programme, *Report on the National KABP Survey* (2005).

Similar improvement in attitudes was also reported among university students in Sudan.[61]

Sources of HIV/AIDS knowledge

Television is by far the main source of HIV/AIDS knowledge in MENA. The percentage of different populations who identified television as the main source of their HIV/AIDS knowledge was 98% in Egypt,[62] 83.6% in the Islamic Republic of Iran,[63] 92% in Pakistan,[64] and 90% in Sudan.[65] This has been seen in many other studies (table E.5 in appendix E). Radio is also a major source of HIV/AIDS information in resource-limited parts of the region, such as Sudan.[66] Mass media is undoubtedly the most effective method of disseminating HIV/AIDS knowledge in this region, but messages cannot be sexually explicit due to cultural sensitivities.[67] Television has already proven to be an effective tool in disseminating birth control information during family planning campaigns in MENA.[68] Television has also been reported as a preferred mode of disseminating information, particularly among youth.[69]

Educational institutions are seldom a main source of HIV/AIDS knowledge. Only 24% of high school students in the Islamic Republic of Iran reported educational programs,[70] and only 15% reported schoolbooks,[71] as a source of HIV/AIDS information. In the Republic of Yemen, only 29% heard about HIV/AIDS from their teachers.[72] However, two studies from the Republic of Yemen provide rare examples where schools were the main source of knowledge: 63%[73] and 71.3%[74] of high school students identified schools as a main source of HIV/AIDS knowledge, indicating a potential role for schools in disseminating correct knowledge about HIV/AIDS to youth. Still, 60%[75] and 88.4%[76] of the students also identified television as a main source of knowledge.

Religious leaders are not a main source of HIV/AIDS information in MENA, although strong preference has been reported for them to be the source of HIV/AIDS knowledge.[77] In Jordan, only 7.3%[78] and 11.6%[79] of youth reported religious leaders as a source of information about HIV/AIDS. Parents are also not a main source of HIV/AIDS knowledge. Only 27% of Iranian adolescents reported parents as a source of HIV/AIDS information.[80]

Differentials in HIV/AIDS knowledge

Research in MENA has identified differentials in HIV/AIDS knowledge. Gender differential varies across populations, though males tend to have better knowledge than females. Women appear to have inferior access to HIV/AIDS sources of information compared to men.[81] They may also have limited knowledge about their bodies and reproductive health, leading to feelings of helplessness.[82] In Egypt, female IDUs were found to have significantly less knowledge about HIV/AIDS than male IDUs.[83] In Pakistan,[84] Turkey,[85] and the Republic of Yemen,[86] male youth had better knowledge of HIV/AIDS than female youth. In the Republic of Yemen, 94.3% and 55.6% of males had ever heard of HIV/AIDS and condoms, respectively, but for females, the corresponding percentages were 80.8 and 41, respectively.[87]

[61] Sudan National HIV/AIDS Control Program, *HIV/AIDS/STIs Prevalence.*
[62] Measure DHS, "Egypt: Demographic and Health Survey 2005."
[63] Karimi and Ataei, "The Assessment of Knowledge."
[64] Khan et al., "Awareness about Common Diseases."
[65] SNAP, UNICEF, and UNAIDS, "Baseline Study on Knowledge."
[66] Yousif, "Health Education Programme"; Ahmed, *Sex Sellers;* Ahmed, *Antenatal;* Ahmed, *Tea Sellers;* Ahmed, *Military;* Ahmed, *Truck Drivers;* Ahmed, *Prisoners;* Sudan National HIV/AIDS Control Program, *HIV/AIDS/STIs Prevalence;* UNHCR, "HIV Behavioural Surveillance Survey"; Ahmed, *University Students;* Ahmed, *TB Patients;* Ahmed, *Internally Displaced People;* Ahmed, *Street Children;* Ahmed, *STDs;* Ahmed, *AIDS Patients.*
[67] Lynn, "Pakistan Launches Media Blitz on AIDS."
[68] El-Bakly and Hess, "Mass Media Makes a Difference."
[69] Sudan National HIV/AIDS Control Program, *HIV/AIDS/STIs Prevalence.*
[70] Karimi and Ataei, "The Assessment of Knowledge."
[71] Yazdi et al., "Knowledge, Attitudes and Sources of Information."
[72] Al-Serouri, "Assessment of Knowledge."
[73] Gharamah and Baktayan, "Exploring HIV/AIDS Knowledge."
[74] Raja and Farhan, "Knowledge and Attitude."

[75] Gharamah and Baktayan, "Exploring HIV/AIDS Knowledge."
[76] Raja and Janjua, "Epidemiology of Hepatitis C."
[77] Ibid.
[78] Jordan National AIDS Control Programme, *Report on the National KABP Survey* (2004).
[79] Jordan National AIDS Control Programme, *Report on the National KABP Survey* (2005).
[80] Yazdi et al., "Knowledge, Attitudes and Sources of Information."
[81] Manhart et al., "Sexually Transmitted Diseases in Morocco."
[82] Boyacioglu and Turkmen, "Social and Cultural Dimensions."
[83] Salama et al., "HIV/AIDS Knowledge and Attitudes."
[84] Raza et al., "Knowledge, Attitude and Behaviour."
[85] Savaser, "Knowledge and Attitudes."
[86] Yemen Central Statistical Organization, *Yemen Demographic, Maternal and Child Health Survey 1997.*
[87] Busulwa, "HIV/AIDS Situation Analysis Study."

Bucking the trend, several studies have documented the opposite tendency, probably reflecting female mass education gains over the last few decades.[88] In Afghanistan, female university students were more knowledgeable than males.[89] In the Islamic Republic of Iran, HIV/AIDS knowledge among female high school students,[90] youth,[91] teachers,[92] and prisoners[93] was found to be higher than that of males. In further studies of college students[94] and the general population[95] in the Islamic Republic of Iran, of high school students[96] in Libya, and of high school students[97] in the Republic of Yemen, no gender differential in knowledge was found.

Other common differentials in knowledge are those of urban versus rural populations, and refugees, internally displaced populations, or minorities versus the bulk of the general population. Rural residents have been found, such as in Egypt[98] and Jordan,[99] to have inferior HIV/AIDS knowledge compared to urban populations. Refugees in the Republic of Yemen were found to have lower knowledge than a marginalized minority (Al-Akhdam), and Al-Akhdam were found to have lower knowledge than the rest of the general population.[100]

Other aspects of HIV/AIDS knowledge

It appears that a considerable fraction of women who have heard of HIV/AIDS also know of the risk of transmission from mothers to their babies. In Egypt, 75.8%, 70.4%, and 51.7% of general population women knew that HIV can be transmitted during pregnancy, delivery, and breastfeeding, respectively.[101] In Jordan these percentages were 70.1, 54.6, and 42.3, respectively.[102] In Morocco, 58% knew of the risk of

transmission through breastfeeding.[103] However, in Sudan, only 4.3% to 39.8% of diverse population groups reported knowing about the risk of mother-to-child transmission.[104] Yet in a more recent study, 80% of a general population group in Southern Sudan knew of the risk of mother-to-child transmission during pregnancy and birth, and 71% knew of the risk through breastfeeding.[105]

Finally, it appears that knowledge of STIs other than HIV is substantially lower than that of HIV/AIDS.[106] While 98% of women in Egypt knew of HIV/AIDS, only 21.8% knew of other STIs.[107] In Jordan, only 27.4% of women knew of other STIs,[108] and in Morocco, 69% of general population women declared that they do not know of other STIs.[109] However, a study among a general population in Southern Sudan found that 90% have heard of STIs.[110]

Analytical summary

MENA countries have made considerable gains in increasing HIV/AIDS basic awareness and knowledge in recent years. The vast majority of the populations are aware of HIV/AIDS and some of its transmission modes. Seventy-five percent of university students in Sudan have been exposed to HIV/AIDS education.[111] Substantial gains in knowledge and prevention practices have been reported in Pakistan among priority populations, partially due to an expansion of prevention programs in recent years.[112] Yet, comprehensive and proper knowledge of HIV/AIDS remains elusive, and misinformation, misconceptions, and myths abound. Most people appear to perceive greater risk for others than for themselves, and behavioral practices may be combining a low level of partner

[88] Roudi-Fahimi and Moghadam, "Empowering Women, Developing Society."

[89] Mansoor et al., "Gender Differences in KAP."

[90] Karimi and Ataei, "The Assessment of Knowledge."

[91] Yazdi et al., "Knowledge, Attitudes and Sources of Information."

[92] Mazloomy and Baghianimoghadam, "Knowledge and Attitude."

[93] Nakhaee, "Prisoners' Knowledge."

[94] Simbar, Tehrani, and Hashemi, "Reproductive Health Knowledge."

[95] Montazeri, "AIDS Knowledge."

[96] El-Gadi, Abudher, and Sammud, "HIV-Related Knowledge and Stigma."

[97] Gharamah and Baktayan, "Exploring HIV/AIDS Knowledge."

[98] Measure DHS, "Egypt: Demographic and Health Survey 2005."

[99] Measure DHS, "Jordan: Demographic and Health Survey 2002."

[100] Al-Serouri, "Assessment of Knowledge."

[101] Measure DHS, "Egypt: Demographic and Health Survey 2005."

[102] Measure DHS, "Jordan: Demographic and Health Survey 2002."

[103] Zidouh, "VIH/SIDA et Infections sexuellement transmissibles."

[104] Ahmed, Sex Sellers; Ahmed, Antenatal; Ahmed, Tea Sellers; Ahmed, Military; Ahmed, Truck Drivers; Ahmed, Prisoners; Ahmed, University Students; Ahmed, TB Patients; Ahmed, Internally Displaced People; Ahmed, Street Children; Ahmed, STDs; Ahmed, AIDS Patients.

[105] UNHCR, "HIV Behavioural Surveillance Survey."

[106] SNAP, UNICEF, and UNAIDS, "Baseline Study on Knowledge."

[107] Measure DHS, "Egypt: Demographic and Health Survey 2005."

[108] Measure DHS, "Jordan: Demographic and Health Survey 2002."

[109] Zidouh, "VIH/SIDA et Infections sexuellement transmissibles."

[110] UNHCR, "HIV Behavioural Surveillance Survey."

[111] Sudan National HIV/AIDS Control Program, HIV/AIDS/STIs Prevalence.

[112] Pakistan National AIDS Control Program, HIV Second Generation Surveillance (Rounds I, II, and III).

exchange with widespread disregard for safe sex.[113] There are, however, some encouraging trends, such as in the Islamic Republic of Iran, where more emphasis is placed on safe sex.[114]

Of particular concern is the limited HIV/AIDS knowledge among priority populations, because these are the populations where HIV has the greatest potential for spread. Illiteracy is a barrier to expanding HIV/AIDS knowledge in some countries, such as Afghanistan, where only 47% of males and 15% of females can read.[115] Stakeholders continue to view reproductive health and sex education as encouraging high-risk activities, though increased knowledge has been associated with less risky behavior.[116] HIV/AIDS information is normally acquired through mass media or personal experiences rather than awareness programs.[117] Media and peers may not provide accurate information on sexual health.[118]

There is immense stigma and human rights issues surrounding HIV in MENA. Attitudes toward PLHIV are generally negative and discriminatory. Encouragingly, there appears to be a trend of decreasing discrimination and stigmatization, but the region as a whole is still far from addressing this challenge.

Media and religious scholars are often cited as preferred sources of HIV/AIDS knowledge.[119] Peers, teachers, and HCWs are also cited as preferred sources of HIV/AIDS knowledge.[120] Proper HIV/AIDS knowledge and stigma reduction programs can be expanded by taking advantage of mass media, especially television, and by involving religious scholars in educational campaigns. Educational programs can also contribute to the expansion of knowledge. Even a single educational session has been found to be useful in significantly increasing HIV/AIDS knowledge and awareness in a MENA context.[121] Group education

and individual counseling programs have been proven useful in increasing knowledge in Egypt,[122] the Islamic Republic of Iran,[123] Saudi Arabia,[124] and Sudan.[125] Education should be expanded in schools, colleges, and universities because these institutions are currently far below their potential of being among the main sources and disseminators of HIV/AIDS knowledge.[126] Well-designed peer education programs may also be effective considering the dense social and family networks in MENA.[127] Peer group education has been found effective among prisoners in the Islamic Republic of Iran.[128]

BIBLIOGRAPHY

Aaraj, E. Unknown. "Report on the Situation Analysis on Vulnerable Groups in Beirut, Lebanon." Grey Report.

Abdelwahab, O. 2006. "Prevalence, Knowledge of AIDS and HIV Risk-Related Sexual Behaviour among Police Personnel in Khartoum State, Sudan 2005." XVI International AIDS Conference, Toronto, August 13–18, abstract CDC0792.

Abolfotouh, M. A. 1995. "The Impact of a Lecture on AIDS on Knowledge, Attitudes and Beliefs of Male School-Age Adolescents in the Asir Region of Southwestern Saudi Arabia." *J Community Health* 20: 271–81.

ACORD. 2006. "Qualitative Socio Economic Research on Female Sex Workers and Their Vulnerability to HIV/AIDS in Khartoum State." Agency for Co-operation and Research in Development.

Afshar, P. Unknown. "From the Assessment to the Implementation of Services Available for Drug Abuse and HIV/AIDS Prevention and Care in Prison Setting: The Experience of Iran." PowerPoint presentation.

Agha, S. 2000. "Potential for HIV Transmission among Truck Drivers in Pakistan." *AIDS* 14: 2404–6.

Ahmed, S. M. 2004a. *AIDS Patients: Situation Analysis-Behavioral Survey Results & Discussions*. Report. Sudan National AIDS Control Program.

———. 2004b. *Antenatal: Situation Analysis-Behavioral Survey Results & Discussions*. Report. Sudan National AIDS Control Program.

———. 2004c. *Internally Displaced People: Situation Analysis-Behavioral Survey Results & Discussions*. Report. Sudan National AIDS Control Program.

[113] Chemtob et al., "Getting AIDS."

[114] Kalkhoran and Hale, "AIDS Education in an Islamic Nation."

[115] World Bank, *HIV/AIDS in Afghanistan.*

[116] Grunseit, "Impact of HIV."

[117] Tehrani and Malek-Afzalip, "Knowledge, Attitudes and Practices."

[118] El-Kak et al., "High School Students."

[119] Farah and Hussein, "HIV Prevalence"; Al-Serouri, "Assessment of Knowledge."

[120] Al-Serouri, "Assessment of Knowledge"; Mohammadi et al., "Reproductive Knowledge."

[121] Ergene et al., "A Controlled-Study"; Khan, "Country Watch: Pakistan."

[122] Salama et al., "HIV/AIDS Knowledge and Attitudes."

[123] Jodati et al., "Impact of Education."

[124] Saleh et al., "Impact of Health Education."

[125] Yousif, "Health Education Programme."

[126] Yazdi et al., "Knowledge, Attitudes and Sources of Information"; Jodati et al., "Impact of Education."

[127] Ergene et al., "A Controlled-Study"; Jodati et al., "Impact of Education."

[128] Afshar, "From the Assessment to the Implementation of Services."

———. 2004d. *Military: Situation Analysis-Behavioral Survey Results & Discussions*. Report. Sudan National AIDS Control Program.

———. 2004e. *Prisoners: Situation Analysis-Behavioral Survey Results & Discussions*. Report. Sudan National AIDS Control Program.

———. 2004f. *Sex Sellers: Situation Analysis-Behavioral Survey Results & Discussions*. Report. Sudan National AIDS Control Program.

———. 2004g. *STDs: Situation Analysis-Behavioral Survey Results & Discussions*. Report. Sudan National AIDS Control Program.

———. 2004h. *Street Children: Situation Analysis-Behavioral Survey Results & Discussions*. Report. Sudan National AIDS Control Program.

———. 2004i. *TB Patients: Situation Analysis-Behavioral Survey Results & Discussions*. Report. Sudan National AIDS Control Program.

———. 2004j. *Tea Sellers: Situation Analysis-Behavioral Survey Results & Discussions*. Report. Sudan National AIDS Control Program.

———. 2004k. *Truck Drivers: Situation Analysis-Behavioral Survey Results & Discussions*. Report. Sudan National AIDS Control Program.

———. 2004l. *University Students: Situation Analysis-Behavioral Survey, Results & Discussions*. Report. Sudan National AIDS Control Program.

Alami, K. 2009. "Tendances récentes de l'épidémie à VIH/SIDA en Afrique du nord." Presentation, Research and AIDS Workshop in North Africa/Marrakech, Morocco.

Al-Mutairi, N., A. Joshi, O. Nour-Eldin, A. K. Sharma, I. El-Adawy, and M. Rijhwani. 2007. "Clinical Patterns of Sexually Transmitted Diseases, Associated Sociodemographic Characteristics, and Sexual Practices in the Farwaniya Region of Kuwait." *Int J Dermatol* 46: 594–99.

Al-Serouri, A. W. 2005. "Assessment of Knowledge, Attitudes and Beliefs about HIV/AIDS among Young People Residing in High Risk Communities in Aden Governatore, Republic of Yemen." Society for the Development of Women & Children (SOUL), Education, Health, Welfare; United Nations Children's Fund, Yemen Country Office, HIV/AIDS Project.

Altaf, A., S. A. Shah, N. A. Zaidi, A. Memon, R. Nadeem ur, and N. Wray. 2007. "High Risk Behaviors of Injection Drug Users Registered with Harm Reduction Programme in Karachi, Pakistan." *Harm Reduct J* 4: 7.

Anonymous. 2007. "Improving HIV/AIDS Response among Most at Risk Population in Sudan." Orientation Workshop, 16 April 2007.

Ardalan, A., K. H. Na'ini, A. M. Tabrizi, and A. Jazayeri. 2002. "Sex for Survival: The Future of Runaway Girls." *Social Welfare Research Quarterly* 2: 187–219.

Askarian, M., Z. Hashemi, P. Jaafari, and O. Assadian. 2006. "Knowledge about HIV Infection and Attitude of Nursing Staff toward Patients with AIDS in Iran." *Infect Control Hosp Epidemiol* 27: 48–53.

Asouab, F. 2005. "Risques VIH/SIDA chez UDI et plan d'action 2006–2010." Grey Report.

Assal, M. 2006. "HIV Prevalence, Knowledge, Attitude, Practices, and Risk Factors among Prisoners in Khartoum State, Sudan." Grey Report.

Ati, H. A. 2005. "HIV/AIDS/STIs Social and Geographical Mapping of Prisoners, Tea Sellers and Commercial Sex Workers in Port Sudan Town, Red Sea State." Draft 2, Ockenden International, Sudan.

Badahdah, A. 2005. "Saudi Attitudes towards People Living with HIV/AIDS." *Int J STD AIDS* 16: 837–38.

Baqi, S., S. A. Shah, M. A. Baig, S. A. Mujeeb, and A. Memon. 1999. "Seroprevalence of HIV, HBV, and Syphilis and Associated Risk Behaviours in Male Transvestites (Hijras) in Karachi, Pakistan." *Int J STD AIDS* 10: 300–4.

Basha, H. M. 2006. "Vulnerable Population Research in Darfur." Grey Report.

Blanchard, J. F., A. Khan, and A. Bokhari. 2008. "Variations in the Population Size, Distribution and Client Volume among Female Sex Workers in Seven Cities of Pakistan." *Sex Transm Infect* 84 Suppl 2: ii24–27.

Bokhari, A., N. M. Nizamani, D. J. Jackson, N. E. Rehan, M. Rahman, R. Muzaffar, S. Mansoor, H. Raza, K. Qayum, P. Girault, E. Pisani, and I. Thaver. 2007. "HIV Risk in Karachi and Lahore, Pakistan: An Emerging Epidemic in Injecting and Commercial Sex Networks." *Int J STD AIDS* 18: 486–92.

Boyacioglu, A. O., and A. Turkmen. 2008. "Social and Cultural Dimensions of Pregnancy and Childbirth in Eastern Turkey." *Cult Health Sex* 10: 277–85.

Busulwa, R. 2003. "HIV/AIDS Situation Analysis Study." Conducted in Hodeidah, Taiz and Hadhramut, Republic of Yemen.

Chaouki, N., F. X. Bosch, N. Munoz, C. J. Meijer, B. El Gueddari, A. El Ghazi, J. Deacon, X. Castellsague, and J. M. Walboomers. 1998. "The Viral Origin of Cervical Cancer in Rabat, Morocco." *Int J Cancer* 75: 546–54.

Chemtob, D., B. Damelin, N. Bessudo-Manor, R. Hassman, Y. Amikam, J. M. Zenilman, and D. Tamir. 2006. "Getting AIDS: Not in My Back Yard: Results from a National Knowledge, Attitudes and Practices Survey." *Isr Med Assoc J* 8: 610–14.

DeJong, J., R. Jawad, I. Mortagy, and B. Shepard. 2005. "The Sexual and Reproductive Health of Young People in the Arab Countries and Iran." *Reprod Health Matters* 13: 49–59.

Dewachi, O. 2001. "Men Who Have Sex with Other Men and HIV AIDS: A Situation Analysis in Beirut, Lebanon: HIV/AIDS Prevention through Outreach to Vulnerable Populations." Grey Report, April 29.

Duyan, V., F. Agalar, and I. Sayek. 2001. "Surgeons' Attitudes toward HIV/AIDS in Turkey." *AIDS Care* 13: 243–50.

Eftekhar, M., M.-M. Gouya, A. Feizzadeh, N. Moshtagh, H. Setayesh, K. Azadmanesh, and A.-R. Vassigh. 2008. "Bio-Behavioural Survey on HIV and Its Risk Factors among Homeless Men Who Have Sex with Men in Teharan, 2006–07."

Egypt MOH (Ministry of Health), and Population National AIDS Program. 2006. *HIV/AIDS Biological and Behavioral Surveillance Survey*. Summary report.

El-Bakly, S., and R. W. Hess. 1994. "Mass Media Makes a Difference." *Integration* 13–15.

El Ghrari, K., Z. Terrab, H. Benchikhi, H. Lakhdar, I. Jroundi, and M. Bennani. 2007. "Prevalence of Syphilis and HIV Infection in Female Prison Population in Morocco." *East Mediterr Health J* 13: 774–79.

El-Gadi, S., A. Abudher, and M. Sammud. 2008. "HIV-Related Knowledge and Stigma among High School Students in Libya." *Int J STD AIDS* 19: 178–83.

El-Kak, F. H., R. A. Soweid, C. Taljeh, M. Kanj, and M. C. Shediac-Rizkallah. 2001. "High School Students in Postwar Lebanon: Attitudes, Information Sources, and Perceived Needs Related to Sexual and Reproductive Health." *J Adolesc Health* 29: 153–55.

El-Rahman, A. 2004. "Risky Behaviours for HIV/AIDS Infection among a Sample of Homosexuals in Cairo City, Egypt." XV International AIDS Conference, Bangkok, July 11–16. Abstract WePeC6146.

Elrashied, S. M. 2006. "Generating Strategic Information and Assessing HIV/AIDS Knowledge, Attitude and Behaviour and Practices as well as Prevalence of HIV1 among MSM in Khartoum State, 2005." A draft report submitted to Sudan National AIDS Control Programme. Together Against AIDS Organization (TAG), Khartoum, Sudan.

El-Sayed, N., M. Abdallah, A. Abdel Mobdy, A. Abdel Sattar, E. Aoun, F. Beths, G. Dallabetta, M. Rakha, C. Soliman, and N. Wasef. 2002. "Evaluation of Selected Reproductive Health Infections in Various Egyptian Population Groups in Greater Cairo." MOHP, IMPACT/FHI/USAID.

El-Sayed, N., A. Darwish, and M. El Geneidy. 1994. "Knowledge, Attitude, and Practice of Homosexuals regarding HIV in Egypt." National AIDS Program, Ministry of Health and Population, Egypt.

El-Sayed, N. M., P. J. Gomatos, G. R. Rodier, T. F. Wierzba, A. Darwish, S. Khashaba, and R. R. Arthur. 1996. "Seroprevalence Survey of Egyptian Tourism Workers for Hepatitis B Virus, Hepatitis C Virus, Human Immunodeficiency Virus, and Treponema Pallidum Infections: Association of Hepatitis C Virus Infections with Specific Regions of Egypt." *Am J Trop Med Hyg* 55: 179–84.

El-Sayyed, N., I. A. Kabbash, and M. El-Gueniedy. 2008. "Knowledge, Attitude and Practices of Egyptian Industrial and Tourist Workers towards HIV/AIDS." *East Mediterr Health J* 14: 1126–35.

Elshimi, T., M. Warner-Smith, and M. Aon. 2004. "Blood-Borne Virus Risks of Problematic Drug Users in Greater Cairo." UNAIDS and UNODC, Geneva.

El-Tawila, S., O. El-Gibaly, B. Ibrahim, et al. 1999. *Transitions to Adulthood: A National Survey of Adolescents in Egypt.* Cairo, Egypt: Population Council.

Emmanuel, F., and M. Fatima. 2008. "Coverage to Curb the Emerging HIV Epidemic among Injecting Drug Users in Pakistan: Delivering Prevention Services Where Most Needed." *Int J Drug Policy* 19 Suppl 1: S59–64.

Ergene, T., F. Cok, A. Tumer, and S. Unal. 2005. "A Controlled-Study of Preventive Effects of Peer Education and Single-Session Lectures on HIV/AIDS Knowledge and Attitudes among University Students in Turkey." *AIDS Educ Prev* 17: 268–78.

Faisel, A., and J. Cleland. 2006. "Study of the Sexual Behaviours and Prevalence of STIs among Migrant Men in Lahore, Pakistan." Arjumand and Associates, Centre for Population Studies, London School of Hygiene and Tropical Medicine.

Farah, M. S., and S. Hussein. 2006. "HIV Prevalence, Knowledge, Attitude, Practices and Risk Factors among Truck Drivers in Karthoum State." Sudan National AIDS Program.

Farghaly, A. G., and M. M. Kamal. 1991. "Study of the Opinion and Level of Knowledge about AIDS Problem among Secondary School Students and Teachers in Alexandria." *J Egypt Public Health Assoc* 66: 209–25.

Farhoudi, B., A. Montevalian, M. Motamedi, M. M. Khameneh, M. Mohraz, M. Rassolinejad, S. Jafari, P. Afshar, I. Esmaili, and L. Mohseni. 2003. "Human Immunodeficiency Virus and HIV-Associated Tuberculosis Infection and Their Risk Factors in Injecting Drug Users in Prison in Iran."

Fido, A., and R. Al Kazemi. 2002. "Survey of HIV/AIDS Knowledge and Attitudes of Kuwaiti Family Physicians." *Fam Pract* 19: 682–84.

Genc, M., G. Gunes, L. Karaoglu, and M. Egri. 2005. "AIDS Awareness and Knowledge among Married Women Living in Malatya (Turkey): Implications for Province-Based Prevention Programs." *New Microbiol* 28: 161–64.

Gharamah, F. A., and N. A. Baktayan. 2006. "Exploring HIV/AIDS Knowledge and Attitudes of Secondary School Students (10th & 11th grade) in Al-Tahreer District, Sana'a City." Republic of Yemen, March–April.

Grunseit, A. 1997. "Impact of HIV and Sexual Health Education on the Sexual Behavior of Young People: A Review Update." UNAIDS, Geneva.

Gul, U., A. Kilic, B. Sakizligil, S. Aksaray, S. Bilgili, O. Demirel, and C. Erinckan. 2008. "Magnitude of Sexually Transmitted Infections among Female Sex Workers in Turkey." *J Eur Acad Dermatol Venereol* 22: 1123–24.

Haider, G., N. Zohra, N. Nisar, and A. A. Munir. 2009. "Knowledge about AIDS/HIV Infection among Women Attending Obstetrics and Gynaecology Clinic at a University Hospital." *J Pak Med Assoc* 59: 95–98.

Hajiabdolbaghi, M., N. Razani, N. Karami, P. Kheirandish, M. Mohraz, M. Rasoolinejad, K. Arefnia, Z. Kourorian, G. Rutherford, and W. McFarland. 2007. "Insights from a Survey of Sexual Behavior among a Group of At-Risk Women in Tehran, Iran, 2006." *AIDS Educ Prev* 19: 519–30.

Haque, N., T. Zafar, H. Brahmbhatt, G. Imam, S. ul Hassan, and S. A. Strathdee. 2004. "High-Risk Sexual Behaviours among Drug Users in Pakistan: Implications for Prevention of STDs and HIV/AIDS." *Int J STD AIDS* 15: 601–7.

Hassen, E., A. Chaieb, M. Letaief, H. Khairi, A. Zakhama, S. Remadi, and L. Chouchane. 2003. "Cervical Human Papillomavirus Infection in Tunisian Women." *Infection* 31: 143–48.

Hawkes, S., M. Collumbien, L. Platt, N. Lalji, N. Rizvi, A. Andreasen, J. Chow, R. Muzaffar, H. ur-Rehman, N. Siddiqui, S. Hasan, and A. Bokhari. 2009. "HIV and Other Sexually Transmitted Infections among Men, Transgenders and Women Selling Sex in Two Cities in Pakistan: A Cross-Sectional Prevalence Survey." *Sex Transm Infect* 85 Suppl 2: ii8–16.

Hedayati-Moghaddam, M. R. 2008. "Knowledge of and Attitudes towards HIV/AIDS in Mashhad, Islamic Republic of Iran." *East Mediterr Health J* 14: 1321–32.

Hermez, J. "HIV/AIDS Prevention through Outreach to Vulnerable Populations in Beirut, Lebanon." Final Report, Beirut, Lebanon. Lebanon National AIDS Program.

Hermez, J., E. Aaraj, O. Dewachi, and N. Chemaly. "HIV/AIDS Prevention among Vulnerable Groups in Beirut, Lebanon." PowerPoint presentation, Beirut, Lebanon, Lebanon National AIDS Program.

Holt, B. Y., P. Effler, W. Brady, J. Friday, E. Belay, K. Parker, and M. Toole. 2003. "Planning STI/HIV Prevention among Refugees and Mobile Populations: Situation Assessment of Sudanese Refugees." *Disasters* 27: 1–15.

Hsairi, M., and S. Ben Abdallah. 2007. "Analyse de la situation de vulnérabilité vis-à-vis de l'infection à VIH des hommes ayant des relations sexuelles avec des hommes." For ATL MST sida NGO–Tunis Section, National AIDS Programme/DSSB, UNAIDS. Final report, abridged version.

IGAD (Intergovernmental Authority on Development). 2006. "IGAD/World Bank Cross Border Mobile Population Mapping Exercise." Sudan, draft report.

Ingold, R. 1994. "Rapid Assessment on Illicit Drug Use in Great Beirut." UNDCP.

IRIB. 2006. "Poll of Tehran Public on AIDS." Unpublished.

Jahani, M. R., S. M. Alavian, H. Shirzad, A. Kabir, and B. Hajarizadeh. 2005. "Distribution and Risk Factors of Hepatitis B, Hepatitis C, and HIV Infection in a Female Population with 'Illegal Social Behaviour.'" *Sex Transm Infect* 81: 185.

Jodati, A. R., G. R. Nourabadi, S. Hassanzadeh, S. Dastgiri, and K. Sedaghat. 2007. "Impact of Education in Promoting the Knowledge of and Attitude to HIV/AIDS Prevention: A Trial on 17,000 Iranian Students." *Int J STD AIDS* 18: 407–9.

Jordan National AIDS Control Programme. 1994. *Report on the National KABP Survey on HIV/AIDS among Jordanian Youth*. NAP Jordan.

———. 1999. *Report on the National KABP Survey on HIV/AIDS among Jordanian Youth*. NAP Jordan.

———. 2004. *Report on the National KABP Survey on HIV/AIDS among Jordanian Youth*. NAP Jordan.

———. 2005. *Report on the National KABP Survey on HIV/AIDS among Jordanian Youth*. NAP Jordan.

Jurjus, A. R., J. Kahhaleh, National AIDS Program, and WHO/EMRO (World Health Organization/Eastern Mediterranean Regional Office). 2004. "Knowledge, Attitudes, Beliefs, and Practices of the Lebanese concerning HIV/AIDS." Beirut, Lebanon.

Kabbash, I. A., M. El-Gueneidy, A. Y. Sharaf, N. M. Hassan, and N. Al-Nawawy. 2008. "Needs Assessment and Coping Strategies of Persons Infected with HIV in Egypt." *East Mediterr Health J* 14: 1308–20.

Kabbash, I. A., N. M. El-Sayed, A. N. Al-Nawawy, I. K. Shady, and M. S. Abou Zeid. 2007. "Condom Use among Males (15–49 Years) in Lower Egypt: Knowledge, Attitudes and Patterns of Use." *East Mediterr Health J* 13: 1405–16.

Kalkhoran, S., and L. Hale. 2008. "AIDS Education in an Islamic Nation: Content Analysis of Farsi-Language AIDS-Education Materials in Iran." *Promot Educ* 15: 21–25.

Karimi, I., and B. Ataei. 2007. "The Assessment of Knowledge about AIDS and Its Prevention on Isfahan High School Students." 17th European Congress of Clinical Microbiology and Infectious Diseases, and 25th International Congress of Chemotherapy, Munich, Germany.

Khan, A. A., N. Rehan, K. Qayyum, and A. Khan. 2008. "Correlates and Prevalence of HIV and Sexually Transmitted Infections among Hijras (Male Transgenders) in Pakistan." *Int J STD AIDS* 19: 817–20.

Khan, S. J., Q. Anjum, N. U. Khan, and F. G. Nabi. 2005. "Awareness about Common Diseases in Selected Female College Students of Karachi." *J Pak Med Assoc* 55: 195–98.

Khan, T. M. 1995. "Country Watch: Pakistan." *AIDS STD Health Promot Exch* 7–8.

Khawaja, Z. A., L. Gibney, A. J. Ahmed, and S. H. Vermund. 1997. "HIV/AIDS and Its Risk Factors in Pakistan." *AIDS* 11: 843–48.

Kulczycki, A. 2004. "The Sociocultural Context of Condom Use within Marriage in Rural Lebanon." *Stud Fam Plann* 35: 246–60.

Kuo, I., S. ul-Hasan, N. Galai, D. L. Thomas, T. Zafar, M. A. Ahmed, and S. A. Strathdee. 2006. "High HCV Seroprevalence and HIV Drug Use Risk Behaviors among Injection Drug Users in Pakistan." *Harm Reduct J* 3: 26.

Lazarus, J. V., H. M. Himedan, L. R. Ostergaard, and J. Liljestrand. 2006. "HIV/AIDS Knowledge and Condom Use among Somali and Sudanese Immigrants in Denmark." *Scand J Public Health* 34: 92–99.

Lebanon National AIDS Control Program. 1996. "General Population Evaluation Survey Assessing Knowledge, Attitudes, Beliefs and Practices Related to HIV/AIDS in Lebanon." Ministry of Public Health.

———. 2008. "A Case Study on Behavior Change among Female Sex Workers." Beirut, Lebanon.

Lynn, W. 1994. "Pakistan Launches Media Blitz on AIDS." *Glob AIDSnews* 1–2.

Mahfouz, A. A., W. Alakija, A. A. al-Khozayem, and R. A. al-Erian. 1995. "Knowledge and Attitudes towards AIDS among Primary Health Care Physicians in the Asir Region, Saudi Arabia." *J R Soc Health* 115: 23–25.

Manhart, L. E., A. Dialmy, C. A. Ryan, and J. Mahjour. 2000. "Sexually Transmitted Diseases in Morocco: Gender Influences on Prevention and Health Care Seeking Behavior." *Soc Sci Med* 50: 1369–83.

Mansoor, A. B., W. Fungladda, J. Kaewkungwal, and W. Wongwit. 2008. "Gender Differences in KAP Related to HIV/AIDS among Freshmen in Afghan Universities." *Southeast Asian J Trop Med Public Health* 39: 404–18.

Mazloomy, S. S., and M. H. Baghianimoghadam. 2008. "Knowledge and Attitude about HIV/AIDS of Schoolteachers in Yazd, Islamic Republic of Iran." *East Mediterr Health J* 14: 292–97.

Measure DHS. 1998. "Jordan: Demographic and Health Survey 1997."

———. 2003. "Jordan: Demographic and Health Survey 2002."

———. 2006. "Egypt: Demographic and Health Survey 2005."

———. 2007. "Pakistan Demographic and Health Survey 2006–7." Preliminary report, National Institute for Population Studies, Measure DHS, and Macro International.

Mehryar, A. H., S. Ahmad-Nia, and S. Kazemipour. 2007. "Reproductive Health in Iran: Pragmatic

Achievements, Unmet Needs, and Ethical Challenges in a Theocratic System." *Stud Fam Plann* 38: 352–61.

Ministry of Health and Medical Education of Iran. 2004. *AIDS/HIV Surveillance Report*, Fourth Quarter. Tehran.

Mishwar. 2008. "An Integrated Bio-Behavioral Surveillance Study among Four Vulnerable Groups in Lebanon: Men Who Have Sex with Men; Prisoners; Commercial Sex Workers and Intravenous Drug Users." Final report, Beirut, Lebanon

Mobeireek, A. F., F. Al-Kassimi, K. Al-Zahrani, A. Al-Shimemeri, S. al-Damegh, O. Al-Amoudi, S. Al-Eithan, B. Al-Ghamdi, and M. Gamal-Eldin. 2008. "Information Disclosure and Decision-Making: The Middle East versus the Far East and the West." *J Med Ethics* 34: 225–29.

Mohammad, K., F. K. Farahani, M. R. Mohammadi, S. Alikhani, M. Zare, F. R. Tehrani, A. Ramezankhani, A. Hasanzadeh, and H. Ghanbari. 2007. "Sexual Risk-Taking Behaviors among Boys Aged 15–18 Years in Tehran." *J Adolesc Health* 41: 407–14.

Mohammadi, M. R., K. Mohammad, F. K. Farahani, S. Alikhani, M. Zare, F. R. Tehrani, A. Ramezankhani, and F. Alaeddini. 2006. "Reproductive Knowledge, Attitudes and Behavior among Adolescent Males in Tehran, Iran." *Int Fam Plan Perspect* 32: 35–44.

Montazeri, A. 2005. "AIDS Knowledge and Attitudes in Iran: Results from a Population-Based Survey in Tehran." *Patient Educ Couns* 57: 199–203.

Morocco MOH. 2004. "Survey on Population and Family Health."

———. 2007. "Survey of Knowledge, Attitude, and Practices of Sex Workers on STD and AIDS." National Programme of Fight against AIDS.

———. Unknown. "Situation épidémiologique actuelle du VIH/SIDA au Maroc."

Morocco MOH, with the support of GTZ. 2007. "Knowledge, Attitudes, and Practices of Youth Regarding STDs and AIDS."

Moszynski, P. 2008. "Egyptian Doctors Who Took Part in Forced HIV Testing 'Violated Medical Ethics.'" *BMJ* 336: 855.

Nakhaee, F. H. 2002. "Prisoners' Knowledge of HIV/AIDS and Its Prevention in Kerman, Islamic Republic of Iran." *East Mediterr Health J* 8: 725–31.

Narenjiha, H., H. Rafiey, A. Baghestani, et al. 2005. "Rapid Situation Assessment of Drug Abuse and Drug Dependence in Iran." DARIUS Institute (draft version, in Persian).

NSNAC (New Sudan AIDS Council), and UNAIDS (United Nations Joint Programme on HIV/AIDS). 2006. *HIV/AIDS Integrated Report South Sudan, 2004–2005*. With United Nations General Assembly Special Session on HIV/AIDS Declaration of Commitment.

Oman MOH (Ministry of Health). 2006. "HIV Risk among Heroin and Injecting Drug Users in Muscat, Oman." Quantitative Survey, Preliminary Data.

Pakistan National AIDS Control Program. 2005. *HIV Second Generation Surveillance in Pakistan*. National Report Round 1. Ministry of Health, Pakistan, and Canada-Pakistan HIV/AIDS Surveillance Project.

———. 2006–7. *HIV Second Generation Surveillance in Pakistan*. National Report Round II. Ministry of Health, Pakistan, and Canada-Pakistan HIV/AIDS Surveillance Project.

———. 2008. *HIV Second Generation Surveillance in Pakistan*. National Report Round III. Ministry of Health, Pakistan, Canada-Pakistan HIV/AIDS Surveillance Project.

Paruk, Z., S. D. Mohamed, C. Patel, and S. Ramgoon. 2006. "Compassion or Condemnation? South African Muslim Students' Attitudes to People with HIV/AIDS." *Sahara J* 3: 510–15.

Parviz, S., Z. Fatmi, A. Altaf, J. B. McCormick, S. Fischer-Hoch, M. Rahbar, and S. Luby. 2006. "Background Demographics and Risk Behaviors of Injecting Drug Users in Karachi, Pakistan." *Int J Infect Dis* 10: 364–71.

PFPPA. 2005. "Assessment of Palestinian Students' Knowledge about AIDS and Their Attitudes toward the AIDS Patient." Jerusalem, Palestine.

Platt, L., P. Vickerman, M. Collumbien, S. Hasan, N. Lalji, S. Mayhew, R. Muzaffar, A. Andreasen, and S. Hawkes. 2009. "Prevalence of HIV, HCV and Sexually Transmitted Infections among Injecting Drug Users in Rawalpindi and Abbottabad, Pakistan: Evidence for an Emerging Injection-Related HIV Epidemic." *Sex Transm Infect* 85 Suppl 2: ii17–22.

Population Studies Research Institute. 2000. "Baseline Survey on Reproductive Health and Family Planning in Northeast and Northwest Regions of Somalia." University of Nairobi, WHO.

Rady, A. 2005. "Knowledge, Attitudes and Prevalence of Condom Use among Female Sex Workers in Lebanon: Behavioral Surveillance Study." UNFPA.

Raja, N. S., and K. A. Janjua. 2008. "Epidemiology of Hepatitis C Virus Infection in Pakistan." *J Microbiol Immunol Infect* 41: 4–8.

Raja, Y., and A. Farhan. 2005. "Knowledge and Attitude of 10th and 11th Grade Students towards HIV/AIDS in Aden Governorate." Republic of Yemen, Grey Report.

Rajabali, A., S. Khan, H. J. Warraich, M. R. Khanani, and S. H. Ali. 2008. "HIV and Homosexuality in Pakistan." *Lancet Infect Dis* 8: 511–15.

Raza, M. I., A. Afifi, A. J. Choudhry, and H. I. Khan. 1998. "Knowledge, Attitude and Behaviour towards AIDS among Educated Youth in Lahore, Pakistan." *J Pak Med Assoc* 48: 179–82.

Refaat, A. 2004. "Practice and Awareness of Health Risk Behaviour among Egyptian University Students." *East Mediterr Health J* 10: 72–81.

Rodier, G. R., J. J. Morand, J. S. Olson, D. M. Watts, and S. Said. 1993. "HIV Infection among Secondary School Students in Djibouti, Horn of Africa: Knowledge, Exposure and Prevalence." *East Afr Med J* 70: 414–17.

Roudi, F. 1999. "Iran's Revolutionary Approach to Family Planning." *Popul Today* 27: 4–5.

Roudi-Fahimi, F., and V. M. Moghadam. 2003. "Empowering Women, Developing Society: Female Education in the Middle East and North Africa." Population Reference Bureau.

Salama, I. I., N. K. Kotb, S. A. Hemeda, and F. Zaki. 1998. "HIV/AIDS Knowledge and Attitudes among Alcohol and Drug Abusers in Egypt." *J Egypt Public Health Assoc* 73: 479–500.

Saleem, N. H., A. Adrien, and A. Razaque. 2008. "Risky Sexual Behavior, Knowledge of Sexually Transmitted

Infections and Treatment Utilization among a Vulnerable Population in Rawalpindi, Pakistan." *Southeast Asian J Trop Med Public Health* 39: 642–48.

Saleh, M. A., Y. S. al-Ghamdi, O. A. al-Yahia, T. M. Shaqran, and A. R. Mosa. 1999. "Impact of Health Education Program on Knowledge about AIDS and HIV Transmission in Students of Secondary Schools in Buraidah City, Saudi Arabia: An Exploratory Study." *East Mediterr Health J* 5: 1068–75.

Sanders-Buell, E., M. D. Saad, A. M. Abed, M. Bose, C. S. Todd, S. A. Strathdee, B. A. Botros, N. Safi, K. C. Earhart, P. T. Scott, N. Michael, and F. E. McCutchan. 2007. "A Nascent HIV Type 1 Epidemic among Injecting Drug Users in Kabul, Afghanistan Is Dominated by Complex AD Recombinant Strain, CRF35_AD." *AIDS Res Hum Retroviruses* 23: 834–39.

Savaser, S. 2003. "Knowledge and Attitudes of High School Students about AIDS: A Turkish Perspective." *Public Health Nurs* 20: 71–79.

Scott, D. A., A. L. Corwin, N. T. Constantine, M. A. Omar, A. Guled, M. Yusef, C. R. Roberts, and D. M. Watts. 1991. "Low Prevalence of Human Immunodeficiency Virus-1 (HIV-1), HIV-2, and Human T Cell Lymphotropic Virus-1 Infection in Somalia." *American Journal of Tropical Medicine and Hygiene* 45: 653.

Shouman, A. E., and A. A. Fotouh. 1995. "The Impact of Health Education on the Knowledge and Attitude of Egyptian Nurses towards Occupational HIV Infection." *J Egypt Public Health Assoc* 70: 25–35.

Simbar, M., F. R. Tehrani, and Z. Hashemi. 2005. "Reproductive Health Knowledge, Attitudes and Practices of Iranian College Students." *East Mediterr Health J* 11: 888–97.

SNAP (Sudan National AIDS Program), UNICEF (United Nations Children's Fund), and UNAIDS (United Nations Joint Programme on HIV/AIDS). 2005. "Baseline Study on Knowledge, Attitudes, and Practices on Sexual Behaviors and HIV/AIDS Prevention amongst Young People in Selected States in Sudan." HIV/AIDS KAPB Report, Projects and Research Department (AFROCENTER Group).

Somaliland Ministry of Health and Labour. 2007. *Somaliland 2007 HIV/Syphilis Seroprevalence Survey: A Technical Report.* Ministry of Health and Labour in collaboration with WHO, UNAIDS, UNICEF/GFATM, and SOLNAC.

Štulhofer, A., and I. Božicevic. 2008. "HIV Bio-Behavioural Survey among FSWs in Aden, Yemen." Grey Report.

Sudan National HIV/AIDS Control Program. 2004. *HIV/AIDS/STIs Prevalence, Knowledge, Attitude, Practices and Risk Factors among University Students and Military Personnel.* Federal Ministry of Health, Khartoum.

Syria Mental Health Directorate. 2008. "Assessment of HIV Risk and Sero-Prevalence among Drug Users in Greater Damascus." Programme SNA, Syrian Ministry of Health, UNODC, UNAIDS.

Syria MOH (Ministry of Health). 2004. "HIV/AIDS Female Sex Workers KABP in Syria." National AIDS Program.

Tavoosi, A., A. Zaferani, A. Enzevaei, P. Tajik, and Z. Ahmadinezhad. 2004. "Knowledge and Attitude towards HIV/AIDS among Iranian Students." *BMC Public Health* 4: 17.

Tehrani, F. R., and H. Malek-Afzalip. 2008. "Knowledge, Attitudes and Practices concerning HIV/AIDS among Iranian At-Risk Sub-Populations." *Eastern Mediterranean Health Journal* 14.

Todd, C. S., M. Ahmadzai, F. Atiqzai, H. Siddiqui, P. Azfar, S. Miller, J. M. Smith, S. A. S. Ghazanfar, and S. A. Strathdee. 2007. "Seroprevalence and Correlates of HIV, Syphilis, and Hepatitis B and C Infection among Antenatal Patients and Testing Practices and Knowledge among Obstetric Care Providers in Kabul." PowerPoint presentation.

UNAIDS (United Nations Joint Programme on HIV/AIDS). 2007. "Key Findings on HIV Status in the West Bank and Gaza." Working document, RST, MENA.

UNAIDS, and WHO (World Health Organization). 2005. *AIDS Epidemic Update 2005.* Geneva.

UNHCR (United Nations High Commissioner for Refugees). 2007. "HIV Behavioural Surveillance Survey Juba Municipality, South Sudan." Grey Report.

Wassef, H. H., E. Fox, E. A. Abbatte, J. F. Toledo, and G. Rodier. 1989. "Knowledge of Sexually Transmitted Diseases and Attitudes towards Them in Populations at Risk in Djibouti." *Bull World Health Organ* 67: 549–53.

WHO (World Health Organization). 2004. *The 2004 First National Second Generation HIV/AIDS/STI Sentinel Surveillance Survey, Somalia: A Technical Report.* Grey Report.

WHO/EMRO (Eastern Mediterranean Regional Office). 2000. "Presentation of WHO Somalia's Experience in Supporting the National Response." Regional Consultation towards Improving HIV/AIDS & STD Surveillance in the Countries of EMRO, Beirut, Lebanon, Oct. 30–Nov. 2.

World Bank. 2006. *HIV/AIDS in Afghanistan.* South Asia Region.

———. 2008. "Mapping and Situation Assessment of Key Populations at High Risk of HIV in Three Cities of Afghanistan." Human Development Sector, South Asia Region (SAR) AIDS Team, World Bank.

Yazdi, C. A., K. Aschbacher, A. Arvantaj, H. M. Naser, E. Abdollahi, A. Asadi, M. Mousavi, M. R. Narmani, M. Kianpishe, F. Nicfallah, and A. K. Moghadam. 2006. "Knowledge, Attitudes and Sources of Information regarding HIV/AIDS in Iranian Adolescents." *AIDS Care* 18: 1004–10.

Yemen Central Statistical Organization. 1998. *Yemen Demographic, Maternal and Child Health Survey 1997.* Macro International. Calverton, MD: Central Statistical Organization and Macro International.

Yousif, M. E. A. 2006. "Health Education Programme among Female Sex Workers in Wad Medani Town-Gezira State." Final report.

Zamani, S., M. Kihara, M. M. Gouya, M. Vazirian, M. Ono-Kihara, E. M. Razzaghi, and S. Ichikawa. 2005. "Prevalence of and Factors Associated with HIV-1 Infection among Drug Users Visiting Treatment Centers in Tehran, Iran." *AIDS* 19: 709–16.

Zargooshi, J. 2002. "Characteristics of Gonorrhoea in Kermanshah, Iran." *Sex Transm Infect* 78: 460–61.

Zidouh, A. Unknown. "VIH/SIDA et Infections sexuellement transmissibles: connaissance et attitudes." Grey Report.

Chapter 9

HIV/AIDS and Vulnerability Settings

Vulnerable populations are defined in our conceptual framework as subpopulations within the general population who are in principle not at high risk of human immunodeficiency virus (HIV) infection, such as prisoners, youth, and mobile populations, but are vulnerable, because of the nature of their living experiences, to practices that may expose them to HIV. Once these vulnerable populations adopt high-risk practices, they are no longer part of our definition of the general population, but become part of the high-risk priority or bridging populations.

The settings of vulnerabilities in the Middle East and North Africa (MENA) are diverse and a large fraction of the population belongs to one or multiple vulnerability settings. A number of populations have been widely identified as vulnerable in the MENA context including prisoners, youth, refugees, internally displaced persons (IDPs), migrant workers, industrial zone workers, fishermen, road builders, the unemployed, sexual partners of injecting drug users (IDUs), tea and *qat* sellers, *geeza* women (serve men who chew *qat*)[1], domestic maids, noninjecting drug users, frequent travelers, tourism workers, health care workers (HCWs), street children, runaway and divorced women, minorities (such as the 200,000 Al-Akhdam in the Republic of Yemen[2]), and temporary and casual workers.

A number of general vulnerability factors have also been identified in the region. These include weak systems of surveillance for all sexually transmitted infections (STIs), a seasonal influx of tourists from both within and outside the region, migrant workers engaging in risky behavior while abroad, a low level of condom knowledge and use, and a lack of adequate knowledge of HIV/AIDS.

Considering the established evidence in other regions of vulnerabilities driving HIV transmission,[3] this chapter discusses the settings of vulnerability from the angle of how these vulnerabilities may contribute as drivers of the region's HIV epidemic. This chapter focuses on the three key vulnerable populations: prisoners, youth, and mobile populations.

PRISONERS AND HIV

The prison environment is conducive to high-risk behaviors, and priority groups, such as IDUs, are often vastly overrepresented among prison inmates.[4] Imprisonment and repeated imprisonments are common among IDUs.[5] Outbreaks of HIV among prisoners driven by

---

[1] Tchupo, *Les maladies sexuellement transmissibles.*
[2] Busulwa, "HIV/AIDS Situation Analysis Study"; Al Ahmadi and Beatty, "Participatory-Socio Economic Needs Survey."

[3] Parker, Easton, and Klein, "Structural Barriers and Facilitators in HIV Prevention."
[4] Gaughwin, Douglas, and Wodak, "Behind Bars."
[5] Dolan et al., "HIV in Prison."

IDU have been reported in different countries around the globe.[6]

The prison population is dynamic, with prisoners and staff moving in and out on a frequent basis.[7] There is extensive evidence of a higher risk of HIV infection among prisoners in both developing[8] and developed settings.[9] In the United States, one-fourth of the people living with HIV (PLHIV) pass through a correctional facility every year.[10] Also in the United States, having sex with a partner who has been incarcerated is a major HIV risk factor for African American women.[11]

The proportion of people who engage in high-risk behavior in prisons is known to be higher than that in the rest of the population.[12] There is a history of prisons serving as a "social petri dish" for increasing the HIV epidemic.[13] The evidence reviewed below suggests that the prisoner population in MENA is a key HIV vulnerable population.

HIV prevalence among prisoners

Different levels of HIV prevalence have been documented among prisoners in MENA. HIV prevalence among prisoners is generally found to be much higher than that of the general population.[14] Outbreaks of HIV infection in prisons have been documented in several MENA countries.[15] HIV incidence among IDUs in a detention center was found to be at very high levels of 16.8% per person per year, in a study in the Islamic Republic of Iran.[16] HIV prevalence among prisoners in Sudan increased from 2% in 2002[17] to 8.6% in 2006.[18] Country surveillance reports of notified HIV/AIDS cases repeatedly document HIV infection among prisoners.[19] High levels of

hepatitis C virus (HCV) prevalence, a proxy of IDU, of as much as 78% were found among prisoners in MENA, suggesting the prevalence of current or previous injecting drug use.[20]

HIV prevalence among prisoners in select MENA countries can be found in table 9.1.[21] Though overall HIV prevalence levels are lower than those found among prisoners in Latin America, South Asia, and sub-Saharan Africa,[22] they are still substantial in several countries.

Imprisonment rates

Imprisonment rates in MENA are not as high as in some other regions, with some notable exceptions.[23] Table 9.1 shows imprisonment rates in several countries for which there are data.[24] The prison population in MENA appears to be dynamic. In the Islamic Republic of Iran, during the 2004–5 Persian fiscal year, there were on average 135,000 prisoners in 230 prisons, but 600,000 persons entered and exited prisons at this time.[25] The Islamic Republic of Iran has made efforts to reduce the prison population by 25% through a comprehensive approach including reducing the terms for drug-related charges, faster prosecution procedures, and alternative penalties to imprisonment for drug-related crimes, but still the rate is high at 185 per 100,000 persons.[26] About half of the prisoners in the Islamic Republic of Iran are first-time offenders and about half spend under 11 days incarcerated.[27]

Risk behaviors and prisons

The risk and vulnerability factors cited for prisons in MENA include injecting and noninjecting drug use, tattooing, sharing of razors, unprotected

[6] Dolan and Wodak, "HIV Transmission"; Bobrik et al., "Prison Health in Russia"; Taylor et al., "Outbreak of HIV Infection in a Scottish Prison."
[7] Dolan et al., "HIV in Prison."
[8] Ibid.
[9] Dolan and Wodak, "HIV Transmission "; Pont et al., "HIV Epidemiology and Risk Behavior."
[10] Spaulding et al., "Human Immunodeficiency Virus."
[11] Ibid.
[12] Bray and Marsden, "Drug Use in Metropolitan America."
[13] Mutter, Grimes, and Labarthe, "Evidence of Intraprison Spread of HIV."
[14] Spaulding et al., "Human Immunodeficiency Virus."
[15] Dolan et al., "HIV in Prison."
[16] Jahani et al., "HIV Seroconversion."
[17] Ahmed, Prisoners.
[18] Assal, "HIV Prevalence."
[19] WHO/EMRO Regional Database on HIV/AIDS.

[20] Khani and Vakili, "Prevalence and Risk Factors of HIV"; Alizadeh et al., "Prevalence of Hepatitis C"; Nassirimanesh, "Proceedings of the Abstract"; Zali et al., "Anti-HCV Antibody among Iranian IV Drug Users"; Quinti et al., "Seroprevalence of HIV and HCV "; Afshar, "From the Assessment to the Implementation of Services"; Mutter, Grimes, and Labarthe, "Evidence of Intraprison Spread of HIV"; Javadi, Avijgan, and Hafizi, "Prevalence of HBV and HCV Infections."
[21] Dolan et al., "HIV in Prison."
[22] Ibid.
[23] Dolan et al., "HIV in Prison."
[24] Dolan et al., "HIV in Prison"; International Centre for Prison Studies, World Prison Brief Country Profiles.
[25] Iran Prison Organization, "Health and Treatment Headquarter."
[26] Burrows, Wodak, and WHO, Harm Reduction in Iran; S. Zamani personal communication (2008).
[27] Mostashari, UNODC, and Darabi, "Summary of the Iranian Situation on HIV Epidemic."

Table 9.1 Imprisonment Rates and HIV Prevalence in Select MENA Countries

Country	Imprisonment (per 100,000)	HIV prevalence in prisons
Afghanistan	30 (International Centre for Prison Studies 2006)	
Algeria	158 (International Centre for Prison Studies 2006)	
Bahrain	95 (International Centre for Prison Studies 2006)	
Djibouti	61 (Dolan et al. 2007; International Centre for Prison Studies 2006)	6.1% (Shrestha 1999)
Egypt, Arab Republic of	About 121 (Dolan et al. 2007; International Centre for Prison Studies 2006)	0.0% (El-Ghazzawi, Hunsmann, and Schneider 1987) 0.0% (Egypt Ministry of Health and Population 2001) 1.6% (Quinti et al. 1995)
Iran, Islamic Republic of	191 (Dolan et al. 2007; International Centre for Prison Studies 2006) 185 (Burrows, Wodak, and WHO 2005)	2% (UNAIDS and WHO 2002; UNAIDS 2002) 1.4% (UNAIDS and WHO 2001) 2.3% (UNAIDS and WHO 2001) 12% (UNAIDS and WHO 2002) 2.1% (mostly IDUs; Afshar [unknown (a)]) 2.3% (mostly IDUs; Afshar [unknown (a)]) 3.3% (mostly IDUs; Afshar [unknown (a)]) 0.9% (injecting and noninjecting drug users; Alizadeh et al. 2005) 24.4% (IDUs; Jahani et al. 2009) 7.0% (IDUs; Rahbar, Rooholamini, and Khoshnood 2004) 22.0% (IDUs; Farhoudi et al. 2003) 24.0% (IDUs; Farhoudi et al. 2003) 12.0% (UNAIDS and WHO 2002) Up to 63.0% (UNAIDS 2002) 22–24% (Spaulding et al. 2002) 6% (Spaulding et al. 2002) 2.5% (Ghannad et al. 2009) 2.4% (Ghannad et al. 2009) 1.9% (Ghannad et al. 2009) 2.3% (Ghannad et al. 2009)
Iraq	About 60 (Dolan et al. 2007; International Centre for Prison Studies 2006)	0.0% (Shrestha 1999) 0.0% (Jordan National AIDS Program, personal communication)
Jordan	104 (International Centre for Prison Studies 2006)	0.0% (Jordan National AIDS Program, personal communication)
Kuwait	130 (International Centre for Prison Studies 2006)	
Lebanon	145 (Dolan et al. 2007; International Centre for Prison Studies 2006)	0.7% (Shrestha 1999) 0.16% (Mishwar 2008)
Libya	207 (Dolan et al. 2007; International Centre for Prison Studies 2006)	18.0% (Sammud 2005) 60.0% (detention for treatment; Dolan et al. 2007)

(continued)

Table 9.1 *(Continued)*

Country	Imprisonment (per 100,000)	HIV prevalence in prisons
Morocco	174 (Dolan et al. 2007; International Centre for Prison Studies 2006)	0.8% (Ministère de la Santé Maroc 2003–04) 0.7% (Elharti et al. 2002) 0.0% (women; Elharti et al. 2002) 2.0% (women; El Ghrari et al. 2007) 0.0% (women; Khattabi and Alami 2005) 0.72% (women; Khattabi and Alami 2005) 0.0% (women; Khattabi and Alami 2005) 1.2% (women; Khattabi and Alami 2005) 2.11% (women; Morocco MOH 2007) 0.9% (female prisoners imprisoned for sex work; Khattabi and Alami 2005) 0.70% (men; Khattabi and Alami 2005) 1.18% (men; Khattabi and Alami 2005) 0.80% (men; Khattabi and Alami 2005) 0.61% (men; Khattabi and Alami 2005) 0.53% (men; Morocco MOH 2007)
Oman	81 (Dolan et al. 2007; International Centre for Prison Studies 2006)	0.2% (Shrestha 1999) 0.14% (UNAIDS 2008)
Pakistan	55 (International Centre for Prison Studies 2006)	0.3% (Baqi et al. 1998) 1.1% (women; Baqi et al. 1998) 1.64% (Mujeeb and Hafeez 1993) 2.8% (Safdar, Mehmood, and Abbas 2009) 0.7% (Safdar, Mehmood, and Abbas 2009) 10% (Safdar, Mehmood, and Abbas 2009) 0.5% (Safdar, Mehmood, and Abbas 2009) 0.4% (Safdar, Mehmood, and Abbas 2009) 0.5% (Safdar, Mehmood, and Abbas 2009) 0.3% (Safdar, Mehmood, and Abbas 2009) 2.1% (Safdar, Mehmood, and Abbas 2009) 0.7% (Safdar, Mehmood, and Abbas 2009) 1.0% (Safdar, Mehmood, and Abbas 2009)
Qatar	55 (International Centre for Prison Studies 2006)	
Somalia		0.0% (Ahmed 1997)
Sudan	About 36 (International Centre for Prison Studies 2006)	0.0% (Burans et al. 1990) 2.0% (UNAIDS 2008) 8.63% (Assal 2006) 27.1% (women; Assal 2006)
Syrian Arab Republic	93 (Dolan et al. 2007; International Centre for Prison Studies 2006)	0–0.2% (Shrestha 1999)
Tunisia	253 (Dolan et al. 2007; International Centre for Prison Studies 2006)	0.0% (Shrestha 1999)
United Arab Emirates	288 (International Centre for Prison Studies 2006)	
Yemen, Republic of	83 (Dolan et al. 2007; International Centre for Prison Studies 2006)	26.5% (Shrestha 1999)

Note: Table adapted from Dolan et al. (2007). Data not available for empty cells.

sex, overcrowding, poor medical facilities, an unhealthy environment, inadequate awareness and education programs, and bullying.[28]

Imprisonment as a risk factor for HIV infection

Several studies have documented the link between HIV infection and incarceration in MENA, mainly in the Islamic Republic of Iran. This link arises from the vulnerability of prisoners to risky practices such as using nonsterile drug-injecting equipment and having unprotected sex while in prison. HIV prevalence among repeat prisoners in the Islamic Republic of Iran was 22%–24%, which is much higher than that of first-time prisoners at 6%.[29] Among HIV and tuberculosis (TB) coinfected persons in the Islamic Republic of Iran, 80% reported a history of imprisonment.[30] HIV infection was significantly associated with imprisonment and the use of nonsterile injecting equipment in prison in several studies in the Islamic Republic of Iran.[31] Among PLHIV in the Islamic Republic of Iran, 74% reported a history of incarceration.[32]

Drug use and incarceration

Ample evidence suggests a strong link between drug use and incarceration in MENA. Fifty-seven percent of IDUs in Afghanistan have been incarcerated, of whom 71.6% were incarcerated for drug-related offenses.[33] Forty-eight percent of prisoners in the Islamic Republic of Iran enter prison for drug-related crimes and 64% of them have a history of drug use.[34] In 2001, the Islamic Republic of Iran reported that more than 300,000 people were arrested on drug-related charges and 47% of the prison population was incarcerated for drug-related offenses.[35] Almost 64% (treatment centers) and 94% (community-based) of IDUs in the Islamic Republic of Iran reported a history of incarceration.[36] In further

studies in the Islamic Republic of Iran, 41%,[37] 75%,[38] and 74.3%[39] of IDUs reported being previously imprisoned, and 6% of prisoners reported starting drug injection while in prison.[40]

Among prisoners in Lebanon, 12% reported a history of injecting drugs.[41] Two percent of female prisoners in Morocco reported IDU.[42] Between 61% and 83% of IDUs in Oman reported ever being arrested for drug-related offenses.[43] One-third of IDUs in one study in Pakistan have been incarcerated in the previous year,[44] and 14% and 40% of IDUs in two other settings reported a history of imprisonment.[45] Twenty-six percent of prisoners in Sudan reported drug use, of whom 8.4% injected drugs prior to incarceration.[46] In the Syrian Arab Republic, 55% of a group, half of which are IDUs, reported a history of imprisonment, and in 68% of the cases, the imprisonment was due to drug-related offenses.[47]

Injecting drug use in prisons

Injecting drug use in prisons appears to be present in several MENA countries. Evidence for this practice in the Islamic Republic of Iran has been firmly established through multiple studies. Drugs are easily available in prisons, although five to eight times as expensive.[48] Between 27.6% and 53.6% of IDUs reported ever injecting drugs in prison,[49] and about 10% of prisoners are believed to inject drugs.[50] Fifty-two percent of inmates confirmed the occurrence of injections in prisons.[51] One study found that one-third of IDUs

---

[28] Assal, "HIV Prevalence, Knowledge, Attitude, Practices, and Risk Factors among Prisoners in Khartoum State, Sudan."

[29] Spaulding et al., "Human Immunodeficiency Virus in Correctional Facilities."

[30] Tabarsi et al., "Clinical and Laboratory Profile."

[31] Zamani et al., "Prevalence of and Factors Associated with HIV-1 Infection"; Zamani et al., "High Prevalence of HIV"; Kheirandish et al., "Prevalence and Correlates of Hepatitis C "; Zamani et al., "Shared Drug Injection inside Prison."

[32] Ramezani, Mohraz, and Gachkar, "Epidemiologic Situation."

[33] Todd et al., "HIV, Hepatitis C, and Hepatitis B Infections."

[34] Afshar, "Health and Prison."

[35] UNODC, "Drug Situation in the I.R. of Iran."

[36] Zamani et al., "Shared Drug Injection inside Prison."

[37] Day et al., "Patterns of Drug Use."

[38] Razzaghi, Rahimi, and Hosseini, *Rapid Situation Assessment (RSA) of Drug Abuse.*

[39] Kheirandish et al., "Prevalence and Correlates of Hepatitis C."

[40] Farhoudi et al., "Human Immunodeficiency Virus and HIV-Associated Tuberculosis Infection."

[41] Mishwar, "An Integrated Bio-Behavioral Surveillance Study."

[42] El Ghrari et al., "Prevalence of Syphilis and HIV."

[43] Oman MOH, "HIV Risk among Heroin and Injecting Drug Users."

[44] Pakistan National AIDS Control Program, *National Study of Reproductive Tract.*

[45] Platt et al., "Prevalence of HIV, HCV, and Sexually Transmitted Infections."

[46] Ati, "HIV/AIDS/STIs Social and Geographical Mapping."

[47] Syria Mental Health Directorate, "Assessment of HIV Risk and Sero-Prevalence."

[48] Zamani, "Methadone Maintenance Treatment (MMT)."

[49] Farhoudi et al., "Human Immunodeficiency Virus and HIV-Associated Tuberculosis Infection."

[50] UNAIDS and WHO, *AIDS Epidemic Update 2002.*

[51] Bolhari and Mirzamani, "Assessment of Substance Abuse in Iran's Prisons."

continue their drug use in prison,[52] while another reported that 85% of IDUs used drugs in prison.[53] A study found that 28% of community-based IDUs with a history of incarceration have injected drugs in prisons,[54] and another reported that 9.7% of drug-using inmates continued to use drugs, mostly heroin, while in prison.[55]

Also in the Islamic Republic of Iran, opioid use prevalence while in prison was found to be 30.7%, though 54.3% of inmates used drugs before incarceration, indicating a reduction in drug use during incarceration.[56] About 25%–30% of prisoners used drugs in prison in one study,[57] with another study indicating that about 30% of prisoners attempt to use drugs in prison and 17%–23% of prisoners use drugs by injection.[58] In further studies, 91% of IDUs and non-injecting drug users ever imprisoned reported using drugs while in prison,[59] and 18.9% and 6.1% reported using opioid and injecting drugs while in prison, respectively.[60]

Other studies have also observed IDU in prisons in other MENA countries. In Algeria, 67% of those incarcerated reported using drugs in prison.[61] In the Arab Republic of Egypt, about 25% of IDUs who had been incarcerated reported injecting drugs in prison.[62] In Lebanon, only 0.16% of prisoners, including IDUs, reported injecting while in prison.[63] In Oman, 26%–44% of IDUs reported drug use in prison and 5%–11% reported injecting drugs in prison.[64] In Syria, 11% of imprisoned IDUs injected drugs in prison.[65]

The prison environment is possibly compelling noninjecting drug users to inject while in prison due to the difficulty of clandestine smoking and scarcity of raw opium.[66] The higher cost of obtaining drugs in prison has also been cited as a reason for injecting drugs because it is the most cost-effective method of using drugs.[67] Inmates find multiple ways of paying for drugs in prison, such as through family financial support, drug dealing, prison work, sex work, forcing their wives to do sex work, selling food and personal effects, gambling, credit, and extortion.[68]

Use of nonsterile injecting equipment in prisons

Although predominantly from the Islamic Republic of Iran, evidence indicates the use of nonsterile injecting equipment in prisons. Studies in the Islamic Republic of Iran found, respectively, that 19%,[69] 29.9%,[70] and 37.1%[71] of IDUs reported using nonsterile injection equipment in prison. In further studies in the Islamic Republic of Iran, 82% of those with a history of IDU in prison have injected drugs using nonsterile utensils,[72] and 23% of community-based IDUs reported using nonsterile drug injection utensils in prison.[73] Twenty-three percent of prisoners in another study used drugs mostly with nonsterile and handmade utensils.[74]

There is also evidence from other countries of using nonsterile injecting equipment in prisons. In Afghanistan, 30% of IDUs in prison reported using nonsterile needles or injection equipment.[75] In Oman, 3%–11% reported using nonsterile needles in prison.[76] In Sudan, 3.2% of prisoners reported using nonsterile syringes while in prison.[77] In Syria, the majority of IDUs who injected in prison did so by using a nonsterile syringe or a needle.[78]

[52] Ibid.

[53] Day et al., "Patterns of Drug Use."

[54] Zamani et al., "High Prevalence of HIV"; Zamani et al., "Shared Drug Injection inside Prison."

[55] Bolhari and Mirzamani, "Assessment of Substance Abuse in Iran's Prisons."

[56] Ibid.

[57] Mostashari, UNODC, and Darabi, "Summary of the Iranian Situation on HIV Epidemic."

[58] Afshar, "From the Assessment to the Implementation of Services"; Afshar, "Health and Prison."

[59] Day et al., "Patterns of Drug Use"; Zamani et al., "Needle and Syringe Sharing."

[60] Zamani et al., "Needle and Syringe Sharing."

[61] Mimouni and Remaoun, "Etude du Lien Potentiel entre l'Usage Problématique de Drogues et le VIH/SIDA."

[62] Elshimi, Warner-Smith, and Aon, "Blood-Borne Virus Risks."

[63] Mishwar, "An Integrated Bio-Behavioral Surveillance Study."

[64] Oman MOH, "HIV Risk among Heroin and Injecting Drug Users."

[65] Syria Mental Health Directorate, "Assessment of HIV Risk and Sero-Prevalence."

[66] Day et al., "Patterns of Drug Use"; Kheirandish et al., "Prevalence and Correlates of Hepatitis C."

[67] Zamani et al., "Shared Drug Injection inside Prison"; Zamani, "Methadone Maintenance Treatment (MMT)."

[68] S. Zamani, personal communication (2008); Bolhari and Mirzamani, "Assessment of Substance Abuse in Iran's Prisons."

[69] Day et al., "Patterns of Drug Use."

[70] Zamani et al., "Needle and Syringe Sharing."

[71] Ibid.

[72] Zamani et al., "High Prevalence of HIV."

[73] Zamani et al., "Shared Drug Injection inside Prison."

[74] Afshar, "Health and Prison."

[75] UNAIDS, "Notes on AIDS in the Middle East and North Africa."

[76] Oman MOH, "HIV Risk among Heroin and Injecting Drug Users."

[77] Assal, "HIV Prevalence."

[78] Syria Mental Health Directorate, "Assessment of HIV Risk and Sero-Prevalence."

This evidence of nonsterile injection equipment use in prison is further supported by the repeated confiscation of injecting equipment in MENA prisons.[79] Prison authorities could also be forcing prisoners to increase the use of nonsterile equipment by limiting their access to safe injecting utensils. In the Islamic Republic of Iran, incarcerated IDUs reported using nonsterile injecting equipment at a rate close to three times as high as the rate among nonincarcerated IDUs.[80] It has been reported that syringes are used at least 30 to 40 times in Iranian prisons before disposal.[81]

Tattooing is a risk factor for HIV infection,[82] and there is evidence of tattooing using nonsterile utensils in Iranian prisons.[83] About 65% of imprisoned IDUs have tattoos,[84] and tattooing was reported by 24.9%–25.1% of Iranian prisoners.[85] Two studies in the Islamic Republic of Iran have also identified tattooing as a risk factor for HCV infection for incarcerated IDUs.[86]

Sexual risk behavior and prisoners

Several studies have documented risky sexual behavior among prisoners in MENA. In the Islamic Republic of Iran, 17% of incarcerated drug users reported paying for drugs in prison through sex work,[87] and 5.4% of incarcerated male IDUs reported sex with another male while in prison.[88] Sexual abuse of prisoners by other prisoners has also been reported in the Islamic Republic of Iran.[89] In Lebanon, 2.6% of male prisoners reported anal sex with another male while in prison.[90] In Oman, 6%–18% of male IDUs reported having sex in prison without condoms.[91] In Pakistan, 4% of male prisoners

reported having sex with other males.[92] In Sudan, 1.4% of male prisoners reported having sex with other males in one prison, but social workers in this prison estimated that about 20% of prisoners engage in such activity.[93] The latter assertion is corroborated by the fact that 14.5% of prisoners have been diagnosed with gonorrhea while incarcerated.[94] In Syria, 5% of imprisoned drug users reported ever having sex in prison.[95]

Anecdotal evidence in Sudan suggests the occurrence of sexual acts between female prisoners and their guards in exchange for better treatment in prison.[96] Prisoners also generally report higher levels of sexual risk behavior than the rest of the general population even prior to incarceration. In Morocco, only 9% of female prisoners reported using condoms and the average number of lifetime sexual partners was 5.17.[97] In Sudan, only 4% of male prisoners reported ever using a condom, 41.9% reported premarital and extramarital sex, and 8.6% had paid for sex.[98] Also in Sudan among male prisoners, 23.7%, 2.8%, 4.7%, and 17.7% reported having one, two, three, and more than three lifetime sexual partners, respectively; 11.4% reported having sex before marriage; and 2.2% reported having sex with another male.[99] Another study in Sudan found that 65.2% of prisoners had extramarital relations prior to incarceration.[100] Though by law prisoners in Sudan have the right to conjugal visits, this right is rarely practiced.[101]

Analytical summary

Prisoners are a large share of the population vulnerable to HIV in MENA. History of imprisonment was demonstrated to be linked to higher risk of HIV infection in the Islamic Republic of Iran and may have contributed to the HIV epidemics in other countries. High HIV prevalence levels and HIV outbreaks have been documented among prisoners in MENA. High levels of injecting

---

[79] Bolhari and Mirzamani, "Assessment of Substance Abuse in Iran's Prisons."

[80] Rahbar, Rooholamini, and Khoshnood, "Prevalence of HIV Infection."

[81] Nassirimanesh, Trace, and Roberts, "The Rise of Harm Reduction."

[82] Martin et al., "Predictive Factors of HIV-Infection"; Buavirat et al., "Risk of Prevalent HIV."

[83] Zamani et al., "High Prevalence of HIV."

[84] Afshar, "From the Assessment to the Implementation of Services."

[85] Farhoudi et al., "Human Immunodeficiency Virus."

[86] Khani and Vakili, "Prevalence and Risk Factors of HIV"; Kheirandish et al., "Prevalence and Correlates of Hepatitis C Infection."

[87] Bolhari and Mirzamani, "Assessment of Substance Abuse in Iran's Prisons."

[88] Zamani et al., "Needle and Syringe Sharing Practices."

[89] Afshar, "From the Assessment to the Implementation of Services."

[90] Mishwar, "An Integrated Bio-Behavioral Surveillance Study."

[91] Oman MOH, "HIV Risk among Heroin and Injecting Drug Users."

[92] Khawaja et al., "HIV/AIDS and Its Risk Factors in Pakistan."

[93] Ati, "HIV/AIDS/STIs Social and Geographical Mapping."

[94] Ibid.

[95] Syria Mental Health Directorate, "Assessment of HIV Risk and Sero-Prevalence."

[96] Ati, "HIV/AIDS/STIs Social and Geographical Mapping."

[97] El Ghrari et al., "Prevalence of Syphilis and HIV."

[98] Ahmed, Prisoners.

[99] Assal, "HIV Prevalence."

[100] Ati, "HIV/AIDS/STIs Social and Geographical Mapping."

[101] Assal, "HIV Prevalence."

drug and sexual risk behaviors have also been observed in MENA prisons.

Prevention efforts are needed to combat HIV infection in prisons; the Islamic Republic of Iran provides an example of what can be achieved in the MENA context by incorporating effective harm reduction in prisons.[102]

YOUTH AND HIV

MENA is distinctively characterized by a "tidal wave" of youth; one-fifth of the population, 95 million people,[103] are in the 15–24 years age group,[104] the average age range of initiation of sexual activities.[105] This is the largest youth cohort in the region's history and the largest vulnerable population in MENA.[106]

Youth are experiencing high rates of unemployment, delayed marital age, increased premarital sex, conflict morbidity and mortality, increased mobility, peer pressure to engage in risky behavior, and changing lifestyle norms.[107] The increasing high educational attainment of youth, coupled with high unemployment, is leading to a structural vulnerability of rising expectations but declining opportunities.[108] There is a widening generation gap between young people on one hand, and their parents and decision makers on the other hand.[109]

Youth play a central role in the HIV epidemic. About half of all HIV infections in sub-Saharan Africa, Eastern Europe, and Central Asia are among those younger than 25 years of age.[110] In most regions, most IDUs, men who have sex with men (MSM), and female sex workers (FSWs) and their clients are young, or if older, they would have started at-risk behavior at a young age.[111] Young people bridge HIV infection between different population groups, such as young, sexually active IDUs exchanging sex for money with MSM and exchanging money for sex with FSWs.[112] Young people are also the best vehicle for change if they can be reached with appropriate interventions.[113] The countries that reported the largest declines in risky behavior and HIV prevalence, such as Uganda, observed the biggest changes among youth.[114]

Demography

The share of youth 15–24 years of age ranges between 15% and 25% among the countries of the region.[115] In Egypt and Morocco, about one-third of the population is between 15 and 29 years of age.[116] In Jordan, 70% of the population is below the age of 25.[117] In the West Bank and Gaza, 52% of the population is below the age of 18.[118] In Sudan, 45% of the population is under the age of 15.[119] In the Republic of Yemen, 46.2% of the population is below age 15 and 58.3% is below age 19.[120]

Though the demographic transition is progressing rapidly and fertility has been in sharp decline in much of the region in recent years, with several countries being even below the replacement level,[121] youth will continue to be the largest vulnerable population as well as the population that has the greatest potential to drive the socioeconomic dynamics in the region.[122] Regrettably, this region as a whole is largely failing to take advantage of this "demographic bonus" by using this window of opportunity for economic growth. MENA youth today are the first generation of young people in recent history that are unlikely to fare better than their parents, despite having higher educational levels than their parents.[123]

[102] Zamani et al., "Prevalence of and Factors Associated with HIV-1 Infection"; Ministry of Health and Medical Education of Iran, "Treatment and Medical Education"; Afshar, "From the Assessment to the Implementation of Services"; Afshar and Kasraee, "HIV Prevention Experiences."

[103] Assaad and Roudi-Fahimi, "Youth in the Middle East and North Africa."

[104] UNAIDS, "Notes on AIDS in the Middle East and North Africa"; Roudi-Fahimi and Ashford, "Sexual & Reproductive Health."

[105] Roudi-Fahimi and Ashford, "Sexual & Reproductive Health"; UNAIDS, Report on the Global AIDS Epidemic.

[106] Assaad and Roudi-Fahimi, "Youth in the Middle East and North Africa."

[107] Busulwa, "HIV/AIDS Situation Analysis Study"; UNAIDS, "Notes on AIDS in the Middle East and North Africa."

[108] Jenkins and Robalino, "HIV in the Middle East and North Africa."

[109] Assaad and Roudi-Fahimi, "Youth in the Middle East and North Africa."

[110] Monasch and Mahy, "Young People."

[111] Ibid.

[112] Michael, Ahmed, and Lemma, "HIV/AIDS Behavioral Surveillance Survey."

[113] Monasch and Mahy, "Young People."

[114] Ibid.

[115] Assaad and Roudi-Fahimi, "Youth in the Middle East and North Africa."

[116] Jenkins and Robalino, "HIV in the Middle East and North Africa."

[117] UNAIDS, "HIV Prevention in Jordan."

[118] UNAIDS, "Key Findings on HIV Status."

[119] Gutbi and Eldin, "Women Tea-Sellers in Khartoum and HIV/AIDS."

[120] Lambert, "HIV and Development Challenges in Yemen."

[121] Rashad, "Demographic Transition in Arab Countries."

[122] Assaad and Roudi-Fahimi, "Youth in the Middle East and North Africa."

[123] Rashad, Osman, and Roudi-Fahimi, Marriage in the Arab World.

Unemployment

The region has the highest youth unemployment rate of all regions at 26%,[124] twice that of South Asia. About 43 million youth are expected to enter the labor force between 2000 and 2010, compared with 47 million who entered the labor market during the four decades from 1950 to 1990.[125] Three-quarters of those unemployed in a country, such as Syria, are youth.[126] The unemployment rate in the West Bank and Gaza is at 26.8%, and most of those unemployed are young adults.[127] Among rural youth in Sudan, 63.5% were found unemployed.[128] The high unemployment among youth has left young people with ample spare time to spend in cafés and entertainment centers, thereby potentially exposing them to pressures for risky behaviors.

Marriage

The rising costs of marriage are a large barrier toward marriage in the region.[129] High dowries have made it difficult if not impossible for youth to marry, thereby preventing them from having the opportunity for sanctioned sex.[130] It is not uncommon for families to spend as much as 15 times the annual household expenditure per capita on marriage-related costs.[131] Consumerism and rising expectations have contributed substantially to the rising cost of marriage.[132] The difficulties facing youth in marriage may have contributed to the large gap in age between spouses: 25% of recent marriages in Egypt and Lebanon included a husband at least 10 years older than his wife.[133] Also, more and more people are adopting modern lifestyles and delaying marriage for education or work outside the home.[134]

The gap between biological adulthood and marriage is conducive to premarital sex.[135] Studies have shown that paying for sex is higher among never married or formerly married men.[136] The age of marriage is steadily rising in MENA.[137] In more than a third of MENA countries, the average age at first marriage has increased between 4.7 and 7.7 years over a span of 20 years.[138] In the Islamic Republic of Iran, it increased from 19.8 years for females and 23.6 years for males in 1986 to 22.4 years and 25.6 years in 1996, respectively.[139] In Jordan, the average marriage age increased for females from 19.6 years in 1990 to 21.8 years in 2002.[140] In Lebanon, the average marriage age is 30.9 years for males and 27.5 years for females,[141] and has increased by 3.9 years from 1989 to 1996.[142] In Saudi Arabia, the average marriage age has increased from 18.22 to 19.90 years over 20 years.[143] In Tunisia, the average marriage age is at 33 years for men and 29 years for women.[144]

MENA is experiencing the phenomenon of marriage squeeze, defined as an imbalance between the numbers of males and females in the prime age for marriage.[145] Marriage squeeze has been documented in Lebanon among both Lebanese and Palestinian refugees, where it is forcing many to delay or forego marriage.[146] Marriage squeeze also seems to be occurring in many other countries around MENA because the mate availability ratios are distorted by demographic stresses driven by delayed age at marriage, high male migration, and conflict-related morbidity and mortality.[147]

The large cohort of single young women is a recent phenomenon in MENA.[148] By 1990, the proportion of women in the sexually active population of 15–49 years of age who are not currently married has reached between 24% and 46% in most countries.[149] Between 7% and

[124] Assaad and Roudi-Fahimi, "Youth in the Middle East and North Africa."
[125] Ibid.
[126] Ibid.
[127] UNAIDS, "Key Findings on HIV Status in the West Bank and Gaza."
[128] SNAP, UNICEF, and UNAIDS, "Baseline Study on Knowledge."
[129] Rashad et al., *Marriage in the Arab World.*
[130] Busulwa, "HIV/AIDS Situation Analysis Study."
[131] Rashad et al., *Marriage in the Arab World.*
[132] Ibid.
[133] Ibid.
[134] Roudi-Fahimi and Ashford, "Sexual & Reproductive Health."
[135] DeJong et al., "The Sexual and Reproductive Health of Young People."
[136] Carael, Cleland, and Adeokun, "Overview"; Carael, "Urban-Rural Differentials."
[137] Rashad and Osman, "Nuptiality in Arab Countries"; Fargues, "Terminating Marriage."
[138] Rashad, "Demographic Transition in Arab Countries."
[139] Mohammadi et al., "Reproductive Knowledge, Attitudes and Behavior."
[140] Naffa, "Jordanian Women: Past and Present."
[141] El-Kak et al., "High School Students in Postwar Lebanon."
[142] Saxena, Kulczycki, and Jurdi, "Nuptiality Transition."
[143] Babay et al., "Age at Menarche."
[144] Fargues, "Terminating Marriage."
[145] Akers, "On Measuring the Marriage Squeeze"; Schoen, "Measuring the Tightness of a Marriage Squeeze."
[146] Saxena, Kulczycki, and Jurdi, "Nuptiality Transition."
[147] Ibid.
[148] DeJong et al., "The Sexual and Reproductive Health of Young People."
[149] Rashad, "Demographic Transition in Arab Countries."

21% of women in MENA are not married by age 30–39.[150] In nearly half of the countries, women spend about one-third of their sexual activity lifespan (15–49 years of age) in an unmarried state.[151] In Lebanon, about one out of five men and women aged 35–39 years was still single in 1996.[152] In Algeria, Jordan, Kuwait, Lebanon, Libya, Morocco, Qatar, Syria, Tunisia, and the West Bank and Gaza, between 10% and 25% of women are never married.[153] Even in a highly traditional and underdeveloped country such as the Republic of Yemen, marriage among women 15–19 years old declined from 27% to 17% between 1997 and 2003.[154]

Early and near universal marriage, where almost all adults spend most of their sexual activity lifetime being married, was once the highlight of this region. Yet, it will soon become the exception rather than the norm.[155] In large part, the demographic transition in MENA is driven by stark changes in nuptiality.[156]

Youth and priority populations

Youth contribute disproportionately to the priority populations in MENA, attesting to the vulnerability of this population group. Being an unemployed youth is a frequent characteristic of IDUs.[157] Drug use in different forms appears to be considerable and probably increasing among youth in MENA.[158] The profile of IDUs in a Tunisian study was that of young men raised in large families shattered by urban-rural migration.[159] Among young prisoners in the Islamic Republic of Iran, 33.9% of inmates used opioid while in prison.[160] IDUs in Oman reported hashish as their first drug at a mean age of 18, and then IDU of heroin at age 22.[161]

The largest burden of drug use in the West Bank and Gaza is in the 31–40 years age group, with a notable increase in drug use among youth.[162] Among high school students, marijuana was used by 2%–2.9% of males and 0.7%–1% of females, and heroin was used by 0.8%–1% of males and 0.4%–0.6% of females.[163] The average age at first use of different forms of drugs ranged between 12.8 and 14.75 years for males and 12 and 16 years for females.[164] Peer pressure was found to be a key determinant of starting drug use among these adolescents.[165] The knowledge of harm was generally poor and multiple use of different drugs was reported by a considerable share of these users.[166]

The lack of engagement in meaningful activities is conducive to risky behavior in MENA. Of high school students in the West Bank and Gaza, 38.2% of males and 5.2% of females spend evenings hanging in streets, and among heroin users, these percentages were 66.7% for males and 42.9% for females.[167]

For MSM, more than half of the participants in a study in Sudan (60.1%) were between 15 and 24 years of age, and 85.5% of them had their first anal experience between the ages of 15 and 25.[168] MSM tend to start having sex at a younger age compared to males who have sex with females.[169] In Lebanon, 54% of MSM reported having their first anal sex at under the age of 18 years.[170] In Egypt, young MSM were the group that changed their sexual partners most often among MSM.[171] Also in Egypt, young MSM were found to be the most sexually active, with a frequency of sexual acts greater than one per day.[172] In studies in Pakistan, male sex workers (MSWs) had an average age of 22.3,[173] 21.3,[174] and 21.7[175] years, and started

[150] Ibid.
[151] Ibid.
[152] Saxena, Kulczycki, and Jurdi, "Nuptiality Transition."
[153] Roudi-Fahimi and Ashford, "Sexual & Reproductive Health."
[154] Ibid.
[155] Rashad, "Demographic Transition in Arab Countries."
[156] Ibid.
[157] Zamani et al., "High Prevalence of HIV."
[158] Ibid.
[159] Tiouiri et al., "Study of Psychosocial Factors."
[160] Bolhari and Mirzamani, "Assessment of Substance Abuse in Iran's Prisons."
[161] Oman MOH, "HIV Risk among Heroin and Injecting Drug Users."

[162] Shareef et al., "Drug Abuse Situation."
[163] Afifi and El-Sousi, "Drug Abuse and Related Behaviors."
[164] Ibid.
[165] Ibid.
[166] Ibid.
[167] Ibid.
[168] Elrashied, "Generating Strategic Information."
[169] Monasch and Mahy, "Young People."
[170] Mishwar, "An Integrated Bio-Behavioral Surveillance Study."
[171] El-Rahman, "Risky Behaviours for HIV/AIDS Infection."
[172] El-Sayyed, Kabbash, and El-Gueniedy, "Risk Behaviours for HIV/AIDS Infection."
[173] Pakistan National AIDS Control Program, *HIV Second Generation Surveillance* (Round I).
[174] Pakistan National AIDS Control Program, *HIV Second Generation Surveillance* (Round II).
[175] Pakistan National AIDS Control Program, *HIV Second Generation Surveillance* (Round III).

commercial sex at an average age of 16.9,[176] 15.9,[177] and 16.2[178] years, respectively.

As for FSWs, 71.4% of FSWs in one study in Sudan were below 30 years of age, including 8.4% who were under 18 years of age.[179] Further studies among FSWs in Sudan have found that the majority are under 30 years of age,[180] 19.6% are less than 18 years of age,[181] and the majority are younger than 28 years and started sex work before 22 years of age.[182] Fifty-three percent of FSWs in a study in Syria were 25 years of age or younger.[183] In Djibouti, 63% of FSWs reported their first commercial sex at under 20 years of age.[184] In Lebanon, 57% of FSWs reported first sex at ages between 11 and 18 years.[185] In Pakistan, young FSWs were found to have the highest client volume.[186] Also in Pakistan, the median age of initiating sex work was reported to be 22 years of age.[187]

Youth and STIs

Youth contribute disproportionately to the disease burden of STIs in MENA. Fifty-nine percent of sexually transmitted disease (STD) cases in Egypt were among young and predominantly single adults.[188] Almost 41% of HIV infections in the Islamic Republic of Iran are found in the 25–34 years age group,[189] and 27.9% of youth report a previous history of STDs.[190] Almost half (45%) of reported STD cases in the Islamic Republic of Iran occurred in the 20–29 years age group, and 10% of all cases involved

teenagers.[191] Most reported STDs among STD clinic attendees in Kuwait were in the age range of 21–30 years.[192] The age group most affected by HIV in Jordan is the 15–35 years age group.[193]

The majority of reported HIV/AIDS cases in the West Bank and Gaza are in the 20–40 years age group, with 31% among the 20–29 years age group.[194] Women under 25 years of age in Oman were twice as likely to acquire an STI compared to women older than 25 years of age.[195] Forty percent of recorded STD cases in Morocco were among youth ages 15–29 years.[196] Most HIV infections in Morocco (63%) and Tunisia (93%) are among single and often young persons.[197]

The highest prevalence of both HIV and syphilis in Somalia (4%) was in the 15–24 years age group.[198] Forty-seven percent of HIV cases in the ANC HIV sentinel sero-survey in Sudan were in the 20–24 years age group.[199] Also in Sudan, HIV prevalence among youth is estimated to be 1% among females and 0.3% among males.[200] The dominant profile of STD clinic attendees in Tunisia was that of young single men with multiple sexual partners.[201]

Sexual behavior among youth

Despite data limitations, several studies have documented the nature of sexual behavior among youth in MENA. The outcomes of behavioral surveys show substantial variability within the region.

In Afghanistan, 14.6% of university students were sexually active, with risk behaviors more prevalent among males than females.[202] In Djibouti, 22% of high school students reported

[176] Pakistan National AIDS Control Program, *HIV Second Generation Surveillance* (Round I).

[177] Pakistan National AIDS Control Program, *HIV Second Generation Surveillance* (Round II).

[178] Pakistan National AIDS Control Program, *HIV Second Generation Surveillance* (Round III).

[179] Ati, "HIV/AIDS/STIs Social and Geographical Mapping."

[180] ACORD, "Socio Economic Research on HIV/AIDS Prevention."

[181] Yousif, *Health Education Programme*.

[182] ACORD, "Qualitative Socio Economic Research."

[183] Syria National AIDS Programme, "HIV/AIDS Female Sex Workers KABP Survey in Syria."

[184] Michael, Ahmed, and Lemma, "HIV/AIDS Behavioral Surveillance Survey."

[185] Mishwar, "An Integrated Bio-Behavioral Surveillance Study."

[186] Pakistan National AIDS Control Program, *HIV Second Generation Surveillance* (Round I).

[187] Pakistan National AIDS Control Program, *HIV Second Generation Surveillance* (Round II).

[188] Ali et al., "Prevalence of Certain Sexually Transmitted Diseases in Egypt."

[189] Iran Center for Disease Management, *Country Report on UNGASS*.

[190] Tehrani and Malek-Afzalip, "Knowledge, Attitudes and Practices concerning HIV/AIDS."

[191] Iran Center for Disease Management, Three Month Statistics of the MoH AIDS Office.

[192] Al-Mutairi et al., "Clinical Patterns."

[193] Anonymous, *Scaling Up the HIV Response*.

[194] UNAIDS, "Key Findings on HIV Status."

[195] Roudi-Fahimi and Ashford, "Sexual & Reproductive Health."

[196] Roudi-Fahimi and Ashford, "Sexual & Reproductive Health"; Jenkins and Robalino, "HIV in the Middle East and North Africa."

[197] Jenkins and Robalino, "HIV in the Middle East and North Africa."

[198] WHO, *The 2004 First National Second Generation HIV/AIDS/STI Sentinel Surveillance Survey.*

[199] Sudan National AIDS/STIs Program, *2007 ANC HIV Sentinel Sero-Survey.*

[200] SNAP, "Update on the HIV Situation in Sudan."

[201] Sellami et al., "Epidemiologic Profile."

[202] Mansoor et al., "Gender Differences in KAP."

being sexually active (40.8% of males and 2.7% of females).[203] Another study in Djibouti reported that 71% of young males and females reported sexual relations without defining the kind of relations, and 39% reported ever using condoms.[204]

In Egypt, 26% of male and 3% of female university students reported having sexual intercourse.[205] In another study, 16.5% of university students engaged in sexual intercourse,[206] and in a third, 18% of the students reported engaging in risky sexual behavior.[207] Low condom use was reported among university students.[208]

In the Islamic Republic of Iran, 12.4% of young males reported premarital or extramarital sex in one study,[209] and in a second study, 28% of males aged 15–18 years reported sexual experience, with 73% of them having more than one lifetime sexual partner.[210] Condom nonuse was associated with poor access to the Internet (reflecting poorer knowledge), feeling regretful at first sex, and one lifetime sexual partner.[211] Meanwhile, multiple sexual partnerships were associated with alcohol consumption, older ages, and poor knowledge of reproductive physiology.[212] Close to half of the adolescents in this sample were unfamiliar with condoms and their protective effect against STIs, including HIV.[213] Eight percent of college students (16% of males and 0.6% of females) reported having sexual intercourse before marriage and 48% had used condoms.[214] Yet another study of adolescents found that 47% were not aware that condoms protect against HIV infection.[215] Finally, from the Islamic Republic of Iran, a study of college students reported that 20% of the respondents had a history of sexual contact.[216]

In Jordan, a survey of youth found casual sex to be rare and condom use to be moderately high among those who engaged in nonmarital sex.[217] Another study reported that 7% of college students and 4% of the general population in the 15–30 years age range admitted to engaging in nonmarital sex.[218] About 90% of the youth who reported sexual partnerships reported opposite sex partners only, while 10% reported sex with the same sex or both sexes.[219] About 10% of the youth reported nonmarital sexual contacts in the last year.[220]

In Lebanon, behavioral surveys suggest increased risky behavior among youth.[221] About 50% of young conscripts reported any lifetime heterosexual experience and about 50% reported consistent condom use.[222] In Mauritania, 40% of male school students reported sexual activity, with 41% of them reporting multiple sexual partnerships and 38% reporting unprotected sexual intercourse.[223] In Pakistan, 80% of young men masturbated and 94% had experienced nocturnal emissions.[224]

In Somalia, 7% of youth acknowledged sexual activity in the last year, 17.8% reported that they had ever had sex, and only 6.5% of them used a condom during the most recent sexual activity.[225] About 23% of women under age 24 had knowledge of condoms.[226]

In Sudan, 6.9% of university students reported having sex and 5.5% engaged in premarital sex.[227] Almost half (48.6%) of sexually active students had one sexual partner, 14.5% had two partners, 10.9% had three partners, and 23.2% had more than three partners.[228] In another study of university students, 6.2% reported ever using a condom, and 14.4% reported extramarital sex.[229] In a study of youth, 0.6% reported condom use, 2% reported

[203] Rodier et al., "HIV Infection among Secondary School Students."
[204] Ministére de la Santé-PNLS et al., "Etude des connaissances attitudes-practiques des jeunes."
[205] El-Zanaty and El-Daw, "Behavior Research."
[206] NAMRU-3, "Young People and HIV/AIDS."
[207] Refaat, "Practice and Awareness of Health Risk Behaviour."
[208] Ibid.
[209] Tehrani and Malek-Afzalip, "Knowledge, Attitudes and Practices concerning HIV/AIDS."
[210] Mohammad et al., "Sexual Risk-Taking Behaviors"; Mohammadi et al., "Reproductive Knowledge, Attitudes and Behavior."
[211] Mohammad et al., "Sexual Risk-Taking Behaviors."
[212] Ibid.
[213] Mohammadi et al., "Reproductive Knowledge, Attitudes and Behavior."
[214] Simbar, Tehrani, and Hashemi, "Reproductive Health Knowledge."
[215] Yazdi et al., "Knowledge, Attitudes and Sources of Information."
[216] Shirazi and Morowatisharifabad, "Religiosity and Determinants of Safe Sex."

[217] UNAIDS and WHO, AIDS Epidemic Update 2005.
[218] Johns Hopkins University, "Youth Survey."
[219] Jenkins and Robalino, "HIV in the Middle East and North Africa."
[220] Jordan National AIDS Control Programme, Report on the National KABP Survey (2005).
[221] Kassak et al., "Final Working Protocol."
[222] Adib et al., "Heterosexual Awareness and Practices."
[223] Ndiaye et al., "Evaluation of Condom Use."
[224] Qidwai, "Sexual Knowledge."
[225] WHO/EMRO, "Presentation of WHO Somalia's Experience."
[226] Population Studies Research Institute, "Baseline Survey."
[227] Sudan National HIV/AIDS Control Program, HIV/AIDS/STIs Prevalence.
[228] Ibid.
[229] Ahmed, University Students.

condom use with commercial sex workers (CSWs), and 9.5% reported nonregular partners in the last year.[230]

While not part of this report's definition of the MENA region, 19% of college students in Turkey reported having had sexual intercourse and 30% reported using a condom during the last sex.[231] In another study, 61.2% of males and 18.3% of females reported sexual intercourse among final-year university students aged 20–25 years.[232] In a third study, 36.6% of college students were sexually active, with males being more sexually active than females, but using condoms less frequently.[233] In a fourth study, 46% of male adolescents and 3% of female adolescents had sexual intercourse.[234] The median age at first intercourse was 17 years for males and 16 years for females.[235] Among those who had intercourse, 44% of the males and 67% of the females had their first experience with their lovers.[236] The rates of sexual activity among high school students were found in yet another study to be much higher among males compared to females, with generally low condom use.[237] Also among high school students, the percentage of people who reported having sexual experiences increased from 11.3% in 1997 to 22.8% in 2004.[238]

Other issues related to sexual behavior of youth

The rapid cultural and socioeconomic transformation in MENA is particularly affecting youth, who are experiencing enormous strains with the rapid social changes, urbanization, and generation gap induced in part by mass education. Among youth who have lived abroad, higher levels of sexual intercourse have been reported, suggesting the influence of cultural exchanges on sexual behavior.[239] Youth emigration is prevalent in MENA, and in Lebanon, a third of the population emigrated for at least some time during the civil war.[240] Students in Lebanon are increasingly

found to embrace Western values, associated with liberal attitudes toward sexuality,[241] rather than traditional values, and appear to have relaxed attitudes toward sexuality.[242]

Youth in MENA do not seem to be concerned about HIV infection. Only 14.2% in Iran[243] and 20% in Djibouti[244] reported concern about HIV infection. Furthermore, the lack of meaningful engagements among youth, coupled with the availability of financial resources, appears to lead to riskier behaviors. A higher allowance in Egypt has been associated with risky sexual behavior among youth.[245] There are no satisfactory data that clarify the engagement of youth in nonconventional forms of marriage,[246] but there is evidence of significantly higher approval of such marriage forms among youth compared to older age groups.[247] More than a quarter of Iranian youth approve of temporary marriages.[248]

Reproductive knowledge among youth, specifically in the Islamic Republic of Iran, has been associated with lower sexual risk behavior and increased condom use,[249] just as in other regions.[250] This highlights the utility of increasing HIV knowledge among youth. Only the Islamic Republic of Iran and Tunisia have national programs on young people's sexual and reproductive health.[251] Some young populations in the Islamic Republic of Iran appear to have higher levels of knowledge than even priority populations. Youth in the Islamic Republic of Iran were found to be more knowledgeable about HIV and prevention measures than FSWs and truck drivers.[252]

The limited behavioral evidence among youth should be interpreted with caution. Considering cultural barriers, youth are not often asked specifically about the kind of sexual contacts they engage in and therefore their responses

[230] Sudan National AIDS Control Program, *Situation Analysis*.

[231] Ungan and Yaman, "AIDS Knowledge and Educational Needs."

[232] Aras et al., "Sexual Behaviours and Contraception."

[233] Gokengin et al., "Sexual Knowledge."

[234] Dagdeviren, Set, and Akturk, "Sexual Activity among Turkish Adolescents."

[235] Ibid.

[236] Ibid.

[237] Aras et al., "Sexual Attitudes and Risk-Taking Behaviors."

[238] Yamazhan et al., "Attitudes towards HIV/AIDS."

[239] El-Kak et al., "High School Students in Postwar Lebanon."

[240] Ibid.

[241] Sigusch, "The Neosexual Revolution."

[242] El-Kak et al., "High School Students in Postwar Lebanon."

[243] Tehrani and Malek-Afzalip, "Knowledge, Attitudes and Practices concerning HIV/AIDS."

[244] Rodier et al., "HIV Infection among Secondary School Students."

[245] Refaat, "Practice and Awareness of Health Risk Behaviour."

[246] Haeri, "Temporary Marriage."

[247] Mohammad et al., "Sexual Risk-Taking Behaviors."

[248] Tehrani and Malek-Afzalip, "Knowledge, Attitudes and Practices concerning HIV/AIDS."

[249] Mohammad et al., "Sexual Risk-Taking Behaviors."

[250] Rock, Ireland, and Resnick, "To Know That We Know What We Know."

[251] DeJong et al., "The Sexual and Reproductive Health of Young People."

[252] Tehrani and Malek-Afzalip, "Knowledge, Attitudes and Practices concerning HIV/AIDS."

may include nonpenetrative sexual activities, which are less of a concern in relation to HIV.[253] Though 28% of males aged 15–18 years reported sexual experiences in the Islamic Republic of Iran,[254] this sexual activity may not have included sexual intercourse. The definition of sexual activity is broad enough in many studies to encompass even kissing or touching.[255] This limitation in behavioral data, in addition to the need to monitor changes in sexual risk behavior among youth, suggests the utility of using biomarkers such as herpes simplex virus type 2 (HSV-2) prevalence and incidence to monitor levels and trends of sexual activity among youth in MENA.

Recent increases in risky behavior

One of the concerning trends in MENA is that of increases in risky behavior, particularly among the youth. Attention needs to focus on identifying trends in risky behavior among this population group.[256] Increases in sexual risk behavior have been observed in other regions, such in Latin America and Asia, due to the changes in the socioeconomic conditions.[257]

Anecdotal observations suggest that risky behaviors and sexual activity are increasing among both male and female youth in MENA.[258] These observations are supported by a trend of increasing HIV incidence in the younger age groups.[259] Other trends also seem to suggest recent increases in risky behavior. In Afghanistan, risky behavior in terms of injecting drug use and commercial sex appears to have considerably increased since the Afghanistan war in 2001.[260] In the Islamic Republic of Iran, reported STD cases have grown by 38% annually since 1998, and the number of cases has quadrupled between 1992 and 2004.[261] Genital ulcers have grown by a factor of 6.2 over the same period, with 45% of

the cases occurring in the 20–29 years age group.[262]

In Kuwait, STI incidence has been steadily increasing,[263] and there appears to be an increase in precancerous cervical lesions in women, with appearance of these lesions at a younger age.[264] In Lebanon, a similar trend of increases in precancerous lesions has been reported over the years from 2002 to 2006, also at younger ages.[265] Also in Lebanon, repeated behavioral surveys have indicated increased risky behavior among youth.[266] In Saudi Arabia, the percentage of abnormal Pap smears appears to be increasing.[267] In Turkey, the share of high school students who reported having sexual experiences increased from 11.3% in 1997 to 22.8% in 2004.[268] Also in Turkey, the prevalence of syphilis among blood donors, though still at low levels, has increased fivefold between 1987 and 2002 in one study,[269] and tenfold in another study between 1998 and 2007.[270]

Analytical summary

Youth form the largest vulnerable population in MENA and are facing enormous challenges that could expose them to HIV infection. Traditional forms of managing youth sexuality are in decline and are not of much use with the rapidly changing socioeconomic realities. Because youth do not appreciate the importance of safe sex, and they have no other sexual outlets, they are increasingly engaging in risky sexual behavior to dissipate their sexual energy.

Youth disproportionately contribute to the HIV epidemic in MENA and behavioral data suggest considerable and increasing levels of sexual and injecting drug risk behaviors among them. Much research is needed to track the trends of risky behavior and STIs of the youth population. Effective HIV prevention interventions for youth that focus specifically on the behaviors that can lead to HIV exposure need to be formulated.

[253] Mohammad et al., "Sexual Risk-Taking Behaviors."

[254] Mohammad et al., "Sexual Risk-Taking Behaviors"; Mohammadi et al., "Reproductive Knowledge, Attitudes and Behavior."

[255] Mohammadi et al., "Reproductive Knowledge, Attitudes and Behavior."

[256] Pisani et al., "HIV Surveillance."

[257] Curtis and Sutherland, "Measuring Sexual Behaviour in the Era of HIV/ AIDS"; Gammeltoft, "Seeking Trust and Transcendence"; Ono-Kihara and Kihara, "The First Nationwide Sexual Behavior Survey in Japan."

[258] Busulwa, "HIV/AIDS Situation Analysis Study."

[259] UNAIDS, and WHO, AIDS Epidemic Update 2005.

[260] World Bank, "Mapping and Situation Assessment."

[261] Iran Center for Disease Management, Three Month Statistics of the MoH AIDS Office; Iran Center for Disease Management, HIV/AIDS and STIs Surveillance Report.

[262] Iran Center for Disease Management, Three Month Statistics of the MoH AIDS Office.

[263] Al-Fouzan and Al-Mutairi, "Overview."

[264] Kapila et al., "Changing Spectrum of Squamous Cell Abnormalities."

[265] Karam et al., "Prevalence of Sexually Transmitted Infections."

[266] Kassak et al., "Final Working Protocol."

[267] Altaf, "Cervical Cancer Screening."

[268] Yamazhan et al., "Attitudes towards HIV/AIDS."

[269] Kocak et al., "Trends in Major Transfusion-Transmissible Infections."

[270] Coskun et al., "Prevalence of HIV and Syphilis."

POPULATION MOBILITY AND HIV

One of the most vulnerable groups in MENA is that of mobile populations, including voluntary or economic migrants, refugees, internally displaced persons, individuals who move for other compelling reasons, nomads, and pastoralists.[271] Other groups such as truck drivers, seafarers, and uniformed personnel are also mobile populations, but here these groups are classified as potential bridging populations (see chapter 6).

The vulnerability of mobile populations stems from poverty, separation from family and regular sexual partners, differences in language and culture leading to isolation, separation from native sociocultural background, lack of community support, lack of access to health and social services, and a sense of anonymity.[272] Displacement, migration, and high urban poverty provide fertile grounds for the establishment of sex work.[273] The loneliness and anonymity associated with living in a foreign country can be conducive to practicing high-risk behavior.[274]

Complex emergencies are prevalent in MENA, such as in Afghanistan, Iraq, Lebanon, Somalia, and the West Bank and Gaza, and these emergencies are key drivers of population mobility. Emergencies can lead to rapid changes in risk behavior and may facilitate HIV infectious spread.[275] The presence of foreign troops and military occupations can complicate HIV efforts. The presence of a large number of foreign troops in Afghanistan has been associated with rapid economic development, but has yielded more opportunities for risky behavior such as IDU and female sex work.[276] The presence of the African Peace Keepers in Darfur has added another risk factor for HIV infection, particularly among women.[277]

There is evidence in MENA that HIV patients are mobile and have crossed national boundaries. Half of the reported HIV cases in Tunisia were believed to have at some point crossed the border into Tunisia, mainly from Libya, to seek antiretroviral treatment or to undergo drug rehabilitation.[278]

Migrants

In this section we discuss migration as vulnerability for HIV infection.

Prevalence of migration

The Arab Middle East has received more than 10% of the world's migrants,[279] with the Persian Gulf region hosting the largest share of guest workers to indigenous populations anywhere.[280] The International Organization for Migration (IOM) estimates that there are 14 million international migrants in the Arab Middle East.[281] Saudi Arabia is the leading source of remittances in MENA, and second only to the United States as a source of migrant worker remittances globally.[282] Three MENA countries, Egypt, Lebanon, and Jordan, are among the nine largest recipients of remittances from migrant workers among developing countries.[283]

Migration has enormously affected demographics in MENA. It is estimated that a million Afghanis leave Afghanistan every year to work abroad.[284] Seasonal economic migration also appears to be high in Afghanistan.[285] The migrant workforce accounted for 4.7% of the total population in the Republic of Yemen in 1994.[286] There are 875,000 Yemenis registered as living abroad.[287] It is estimated that there are 2 million economic migrants[288] and 16 million pastoralists[289] in the Horn of Africa region. Migration and being away from family are associated with higher exposure to STIs.[290]

Structural factors related to migration

There are structural problems in MENA that drive the high levels of migration. The Arab

[271] IGAD, *IGAD/World Bank Cross Border Mobile Population Mapping Exercise.*

[272] Ibid.

[273] Ati, "HIV/AIDS/STIs Social and Geographical Mapping."

[274] Al-Mutairi et al., "Clinical Patterns."

[275] Salama and Dondero, "HIV Surveillance in Complex Emergencies."

[276] World Bank, "Mapping and Situation Assessment."

[277] Basha, "Vulnerable Population Research in Darfur."

[278] UNAIDS, and WHO, *AIDS Epidemic Update 2003.*

[279] Jaber, Métral, and Doraï, "Migration in the Arab Middle East."

[280] IOM, "World Migration."

[281] Ibid.

[282] Ibid.

[283] Ibid.

[284] Ryan, "Travel Report Summary."

[285] World Bank, "Mapping and Situation Assessment."

[286] Yemen Ministry of Planing and Development, *Yemen Human Development Report 1998.*

[287] Yemen MOH, *National Strategic Framework.*

[288] HOAP, "Regional Partnership on HIV Vulnerability."

[289] Morton, "Conceptualising the Links."

[290] Carael, Cleland, and Adeokun, "Overview"; Obasi et al., "Antibody to Herpes Simplex Virus Type 2."

Middle East has the highest unemployment rate in the world at an average of 15%,[291] three times the global average.[292] There are currently 6 million new entrants to the labor market every year in a flow that is proportionately greater than that of any other region in the world.[293] Economic hardship and poor economic development are forcing many to emigrate in search of employment. The industrial labor productivity per worker has been in decline since the 1980s, with the level in 1990 comparable to that in 1970.[294]

The large gap in income across countries and the pockets of wealth created by oil and gas revenues are also major drivers of migration. Rapid an economic development in oil-rich states, in addition to rising personal wealth, has created an enormous demand for migrant labor in the construction and services sectors.

Although women's share of employment is only 29% of the regional labor force, women from countries outside the region, principally from Bangladesh, Ethiopia, India, Indonesia, Pakistan, the Philippines, Sri Lanka, and Thailand, are recruited to fill positions not filled by indigenous women.[295] These women are filling positions as domestic workers or in the service sector in a trend that has contributed to increasing the percentage of women among migrants in recent years.[296]

Domestic workers in MENA are vulnerable to marginalization, gender-based discrimination, and exploitation[297] and some are experiencing sexual abuse or are being forced into sex work.[298] Abundant articles in the media document cases of harassment, sexual abuse, and violence against domestic workers, who on occasion can find no escape from their employers and jump out of windows or off of balconies to their death or injury.[299] Trafficking in persons is another aspect of migration in MENA.[300]

The segmentation of the labor market is one of the key structural trends that are contributing to heavy dependence on migrant workers. Indigenous populations are reluctant to work in certain sectors of the economy, relegating those sectors to migrant workers. Some countries are both exporters and importers of migrant workers. Migrant workers constitute about 20% of the resident labor force in Jordan, even though millions of Jordanians are working abroad and over 400,000 net emigrants have left the country between 1999 and 2003.[301] The growth of the Qualifying Industrial Zones in Jordan has also created more demand for migrant workers.[302]

The rural-urban and urban-urban migrations are also structural challenges in MENA.[303] In Sudan, large percentages of different population groups reported living in a place other than their place of birth, including 59.3% of university students,[304] 91.7% of military personnel,[305] 76.9% of prisoners,[306] 78.2% of truck drivers,[307] 58.4% of tea sellers,[308] 66.5% of street children,[309] 51.4% of ANC attendees,[310] 62.6% of FSWs,[311] 56.3% of TB patients,[312] 55.9% of STD clinic attendees,[313] and 78.3% of suspected AIDS patients.[314] The main reported causes of movement were work, marriage, war, education, treatment, and drought. Women are especially vulnerable in this kind of migration because it exposes them to the risk of being trapped into sex work.[315] Among FSWs in the Red Sea State in Sudan, 59% were migrants from outside of this state[316]; and among FSWs in Khartoum State, only about one-quarter were born in this state.[317] In Pakistan, 40%–70% of different priority populations reported having emigrated

[291] Fergany, *Aspects of Labor Migration.*
[292] UNDP, *The Arab Human Development Report 2002.*
[293] IOM, "World Migration."
[294] Fergany, *Aspects of Labor Migration.*
[295] IOM, "World Migration."
[296] Ibid.
[297] Ibid.
[298] Jenkins and Robalino, "HIV in the Middle East and North Africa"; Al-Najjar, "Women Migrant Domestic Workers in Bahrain"; Sabban, "United Arab Emirates: Migrant Women"; UNDP, "HIV Vulnerabilities of Migrant Women."
[299] IOM, "World Migration."
[300] Ibid.

[301] Ibid.
[302] Ibid.
[303] Ibid.
[304] Ahmed, *University Students.*
[305] Ahmed, *Military.*
[306] Ahmed, *Prisoners.*
[307] Ahmed, *Truck Drivers.*
[308] Ahmed, *Tea Sellers.*
[309] Ahmed, *Street Children.*
[310] Ahmed, *Antenatal.*
[311] Ahmed, *Sex Sellers.*
[312] Ahmed, *TB Patients.*
[313] Ahmed, *STDs.*
[314] Ahmed, *AIDS Patients.*
[315] Taha, "Sudanese Women Carry a Double Burden."
[316] Ati, "HIV/AIDS/STIs Social and Geographical Mapping."
[317] ACORD, "Qualitative Socio Economic Research."

from other cities.[318] In the Islamic Republic of Iran, 14.5% of the population had migrated within the country.[319]

The immigration systems in MENA are generally those of guest-worker-based·labor systems where a large fraction of migrants are single or without their spouses.[320] These workers are vulnerable to practices that increase the risk of exposure to HIV.[321] There is a large male-to-female disparity among migrant workers. In Saudi Arabia, 69.5% of migrant workers are males while 30.5% are females, and the vast majority of these workers are single or away from spouses.[322] A large share of the population in some MENA countries, if not the majority of the population, is made up of migrants, such as 23% in Oman,[323] 76% in the United Arab Emirates,[324] and 62% in Kuwait.[325] The ratio of nonnationals among the adult population is even higher, such as in Kuwait, where it is 70% and almost half of nonnationals are single.[326]

The sizable contribution of migrants in the labor force is not limited to the oil-rich economies. Even in a country like Jordan, with a resident labor force of 1,150,000 people, there were around 125,000 documented migrant workers in 2003 and as many undocumented migrants.[327] In the Maghreb region of MENA, the dominant pattern of migration is to Western Europe.[328] The Maghreb region is also increasingly used as a transit route toward Europe, or as a destination of sub-Saharan African migrants.[329]

Sexual and injecting risk behaviors among migrants

Several studies have documented some aspects of sexual and injecting drug behaviors among migrants. About 73% of IDUs in Afghanistan lived or worked outside of Afghanistan,[330] and 66% reported starting drug use while living in the Islamic Republic of Iran.[331] Among married STD clinic attendees in Kuwait, 70% were living alone and the average number of sexual partners was 2.3.[332]

Over 55% of single migrant men in Pakistan reported sexual experiences and 36% of married migrant men reported premarital sex.[333] Over the preceding 12 months, 13% of single migrant men reported nonmarital female sexual partners, 7% reported contacts with FSWs, and 2% reported sexual contacts with other males.[334] Among Pakistani workers in the Middle East, there is evidence of high-risk behaviors such as contacts with sex workers.[335]

Women from the former Soviet Union represent the majority of FSWs in the United Arab Emirates.[336] FSWs come to the Persian Gulf region through a manipulation of immigration laws that makes it possible for these women to stay as irregular migrants.[337] Official efforts continue to focus on drug smuggling and money laundering in the entertainment industry rather than on sex trade.

HIV spread among migrants

The Persian Gulf countries have instituted a policy of mandatory and periodic HIV testing of migrant workers since at least 2002.[338] Most often the testing happens without counseling or informed consent.[339] Migrant workers who test positive for HIV are deported. Already this policy has resulted in the deportation of over 400 HIV-positive people from Bahrain alone.[340]

The rate of positive HIV testing among migrant workers has been hovering around 0.021%, with a range of 0.011% to 0.031% over several years in Kuwait,[341] 0.05% in Qatar,[342] 0.1% to 0.2% in Saudi Arabia,[343] and

---

[318] Pakistan National AIDS Control Program, "Report of the Pilot Study in Karachi & Rawalpindi."

[319] Iranian Statistics Center, "Iran as Reflected by Statistics."

[320] IOM, "World Migration."

[321] UNAIDS, "Notes on AIDS in the Middle East and North Africa."

[322] Madani, "Sexually Transmitted Infections in Saudi Arabia."

[323] UNAIDS, "Notes on AIDS in the Middle East and North Africa."

[324] Ibid.

[325] Al-Fouzan and Al-Mutairi, "Overview."

[326] Ibid.

[327] IOM, "World Migration."

[328] Ibid.

[329] Ibid.

[330] World Bank, "Mapping and Situation Assessment."

[331] Action Aid Afghanistan, "HIV AIDS in Afghanistan."

[332] Al-Mutairi et al., "Clinical Patterns."

[333] Faisel and Cleland, "Migrant Men."

[334] Ibid.

[335] Khawaja et al., "HIV/AIDS and Its Risk Factors in Pakistan"; Shah et al., "HIV-Infected Workers Deported"; Baqi, Kayani, and Khan, "Epidemiology and Clinical Profile."

[336] IOM, "World Migration."

[337] Ibid.

[338] Khoja, "Rules & Regulations."

[339] UNDP, "HIV Vulnerabilities of Migrant Women."

[340] S. A. Jowder, Director, National HIV/AIDS/STI Program, personal communication (2007).

[341] Akhtar and Mohammad, "Spectral Analysis of HIV Seropositivity."

[342] Saeed, "Thirty-Two HIV/AIDS Cases Detected in June."

[343] T. A. Madani, personal communication (2007).

0.06% in the United Arab Emirates.[344] Many of the migrant workers who tested positive and were then deported had negative serology results for HIV when their residencies were initially granted. This suggests an ongoing HIV transmission within the Persian Gulf region and is confirmed by HIV case reports among migrants from countries that send their migrants primarily to the Arab world. There is evidence of HIV infection in the Persian Gulf region among migrants from Afghanistan,[345] Egypt,[346] Indonesia,[347] Lebanon,[348] the Philippines,[349] Sri Lanka,[350] Sudan,[351] and the Republic of Yemen.[352] Most exposures to STDs among migrant STD clinic attendees in Kuwait (92%) occurred in Kuwait.[353]

In Bangladesh, 51% of the reported cumulative HIV cases in 2002 were among returning migrant workers and 47 out of 259 HIV infections between 2002 and 2004 occurred while being away as migrants.[354] Among the newly identified infections in 2004, 56% were among returning migrants.[355] Most diagnosed HIV infections among Pakistanis for the first two decades following discovery of HIV/AIDS were attributed to deported HIV-positive migrants from the Persian Gulf states.[356] These workers represented 61% to 86% of reported cases every year in Pakistan during the 1996–98 period.[357] In the Philippines, 34% of PLHIV were overseas Filipino workers and 17% of them were domestic workers, while only 8% were entertainers.[358] In Sri Lanka, about 40% of identified HIV infections among women have been linked to working in the Persian Gulf region, mostly as domestic workers.[359]

Due to the hostile environment endured by HIV-positive migrant workers, including the threat of immediate deportation, there is a constant fear of persecution that creates challenges in supporting HIV efforts to aid migrants in MENA.[360]

Refugees and internally displaced persons

This section discusses population displacement as a vulnerability for HIV infection.

Numbers of refugees and internally displaced persons

There were some 42 million forcibly displaced people worldwide at the end of 2008.[361] This includes 15.2 million refugees, 827,000 asylum seekers, and 26 million IDPs.[362] Pakistan is host to the largest number of refugees worldwide (1.8 million), followed by Syria (1.1. million), and the Islamic Republic of Iran (980,000).[363] Afghan and Iraqi refugees account for almost half of all refugees under the United Nations High Commissioner for Refugees (UNHCR) responsibility worldwide.[364] In addition, there are 4.7 million Palestinian refugees under the responsibility of the United Nations Relief and Works Agency for Palestine Refugees in the Near East (UNRWA).[365]

MENA continues to have high numbers of internally displaced persons in Afghanistan, Iraq, Somalia, and Sudan. There are 2.6 million IDPs in Iraq.[366] The Iraqi diaspora involves more than 4 million people who are living abroad as refugees, asylum seekers, illegal migrants, migrant workers, or naturalized citizens of other countries.[367] Sudan is ranked among the leading countries in the world in terms of the number of IDPs.[368] There are about 4 million IDPs living in Khartoum and other states.[369] During the civil war in Lebanon, almost a third of the population was displaced.[370]

[344] U.A.E. MOH, "United Arab Emirates: Migrant Women."

[345] Ryan, "Travel Report Summary"; Todd et al., "Seroprevalence and Correlates of HIV."

[346] Jenkins and Robalino, "HIV in the Middle East and North Africa."

[347] UNDP, "HIV Vulnerabilities of Migrant Women."

[348] Pieniazek et al., "Introduction of HIV-2."

[349] UNDP, "HIV Vulnerabilities of Migrant Women."

[350] Ibid.

[351] Hierholzer et al., "HIV Type 1 Strains from East and West Africa."

[352] Saad et al., "HIV Type 1 Strains."

[353] Al-Mutairi et al., "Clinical Patterns."

[354] UNDP, "HIV Vulnerabilities of Migrant Women."

[355] Ibid.

[356] Khawaja et al., "HIV/AIDS and Its Risk Factors in Pakistan"; Rai et al., "HIV/AIDS in Pakistan"; Shah et al., "HIV-Infected Workers Deported"; Kayani et al., "A View of HIV-I Infection in Karachi."

[357] UNDP, "HIV Vulnerabilities of Migrant Women."

[358] Ibid.

[359] Jenkins and Robalino, "HIV in the Middle East and North Africa."

[360] AIDS Policy Law, "Fear of Persecution."

[361] UNHCR, "2008 Global Trends."

[362] Ibid.

[363] Ibid.

[364] Ibid.

[365] Ibid.

[366] Ibid.

[367] IOM, "World Migration."

[368] IGAD, IGAD/World Bank Cross Border Mobile Population Mapping Exercise.

[369] Sudan Government of National Unity, United Nations National Integrated Annual Action Plan 2007; Hampton, "Internally Displaced People."

[370] IOM, "World Migration."

Vulnerability to HIV

The characteristics that define a complex emergency, such as conflict, social instability, increased poverty, environmental destruction, and powerlessness, can increase vulnerability to HIV by reducing access to HIV prevention services, breaking down health infrastructure, disrupting social support networks, increasing exposure to sexual violence (rape, sexual abuse, and exploitation), increasing the number of persons having sex in return for food and shelter, and forcing population movement to an area of higher HIV prevalence.[371]

Studies have shown that the factors that affect HIV transmission during humanitarian emergencies are complex, depending upon many dynamic and interacting factors, including HIV prevalence rates in the area of origin and that of the host population, level of interaction between the displaced and surrounding populations, length of time of displacement, and location of displacements (for example, urban camps versus isolated camps).[372]

Levels of HIV knowledge tend to differ among displaced persons, and the location of refuge affects the level of knowledge. Among IDUs in Pakistan, Afghani refugees had lower HIV/AIDS knowledge than Pakistani nationals.[373] Among refugees returning to Afghanistan, 79% of returnees from the Islamic Republic of Iran reported receiving information about HIV, but only 51% of returnees from Pakistan reported receiving such information.[374] Low levels of knowledge were found among IDPs in Sudan in comparison to other population groups.[375] Refugees in the Republic of Yemen were found to have lower knowledge than both citizen and marginalized populations.[376] This may be due to lack of access to appropriate HIV awareness messages in languages refugees can understand.

Risky behavior and risk of HIV infection

A few studies in MENA have attempted to document sexual behavior among refugees and compare this to the surrounding host communities.

In Sudan, 9.1% of refugees reported extramarital affairs,[377] and among IDPs, 5.0% reported ever using a condom, 21.3% reported premarital and extramarital sex, 2.4% reported premarital sex, and 1.9% exchanged sex for money.[378] Also in Sudan, 41% of unmarried male refugees had casual sex in the last year and 0% had ever had transactional sex partners.[379] Among IDPs as well as the nondisplaced population, these percentages were 18% and 2%, respectively.[380] Condom use was found to be much higher among refugees (35%) than among IDPs and those not displaced (8%).[381]

A systematic review of HIV infection in conflict-affected and displaced people in seven sub-Saharan African countries found insufficient data to support the assertion that conflict, forced displacement, and wide-scale rape increase HIV prevalence.[382] There is evidence in MENA that does not support a link between increased HIV risk and population displacement such as among Somali and Sudanese refugees and IDPs.[383] There is also evidence that suggests better HIV knowledge and prevention practices among refugees. A behavioral surveillance study in Juba, Southern Sudan, showed that returning refugees compared to settled populations had greater HIV knowledge and better HIV prevention practices, such as condom use.[384]

However, there is also some evidence in MENA that seems to suggest some link between displacement and risk of exposure to HIV. Yet, it is not clear whether this merely reflects the influence of home country risk factors and HIV prevalence, or HIV risks specific to the refugees in the host country. For instance, Afghani IDUs in Pakistan reported higher injecting drug use (18.8% versus 12.3%) and nonsterile needle use (72.2% versus 48.2%) compared to Pakistani IDUs.[385] A survey in Somalia showed that women in IDP camps have higher HIV prevalence than

[371] UNAIDS and UNHCR, "Strategies."
[372] Spiegel et al., "Prevalence of HIV."
[373] Zafar et al., "HIV Knowledge and Risk Behaviors."
[374] Action Aid Afghanistan, "HIV AIDS in Afghanistan."
[375] Ahmed, *Internally Displaced People.*
[376] Al-Serouri, "Assessment of Knowledge."

[377] Elkarim et al., *The National Strategic Plan.*
[378] Ahmed, *Internally Displaced People.*
[379] UNHCR, "HIV Behavioural Surveillance Survey."
[380] Ibid.
[381] Ibid.
[382] Spiegel et al., "Prevalence of HIV."
[383] UNHCR, *HIV Sentinel Surveillance among Antenatal Clients and STI Patients;* UNHCR, "HIV Behavioural Surveillance Survey."
[384] UNHCR, "HIV Behavioural Surveillance Survey."
[385] Zafar et al., "HIV Knowledge and Risk Behaviors."

women in the general population.[386] In Southern Sudan, HIV prevalence was 4.4% in Yei town, where half of the respondents were internally displaced, but only 0.4% in Rumbek town, where the level of displacement is considerably lower.[387] In North Sudan, the prevalence among ANC women who were internally displaced (1.6%) was much higher than that of other pregnant women (0.3%).[388]

No evidence has been found in MENA to support the claim that refugees spread HIV infection in host communities.[389]

HIV spread among refugees and internally displaced persons

Several other point-prevalence surveys documented the level of HIV spread among displaced populations in MENA. Among Afghani refugees in the Islamic Republic of Iran, HIV prevalence was 0.2%.[390] Among Sudanese refugees, separate studies reported that HIV prevalence was 5.0% and 1.2% for ANC attendees and 0.8% for prevention of mother-to-child transmission (PMTCT) attendees in Kenya[391]; 5% for men and 2% for women in Ethiopia[392]; and 1% and 2.7% in Uganda.[393] In several studies in Sudan, HIV prevalence among IDPs or refugees was 1.57%,[394] 1%,[395] 4%,[396] 1%,[397] 0.26%,[398] and 0.27%.[399] Among Somali refugees attending ANCs in Kenya, HIV prevalence was 0.7% in 2003,[400] 1.4% in 2005,[401] and 1% in 2006.[402] Also at this location, studies found that HIV prevalence was 0.1% among Somali refugees attending ANCs who were offered PMTCT services, and 2.0% (2003), 1.7% (2005), and 0.9% (2006) among Somali refugees attending STI clinics.[403]

Analytical summary

Population mobility is a key HIV risk factor in MENA due to the sheer size of the mobile populations and the extensive presence of this vulnerability across MENA countries. The complex emergencies that continue to be present in the region lead to increased vulnerability to HIV. It is therefore important that forcibly displaced populations are included in national HIV programs and have universal access to prevention, treatment, and care programs.

STREET CHILDREN

Though prisoners, youth, and mobile populations are the key vulnerable populations in MENA, another important vulnerable population is that of "street children."

The presence of street children is an increasingly emerging phenomenon in several MENA countries, as well as globally.[404] Causes of this phenomenon in MENA include poverty, family disruption, natural and manmade disasters, following friends, and desiring drugs.[405] There are two types of street children: "home-based," where children spend most of the day on the street but still return home at night and may have some family support; and "street-based," where children spend most of day and night on the street and are functionally without family.[406]

Boys often engage in odd jobs, begging, theft, and sex work.[407] Girls, who have fewer work opportunities, obtain money primarily through begging and sex work.[408] Street girls in Sudan reported being frequently raped by street boys,

[386] Somaliland Ministry of Health and Labour, *Somaliland 2007 HIV/ Syphilis Seroprevalence Survey.*

[387] Kaiser et al., "HIV, Syphilis, Herpes Simplex Virus 2, and Behavioral Surveillance."

[388] Sudan Ministry of Health, *Sudan National HIV/AIDS Surveillance Unit.*

[389] UNHCR, "HIV Behavioural Surveillance Survey"; Spiegel et al., "Prevalence of HIV."

[390] SeyedAlinaghi, "Assessing the Prevalence of HIV."

[391] UNHCR, *HIV Sentinel Surveillance among Conflict Affected Populations.*

[392] Holt et al., "Planning STI/HIV Prevention."

[393] UNHCR, *HIV Sentinel Surveillance Report;* Uganda MOH, *STD/HIV/ AIDS Surveillance Report.*

[394] SNAP and UNAIDS, "HIV/AIDS Integrated Report North Sudan, 2004–5."

[395] Ahmed, *Internally Displaced People.*

[396] SNAP, "HIV Sentinel Surveillance."

[397] Ahmed, *Internally Displaced People.*

[398] Sudan National AIDS/STIs Program, *2007 ANC HIV Sentinel Sero-Survey.*

[399] Ibid.

[400] UNHCR, "HIV Sentinel Surveillance in Dadaab Refugee Camps" (2003).

[401] UNHCR, "Sentinel Surveillance Report Dadaab Refugee Camps" (2005).

[402] UNHCR, *HIV Sentinel Surveillance among Antenatal Clients and STI Patients.*

[403] Ibid.

[404] Dallape, "Urban Children"; UNICEF, *The State of the World's Children 2006.*

[405] Khalil, *Street Children and HIV/AIDS;* Kudrati et al., "Sexual Health and Risk Behaviour."

[406] Khalil, *Street Children and HIV/AIDS.*

[407] Kudrati, Plummer, and Yousif, "Children of the Sug."

[408] Ibid.

police, or other men, particularly at night.[409] Seventeen percent of these girls report sex work as their main means of earning money.[410] Street children are especially threatened by police.[411] Gang rape and substance abuse are common and 14% of street girls and 1% of street boys reported that sexual abuse is their greatest danger on the street.[412]

The number of street children appears to be growing in Sudan as a consequence of high rates of population mobility resulting from civil strife, political conflict, and economic hardship, particularly in rural areas.[413] It is estimated that there are 70,000 working and street children in Sudan, of which 86% are males.[414] It is also estimated that there are 200,000 street children in Egypt,[415] and 5,000–7,000 street children[416] in Lahore, Pakistan.

Child prostitution appears to be a growing problem in Morocco where street children approach tourists offering their sexual services.[417] A study of male street children in Pakistan found that 40% of the boys had exchanged sex for money, drugs, or goods over the last three months.[418]

An integrated biological and behavioral surveillance survey was conducted among street children 12–17 years old in Egypt.[419] Substantial levels of sexual activity were found, with 54.7% of males and 50% of females reporting previous sexual activity. Of these, 75.3% of the males and 71.9% of the females reported sexual activity within the 12 months preceding the survey. Alarmingly, 14.9% of these males and 33.3% of these females reported commercial sexual activity. Thirty-seven percent of the males reported being forced to have sex with males, and 6% reported being forced to have sex with females. Among females, 44.9% reported being forced to have sex with males.

Among males, 77.4% reported engaging in sex with other males.

Condom use was low among both males and females: 12% with commercial sex partners and 2% with noncommercial partners among males, and 13% with commercial sex partners and 6% with noncommercial partners among females. IDU was also reported by 1% of the males and 13.5% of the females. Other forms of substance abuse were reported by 67.9% of the males and 71.4% of the females. Knowledge of HIV/AIDS, STIs, and condoms was low among the surveyed street children.[420]

Among street children in Sudan, 5.8% reported ever using a condom, 56.3% reported premarital and extramarital sex, and 11.1% exchanged sex for money.[421] In the Islamic Republic of Iran, 60% of runaway girls are reported to become victims of sexual abuse within one week of leaving home, as well as having a substance abuse rate of 80%.[422]

These studies suggest a high-risk environment for street children in several MENA countries and provide clear evidence of how the vulnerability of this group is leading to high levels of risky behavior. Although no HIV cases were found in one of the studies in Egypt,[423] the levels of reported risk behavior suggest potential HIV transmission if the infection enters this population. Indeed, there is documented evidence for some HIV prevalence among street children in MENA; HIV prevalence was reported to be 1.3%[424] and 0%[425] by two studies in Egypt, and by other studies as 0%[426] in the Islamic Republic of Iran and 2.2%[427] in Sudan.

VULNERABILITY SETTINGS: ANALYTICAL SUMMARY

MENA has several vulnerability factors and the vulnerable populations are diverse, with a large fraction of the population belonging to one or

[409] Kudrati, Plummer, and Yousif, "Children of the Sug"; Lalor et al., "Victimisation amongst Street Children."

[410] Kudrati et al., "Sexual Health and Risk Behaviour."

[411] Awad, "Sudanese Street Children."

[412] Kudrati, Plummer, and Yousif, "Children of the Sug"; Plummer et al., "Beginning Street Life."

[413] Khalil, Street Children and HIV/AIDS.

[414] Consortium for Street Children, "A Civil Society Forum."

[415] Jenkins and Robalino, "HIV in the Middle East and North Africa."

[416] Towe et al., "Street Life and Drug Risk Behaviors."

[417] Kandela, "Child Prostitution and the Spread of AIDS."

[418] Towe et al., "Street Life and Drug Risk Behaviors."

[419] Egypt Ministry of Health and Population, and National AIDS Program, HIV/AIDS Biological and Behavioral Surveillance Survey.

[420] Egypt Ministry of Health and Population, and National AIDS Program, HIV/AIDS Biological and Behavioral Surveillance Survey.

[421] Ahmed, Street Children.

[422] Navipour and Mohebbi, "Street Children."

[423] Egypt Ministry of Health and Population, and National AIDS Program, HIV/AIDS Biological and Behavioral Surveillance Survey.

[424] SNAP, UNICEF, and UNAIDS, "Baseline Study on Knowledge."

[425] Egypt Ministry of Health and Population, and National AIDS Program, HIV/AIDS Biological and Behavioral Surveillance Survey.

[426] Vahdani et al., "Prevalence of Hepatitis."

[427] Ahmed, Street Children.

BOX **9.1**

Youth, Drug Use, and Marginalization in Lebanon

"The drug user is exposed to HIV/AIDS, suicide, and death most of the times . . . there should be someone giving him support." —Ramy

Ramy discussed several problems that face drug users, especially those of being exposed to HIV and other sexually transmitted infections, depression, and marginalization by family members, society, and law enforcement officers.

Ramy stated the example of "female drug users, who are engaged in sex work in order to purchase drugs, [and] cannot oblige their sexual partners to use condoms as prevention from HIV/AIDS and other STIs." He added: "I guarantee that more than 90% of people who use drugs would seek opioid substitution therapy if provided at low-prices and available within specialized centers [drop-in centers] that offer health, social and counseling services."

Ramy continued the story of the despair that he lived and that took over his life after 10 years of drug use. This led him to search for a solution, a way out of a worse situation—suicide—a solution [that] would stop his long suffering with drugs.

Then, Ramy met a social worker who introduced him to Soins Infirmiers et Développement Communautaire (SIDC) while visiting his friends in prison. SIDC was the NGO [nongovernmental organization] that led him down the road of reducing the harms that drugs were exposing

him to, and eventually to make the "life-changing" decision to stop using drugs.

Two years after health and psychological treatment and follow-up for Ramy, in addition to his work of outreach and peer education, he is transformed from being a drug user to a companion and supporting figure for his drug users friends.

They [drug users] have confidence in ex-drug users who are cured and who give them hope of becoming cured themselves, and who also help them to be prevented from HIV and hepatitis . . . those people [drug users] are exposed to several kinds of marginalization within their families, the society where they live, some of the health and medical centers, and law enforcement officers who specifically contribute to their unemployment because of their judicial record as a drug user.

Finally for Ramy, [a] "drug abuser is not a criminal, but a victim, and others have to accept him in the society without any discrimination, an attitude which helps to improve his health and helps him to be cured from drugs and thus he will become a productive and effective person in his society far from being marginalized and judged."

Source: Middle East and North Africa Harm Reduction Network 2008.

multiple vulnerability settings. There are three key vulnerable populations in MENA: prisoners, youth, and mobile populations. The above evidence highlights the vulnerability of these populations to HIV infection.

Prisoners are the most vulnerable group and prevention efforts need to focus on this population. Youth are enduring immense challenges that may compel them to engage in risky

behavior. There appears to be increasingly risky behavior among the youth population and it would be useful for surveillance efforts to monitor trends of youth behavior and STI incidence. Mobile populations have an extensive presence across the region, but their vulnerability to risk practices is not widely acknowledged.

Vulnerability settings will continue to be among the drivers of HIV transmission for the

Iraqi Women Refugees and Commercial Sex in Syria

Human rights organizations, UNHCR, and the international press have documented anecdotes of a thriving industry of Iraqi girls as young as age 12 working in night clubs in Damascus following the invasion of Iraq in 2003. Reliable statistics of Iraqi girls engaged in sex work are not available.

"Nada, 16, was dumped by her father at the Iraq-Syria border after her cousin had raped her. Five Iraqi men took her from the border to Damascus, where they raped her and sold her to a woman who forced her to work in night clubs and private villas."

Women picked up by the police are taken to government protection centers from where they frequently escape, are bailed out, or are sent to prison. Those deported to Iraq often make their way back to Syria.

In 2007, UNHCR reported 1.2 million Iraqi refugees in Syria. Despite the country's relaxed entry policy for its Arab neighbors, refugees, with the exception of Palestinian refugees, are not officially allowed to hold jobs. With the economic conditions declining over the extended period in exile or inside Iraq, aid workers and authorities attested to a marked increase in the numbers of Iraqi women and young girls engaged in sex work.

A United Nations report found that many women-headed families in "severe need" turned to sex work, in secret or with the knowledge or involvement of family members.

"I met three sisters-in-law recently who were living together and all prostituting themselves. They would go out on alternate nights—each woman took her turn—and then divide the money to feed all children" (Sister Marie-Claude, Good Shepherd Convent, Damascus).

The influx of Iraqi refugees to Syria overwhelmed the host country's infrastructure and restrained access to services, particularly to health services, for the vulnerable women and young girls.

Sources: BBC News report, December 2007; *New York Times*, May 2007.

---

years to come unless efforts are created to address them. Nevertheless, addressing these vulnerabilities should not distract us from focusing prevention efforts on priority populations, including IDUs, MSM, and FSWs, which are at the highest risk of HIV infection in MENA.

BIBLIOGRAPHY

ACORD. 2005. "Socio Economic Research on HIV/AIDS Prevention among Informal Sex Workers." Agency for Co-operation and Research in Development, Federal Ministry of Health, Sudan National AIDS Control Program, and the World Health Organization.

———. 2006. "Qualitative Socio Economic Research on Female Sex Workers and Their Vulnerability to HIV/AIDS in Khartoum State." Agency for Co-operation and Research in Development.

Action Aid Afghanistan. 2006. "HIV AIDS in Afghanistan: A Study on Knowledge, Attitude, Behavior, and Practice in High Risk and Vulnerable Groups in Afghanistan."

Adib, S. M., S. Akoum, S. El-Assaad, and A. Jurjus. 2002. "Heterosexual Awareness and Practices among Lebanese Male Conscripts." *East Mediterr Health J* 8: 765–75.

Afifi, M., and S. El-Sousi. 2004. "Drug Abuse and Related Behaviors among High School Student Children in Palestine Authority (2002–2004)."

Afshar, P. Unknown (a). "From the Assessment to the Implementation of Services Available for Drug Abuse and HIV/AIDS Prevention and Care in Prison Setting: The Experience of Iran." PowerPoint presentation.

———. Unknown (b). "Health and Prison." Director General of Health, Office of Iran Prisons Organization.

Afshar, P., and F. Kasraee. 2005. "HIV Prevention Experiences and Programs in Iranian Prisons" [MoPC0057]. Presented at the Seventh International Congress on AIDS in Asia and the Pacific, Kobe.

Ahmed, H. 1997. "STD/HIV Prevalence and Chemotherapy Studies in Somalia." Department of

Medical Microbiology, University of Gothenburg, Gothenburg.

Ahmed, S. M. 2004a. *AIDS Patients: Situation Analysis-Behavioral Survey Results & Discussions.* Report, Sudan National AIDS Control Program.

———. 2004b. *Antenatal: Situation Analysis-Behavioral Survey Results & Discussions.* Report, Sudan National AIDS Control Program.

———. 2004c. *Internally Displaced People: Situation Analysis-Behavioral Survey Results & Discussions.* Report, Sudan National AIDS Control Program.

———. 2004d. *Military: Situation Analysis-Behavioral Survey Results & Discussions.* Report, Sudan National AIDS Control Program.

———. 2004e. *Prisoners: Situation Analysis-Behavioral Survey Results & Discussions.* Report, Sudan National AIDS Control Program.

———. 2004f. *Sex Sellers: Situation Analysis-Behavioral Survey Results & Discussions.* Report, Sudan National AIDS Control Program.

———. 2004g. *STDs: Situation Analysis-Behavioral Survey Results & Discussions.* Report, Sudan National AIDS Control Program.

———. 2004h. *Street Children: Situation Analysis-Behavioral Survey Results & Discussions.* Report, Sudan National AIDS Control Program.

———. 2004i. *TB Patients: Situation Analysis-Behavioral Survey Results & Discussions.* Report, Sudan National AIDS Control Program.

———. 2004j. *Tea Sellers: Situation Analysis-Behavioral Survey Results & Discussions.* Report, Sudan National AIDS Control Program.

———. 2004k. *Truck Drivers: Situation Analysis-Behavioral Survey Results & Discussions.* Report, Sudan National AIDS Control Program.

———. 2004l. *University Students: Situation Analysis-Behavioral Survey, Results & Discussions.* Report, Sudan National AIDS Control Program.

AIDS Policy Law. 2005. "Immigration: Fear of Persecution for Being HIV-Positive in Lebanon Is Valid." *AIDS Policy Law* 20: 7.

Akers, D. S. 1967. "On Measuring the Marriage Squeeze." *Demography* 4: 907–24.

Akhtar, S., and H. G. Mohammad. 2008. "Spectral Analysis of HIV Sero-Positivity among Migrant Workers Entering Kuwait." *BMC Infect Dis* 8: 37.

Al Ahmadi, A., and S. Beatty. 1997. "Participatory-Socio Economic Needs Survey of the Sana'a Urban Settlements Dwellers with Special Reference to Women." Oxfam, Yemen.

Al-Fouzan, A., and N. Al-Mutairi. 2004. "Overview of Incidence of Sexually Transmitted Diseases in Kuwait." *Clin Dermatol* 22: 509–12.

Ali, F., A. A. Aziz, M. F. Helmy, A. A. Mobdy, and M. Darwish. 1996. "Prevalence of Certain Sexually Transmitted Diseases in Egypt." *J Egypt Public Health Assoc* 71: 553–75.

Alizadeh, A. H., S. M. Alavian, K. Jafari, and N. Yazdi. 2005. "Prevalence of Hepatitis C Virus Infection and Its Related Risk Factors in Drug Abuser Prisoners in Hamedan—Iran." *World J Gastroenterol* 11: 4085–89.

Al-Mutairi, N., A. Joshi, O. Nour-Eldin, A. K. Sharma, I. El-Adawy, and M. Rijhwani. 2007. "Clinical Patterns of Sexually Transmitted Diseases, Associated Sociodemographic Characteristics, and Sexual Practices in the Farwaniya Region of Kuwait." *Int J Dermatol* 46: 594–99.

Al-Najjar, S. 2002. "Women Migrant Domestic Workers in Bahrain." International Labour Office, International Migration Branch.

Al-Serouri, A. W. 2005. "Assessment of Knowledge, Attitudes and Beliefs about HIV/AIDS among Young People Residing in High Risk Communities in Aden Governatore, Republic of Yemen." Society for the Development of Women & Children (SOUL), Education, Health, Welfare. United Nations Children's Fund, Yemen Country Office, HIV/AIDS Project.

Altaf, F. J. 2006. "Cervical Cancer Screening with Pattern of Pap Smear: Review of Multicenter Studies." *Saudi Med J* 27: 1498–502.

Anonymous. 2006. *Scaling Up the HIV Response toward Universal Access to Prevention, Treatment, Care and Support in Jordan.* Summary report of the national consultation.

Aras, S., E. Orcin, S. Ozan, and S. Semin. 2007. "Sexual Behaviours and Contraception among University Students in Turkey." *J Biosoc Sci* 39: 121–35.

Aras, S., S. Semin, T. Gunay, E. Orcin, and S. Ozan. 2007. "Sexual Attitudes and Risk-Taking Behaviors of High School Students in Turkey." *J Sch Health* 77: 359–66; quiz 379–81.

Assaad, R., and F. Roudi-Fahimi. 2007. "Youth in the Middle East and North Africa: Demographic Opportunity Or Challenge?" Population Reference Bureau.

Assal, M. 2006. "HIV Prevalence, Knowledge, Attitude, Practices, and Risk Factors among Prisoners in Khartoum State, Sudan."

Ati, H. A. 2005. "HIV/AIDS/STIs Social and Geographical Mapping of Prisoners, Tea Sellers and Commercial Sex Workers in Port Sudan Town, Red Sea State." Draft 2, Ockenden International, Sudan.

Awad, S. S. 2003. "Sudanese Street Children Narrating Their Life Experiences." *Journal of Psychology in Africa* 13: 133–47.

Babay, Z. A., M. H. Addar, K. Shahid, and N. Meriki. 2004. "Age at Menarche and the Reproductive Performance of Saudi Women." *Ann Saudi Med* 24: 354–56.

Baqi, S., N. Kayani, and J. A. Khan. 1999. "Epidemiology and Clinical Profile of HIV/AIDS in Pakistan." *Trop Doct* 29: 144–48.

Baqi, S., N. Nabi, S. N. Hasan, A. J. Khan, O. Pasha, N. Kayani, R. A. Haque, I. U. Haq, M. Khurshid, S. Fisher-Hoch, S. P. Luby, and J. B. McCormick. 1998. "HIV Antibody Seroprevalence and Associated Risk Factors in Sex Workers, Drug Users, and Prisoners in Sindh, Pakistan." *J Acquir Immune Defic Syndr Hum Retrovirol* 18: 73–79.

Basha, H. M. 2006. "Vulnerable Population Research in Darfur."

Bobrik, A., K. Danishevski, K. Eroshina, and M. McKee. 2005. "Prison Health in Russia: The Larger Picture." *J Public Health Policy* 26: 30–59.

Bolhari, J., and S. M. Mirzamani. 2002. "Assessment of Substance Abuse in Iran's Prisons." United Nations Drug Control Program in Cooperation with the Drug Control Headquarters.

Bray, R. M., and M. E. Marsden. 1998. "Drug Use in Metropolitan America." Sage Publications.

Buavirat, A., K. Page-Shafer, G. J. van Griensven, J. S. Mandel, J. Evans, J. Chuaratanaphong, S. Chiamwongpat, R. Sacks, and A. Moss. 2003. "Risk of Prevalent HIV Infection Associated with Incarceration among Injecting Drug Users in Bangkok, Thailand: Case-Control Study." *BMJ* 326: 308.

Burans, J. P., M. McCarthy, S. M. el Tayeb, A. el Tigani, J. George, R. Abu-Elyazeed, and J. N. Woody. 1990. "Serosurvey of Prevalence of Human Immunodeficiency Virus amongst High Risk Groups in Port Sudan, Sudan." *East Afr Med J* 67: 650–55.

Burrows, D., A. Wodak, and WHO (World Health Organization). 2005. *Harm Reduction in Iran: Issues in National Scale-Up.* Report for WHO.

Busulwa, R. 2003. "HIV/AIDS Situation Analysis Study." Conducted in Hodeidah, Taiz, and Hadhramut, Ministry of Health, Republic of Yemen.

Carael, M. 1997. "Urban-Rural Differentials in HIV/STDs and Sexual Behaviour." In *Sexual Cultures and Migration in the Era of AIDS*, ed. G. Herdt, 107–26. Oxford: Oxford University Press.

Carael, M., J. Cleland, and L. Adeokun. 1991. "Overview and Selected Findings of Sexual Behaviour Surveys." *AIDS* 5 Suppl 1: S65–74.

Consortium for Street Children. 2004. "A Civil Society Forum for North Africa and the Middle East on Promoting and Protecting the Rights of Street Children." Consortium for Street Children, London. Cairo, Egypt, March 3–6.

Coskun, O., C. Gul, H. Erdem, O. Bedir, and C. P. Eyigun. 2008. "Prevalence of HIV and Syphilis among Turkish Blood Donors." *Ann Saudi Med* 28: 470.

Curtis, S. L., and E. G. Sutherland. 2004. "Measuring Sexual Behaviour in the Era of HIV/AIDS: The Experience of Demographic and Health Surveys and Similar Enquiries." *Sex Transm Infect* 80 Suppl 2: ii22–27.

Dagdeviren, N., T. Set, and Z. Akturk. 2008. "Sexual Activity among Turkish Adolescents: Once More the Distinguished Male." *Int J Adolesc Med Health* 20: 431–39.

Dallape, F. 1996. "Urban Children: A Challenge and an Opportunity." *Childhood* 3(2): 283–94.

Day, C., B. Nassirimanesh, A. Shakeshaft, and K. Dolan. 2006. "Patterns of Drug Use among a Sample of Drug Users and Injecting Drug Users Attending a General Practice in Iran." *Harm Reduct J* 3: 2.

DeJong, J., R. Jawad, I. Mortagy, and B. Shepard. 2005. "The Sexual and Reproductive Health of Young People in the Arab Countries and Iran." *Reprod Health Matters* 13: 49–59.

Dolan, K., B. Kite, E. Black, C. Aceijas, and G. V. Stimson. 2007. "HIV in Prison in Low-Income and Middle-Income Countries." *Lancet Infect Dis* 7: 32–41.

Dolan, K. A., and A. Wodak. 1999. "HIV Transmission in a Prison System in an Australian State." *Med J Aust* 171: 14–17.

Egypt Ministry of Health and Population. 2001. "HIV/AIDS Surveillance in Egypt, 2001." Proceedings of the WHO 11th Intercountry Meeting of National AIDS Program Managers.

Egypt Ministry of Health and Population, and National AIDS Program. 2006. *HIV/AIDS Biological and Behavioral Surveillance Survey.* Summary report.

El-Ghazzawi, E., G. Hunsmann, and J. Schneider. 1987. "Low Prevalence of Antibodies to HIV-1 and HTLV-I in Alexandria, Egypt." *AIDS Forsch* 2: 639.

El Ghrari, K., Z. Terrab, H. Benchikhi, H. Lakhdar, I. Jroundi, and M. Bennani. 2007. "Prevalence of Syphilis and HIV Infection in Female Prison Population in Morocco." *East Mediterr Health J* 13: 774–79.

Elharti, E. E., Z. A. Zidouh, M. R. Mengad, B. O. Bennani, S. A. Siwani, K. H. Khattabi, A. M. Alami, and E. R. Elaouad. 2002. "Result of HIV Sentinel Surveillance Studies in Morocco during 2001." *Int Conf AIDS*: 14.

El-Kak, F. H., R. A. Soweid, C. Taljeh, M. Kanj, and M. C. Shediac-Rizkallah. 2001. "High School Students in Postwar Lebanon: Attitudes, Information Sources, and Perceived Needs Related to Sexual and Reproductive Health." *J Adolesc Health* 29: 153–55.

Elkarim, M. A. A., H. A. Ahmed, S. M. Ahmed, I. Bashir, and S. Musa. 2003. *The National Strategic Plan for the Prevention and Control of HIV/AIDS in the Sudan, 2003–2007.* Sudan National AIDS Control Program, Federal Ministry of Health, Republic of the Sudan, Khartoum, Sudan.

El-Rahman, A. 2004. "Risky Behaviours for HIV/AIDS Infection among a Sample of Homosexuals in Cairo City, Egypt." XV International AIDS Conference, Bangkok, July 11–16, abstract WePeC6146.

Elrashied, S. M. 2006. "Generating Strategic Information and Assessing HIV/AIDS Knowledge, Attitude and Behaviour and Practices as well as Prevalence of HIV1 among MSM in Khartoum State, 2005." A draft report submitted to Sudan National AIDS Control Programme. Together Against AIDS Organization (TAG), Khartoum, Sudan.

El-Sayyed, N., I. A. Kabbash, and M. El-Gueniedy. 2008. "Risk Behaviours for HIV/AIDS Infection among Men Who Have Sex with Men in Cairo, Egypt." *East Mediterr Health J* 14: 905–15.

Elshimi, T., M. Warner-Smith, and M. Aon. 2004. "Blood-Borne Virus Risks of Problematic Drug Users in Greater Cairo." UNAIDS and UNODC, Geneva.

El-Zanaty, F., and A. El-Daw. 1996. "Behavior Research among Egyptian University Students." International Medical Technology Egypt (MEDTRIC), Family Health International, Behavioural Research Unit, unpublished report.

Faisel, A., and J. Cleland. 2006. "Migrant Men: A Priority for HIV Control in Pakistan?" *Sex Transm Infect* 82: 307–10.

Fargues, P. 2003. "Terminating Marriage." In *The New Arab Family, Cairo, Papers in Social Science, Vol. 24,*

Nos.1–2, ed. N. Hopkins, 247–73. Cairo: American University in Cairo Press.

Farhoudi, B., A. Montevalian, M. Motamedi, M. M. Khameneh, M. Mohraz, M. Rassolinejad, S. Jafari, P. Afshar, I. Esmaili, and L. Mohseni. 2003. "Human Immunodeficiency Virus and HIV-Associated Tuberculosis Infection and Their Risk Factors in Injecting Drug Users in Prison in Iran."

Fergany, N. 2001. *Aspects of Labor Migration and Unemployment in the Arab Region*. Cairo, Egypt: Almishkat Center for Research.

Gammeltoft, T. 2002. "Seeking Trust and Transcendence: Sexual Risk-Taking among Vietnamese Youth." *Soc Sci Med* 55: 483–96.

Gaughwin, M., R. Douglas, and A. Wodak. 1991. "Behind Bars—Risk Behaviours for HIV Transmission in Prisons: A Review." In *HIV/AIDS and Prisons Conference Proceedings*, ed. J. Norberry, S. A. Gerull, and M. D. Gaughwin, 89–108. Canberra: Australian Institute of Criminology.

Ghannad, M. S., S. M. Arab, M. Mirzaei, and A. Moinipur. 2009. "Epidemiologic Study of Human Immunodeficiency Virus (HIV) Infection in the Patients Referred to Health Centers in Hamadan Province, Iran." *AIDS Res Hum Retroviruses* 25: 277–83.

Gokengin, D., T. Yamazhan, D. Ozkaya, S. Aytug, E. Ertem, B. Arda, and D. Serter. 2003. "Sexual Knowledge, Attitudes, and Risk Behaviors of Students in Turkey." *J Sch Health* 73: 258–63.

Gutbi, O. S.-A., and A. M. G. Eldin. 2006. "Women Tea-Sellers in Khartoum and HIV/AIDS: Surviving Against the Odds." Khartoum, Sudan.

Haeri, S. 1994. "Temporary Marriage: An Islamic Discourse on Female Sexuality in Iran." In *The Eye of the Storm: Women in Post-Revolutionary Iran*, ed. M. Afkhami and E. Friedl, 98–114. New York, NY: Tauris Publishers.

Hampton, J. 1998. "Internally Displaced People: A Global Survey." Earthscan/James & James.

Hierholzer, M., R. R. Graham, I. El Khidir, S. Tasker, M. Darwish, G. D. Chapman, A. H. Fagbami, A. Soliman, D. L. Birx, F. McCutchan, and J. K. Carr. 2002. "HIV Type 1 Strains from East and West Africa Are Intermixed in Sudan." *AIDS Res Hum Retroviruses* 18: 1163–66.

HOAP (Horn of Africa Project). 2006. "Regional Partnership on HIV Vulnerability and Cross-Border Mobility in the Horn of Africa. Meeting Report." Hargeisa, Somaliland, November 13–15.

Holt, B. Y., P. Effler, W. Brady, J. Friday, E. Belay, K. Parker, and M. Toole. 2003. "Planning STI/HIV Prevention among Refugees and Mobile Populations: Situation Assessment of Sudanese Refugees." *Disasters* 27: 1–15.

IGAD (Intergovernmental Authority on Development). 2006. "IGAD/World Bank Cross Border Mobile Population Mapping Exercise." Sudan, draft report.

International Centre for Prison Studies. 2006. World Prison Brief Country Profiles, www.prisonstudies.org.

IOM (International Organization for Migration). 2005. "World Migration: Costs and Benefits of International Migration." IOM. Geneva.

Iran Center for Disease Management. Unknown. *Country Report on UNGASS Declaration of Commitment*. Office of Deputy Minister of Health in Health Affairs, Islamic Republic of Iran, in cooperation with UNAIDS Iran and the Iranian Center for AIDS Research.

———. 2004. *HIV/AIDS and STIs Surveillance Report*. Center for Disease Management, Ministry of Health and Medical Education, Tehran.

———. 2005. Three Month Statistics of the MoH AIDS Office. Unpublished.

Iran Prison Organization. 2006. "Health and Treatment Headquarter: An Overview on HIV/AIDS in Prisons of Islamic Republic of Iran" (in Persian).

Iranian Statistics Center. 2005. "Iran as Reflected by Statistics: 2004."

Jaber, H., F. Métral, and M. Doraï. 2000. "Migration in the Arab Middle East: Policies, Networks and Communities in the Context of Globalisation." Research Programme, CERMOC, Beirut/Amman, Konrad Adenauer Foundation.

Jahani, M. R., P. Kheirandish, M. Hosseini, H. Shirzad, S. A. Seyedalinaghi, N. Karami, P. Valiollahi, M. Mohraz, and W. McFarland. 2009. "HIV Seroconversion among Injection Drug Users in Detention, Tehran, Iran." *AIDS* 23: 538–40.

Javadi, A. A., M. Avijgan, and M. Hafizi. 2006. "Prevalence of HBV and HCV Infections and Associated Risk Factors in Addict Prisoners." *Iranian J Publ Health* 35: 33–36.

Jenkins, C., and D. A. Robalino. 2003. "HIV in the Middle East and North Africa: The Cost of Inaction." Orientations in Development Series. Washington, DC: World Bank.

Johns Hopkins University. 2001. "Youth Survey: Knowledge, Attitudes and Practices on Reproductive Health and Life Planning." Center for Communication Programs, National Population Commission, Jordan, Johns Hopkins University.

Jordan National AIDS Control Programme. 2005. *Report on the National KABP Survey on HIV/AIDS among Jordanian Youth*. NAP Jordan.

Kaiser, R., T. Kedamo, J. Lane, G. Kessia, R. Downing, T. Handzel, E. Marum, P. Salama, J. Mermin, W. Brady, and P. Spiegel. 2006. "HIV, Syphilis, Herpes Simplex Virus 2, and Behavioral Surveillance among Conflict-Affected Populations in Yei and Rumbek, Southern Sudan." *AIDS* 20: 942–44.

Kandela, P. 2000. "Child Prostitution and the Spread of AIDS." *Lancet* 356: 1991.

Kapila, K., S. S. George, A. Al-Shaheen, M. S. Al-Ottibi, S. K. Pathan, Z. A. Sheikh, B. E. Haji, M. K. Mallik, D. K. Das, and I. M. Francis. 2006. "Changing Spectrum of Squamous Cell Abnormalities Observed on Papanicolaou Smears in Mubarak Al-Kabeer Hospital, Kuwait, over a 13-year Period." *Med Princ Pract* 15: 253–59.

Karam, W., G. Aftimos, A. Jurjus, S. Khairallah, and N. Bedrossian. 2007. "Prevalence of Sexually Transmitted Infections in Lebanese Women as Revealed by Pap Smear Cytology: A Cross Sectional Study from 2002–2006." WHO/EMRO.

Kassak, K., J. DeJong, Z. Mahfoud, R. Afifi, S. Abdurahim, M. L. Sami Ramia, F. El-Barbir, M. Ghanem, S. Shamra, K. Kreidiyyeh, and D. El-Khoury. 2008. "Final Working Protocol for an Integrated Bio-Behavioral Surveillance Study among Four Vulnerable Groups in Lebanon: Men Who Have Sex with Men; Prisoners; Commercial Sex Workers; and Intravenous Drug Users." Grey Report.

Kayani, N., A. Sheikh, A. Khan, C. Mithani, and M. Khurshid. 1994. "A View of HIV-I Infection in Karachi." *J Pak Med Assoc* 44: 8–11.

Khalil, J. H. 2006. *Street Children and HIV/AIDS*. Report on training of counselors and peer educators. Afrocenter Projects and Research Department, SNAP/UNFPA Joint HIV/AIDS/STIs Project.

Khani, M., and M. M. Vakili. 2003. "Prevalence and Risk Factors of HIV, Hepatitis B Virus, and Hepatitis C Virus Infections in Drug Addicts among Zanjan Prisoners." *Arch Iranian Med* 6: 1–4.

Khattabi, H., and K. Alami. 2005. "Surveillance sentinelle du VIH, Résultats 2004 et tendance de la séro-prévalence du VIH." Morocco Ministry of Health, UNAIDS.

Khawaja, Z. A., L. Gibney, A. J. Ahmed, and S. H. Vermund. 1997. "HIV/AIDS and Its Risk Factors in Pakistan." *AIDS* 11: 843–48.

Kheirandish, P., S. SeyedAlinaghi, M. Jahani, H. Shirzad, M. Seyed Ahmadian, A. Majidi, A. Sharifi, M. Hosseini, M. Mohraz, and W. McFarland. 2009. "Prevalence and Correlates of Hepatitis C Infection among Male Injection Drug Users in Detention, Tehran, Iran." Unpublished, Iranian Center for HIV AIDS Research, Department of Infectious and Tropical Diseases, Tehran University.

Khoja, T. A. 2002. "Rules & Regulations for Medical Examination of Expatriates Recruited for Work in the Arab States of the Gulf Cooperation Council." Executive Board of the Health Ministers' Council for the GCC States.

Kocak, N., S. Hepgul, S. Ozbayburtlu, H. Altunay, M. F. Ozsoy, E. Kosan, Y. Aksu, G. Yilmaz, and A. Pahsa. 2004. "Trends in Major Transfusion-Transmissible Infections among Blood Donors over 17 Years in Istanbul, Turkey." *J Int Med Res* 32: 671–75.

Kudrati, M., M. L. Plummer, and N. D. Yousif. 2008. "Children of the Sug: A Study of the Daily Lives of Street Children in Khartoum, Sudan, with Intervention Recommendations." *Child Abuse Negl* 32: 439–48.

Kudrati, M., M. Plummer, N. Dafaalla El Hag Yousif, A. Mohamed Adam Adham, W. Mohamed Osman Khalifa, A. Khogali Eltayeb, J. Mohamed Jubara, V. Omujwok Apieker, S. Ali Yousif, and S. Mohamed Elnour. 2002. "Sexual Health and Risk Behaviour of Full-Time Street Children in Khartoum, Sudan." International Conference on AIDS, Barcelona, Spain, July 7–12; 14: abstract no. LbOr04.

Lalor, K., M. Taylor, A. Veale, A. H. Ali, and M. E. Bushra. 1993. "Victimisation amongst Street Children in Sudan and Ethiopia: A Preliminary Analysis." In *Understanding Crime: Experiences of Crimes and Crime Control*, ed. A. Frate, U. Zvekic, and J. Dijk, 343–49. United Nations Crime and Justice Research Institute Publication No. 49. Rome: UNICRI.

Lambert, L. 2007. "HIV and Development Challenges in Yemen: Which Grows Fastest?" *Health Policy and Planning* 22: 60.

Madani, T. A. 2006. "Sexually Transmitted Infections in Saudi Arabia." *BMC Infect Dis* 6: 3.

Mansoor, A. B., W. Fungladda, J. Kaewkungwal, and W. Wongwit. 2008. "Gender Differences in KAP Related to HIV/AIDS among Freshmen in Afghan Universities." *Southeast Asian J Trop Med Public Health* 39: 404–18.

Martin, V., J. A. Cayla, M. L. Moris, L. E. Alonso, and R. Perez. 1998. "Predictive Factors of HIV-Infection in Injecting Drug Users upon Incarceration." *Eur J Epidemiol* 14: 327–31.

Michael, T., M. Ahmed, and W. Lemma. 2003. "HIV/AIDS Behavioral Surveillance Survey (BSS): Round One." Djibouti, Ministry of Health.

Middle East and North Africa Harm Reduction Network. 2008. News bulletin, sixth issue, November.

Mimouni, B., and N. Remaoun. 2006. "Etude du Lien Potentiel entre l'Usage Problématique de Drogues et le VIH/SIDA en Algérie 2004–2005." Ministry of Higher Education, Algeria.

Ministère de la Santé Maroc. 2003–4. *Bulletin épidemiologique de surveillance du VIH/SIDA et des infections sexuellement transmissibles*. Rabat, Ministère de la Santé Maroc.

Ministére de la Santé-PNLS, de la Jeunesse, de la Promotion Femme, de l'Education, ADEPF (Association Djiboutienne pour l'Equilibre et la Promotion de la Famille), and UNICEF (United Nations Children's Fund). 2001. "Etude des connaissances attitudes-practiques des jeunes et leurs participations a la promotion de leurs activités et a la prévention des VIH/SIDA/MST a Djiboutiville."

Ministry of Health and Medical Education of Iran. 2006. "Treatment and Medical Education." Islamic Republic of Iran HIV/AIDS Situation and Response Analysis.

Mishwar. 2008. "An Integrated Bio-Behavioral Surveillance Study among Four Vulnerable Groups in Lebanon: Men Who Have Sex with Men; Prisoners; Commercial Sex Workers and Intravenous Drug Users." Internal document, final report, American University of Beirut and World Bank, Beirut, Lebanon.

Mohammad, K., F. K. Farahani, M. R. Mohammadi, S. Alikhani, M. Zare, F. R. Tehrani, A. Ramezankhani, A. Hasanzadeh, and H. Ghanbari. 2007. "Sexual Risk-Taking Behaviors among Boys Aged 15–18 Years in Tehran." *J Adolesc Health* 41: 407–14.

Mohammadi, M. R., K. Mohammad, F. K. Farahani, S. Alikhani, M. Zare, F. R. Tehrani, A. Ramezankhani, and F. Alaeddini. 2006. "Reproductive Knowledge, Attitudes and Behavior among Adolescent Males in Tehran, Iran." *Int Fam Plan Perspect* 32: 35–44.

Mohtasham Amiri, Z., M. Rezvani, R. Jafari Shakib, and A. Jafari Shakib. 2007. "Prevalence of Hepatitis C Virus Infection and Risk Factors of Drug Using Prisoners in Guilan Province." *East Mediterr Health J* 13: 250–56.

Monasch, R., and M. Mahy. 2006. "Young People: The Centre of the HIV Epidemic." *World Health Organ Tech Rep Ser* 938: 15–41.

Morocco MOH (Ministry of Health). 2007. *Surveillance sentinelle du VIH, résultats 2006 et tendances de la séroprévalence du VIH.*

Morton, J. 2003. "Conceptualising the Links between HIV/AIDS and Pastoralist Livelihoods." Paper presented to the Annual Conference of the Development Studies Association, 10-12.09. 03, amended draft 31.10. 03, Natural Resources Institute, University of Greenwich.

Mostashari, G., UNODC (United Nations Office on Drugs and Crime), and M. Darabi. 2006. "Summary of the Iranian Situation on HIV Epidemic." NSP Situation Analysis.

Mujeeb, S. A., and A. Hafeez. 1993. "Prevalence and Pattern of HIV Infection in Karachi." *J Pak Med Assoc* 43: 2–4.

Mutter, R. C., R. M. Grimes, and D. Labarthe. 1994. "Evidence of Intraprison Spread of HIV Infection." *Arch Intern Med* 154: 793–95.

Naffa, S. 2004. "Jordanian Women: Past and Present."

NAMRU-3 (Naval Medical Research Unit). 2004. "Young People and HIV/AIDS." A Qualitative Study in Cairo and Qena, Egypt. UNAIDS Secretariat and the National AIDS Programme, with Ford Foundation Funding.

Nassirimanesh, B. 2002. "Proceedings of the Abstract for the Fourth National Harm Reduction Conference." Harm Reduction Coalition, Seattle, USA.

Nassirimanesh, B., M. Trace, and M. Roberts. 2005. "The Rise of Harm Reduction in the Islamic Republic of Iran." Briefing Paper Eight, for the Beckley Foundation, Drug Policy Program.

Navipour, R., and M. R. Mohebbi. 2004. "Street Children and Runaway Adolescents in Iran." *Indian Pediatr* 41: 1283–84.

Ndiaye, P., H. O. Abdallahi el, A. Diedhiou, A. Tal-Dia, and J. P. Lemort. 2005. "Evaluation of Condom Use among Students of the El Mina Middle School in Nouakchott in the Islamic Republic of Mauritania." *Sante* 15: 189–94.

Obasi, A., F. Mosha, M. Quigley, Z. Sekirassa, T. Gibbs, K. Munguti, J. Todd, H. Grosskurth, P. Mayaud, J. Changalucha, D. Brown, D. Mabey, and R. Hayes. 1999. "Antibody to Herpes Simplex Virus Type 2 as a Marker of Sexual Risk Behavior in Rural Tanzania." *J Infect Dis* 179: 16–24.

Oman MOH (Ministry of Health). 2006. "HIV Risk among Heroin and Injecting Drug Users in Muscat, Oman." Quantitative survey, preliminary data.

Ono-Kihara, M., and M. Kihara. 2001. "The First Nationwide Sexual Behavior Survey in Japan—The Results of 'HIV & Sex in Japan 1999' Survey." *J Asian Sexol* 2.

Pakistan National AIDS Control Program. 2005a. *HIV Second Generation Surveillance in Pakistan.* National Report Round 1. Ministry of Health, Pakistan, and Canada-Pakistan HIV/AIDS Surveillance Project.

———. 2005b. *National Study of Reproductive Tract and Sexually Transmitted Infections: Survey of High Risk Groups in Lahore and Karachi.* Ministry of Health, Pakistan.

———. 2005c. "Report of the Pilot Study in Karachi & Rawalpindi." Ministry of Health Canada-Pakistan HIV/AIDS Surveillance Project, Integrated Biological & Behavioral Surveillance 2004–5.

———. 2006-7. *HIV Second Generation Surveillance in Pakistan.* National Report Round II. Ministry of Health, Pakistan, and Canada-Pakistan HIV/AIDS Surveillance Project.

———. 2008. *HIV Second Generation Surveillance in Pakistan.* National Report Round III. Ministry of Health, Pakistan, Canada-Pakistan HIV/AIDS Surveillance Project.

Parker, R. G., D. Easton, and C. H. Klein. 2000. "Structural Barriers and Facilitators in HIV Prevention: A Review of International Research." *AIDS* 14 Suppl 1: S22–32.

Pieniazek, D., J. Baggs, D. J. Hu, G. M. Matar, A. M. Abdelnoor, J. E. Mokhbat, A. Uwaydah, A. R. Bizri, A. Ramos, L. M. Janini, A. Tanuri, C. Fridlund, C. Schable, L. Heyndrickx, M. A. Rayfield, and W. Heneine. 1998. "Introduction of HIV-2 and Multiple HIV-1 Subtypes to Lebanon." *Emerg Infect Dis* 4: 649–56.

Pisani, E., S. Lazzari, N. Walker, and B. Schwartlander. 2003. "HIV Surveillance: A Global Perspective." *J Acquir Immune Defic Syndr* 32 Suppl 1: S3–11.

Platt, L. P. Vickerman, M. Collumbien, S. Hasan, N. Lalji, S. Mayhew, R. Muzaffar, A. Andreasen, and S. Hawkes. 2009. "Prevalence of HIV, HCV and Sexually Transmitted Infections among Injecting Drug Users in Rawalpindi and Abbottabad, Pakistan: Evidence for an Emerging Injection-Related HIV Epidemic." *Sex Transm Infect* 85 Suppl 2: ii17–22.

Plummer, M. L., M. Kudrati, and N. Dafalla El Hag Yousif. 2007. "Beginning Street Life: Factors Contributing to Children Working and Living on the Streets of Khartoum, Sudan." *Children and Youth Services Review* 29: 1520–36.

Pont, J., H. Strutz, W. Kahl, and G. Salzner. 1994. "HIV Epidemiology and Risk Behavior Promoting HIV Transmission in Austrian Prisons." *Eur J Epidemiol* 10: 285–89.

Population Studies Research Institute. 2000. "Baseline Survey on Reproductive Health and Family Planning in Northeast and Northwest Regions of Somalia." University of Nairobi, WHO.

Qidwai, W. 1999. "Sexual Knowledge and Practice in Pakistani Young Men." *J Pak Med Assoc* 49: 251–54.

Quinti, I., E. Renganathan, E. El Ghazzawi, M. Divizia, G. Sawaf, S. Awad, A. Pana, and G. Rocchi. 1995. "Seroprevalence of HIV and HCV Infections in Alexandria, Egypt." *Zentralbl Bakteriol* 283: 239–44.

Rahbar, A. R., S. Rooholamini, and K. Khoshnood. 2004. "Prevalence of HIV Infection and Other Blood-Borne Infections in Incarcerated and Non-Incarcerated Injection Drug Users (IDUs) in Mashhad, Iran." *International Journal of Drug Policy* 15: 151–55.

Rai, M. A., H. J. Warraich, S. H. Ali, and V. R. Nerurkar. 2007. "HIV/AIDS in Pakistan: The Battle Begins." *Retrovirology* 4: 22.

Ramezani, A., M. Mohraz, and L. Gachkar. 2006. "Epidemiologic Situation of Human Immunodeficiency Virus (HIV/AIDS Patients) in a Private Clinic in Tehran, Iran." *Arch Iran Med* 9: 315–18.

Rashad, H. 2000. "Demographic Transition in Arab Countries: A New Perspective." *Journal of Population Research* 17: 83–101.

Rashad, H., and M. Osman. 2003. "Nuptiality in Arab Countries: Changes and Implications." In *The New Arab Family, Cairo Papers in Social Science, Vol. 24, Nos. 1–2*, ed. N. Hopkins, 20–50. Cairo: American University in Cairo Press.

Rashad, H., M. I. Osman, and F. Roudi-Fahimi. 2005. *Marriage in the Arab World*. Population Reference Bureau.

Razzaghi, E., A. Rahimi, and M. Hosseini. 1999. *Rapid Situation Assessment (RSA) of Drug Abuse in Iran*. Tehran: Prevention Department, State Welfare Organization, Ministry of Health, I.R. of Iran and United Nations International Drug Control Program.

Refaat, A. 2004. "Practice and Awareness of Health Risk Behaviour among Egyptian University Students." *East Mediterr Health J* 10: 72–81.

Rock, E. M., M. Ireland, and M. D. Resnick. 2003. "To Know That We Know What We Know: Perceived Knowledge and Adolescent Sexual Risk Behavior." *J Pediatr Adolesc Gynecol* 16: 369–76.

Rodier, G. R., J. J. Morand, J. S. Olson, D. M. Watts, and S. Said. 1993. "HIV Infection among Secondary School Students in Djibouti, Horn of Africa: Knowledge, Exposure and Prevalence." *East Afr Med J* 70: 414–17.

Roudi-Fahimi, F., and L. Ashford. 2008. "Sexual & Reproductive Health in the Middle East and North Africa. A Guide for Reporters." Population Reference Bureau.

Ryan, S. 2006. "Travel Report Summary." Kabul, Afghanistan. Joint United Nations Programme on HIV/AIDS, February 27 through March 7, 2006.

Saad, M. D., A. Al-Jaufy, R. R. Grahan, Y. Nadai, K. C. Earhart, J. L. Sanchez, and J. K. Carr. 2005. "HIV Type 1 Strains Common in Europe, Africa, and Asia Cocirculate in Yemen." *AIDS Res Hum Retroviruses* 21: 644–48.

Sabban, R. 2002. "United Arab Emirates: Migrant Women in the United Arab Emirates, the Case of Female Domestic Workers." GENPROM Working Paper.

Saeed, Mohamed. "Thirty-Two HIV/AIDS Cases Detected in June," *The Peninsula Qatar*, July 21, 2008. http://thepeninsulaqatar.com/Display_news.asp?section=local_news&month=july2008&file=local_news2008072122852.xml.

Safdar, S., A. Mehmood, and S. Q. Abbas. 2009. "Prevalence of HIV/AIDS among Jail Inmates in Sindh." *J Pak Med Assoc* 59: 111–12.

Salama, P., and T. J. Dondero. 2001. "HIV Surveillance in Complex Emergencies." *AIDS* 15 Suppl 3: S4–12.

Sammud, A. 2005. "HIV in Libya." Ministry of Health, Tripoli, August.

Saxena, P., A. Kulczycki, and R. Jurdi. 2004. "Nuptiality Transition and Marriage Squeeze in Lebanon." *Journal of Comparative Marriage Studies* 35: 241.

Schoen, R. 1983. "Measuring the Tightness of a Marriage Squeeze." Working Papers in Population Studies No. PS 8201.

Sellami, A., M. Kharfi, S. Youssef, M. Zghal, B. Fazaa, I. Mokhtar, and M. R. Kamoun. 2003. "Epidemiologic Profile of Sexually Transmitted Diseases (STD) through a Specialized Consultation of STD." *Tunis Med* 81: 162–66.

SeyedAlinaghi, S. 2009. "Assessing the Prevalence of HIV among Afghani Immigrants in Iran through Rapid HIV Testing in the Field." Personal communication of unpublished document.

Shah, S. A., O. A. Khan, S. Kristensen, and S. H. Vermund. 1999. "HIV-Infected Workers Deported from the Gulf States: Impact on Southern Pakistan." *Int J STD AIDS* 10: 812–14.

Shareef, A., A. J. Burqan, A. Abed, E. Kalloub, and A. Alaiwi. 2006. "Drug Abuse Situation and ANGA Needs Study." PowerPoint presentation.

Shirazi, K. K., and M. A. Morowatisharifabad. 2009. "Religiosity and Determinants of Safe Sex in Iranian Non-Medical Male Students." *J Relig Health* 48: 29–36.

Shrestha, P. 1999. "Forthcoming WER Global Update of AIDS Cases." Reported to WHO, WHO/EMRO/ASD, 9/28/A5/61/2, Sept. 21, document tables. Geneva.

Sigusch, V. 1998. "The Neosexual Revolution." *Archives of Sexual Behavior* 27: 331–59.

Simbar, M., F. R. Tehrani, and Z. Hashemi. 2005. "Reproductive Health Knowledge, Attitudes and Practices of Iranian College Students." *East Mediterr Health J* 11: 888–97.

SNAP (Sudan National AIDS Programme). 2006. "HIV Sentinel Surveillance among Tuberculosis Patients in Sudan." Federal Ministry of Health, General Directorate of Preventive Medicine, SNAP.

———. 2008. "Update on the HIV Situation in Sudan." PowerPoint presentation.

SNAP, and UNAIDS (Joint United Nations Programme on HIV/AIDS). 2006. "HIV/AIDS Integrated Report North Sudan, 2004–2005 (draft)." With United Nations General Assembly Special Session on HIV/AIDS Declaration of Commitment.

SNAP, UNICEF (United Nations Children's Fund), and UNAIDS. 2005. "Baseline Study on Knowledge, Attitudes, and Practices on Sexual Behaviors and HIV/AIDS Prevention amongst Young People in Selected States in Sudan." HIV/AIDS KAPB Report. Projects and Research Department (AFROCENTER Group).

Somaliland Ministry of Health and Labour. 2007. *Somaliland 2007 HIV/Syphilis Seroprevalence Survey: A Technical Report*. Ministry of Health and Labour in collaboration with the WHO, UNAIDS, UNICEF/GFATM, and SOLNAC.

Spaulding, A., B. Stephenson, G. Macalino, W. Ruby, J. G. Clarke, and T. P. Flanigan. 2002. "Human Immunodeficiency Virus in Correctional Facilities: A Review." *Clin Infect Dis* 35: 305–12.

Spiegel, P. B., A. R. Bennedsen, J. Claass, L. Bruns, N. Patterson, D. Yiweza, and M. Schilperoord. 2007. "Prevalence of HIV Infection in Conflict-Affected and Displaced People in Seven Sub-Saharan African Countries: A Systematic Review." *Lancet* 369: 2187–95.

Sudan Government of National Unity. 2007. *United Nations National Integrated Annual Action Plan 2007.* United Nations.

Sudan Ministry of Health. 2005. *Sudan National HIV/AIDS Surveillance Unit, Annual Report.* Khartoum.

Sudan National AIDS/STIs Program. 2008. *2007 ANC HIV Sentinel Sero-survey, Technical Report.* Federal Ministry of Health, Preventive Medicine Directorate, Draft.

Sudan National HIV/AIDS Control Program. 2002. *Situation Analysis: Behavioral & Epidemiological Surveys & Response Analysis.* HIV/AIDS Strategic Planning Process Report, Federal Ministry of Health, Khartoum.

———. 2004. *HIV/AIDS/STIs Prevalence, Knowledge, Attitude, Practices and Risk Factors among University Students and Military Personnel.* Federal Ministry of Health, Khartoum.

Syria Mental Health Directorate. 2008. "Assessment of HIV Risk and Sero-Prevalence among Drug Users in Greater Damascus." Programme SNA, Syrian Ministry of Health, UNODC, UNAIDS.

Syria National AIDS Programme. 2004. "HIV/AIDS Female Sex Workers KABP Survey in Syria."

Tabarsi, P., S. M. Mirsaeidi, M. Amiri, S. D. Mansouri, M. R. Masjedi, and A. A. Velayati. 2008. "Clinical and Laboratory Profile of Patients with Tuberculosis/HIV Coinfection at a National Referral Centre: A Case Series." *East Mediterr Health J* 14: 283–91.

Taha, S. I. 1995. "Sudanese Women Carry a Double Burden: Special Report; Women and HIV." *AIDS Anal Afr* 5: 12.

Taylor, A., D. Goldberg, J. Emslie, J. Wrench, L. Gruer, S. Cameron, J. Black, B. Davis, J. McGregor, E. Follett, et al. 1995. "Outbreak of HIV Infection in a Scottish Prison." *BMJ* 310: 289–92.

Tchupo, J. P. 1998. *Les maladies sexuellement transmissibles en République de Djibouti: Evaluation de la situation et recommandations pour une prise en charge optimale.* Report de mission, UNAIDS.

Tehrani, F. R., and H. Malek-Afzalip. 2008. "Knowledge, Attitudes and Practices concerning HIV/AIDS among Iranian At-Risk Sub-Populations." *Eastern Mediterranean Health Journal* 14.

Tiouiri, H., B. Naddari, G. Khiari, S. Hajjem, and A. Zribi. 1999. "Study of Psychosocial Factors in HIV Infected Patients in Tunisia." *East Mediterr Health J* 5: 903–11.

Todd, C. S., A. M. Abed, S. A. Strathdee, P. T. Scott, B. A. Botros, N. Safi, and K. C. Earhart. 2007. "HIV, Hepatitis C, and Hepatitis B Infections and Associated Risk Behavior in Injection Drug Users, Kabul, Afghanistan." *Emerg Infect Dis* 13: 1327–31.

Todd, C. S., M. Ahmadzai, F. Atiqzai, S. Miller, J. M. Smith, S. A. Ghazanfar, and S. A. Strathdee. 2008. "Seroprevalence and Correlates of HIV, Syphilis, and Hepatitis B and C Virus among Intrapartum Patients in Kabul, Afghanistan." *BMC Infect Dis* 8: 119.

Towe, V. L., S. ul Hasan, S. T. Zafar, and S. G. Sherman. 2009. "Street Life and Drug Risk Behaviors Associated with Exchanging Sex among Male Street Children in Lahore, Pakistan." *J Adolesc Health* 44: 222–28.

U.A.E. MOH (United Arab Emirates/Ministry of Health). 2006. "United Arab Emirates: Migrant Women in the United Arab Emirates."

Uganda MOH (Ministry of Health). 2003. *STD/HIV/AIDS Surveillance Report.* Kampala.

UNAIDS (Joint United Nations Programme on HIV/ AIDS). 2002. "Factsheet 2002: The Middle East and North Africa." UNAIDS, Geneva.

———. 2004. *Report on the Global AIDS Epidemic: 4th Global Report.* Geneva, Switzerland.

———. 2006. "HIV Prevention in Jordan: Common Country Assessment; Key Challenges in Health."

———. 2007. "Key Findings on HIV Status in the West Bank and Gaza." Working document, UNAIDS Regional Support Team (RST) for the Middle East and North Africa.

———. 2008. "Notes on AIDS in the Middle East and North Africa." RST MENA.

UNAIDS, and UNHCR (United Nations High Commissioner on Refugees). 2005. "Strategies to Support the HIV Related Needs of Refugees and Host Populations." Geneva.

UNAIDS, and WHO (World Health Organization). 2001. *AIDS Epidemic Update 2001.* Geneva.

———. 2002. *AIDS Epidemic Update 2002.* Geneva.

———. 2003. *AIDS Epidemic Update 2003.* Geneva.

———. 2005. *AIDS Epidemic Update 2005.* Geneva.

UNDP (United Nations Development Programme). 2002. *The Arab Human Development Report 2002: Creating Opportunities for Future Generations.* United Nations Development Programme, Regional Bureau for Arab States.

———. 2008. "HIV Vulnerabilities of Migrant Women: From Asia to the Arab States; Shifting from Silence, Stigma and Shame to Safe Mobility with Dignity, Equity and Justice." Regional Centre in Colombo.

Ungan, M., and H. Yaman. 2003. "AIDS Knowledge and Educational Needs of Technical University Students in Turkey." *Patient Educ Couns* 51: 163–67.

UNHCR (United Nations High Commissioner on Refugees). 2003. "HIV Sentinel Surveillance in Dadaab Refugee Camps."

———. 2005. "Sentinel Surveillance Report Dadaab Refugee Camps."

———. 2006. *HIV Sentinel Surveillance Report in Two Refugee Settlements in Uganda, 2004.* Kampala: UNHCR.

———. 2006–7a. *HIV Sentinel Surveillance among Antenatal Clients and STI Patients.* Dadaab Refugee Camps, Kenya.

———. 2006–7b. *HIV Sentinel Surveillance among Conflict Affected Populations.* Kakuma Refugee Camp— Refugees and Host Nationals, Great Lakes Initiative on HIV/AIDS.

———. 2007. "HIV Behavioural Surveillance Survey Juba Municipality, South Sudan." UNHCR.

———. 2009. "2008 Global Trends: Refugees, Asylum-Seekers, Returnees, Internally Displaced Persons and Stateless Persons."

UNICEF (United Nations Children's Fund). 2006. *The State of the World's Children 2006: Excluded and Invisible.* New York: UNICEF.

UNODC (United Nations Office on Drugs and Crime). 2002. "Drug Situation in the I.R. of Iran (May 2002)." Tehran, UNODC.

Vahdani, P., S. M. Hosseini-Moghaddam, L. Gachkar, and K. Sharafi. 2006. "Prevalence of Hepatitis B, Hepatitis C, Human Immunodeficiency Virus, and Syphilis among Street Children Residing in Southern Tehran, Iran." *Arch Iran Med* 9: 153–55.

WHO (World Health Organization). 2004. *The 2004 First National Second Generation HIV/AIDS/STI Sentinel Surveillance Survey, Somalia: A Technical Report.*

WHO/EMRO (Eastern Mediterranean Regional Office). 2000. "Presentation of WHO Somalia's Experience in Supporting the National Response." Somalia. Regional Consultation towards Improving HIV/AIDS & STD Surveillance in the Countries of EMRO, Beirut, Lebanon, Oct. 30–Nov. 2.

World Bank. 2008. "Mapping and Situation Assessment of Key Populations at High Risk of HIV in Three Cities of Afghanistan." Human Development Sector, South Asia Region (SAR) AIDS Team, World Bank.

Yamazhan, T., D. Gokengin, E. Ertem, R. Sertoz, S. Atalay, and D. Serter. 2007. "Attitudes towards HIV/AIDS and Other Sexually Transmitted Diseases in Secondary School Students in Izmir, Turkey: Changes in Time." *Trop Doct* 37: 10–12.

Yazdi, C. A., K. Aschbacher, A. Arvantaj, H. M. Naser, E. Abdollahi, A. Asadi, M. Mousavi, M. R. Narmani, M. Kianpishe, F. Nicfallah, and A. K. Moghadam. 2006. "Knowledge, Attitudes and Sources of Information regarding HIV/AIDS in Iranian Adolescents." *AIDS Care* 18: 1004–10.

Yemen Ministry of Planning and Development. 1998. *Yemen Human Development Report 1998.*

Yemen MOH (Ministry of Health). Unknown. *National Strategic Framework for the Control and Prevention of HIV/AIDS in the Republic of Yemen.*

Yousif, M. E. A. 2006. *Health Education Programme among Female Sex Workers in Wad Medani Town-Gezira State.* Final report.

Zafar, T., H. Brahmbhatt, G. Imam, S. ul Hassan, and S. A. Strathdee. 2003. "HIV Knowledge and Risk Behaviors among Pakistani and Afghani Drug Users in Quetta, Pakistan." *J Acquir Immune Defic Syndr* 32: 394–98.

Zali, M. R., R. Aghazadeh, A. Nowroozi, and H. Amir-Rasouly. 2001. "Anti-HCV Antibody among Iranian IV Drug Users: Is It a Serious Problem?" *Arch Iranian Med* 4: 115–19.

Zamani, S. 2008. "Methadone Maintenance Treatment (MMT) for Drug-Using Prisoners in Ghezel Hesar Prison, Karaj, Iran: A Qualitative Study." UNAIDS Collaborating Centre on Socio-Epidemiological HIV Research, Kyoto University, Japan.

Zamani, S., M. Kihara, M. M. Gouya, M. Vazirian, B. Nassirimanesh, M. Ono-Kihara, S. M. Ravari, A. Safaie, and S. Ichikawa. 2006. "High Prevalence of HIV Infection Associated with Incarceration among Community-Based Injecting Drug Users in Tehran, Iran." *J Acquir Immune Defic Syndr* 42: 342–46.

Zamani, S., M. Kihara, M. M. Gouya, M. Vazirian, M. Ono-Kihara, E. M. Razzaghi, and S. Ichikawa. 2005. "Prevalence of and Factors Associated with HIV-1 Infection among Drug Users Visiting Treatment Centers in Tehran, Iran." *AIDS* 19: 709–16.

Zamani, S., G. M. Mehdi, M. Ono-Kihara, S. Ichikawa, and M. Kuhara. 2007. "Shared Drug Injection inside Prison as a Potent Associated Factor for Acquisition of HIV Infection: Implication for Harm Reduction Interventions in Correctional Settings." *Journal of AIDS Research* 9: 217–22.

Zamani, S., M. Vazirian, B. Nassirimanesh, E. M. Razzaghi, M. Ono-Kihara, S. Mortazavi Ravari, M. M. Gouya, and M. Kihara. 2008. "Needle and Syringe Sharing Practices among Injecting Drug Users in Tehran: A Comparison of Two Neighborhoods, One with and One without a Needle and Syringe Program." *AIDS Behav.* DOI 10.1007/s10461-008-9404-2.

Chapter 10

Proxy Biological Markers of Sexual Risk Behavior

Sexual and injecting drug use (IDU) risk behavior measures in the Middle East and North Africa (MENA) tend to be poor, partially due to limited surveillance efforts and partially due to the conservative nature of its societies and the stigma associated with sexual and IDU risk behaviors. Even when such risk behavior measures exist, they may not provide us with a precise or even accurate assessment of the risk of exposure to human immunodeficiency virus (HIV).

Sexual risk behavior, and to some extent injecting drug use, is a complex phenomenon that cannot be directly observed. Only indirect data are available on sexual activity and these data are typically collected from questionnaires, interviews, focus group discussions, and other qualitative methods.[1] The indirect nature of evidence, the private and sensitive nature of sexual behavior, the informational limitations of egocentric sexual behavior data, and the nonrandom biases in sexual behavior reporting, including social desirability and memory, can introduce elements of bias and uncertainty in available measures.[2] Part of the population, such as women, may under-report their sexual activity while another part of the population, such as men, may over-report their

sexual activity.[3] The validity of reported risk behaviors from people whose risk behaviors are illegal, such as those of priority groups, is open to question.[4]

It is also challenging to precisely quantify risky behavior due to the multitude of facets of sexual behavior, from partnership formation to contact with sex workers, to heterogeneity in partner change rates, to assortative and age cohort mixing, among others. Network structure and concurrency of partnerships can further play a major role in HIV transmission.[5] A monogamous person in a stable sexual partnership, who is considered to have low-risk behavior, can still be considered at high risk of infection because she/he can be connected through her/his partner, or the partner of the partner, to a high-risk sexual network. Conversely, a person with frequent partnership changes who is considered to have high-risk behavior, can still be at low risk of infection if his/her network is virtually closed with a low risk of HIV penetration.

Despite some evidence for substantial levels of reported sexual and IDU risk behaviors in some priority groups in MENA, HIV prevalence appears to remain at low levels. This may

---

[1] Obasi et al., "Antibody to Herpes Simplex Virus Type 2."

[2] Lee and Renzetti, "The Problems of Researching Sensitive Topics"; Caldwell and Quiggin, "The Social Context of AIDS"; Wadsworth et al., "Methodology of the National Survey"; Morris, "Telling Tails"; Morris, *Network Epidemiology;* Cleland et al., "Measurement of Sexual Behaviour."

[3] Catania et al., "Methodological Problems."

[4] Pisani et al., "HIV Surveillance."

[5] Kretzschmar and Morris, "Measures of Concurrency in Networks"; Morris, "Sexual Networks and HIV"; Watts and May, "The Influence of Concurrent Partnerships"; Ghani, Swinton, and Garnett, "The Role of Sexual Partnership Networks."

suggest the limited explanatory power of available risk behavior measures. Faced with this dilemma, this chapter focuses on available data for sexually transmitted infections (STIs) with a special focus on herpes simplex virus type 2 (HSV-2) and human papillomavirus (HPV), which are relevant to the dynamics of HIV infectious spread. Biological markers of STIs provide inexpensive and reliable tools to gauge the nature of sexual activity in MENA and its manifestation in terms of the risk of HIV exposure. Most important, these measures provide us with an indication of the potential HIV spread in different population groups.

HSV-2 AS A MARKER OF SEXUAL RISK BEHAVIOR

Why HSV-2?

HSV-2, which causes the disease known as genital herpes, is one of the most infectious and widespread STIs,[6] and is the leading cause of genital ulcer disease (GUD) in both developed and developing countries.[7] It is estimated that there were 536 million people living with this infection in 2003, and 23.6 million people were newly infected in this same year.[8] Genital herpes is almost exclusively transmitted sexually and induces the production of lifelong antibodies.[9]

The strong observed correlations between HSV-2 infection and sexual risk behavior[10] suggested the use of HSV-2 antibodies in the blood as a convenient and objective serological marker of sexual behavior in different populations.[11] In addition to its role as a behavioral biomarker, there is extensive evidence that HSV-2 infection in both its clinical and subclinical forms substantially

increases HIV infection and transmission,[12] and that it had played a leading role in fueling the HIV epidemic in different populations.[13] The vast majority of HIV-positive people are also infected with HSV-2, and HSV-2 is most often acquired before HIV.[14]

Due to the common risk factors between HIV and HSV-2 but the larger infectivity of the HSV-2 infection, HSV-2 spreads faster than HIV along the paths of sexual risk and it delineates the potential avenues of future HIV spread in the population. In a sense, HSV-2 infection acts as a "tour guide" for HIV infection. HSV-2 can quantify the risk of exposure to STIs even when conventional behavioral measures, such as partnership change rates, may fail to quantify the risk posed by the structure of sexual networks.[15]

HSV-2 prevalence levels

Several studies have documented HSV-2 prevalence levels in MENA and in related cultural settings as listed in table 10.1. It is estimated that there are 9.6 million females and 8.6 million males infected with HSV-2 in this region, and that 388,000 and 195,000 new infections occurred in the year 2003 among females and males, respectively.[16] The pattern in table 10.1 is that of low or very low HSV-2 prevalence among general populations groups, but substantial prevalence among groups with identifiable risk factors such as male sex workers (MSWs), female sex workers (FSWs), "bar girls," IDUs, and sexually transmitted disease (STD) clinic attendees.

A few other studies found higher HSV-2 prevalence levels in MENA. In the Arab Republic of Egypt, an HSV-2 prevalence of 32% was reported among female clinic attendees.[17] In the Islamic Republic of Iran, a 28% prevalence was reported among a randomly selected population of women attending nine primary health care centers.[18] In Jordan, a prevalence of 53% for males and 42% for females was reported among

---

[6] O'Farrell, "Increasing Prevalence of Genital Herpes"; Smith and Robinson, "Age-Specific Prevalence of Infection"; Weiss, "Epidemiology of Herpes."

[7] Ahmed et al., "Etiology of Genital Ulcer Disease"; Mertz et al., "Etiology of Genital Ulcers"; Morse, "Etiology of Genital Ulcer Disease."

[8] Looker, Garnett, and Schmid, "An Estimate of the Global Prevalence."

[9] van de Laar et al., "Prevalence and Correlates of Herpes."

[10] Obasi et al., "Antibody to Herpes Simplex Virus Type 2"; van de Laar et al., "Prevalence and Correlates of Herpes"; Cowan et al., "Antibody to Herpes Simplex Virus Type 2"; Cunningham et al., "Herpes Simplex Virus Type 2 Antibody."

[11] Nahmias, Lee, and Beckman-Nahmias, "Sero-Epidemiological and Sociological Patterns."

[12] Freeman et al., "Herpes Simplex Virus 2 Infection."

[13] Abu-Raddad et al., "Genital Herpes"; Corey et al., "The Effects of Herpes."

[14] Corey et al., "The Effects of Herpes."

[15] Nagelkerke et al., "Body Mass Index."

[16] Looker, Garnett, and Schmid, "An Estimate of the Global Prevalence."

[17] El-Sayed, Zaki, and Goda, "Relevance of Parvovirus B19."

[18] Kasraeian, Movaseghii, and Ghiam, "Seroepidemiological Study."

Table 10.1 HSV-2 Prevalence in Different Population Groups

Country	HSV-2 prevalence
Arab Israelis	9.0% (Arab and Jewish non-Soviet immigrants; pregnant women; Dan et al. 2003)
	2.4% (Arabs; STD clinic attendees; Feldman et al. 2003)
Bangladesh	12.0% (women attending basic health care clinic; Bogaerts et al. 2001)
Djibouti	2.0% (general population women; Marcelin et al. 2001)
	5.0% (male blood donors; Marcelin et al. 2001)
	49.0% (luxury bar FSWs; Marcelin et al. 2001)
	81% (street-based FSWs; Marcelin et al. 2001)
Egypt, Arab Republic of	6.2% (STD clinic attendees; Saleh et al. 2000)
Iran, Islamic Republic of	8.25% (pregnant women; Ziyaeyan et al. 2007)
Lebanon	0.027% (general population women; Karam et al. 2007)
Morocco	12.9% (ANC attendees; Cowan et al. 2003)
	16.2% (ANC attendees; WHO/EMRO Regional Database on HIV/AIDS)
	13.0% (general population women; WHO/EMRO Regional Database on HIV/AIDS)
	10.0% (general population men; WHO/EMRO Regional Database on HIV/AIDS)
	26.0% (urban women with a median age of 40 years; Patnaik et al. 2007)
	9.2% (male HIV sentinel surveillance attendees; Cowan et al. 2003)
	6.5% (military personnel; Cowan et al. 2003)
	6.7% (STD clinic attendees; WHO/EMRO Regional Database on HIV/AIDS)
Pakistan	11.0% (IDUs; Platt et al. 2009)
	6.0% (IDUs; Platt et al. 2009)
	8.0% (FSWs; Hawkes et al. 2009)
	4.7% (FSWs; Hawkes et al. 2009)
	7.4% (MSWs; *banthas;* Hawkes et al. 2009)
	2.5% (MSWs; *banthas;* Hawkes et al. 2009)
	14.0% (MSWs; *khotkis;* Hawkes et al. 2009)
	25.0% (MSWs; *khotkis;* Hawkes et al. 2009)
	54.0% (MSWs; *khusras;* Hawkes et al. 2009)
	31.3% (MSWs; *khusras;* Hawkes et al. 2009)
Sudan	5.5% (household cluster survey; Southern Sudan; Kaiser et al. 2006)
	27.0% (male Sudanese refugees in Ethiopia; Holt et al. 2003)
	26.0% (female Sudanese refugees in Ethiopia; Holt et al. 2003)
Syrian Arab Republic	0.0% (pregnant women; Ibrahim, Kouwaitli, and Obeid 2000)
	0.0% (general population women; Ibrahim, Kouwaitli, and Obeid 2000)
	0.3% (general population men; Ibrahim, Kouwaitli, and Obeid 2000)
	0.0% (neonates; Ibrahim, Kouwaitli, and Obeid 2000)
	9.5% (STD clinic attendees; Ibrahim, Kouwaitli, and Obeid 2000)
	8.0% (women with cervical cancer; Ibrahim, Kouwaitli, and Obeid 2000)
	20.0% ("bar girls"; Ibrahim, Kouwaitli, and Obeid 2000)
	34.0% (FSWs; Ibrahim, Kouwaitli, and Obeid 2000)
Turkey	5.0% (pregnant women; Dolar et al. 2006)
	8.0% (women with pregnancy complications; Cengiz et al. 1993)
	5.5% (blood donors; Dolar et al. 2006)
	4.8% (sexually active adults; Dolar et al. 2006)
	8.3% (hotel staff; Dolar et al. 2006)
	17.3% (patients with genital warts; Dolar et al. 2006)
	60.0% (FSWs; Dolar et al. 2006)
	6.15% (IgM; FSWs; Gul et al. 2008)
	80.0% (IgG; FSWs; Gul et al. 2008)
United Arab Emirates	12.0% (migrant workers; N. J. Nagelkerke, personal communication [2007])

Figure 10.1 HSV-2 Prevalence for Selected Populations, by Age Group in Morocco

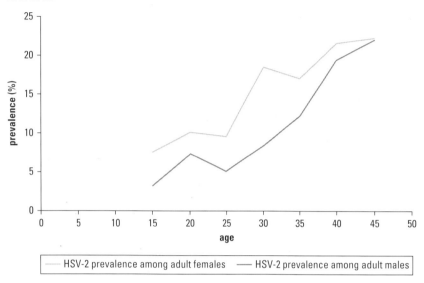

Source: Cowan et al. 2003.

healthy university students aged 18–24 years.[19] In Saudi Arabia, a prevalence of 27% was reported among pregnant women.[20] Finally, in Turkey, a prevalence of 63% was reported among pregnant women,[21] 53.5% was reported among general population women in a rural area,[22] and 26% was reported among men who have sex with men (MSM).[23]

However, some of the results of these studies appear to contradict the results in table 10.1 and need confirmation, because the serology tests used appear to suffer from high levels of cross-reactivity with herpes simplex virus type 1 (HSV-1) antibodies and use of nonspecific serologic assays.[24] HSV-1 infection is predominantly transmitted orally (not sexually), has a very high prevalence in MENA,[25] and shows extensive sequence homology with HSV-2.[26]

The type of tests conducted for HSV-2 serology in these studies was not able to be confirmed or clarified, despite repeated attempts. Some of these studies also tended to convey limited knowledge of HSV-2 epidemiology.

Figure 10.1 shows the age-stratified prevalence in a study from Morocco.[27] The prevalence grows rather slowly for both males and females compared to other regions,[28] suggesting that it takes a long time after sexual debut for the risk of exposure to this STI to be appreciable in magnitude. An alternative explanation might be a changing experience of successive birth cohorts in being exposed to HSV-2 infection in different eras.[29] However, this explanation seems unlikely because recent trends suggest increasing, rather than declining, sexual risk behaviors.

Implications, limitations, and future applications

The above data suggest that HSV-2 prevalence in the general population in MENA is low, and indeed among the lowest globally compared to other regions (table 10.2).[30] This provides an indication that the levels of sexual risk behavior in the general population are low and that HIV infection is likely to have limited inroads into this population. However, HSV-2 prevalence levels in populations with identifiable risk behaviors are considerable, and comparable to those in other regions, though at somewhat lower levels.[31] This suggests the potential for HIV to spread among priority populations.

[19] Abuharfeil and Meqdam, "Seroepidemiologic Study."

[20] Ghazi, Telmesani, and Mahomed, "TORCH Agents in Pregnant Saudi Women."

[21] Duran et al., "Asymptomatic Herpes."

[22] Maral et al., "Seroprevalences of Herpes."

[23] Cengiz et al., "Detection of Herpes"; Cengiz et al., "Demonstration of Herpes."

[24] Ashley et al., "Inability of Enzyme Immunoassays to Discriminate"; R. Ashley, personal communication (2007); Abu-Raddad et al., "HSV-2 Serology."

[25] Smith and Robinson, "Age-Specific Prevalence of Infection"; Cowan et al., "Seroepidemiological Study."

[26] R. Ashley, personal communication (2007); H. Weiss, personal communication (2007).

[27] Cowan et al., "Seroepidemiological Study."

[28] Smith and Robinson, "Age-Specific Prevalence of Infection"; Cowan et al., "Seroepidemiological Study."

[29] Burchell et al., "Chapter 6."

[30] O'Farrell, "Increasing Prevalence of Genital Herpes"; Smith and Robinson, "Age-Specific Prevalence of Infection"; Weiss, "Epidemiology of Herpes"; Pebody et al., "The Seroepidemiology of Herpes"; Paz-Bailey et al., "Herpes Simplex Virus Type 2."

[31] Smith and Robinson, "Age-Specific Prevalence of Infection."

Table 10.2 HSV-2 Prevalence in the General Population in Different Regions of the World Compared to MENA

Region	HSV-2 prevalence
Asia	10% to 30%
Europe	4% to 24%
Latin America	20% to 40%
Middle East and North Africa	0% to 15%
North America	18% to 26%
Sub-Saharan Africa	10% to 80%

Sources: O'Farrell 1999; Smith and Robinson 2002; Pebody et al. 2004; Weiss 2004; Paz-Bailey et al. 2007.

HSV-2 serology is a powerful marker of sexual risk behavior and should be a standard component in any planned or proposed surveillance efforts in MENA. HSV-2 prevalence can also help in identifying subgroups with an elevated risk of exposure to HIV that may benefit most from interventions. For example, in table 10.1, it is manifest that due to substantial HSV-2 prevalence among MSWs, FSWs, "bar girls," and STD clinic attendees, these groups are likely to be at an elevated risk of exposure to HIV and would benefit most from interventions. Given the difficulty of identifying populations at high risk in MENA, HSV-2 prevalence can be helpful in assessing the levels of risky behavior when data are limited or HIV prevalence is still at low levels, particularly among priority populations.

HSV-2 prevalence and incidence data can further be used in MENA for the evaluation of changes in sexual risk behavior or assessing the impact of interventions in different age cohorts over time.[32] Rates of HSV-2 prevalence change most rapidly among adolescents and young adults, suggesting that HSV-2 can be used to gauge recent changes in risky behavior among the young age cohorts.[33] Population-based data of HSV-2 collected sequentially in time would be valuable to determine the trends of sexual risk behavior.[34] This is pertinent given the rapid socioeconomic changes and liberalization of culture that this region is experiencing. HSV-2

prevalence in older age cohorts may not be as informative because the infection may have been acquired long before the serology test was performed. Monitoring of HSV-2 infection should be conducted using serology tests rather than diagnosis of herpetic ulcers because up to 90% of HSV-2 infections are asymptomatic or not clinically apparent.[35] Furthermore, the dominant form of herpetic ulceration may not be due to HSV-2 in MENA, but to HSV-1 (oro-genital transmission rather than purely genital transmission), as has been observed in Israel.[36]

In terms of limitations, HSV-1 infection has near universal prevalence in MENA[37] and may have a protective effect against HSV-2 acquisition,[38] thereby partially contributing to the low prevalence of HSV-2 in MENA. However, the evidence for a protective effect is conflicting,[39] and despite high HSV-1 prevalence in most populations around the globe,[40] this has not tainted the predictive power of HSV-2 as a proxy for sexual risk behavior. Indeed, the overwhelming evidence confirms the utility of HSV-2 as a marker of risky behavior irrespective of HSV-1 prevalence.[41] The near universal male circumcision coverage in MENA is also unlikely to explain the low and limited HSV-2 prevalence because male circumcision does not appear to substantially reduce HSV-2 sero-incidence.[42]

Some of the HSV-2 research work in MENA reflects methodological limitations. HSV-2 serology tests must be conducted carefully to avoid cross-reactivity with HSV-1 infection. Serological assays need to be validated in different populations

[32] van de Laar et al., "Prevalence and Correlates of Herpes"; Slomka, "Seroepidemiology and Control of Genital Herpes."
[33] Obasi et al., "Antibody to Herpes Simplex Virus Type 2."
[34] Looker, Garnett, and Schmid, "An Estimate of the Global Prevalence."

[35] Cowan et al., "Antibody to Herpes Simplex Virus Type 2"; Corey and Handsfield, "Genital Herpes and Public Health"; Fleming et al., "Herpes Simplex Virus Type 2."
[36] Samra, Scherf, and Dan, "Herpes Simplex Virus Type 1."
[37] Smith and Robinson, "Age-Specific Prevalence of Infection"; Cowan et al., "Seroepidemiological Study."
[38] Cowan et al., "Antibody to Herpes Simplex Virus Type 2"; Mertz et al., "Frequency of Acquisition."
[39] Cowan et al., "Seroepidemiological Study"; Brown et al., "The Acquisition of Herpes "; Langenberg et al., "A Prospective Study of New Infections with Herpes."
[40] Smith and Robinson, "Age-Specific Prevalence of Infection"; Cowan et al., "Seroepidemiological Study."
[41] Obasi et al., "Antibody to Herpes Simplex Virus Type 2"; van de Laar et al., "Prevalence and Correlates of Herpes"; Cowan et al., "Antibody to Herpes Simplex Virus Type 2"; Cunningham et al., "Herpes Simplex Virus"; Cowan et al., "Seroepidemiological Study"; Dan et al., "Prevalence and Risk Factors."
[42] Weiss et al., "Male Circumcision"; Bailey, "Scaling Up Circumcision Programmes."

by Western blot assays (WBA), which provide the golden reference standard for measuring HSV-2 serology.[43] This validation appears to have been done only once in MENA on a Moroccan sample using centralized study protocols and laboratory testing.[44] This further highlights the need for research expansion and surveillance work on HSV-2 in MENA.

Analytical summary

HSV-2 prevalence levels in the general population in MENA are low, but are considerable among priority groups. The prevalence level in the general population is among the lowest globally, suggesting that levels of sexual risk behavior in this population are low. HIV infection is unlikely to have substantial inroads into this population, confirming the results of HIV prevalence and behavioral measures (chapter 7). The substantial levels in priority groups suggest a potential for HIV spread among these groups.

HSV-2 serological measurements are underused in MENA despite their utility in indicating the levels of sexual risk behavior and HIV epidemic potential in different population groups. HSV-2 serology can also be used to track the trends of sexual risk behavior among youth. HSV-2 research in MENA needs to be expanded and HSV-2 serology should be included as a standard component of every surveillance effort.

HPV AND CERVICAL CANCER LEVELS AS MARKERS OF SEXUAL RISK BEHAVIOR

Why HPV and cervical cancer?

HPV is one of the most infectious sexually transmitted viruses.[45] It is the leading cause of over 99% of all cervical cancer cases worldwide.[46] HPV is also the causative agent of anogenital warts, which cause substantial health care costs globally,[47] and HPV is a major cause of the

cancers of the vagina, vulva, and penis.[48] HPV infection is the most common STI worldwide and most sexually active individuals, even with low sexual risk behavior, are likely to be exposed to HPV during their lifetime.[49]

Rates of HPV acquisition among women and men are very high following sexual debut as well as with the acquisition of new sexual partners.[50] Numerous studies have demonstrated the association between the number of lifetime sex partners and genital HPV infection,[51] including studies in MENA.[52] HPV, cervical cancer, and genital warts incidence and prevalence can be used as proxies of the levels of sexual risk behavior in the population.[53] HPV infection is not only associated with sexual intercourse, but also with other sexual contacts such as penile-vulvar, oral-penile, or finger-vulvar contacts.[54] HPV prevalence and cervical cancer levels appear to be particularly sensitive to the sexual behavior of the male population and, in particular, to contacts with FSWs.[55]

Cervical cancer levels

A number of studies and international databases[56] have documented cervical cancer levels in MENA. Table 10.3 shows the rates of cervical cancer incidence for each of the MENA countries.[57] These numbers represent national reports and are not necessarily derived using robust methodology. Table 10.4 displays the rates at select surveillance sites derived using sound methodology.[58] Figure 10.2 depicts the age-stratified cervical cancer

[43] Ashley and Wald, "Genital Herpes."

[44] Patnaik et al., "Type-Specific Seroprevalence."

[45] Burchell et al., "Modeling the Sexual Transmissibility."

[46] Bosch et al., "Prevalence of Human Papillomavirus in Cervical Cancer"; Walboomers et al., "Human Papillomavirus."

[47] Lacey, Lowndes, and Shah, "Chapter 4."

[48] Munoz et al., "Chapter 1."

[49] Trottier and Franco, "The Epidemiology of Genital Human Papillomavirus Infection."

[50] Collins et al., "Proximity of First Intercourse to Menarche"; Winer et al., "Genital Human Papillomavirus Infection"; Partridge et al., "Genital Human Papillomavirus Infection in Men."

[51] Baseman and Koutsky, "The Epidemiology of Human Papillomavirus Infections"; Lu et al., "Factors Associated with Acquisition and Clearance."

[52] Chaouki et al., "The Viral Origin of Cervical Cancer"; Hassen et al., "Cervical Human Papillomavirus Infection"; Hammouda et al., "Cervical Carcinoma in Algiers."

[53] Trottier and Franco, "The Epidemiology of Genital Human Papillomavirus Infection"; Chuang et al., "Condyloma Acuminatum."

[54] Burchell et al., "Chapter 6."

[55] Skegg et al., "Importance of the Male Factor."

[56] IARC and WHO, http://www.iarc.fr/.

[57] Ferlay et al., "GLOBOCAN 2002."

[58] Curado et al., *Cancer Incidence in Five Continents*, Volume IX.

Table 10.3 Age-Standardized Rates of Cervical Cancer Incidence and Mortality (per 100,000 women per year)

Country/Region	Incidence ASR	Mortality ASR
Afghanistan	6.9	3.6
Algeria	15.6	12.7
Bahrain	8.5	4.8
Djibouti	42.7	34.6
Egypt, Arab Rep. of	9.7	7.9
Iraq	3.3	1.8
Iran, Islamic Republic of	4.4	2.4
Israel	4.6	2.3
Jordan	4.3	2.4
Kuwait	6.1	3.4
Lebanon	15.4	8.0
Libya	11.9	9.6
Morocco	13.2	10.7
Oman	6.9	3.9
Pakistan	6.5	3.6
Qatar	3.9	2.2
Saudi Arabia	4.6	2.5
Somalia	42.7	34.6
Sudan	15.4	12.7
Syrian Arab Republic	2.0	1.0
Tunisia	6.8	5.5
Turkey	4.5	2.4
United Arab Emirates	9.9	5.3
Yemen, Republic of	8.0	4.6

Source: Ferlay et al. 2004.

Note: ASR = age-standardized rates.

Table 10.4 Age-Standardized Rates of Cervical Cancer Incidence and Mortality at Specific Surveillance Sites or Population Groups (per 100,000 women per year)

Country	ASR
Algeria	
Setif	11.6
Egypt, Arab Rep. of	
Gharbiah	2.1
Tunis	
Centre, Sousse	7.1
Bahrain	
Bahraini	6
Israel	
Non-Jews	2.4
Kuwait	
Kuwaitis	4.5
Non-Kuwaitis	5.3
Malaysia	
Penang	17.9
Sarawak	15.9
Oman	
Omani	6.5
Pakistan	
South Karachi	7.5
Singapore	
Malay	7.3
Turkey	
Antalya	4.4
Izmir	5.4

Source: Curado et al. 2007.

Note: Rates derived using robust methodology; ASR = age-standardized rates.

incidence in select MENA populations compared to the global average.[59]

Globally, the incidence of cervical cancer per country varies widely with rates ranging from 3 to 61 per 100,000 women per year.[60] As evident in the table, the rates in MENA are mostly low, and, in fact, the list of the lowest seven cervical cancer rates in the world (Syrian Arab Republic, Iraq, Turkey, Azerbaijan, Jordan, the Republic of Yemen, and Saudi Arabia) includes five MENA countries.[61] The Middle Eastern region has the lowest cervical cancer incidence rate of all regions at 5.6 per 100,000 women per year.[62] Of the distribution by predominant religion, Muslim states have the lowest cervical cancer rates at 15.6 per 100,000 women per year.[63] The lowest recorded incidence rate of cervical cancer worldwide is 0.4 per 100,000 women per year

in Ardabil, Islamic Republic of Iran.[64] Data from MENA also show a generally low prevalence of cervical intraepithelial neoplasia, the precursor to cervical cancer.[65]

Nonetheless, there is substantial variability in the region, with Djibouti and Somalia recording relatively high levels of cervical cancer. Cervical cancer is the most common cancer in Somalia among women,[66] just as it is the most common cancer in developing countries.[67] It is the second

[59] Parkin et al., *Cancer Incidence in Five Continents*, Vol. VIII.
[60] Drain et al., "Determinants of Cervical Cancer Rates."
[61] Ibid.
[62] Ibid.
[63] Ibid.

[64] Sadjadi et al., "Cancer Occurrence in Ardabil."
[65] El-All, Refaat, and Dandash, "Prevalence of Cervical Neoplastic Lesions"; Hammad, Jones, and Zayed, "Low Prevalence of Cervical Intraepithelial Neoplasia"; Komoditi, "Cervical and Corpus Uterine Cancer"; Altaf, "Pattern of Cervical Smear Cytology."
[66] Elattar, "Cancer in the Arab World."
[67] WHO, "Human Papillomavirus and HPV Vaccination."

Figure 10.2 Age-Stratified Cervical Cancer Incidence in Select MENA Populations Compared to the Global Average

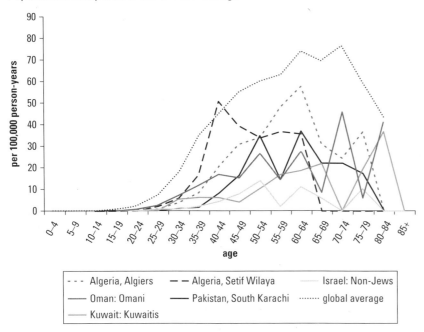

Source: Parkin et al. 2002.

most common cancer in Algeria,[68] Morocco,[69] and Tunisia,[70] but not one of the five leading cancers among women in Egypt, Jordan, Kuwait, Lebanon, and Saudi Arabia.[71] Cervical cancer accounts for 28.4% of cancer cases in Somalia, 16.3% in Algeria, 14.7% in Morocco, and 8.6% in Tunisia, but accounts for less than 6% in Egypt, Iraq, Kuwait, Lebanon, Saudi Arabia, and the Republic of Yemen.[72] In Jordan, cervical cancer accounts for only 2% of female cancers, ranking 13th to 16th among female cancers in the years 2000 to 2004.[73]

HPV prevalence levels

A number of studies have documented HPV prevalence in different population groups. Table 10.5 lists a summary of these studies as measured by DNA detection. These results suggest low-to-intermediate prevalence levels compared to other settings worldwide.[74] Yet,

prevalence levels are considerable and suggest significant HPV infection transmission in MENA.[75] Some studies found high levels of HPV infection, such as in Saudi Arabia,[76] despite low levels of cervical cancer in this country.[77] There is a question as to whether some of these studies are representative of women in the general population and whether they reflect prevalence of cancerous HPV types or not.[78] Well over a hundred HPV types have been identified, with only a minority of them being sexually transmitted.[79]

A few HPV and cervical cancer studies in MENA indicated an association between level of HPV prevalence (or cervical cancer) and socioeconomic status, including rural versus urban environment, type of household and occupation, and hygiene, sanitation, income, and education levels.[80] It is not clear what drives this association and whether it reflects a higher sexual risk behavior with lower socioeconomic status or not.

Implications, limitations, and future applications

HPV and cervical cancer levels in MENA suggest that the average level of sexual risk behavior in MENA populations is considerably less than that in other regions of the globe. However, there is substantial heterogeneity of HPV and cervical cancer levels, indicating variability of sexual risk behavior within MENA. It appears that countries closest to sub-Saharan Africa have the highest levels of risky behavior followed by the Maghreb countries in the western part of MENA. The lowest

[68] Elattar, "Cancer in the Arab World."
[69] Chaouki et al., "The Viral Origin of Cervical Cancer."
[70] Elattar, "Cancer in the Arab World."
[71] Ibid.
[72] Ibid.
[73] Jordan National Cancer Registry, *Cancer Incidence in Jordan;* Mahafzah et al., "Prevalence of Sexually Transmitted Infections."
[74] Curado et al., *Cancer Incidence in Five Continents;* Drain et al., "Determinants of Cervical Cancer Rates."

[75] Munoz et al., "Chapter 1."
[76] Al-Muammar et al., "Human Papilloma Virus-16/18 Cervical Infection."
[77] Jamal and Al-Maghrabi, "Profile of Pap Smear Cytology."
[78] Hamkar et al., "Prevalence of Human Papillomavirus."
[79] Baseman and Koutsky, "The Epidemiology of Human Papillomavirus Infections"; R. Barnabas, personal communication (2007); P. Drain, personal communication (2007); L. Koutsky, personal communication (2007).
[80] Roudi-Fahimi and Ashford, "Sexual & Reproductive Health"; Chaouki et al., "The Viral Origin of Cervical Cancer"; Hammouda et al., "Cervical Carcinoma in Algiers."

Table 10.5 HPV Prevalence in Different Population Groups in MENA

Country	HPV prevalence
Algeria	12.4% (controls in a hospital-based, case control study; Hammouda et al. 2005)
Bahrain	11.0% (women attending health facilities; Hajjaj et al. 2006)
Egypt, Arab Republic of	3.0% (community-based household survey; El-All, Refaat, and Dandash 2007) 15.0% (general population women; Abdel Aziz et al. 2006)
Iran, Islamic Republic of	13.0% (gynecology clinic attendees; Ghaffari et al. 2006) 9.0% (general population women; Hamkar et al. 2002) 3.0% (general population women; Farhadi 2005)
Jordan	0.0% (hospital attendees; Malkawi et al. 2004)
Lebanon	4.9% (gynecological clinic attendees; Mroueh et al. 2002)
Morocco	21.0% (controls in a hospital-based case control study; Chaouki et al. 1998)
Pakistan	33.0% (unspecified cervical specimens; Anwar et al. 1991)
Saudi Arabia	32.0% (family medical clinic attendees; Al-Muammar et al. 2007)
Tunisia	14.0% (national family population office attendees; Hassen, Remadi, and Chouchane 1999)
Turkey	8.0% (adolescent pregnant women; Yildirim, Inal, and Tinar 2005) 6.0% (low-risk hospital attendees; Ozcelik et al. 2003) 2.0% (general population women; Inal et al. 2007) 2.0% (controls in a clinic-based case control study; Cirpan et al. 2007)
West Bank and Gaza	13.0% (pregnant women; Lubbad and Al-Hindi 2007)

levels of risk appear to be in the Mashriq countries in the eastern part of the region.

The apparent differences in the levels of risk behavior across MENA may not be strictly due to substantial differences in how often people acquire new sexual partners, but may reflect the nature of sexual networks in different parts of the region. Cervical cancer rates appear to be determined by male rather than female sexual behavior.[81] A leading cause of this could be contacts with sex workers and the role of commercial sex in linking individuals within sexual networks.[82] Since HPV is very infectious and its transmission probability may be as high as 40% per coital act,[83] HPV can be easily transmitted between men and FSWs even after very few sex acts. Men pass this infection to their spouses who become infected despite practicing strict monogamy.

Accordingly, HPV infection levels provide a "snapshot" of sexual network connectivity in the region. The data suggest that sexual networks tend to be sparser in most countries of MENA compared to other regions, but fairly connected in other countries, perhaps through a higher fraction of men contacting FSWs. This is illustrated in the schematic diagrams in figure 10.3. In these two sexual networks, the number of sexual partnerships is equal, but the distribution of these partnerships is different. In figure 10.3a, the network is sparse, while in figure 10.3b the network has a high degree of connectivity as people are connected to each other through contacts with a node with a large number of partners. HPV could have a high prevalence in network (b), but a much lower prevalence in network (a).

One of the limitations of using cervical cancer as a proxy for sexual risk behavior is that women develop cervical cancer close to 20 years after HPV infection, as can be seen in figure 10.4.[84] The mean age of women with cervical cancer in MENA, as well as globally, is around 50 years.[85] Current levels of cervical cancer reflect levels of exposure among women two decades earlier, which may not be predictive of current risk behavior among young men and women. There could be a cohort effect of changing risk behavior across generations in different eras.[86] Measures

[81] Bosch et al., "Importance of Human Papillomavirus."

[82] Skegg et al., "Importance of the Male Factor."

[83] Burchell et al., "Modeling the Sexual Transmissibility."

[84] Schiffman and Castle, "The Promise of Global Cervical-Cancer Prevention."

[85] Baseman and Koutsky, "The Epidemiology of Human Papillomavirus Infections"; Altaf, "Pattern of Cervical Smear Cytology."

[86] Burchell et al., "Chapter 6."

Figure 10.3 A Schematic Diagram of Two Different Kinds of Sexual Networks with Different Connectivity

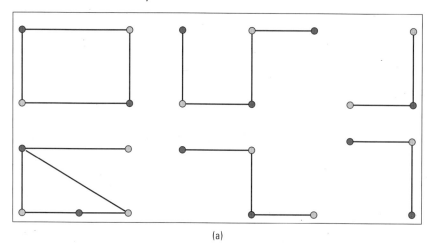

(a)

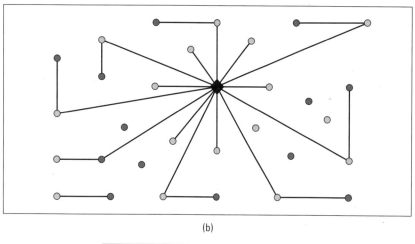

(b)

● Females   ○ Males   ◆ Female sex workers

Source: Author.

of precancerous lesions as well HPV prevalence levels may provide, when well established, better proxies of recent changes in risky behavior. There appears to be an increase in precancerous lesions due to HPV among Kuwaiti women over the years, as well as the appearance of these lesions at a younger age.[87] A similar apparent trend has been reported among women in Lebanon, particularly at younger ages.[88] The percentage of abnormal Pap smears also appears to be increasing in Saudi Arabia.[89] This may suggest an increase in sexual risk behavior among youth in MENA.

Another potential limitation to the use of HPV as a proxy measure is the role of male circumcision, which has been shown to reduce the risk of penile HPV[90] and genital warts[91] and improve clearance of HPV infection among men,[92] thereby reducing the transmission to women. This suggests that HPV prevalence in MENA could be low despite higher levels of risk behavior.

HPV levels can be used to measure recent changes in sexual risk behavior by examining increases in incidence of low-grade and high-grade precancerous lesions and cervical cancer levels among young females 20–30 years of age. HPV prevalence, as measured by direct HPV virus DNA detection, can also be an alternative powerful measure of changes in risky behavior over time.

Though low, our study suggests that levels of cervical cancer are considerable enough to warrant interventions for this health challenge. There are severe limitations in the screening programs and treatment facilities in much of the region; therefore, expansion of screening programs is recommended.[93] Pap smear screening appears to be at low levels, such as at 2% in Egypt[94] and 2.6% in Pakistan.[95] Cervical cancer diagnosis appears to occur in advanced stages where it is associated with a high mortality rate.[96] Despite the availability of screening infrastructure and its free cost in some resource-rich settings, such as in the United Arab Emirates, only 15.4% of women reported ever having a Pap smear test.[97]

[87] Kapila et al., "Changing Spectrum of Squamous Cell Abnormalities."
[88] Karam et al., "Prevalence of Sexually Transmitted Infections."
[89] Altaf, "Cervical Cancer Screening."

[90] Castellsague et al., "Male Circumcision."
[91] Bailey, "Scaling Up Circumcision Programmes."
[92] Lu et al., "Factors Associated with Acquisition and Clearance."
[93] Bennis et al., "Role of Cervical Smear."
[94] El-All, Refaat, and Dandash, "Prevalence of Cervical Neoplastic Lesions."
[95] Imam et al., "Perceptions and Practices."
[96] Chaouki et al., "The Viral Origin of Cervical Cancer"; Hammouda et al., "Cervical Carcinoma in Algiers."
[97] Bener, Denic, and Alwash, "Screening for Cervical Cancer."

In part, this is due to the lack of satisfactory awareness of this health issue among both the population and medical practitioners as well as the lack of a national screening policy for cervical cancer. In Pakistan, only 5% of women knew that screening was available for cervical cancer.[98] Due to the intrusive nature of the test, in conservative societies many women prefer for such a test to be administered by females.[99] In Kuwait, 78.7% of women in one study preferred that a female doctor conduct the test.[100]

On the other hand, it appears that a rather significant proportion of women report having at least one Pap smear in their lifetime in a few countries.[101] In a study in the Islamic Republic of Iran, 68.5% of women reported having undergone at least one Pap test.[102] In a study in Kuwait, 52.3% of women knew of screening, 30.6% had a positive attitude toward it, and 23.8% had the test on a fairly routine basis.[103] There is a need to develop national policies for screening, train female nurses to conduct the screening, and increase awareness of the benefits of screening and the dangers of cervical cancer, despite the relatively low rates in MENA. Once-in-a-lifetime screening of women 30–50 years of age using Pap smears, direct visual inspection, and/or HPV DNA testing may be cost-effective in reducing the mortality of cervical cancer.[104]

HPV vaccination should be considered as a prevention intervention for girls as well as women in MENA, and there is no need to screen for HPV before offering the vaccine because only very few women would have been infected by all four leading cancerous HPV types.[105] The available vaccines protect against the dominant types that cause cervical cancer in MENA (mainly

Figure 10.4 The Natural History of HPV Infection and Cervical Cancer

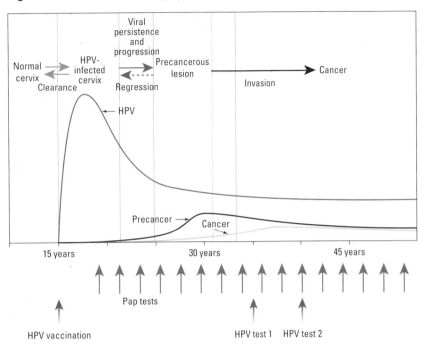

Source: Schiffman and Castle 2005.
Note: Reproduced with permission. Copyright © 2005 Massachusetts Medical Society. All rights reserved.

types 16 and 18).[106] It also appears that there is a positive attitude toward HPV vaccination in at least a few Muslim societies.[107]

Vaccination can reduce the need for Pap smear screening by reducing the age of initiation of screening or its frequency.[108] Considering that screening is limited in MENA, vaccination may offer a cost-effective method to reduce cervical cancer mortality. In Brazil, a middle-income country similar to many countries in MENA, it was estimated that vaccination can reduce cervical cancer incidence by 43%.[109] Combining vaccination with three screening events per lifetime can reduce the incidence by 61%.[110] Several countries in MENA can easily afford such vaccination programs, while other countries should pursue arrangements with vaccine providers to reduce the cost of vaccination and make it affordable to them. In addition to

[98] Imam et al., "Perceptions and Practices."
[99] Bener, Denic, and Alwash, "Screening for Cervical Cancer."
[100] Al Sairafi and Mohamed, "Knowledge, Attitudes, and Practice."
[101] Chaouki et al., "The Viral Origin of Cervical Cancer"; Hammouda et al., "Cervical Carcinoma in Algiers."
[102] Allahverdipour and Emami, "Perceptions of Cervical Cancer."
[103] Al Sairafi and Mohamed, "Knowledge, Attitudes, and Practice."
[104] Goldie et al., "Policy Analysis of Cervical Cancer Screening."
[105] WHO, "Human Papillomavirus and HPV Vaccination."

[106] Chaouki et al., "The Viral Origin of Cervical Cancer"; Hassen et al., "Cervical Human Papillomavirus Infection"; Hammouda et al., "Cervical Carcinoma in Algiers"; Lalaoui et al., "Human Papillomavirus DNA"; Khair et al., "Molecular Detection."
[107] Baykal et al., "Knowledge and Interest."
[108] WHO, "Human Papillomavirus and HPV Vaccination."
[109] Ibid.
[110] Ibid.

protection against cervical cancer, the vaccines, especially the quadrivalent one, may partially protect against genital warts, cancers of the neck, head, anus, vagina, and vulva as well as recurrent respiratory papillomatosis. Even in settings with low HPV prevalence, HPV vaccination has been shown to be cost-effective, very cost-effective, and cost saving, provided the cost per dose can be reduced to $96.85, $50.42, and $27.20, respectively.[111] However, a detailed cost-effectiveness analysis that takes into account the diversity of settings in this region needs to be conducted.

Increasing the level of awareness of cervical cancer and screening may pose challenging ethical issues in conservative cultures.[112] Though women are likely to welcome the possible introduction of HPV testing, they may not be fully aware of the sexually transmitted nature of cervical cancer. This may cause anxiety, confusion, and stigma about HPV as an STI and may raise concerns about women's sexual relationships in terms of trust, fidelity, blame, and protection.[113] Participation in HPV testing may communicate messages of distrust, infidelity, and promiscuity to women's partners, family, and community. These issues should be dealt with in any expansion of HPV testing and awareness in the region. Any anxieties concerning screening should not cause women to forgo screenings.[114]

Analytical summary

Cervical cancer and HPV prevalence levels in MENA are generally lower than those in other regions, suggesting lower levels of sexual risk behavior and limited connectivity of sexual networks. HIV infection is unlikely to have major inroads into the general population in MENA, confirming the results of HIV prevalence and behavioral measures (chapter 6).

Nevertheless, there is substantial heterogeneity of cervical cancer and HPV prevalence levels indicating variability of sexual risk behavior within MENA. It appears that countries closest to sub-Saharan Africa have the highest levels of

risky behavior followed by the Maghreb countries in the western part of MENA. The lowest levels of risk behavior appear to be in the Mashriq countries in the eastern part of the region. These differences may merely reflect differences in the sizes of commercial sex networks and the fraction of men who have sexual contact with FSWs.

Low-grade and high-grade precancerous cervical lesions and HPV prevalence levels can be used in MENA to monitor trends of sexual risk behavior, particularly among youth.

There are severe limitations in HPV screening programs in MENA, and HPV vaccination is virtually nonexistent. Public health authorities need to consider expansion of screening and vaccination programs and the formulation of national screening and vaccination policies.

BACTERIAL STIs AS MARKERS OF SEXUAL RISK BEHAVIOR

In a fashion similar to the use of HSV-2 and HPV to map levels of sexual risk behavior, prevalence levels of bacterial STIs, including syphilis, gonorrhea, and chlamydia, were used to map the presence of sexual risk behaviors. Bacterial STIs are mainly prevalent among populations with high-risk practices, or their partners, and are not common among general population groups.[115] Bacterial STI prevalence levels are specifically indicative of the presence of high-risk behaviors in a small part of the population, compared to HPV and HSV-2 infections, which may propagate in populations with intermediate or even relatively low-risk behaviors.

Different studies have documented bacterial STI prevalence in different population groups. Tables 10.6, 10.7, and 10.8 list summaries of these prevalence levels. These measures suggest that bacterial STIs are present in MENA and are common among priority populations. Nevertheless, prevalence levels outside of priority populations are generally low, and possibly reflect exposures among sexual partners of priority or bridging populations.

In addition to the data in the tables, further data suggest that bacterial STIs are present in

---

[111] Ginsberg et al., "Cost-Utility Analysis."

[112] Matin and LeBaron, "Attitudes toward Cervical Cancer"; Shafiq and Ali, "Sexually Transmitted Infections in Pakistan."

[113] McCaffery et al., "Attitudes towards HPV Testing."

[114] Azaiza and Cohen, "Between Traditional and Modern Perceptions."

[115] Brunham and Plummer, "A General Model."

Table 10.6 Syphilis Prevalence in Different Population Groups

Country	Syphilis prevalence
Afghanistan	0.0% (ANC attendees; Todd et al. 2007; Todd et al. 2008) 1.1% (blood donors; Afghanistan Central Blood Bank 2006) 2.2% (IDUs; Todd et al. 2007)
Algeria	0.8% (pregnant women; Alami 2009) 0.8% (pregnant women; Alami 2009) 0.53% (pregnant women; Aidaoui, Bouzbid, and Laouar 2008) 3.62% (ANC attendees; Unknown, Statut de la réponse nationale) 2.3% (STI clinic attendees; Alami 2009) 5.8% (STI clinic attendees; Alami 2009) 11.9% (FSWs; Alami 2009) 8.4% (FSWs; Alami 2009)
Djibouti	0.0% (high school students; Rowe 2007) 3.1% (pregnant women; WHO and EMRO 1998) 4.0% (ANC attendees; Unknown 2002) 0.4% (blood donors; Massenet and Bouh 1997) 41.0% (FSWs; Rowe 2007) 46.0% (FSWs; Rodier et al. 1993; Rowe 2007)
Egypt, Arab Republic of	0.05% (university students; El-Gilany and El-Fedawy 2006) 0.0% (family planning attendees; El-Sayed et al. 2002) 0.0% (ANC attendees; El-Sayed et al. 2002) 0.3% (tourism workers; El-Sayed et al. 1996) 1.0% (STD clinic attendees; El-Sayed et al. 1996) 1.0% (active syphilis; STD clinic attendees; El-Sayed et al. 1996) 1.3% (IDUs; El-Sayed et al. 2002) 5.8% (FSWs; El-Sayed et al. 2002) 7.5% (MSM; El-Sayed et al. 2002)
Iran, Islamic Republic of	0.0% (street children; Vahdani et al. 2006) 0.1% (general population; Dezfulimanesh and Tehranian 2005) 0.0% (runaways and other women seeking safe haven; Hajiabdolbaghi et al. 2007) 0.0% (blood donors; Khedmat et al. 2007)
Jordan	0.0% (symptomatic hospital attendees; Jordan Ministry of Health 2004) 0.0% (asymptomatic hospital attendees; Jordan Ministry of Health 2004) 0.0% (symptomatic hospital attendees; As'ad 2004) 0.0% (asymptomatic hospital attendees; As'ad 2004) 0.0% (symptomatic hospital attendees; Mahafzah et al. 2008) 0.0% (asymptomatic hospital attendees; Mahafzah et al. 2008)
Kuwait	0.0% (STD clinic attendees; Al-Mutairi et al. 2007)
Lebanon	0.0% (rural population; Deeb et al. 2003)
Morocco	3.4% (family planning center attendees; Ryan et al. 1998) 5.6% (symptomatic primary health care center attendees; Ryan et al. 1998) 2.8% (ANC attendees; WHO/EMRO Regional Database on HIV/AIDS) 3.0% (pregnant women; WHO/EMRO 1998) 1.0% (pregnant women; Khattabi and Alami 2005) 0.73% (pregnant women; Bennani and Alami 2006) 2.8% (general population; WHO/EMRO Regional Database on HIV/AIDS) 1.3% (blood donors; WHO/EMRO 1998) 0.4% (hotel staff; Khattabi and Alami 2005) 0.94% (hotel staff; Bennani and Alami 2006) 2.9% (seasonal female laborers; Khattabi and Alami 2005) 2.17% (seasonal female laborers; Bennani and Alami 2006) 0.0% (male laborers; Khattabi and Alami 2005) 4.51% (male laborers; Bennani and Alami 2006) 9.55% (truck drivers; Khattabi and Alami 2005)

(continued)

Table 10.6 *(Continued)*

Country	Syphilis prevalence
	1.9% (sailors; Khattabi and Alami 2005)
	3.37% (sailors; Bennani and Alami 2006)
	2.3% (TB patients; Khattabi and Alami 2005)
	4.0% (TB patients; Bennani and Alami 2006)
	23.0% (female prisoners; El Ghrari et al. 2007)
	7.8% (female prisoners; Khattabi and Alami 2005)
	16.39% (female prisoners; Bennani and Alami 2006)
	4.8% (male prisoners; Khattabi and Alami 2005)
	4.03% (male prisoners; Khattabi and Alami 2005)
	2.7% (female STD clinic attendees; WHO/EMRO Regional Database on HIV/AIDS)
	13.2% (STD clinic attendees; Heikel et al. 1999)
	18.4% (STD clinic attendees; Ryan et al. 1998)
	4.0% (STD clinic attendees; WHO/EMRO Regional Database on HIV/AIDS)
	3.8% (STD clinic attendees; Khattabi and Alami 2005)
	4.92% (STD clinic attendees; Bennani and Alami 2006)
	9.6% (female prisoners imprisoned for sex work; Khattabi and Alami 2005)
	11.76% (female prisoners imprisoned for sex work; Bennani and Alami 2006)
	12.1% (FSWs; Khattabi and Alami 2005)
	9.0% (FSWs; Khattabi and Alami 2005)
	13.29% (FSWs; Bennani and Alami 2006)
	17% (FSWs; WHO/EMRO Regional Database on HIV/AIDS)
Pakistan	0.4% (ANC attendees; WHO/EMRO 2007)
	0.4% (general population; WHO/EMRO Regional Database on HIV/AIDS)
	0.19%–0.57% (blood donors; Sultan, Mehmood, and Mahmood 2007)
	9.4% (truck drivers; WHO/EMRO 2007)
	1%–4% (truck drivers; Pakistan National AIDS Control Program 2005a)
	7.0% (persons arrested for drug-related crimes; Baqi 1995)
	4%–18% (IDUs; Pakistan National AIDS Control Program 2005a)
	11.0% (IDUs; WHO/EMRO Regional Database on HIV/AIDS)
	7.6% (IDUs; Platt et al. 2009)
	3.9% (IDUs; Platt et al. 2009)
	23.5% (FSWs; WHO/EMRO 2007)
	4–7% (FSWs; Pakistan National AIDS Control Program 2005a)
	1.2% (FSWs; Hawkes et al. 2009)
	2.8% (FSWs; Hawkes et al. 2009)
	6–36% (MSWs; Pakistan National AIDS Control Program 2005a)
	21% (MSWs; WHO/EMRO Regional Database on HIV/AIDS)
	11%–60% *(hijras;* Pakistan National AIDS Control Program 2005a)
	50.0% *(hijras;* Khan et al. 2008)
	36.0% *(hijras;* WHO/EMRO Regional Database on HIV/AIDS)
	4.7% (MSWs; *banthas;* Hawkes et al. 2009)
	4.9% (MSWs; *banthas;* Hawkes et al. 2009)
	9.6% (MSWs; *khotkis;* Hawkes et al. 2009)
	0.0% (MSWs; *khotkis;* Hawkes et al. 2009)
	48.8% (MSWs; *khusras;* Hawkes et al. 2009)
	37.5% (MSWs; *khusras;* Hawkes et al. 2009)
Qatar	1.1% (blood donors; WHO/EMRO 1998)
Somalia	2.0% (ANC attendees; Somaliland Ministry of Health and Labour 2007)
	1.4% (ANC attendees; Somaliland Ministry of Health and Labour 2007)
	3.6% (ANC attendees; Somaliland Ministry of Health and Labour 2007)
	0.0% (ANC attendees; Somaliland Ministry of Health and Labour 2007)
	2.4% (ANC attendees; Somaliland Ministry of Health and Labour 2007)
	1.8% (ANC attendees; Somaliland Ministry of Health and Labour 2007)

Table 10.6 *(Continued)*

Country	Syphilis prevalence
	3.0% (general population; Ismail et al. 1990)
	5.2% (miscellaneous individuals; Scott et al. 1991)
	1.0% (active syphilis; Somali ANC refugee attendees in Kenya; UNHCR 2006–07)
	4.4% (active syphilis; Somali ANC refugee attendees in Kenya; UNHCR 2006–07)
	1.6% (active syphilis; Somali ANC refugee attendees in Kenya; UNHCR 2006–07)
	2.4% (active syphilis; Somali ANC refugee attendees in Kenya; UNHCR 2006–07)
	3.3% (active syphilis; Somali ANC refugee attendees in Kenya; UNHCR 2006–07)
	3.8% (active syphilis; Somali ANC refugee attendees in Kenya; UNHCR 2006–07)
	0.9% (active syphilis; Somali ANC refugee attendees in Kenya; UNHCR 2006–07)
	2.7% (active syphilis; Somali ANC refugee attendees in Kenya; UNHCR 2006–07)
	1.0% (active syphilis; Somali refugees attending STI clinic in Kenya; UNHCR 2006–07)
	4.7% (active syphilis; Somali refugees attending STI clinic in Kenya; UNHCR 2006–07)
	1.3% (active syphilis; Somali refugees attending STI clinic in Kenya; UNHCR 2006–07)
	2.3% (active syphilis; Somali refugees attending STI clinic in Kenya; UNHCR 2006–07)
	2.0% (female STD clinic attendees; WHO 2004)
	0.0% (male STD clinic attendees; WHO 2004)
	1.4% (STD clinic attendees; Somaliland Ministry of Health and Labour 2007)
	10.0% (STD clinic attendees; Ismail et al. 1990)
	12.6% (STD clinic attendees; Scott et al. 1991)
	18.0% (a group of FSWs, STD clinic attendees, male soldiers, and tuberculosis patients; Watts et al. 1994)
	69.0% (FSWs; Ahmed et al. 1991)
	10.0% (FSWs; Corwin et al. 1991)
	5.6% (FSWs; Corwin et al. 1991)
	50.8% (FSWs; Scott et al. 1991)
	3.1% (Testa and Kriitmaa 2009)
Sudan	0.9% (randomly sampled women in a suburban community; Kafi, Mohamed, and Musa 2000)
	2.4% (pregnant women; WHO/EMRO 1998)
	2.0% (ANC attendees; Sudan National AIDS/STIs Program 2008)
	11.2% (ANC attendees; Southern Sudan; Southern Sudan AIDS Commission 2007)
	0%–27% (various locations; ANC attendees; Southern Sudan; Southern Sudan AIDS Commission 2007)
	4.4% (active syphilis; Sudanese ANC refugee attendees in Kenya; UNHCR 2006–07)
	5.6% (blood donors; Sudan National AIDS Program 2008)
	1.8% (refugees; Sudan National AIDS/STIs Program 2008)
	11.0% (female Sudanese refugees in Ethiopia; Holt et al. 2003)
	26.0% (male Sudanese refugees in Ethiopia; Holt et al. 2003)
	6.3% (active syphilis; Sudanese refugees attending STI clinic in Kenya; UNHCR 2006–07)
	17.0% (a population of FSWs, soldiers, truck drivers, outpatients, and Ethiopian refugees; McCarthy et al. 1989)
Turkey	0.1% (engaged couples; Alim et al. 2009)
	0.168% (blood donors; Coskun et al. 2008)
	5.38% (FSWs; Gul et al. 2008)
Yemen, Republic of	2.0% (general population; WHO/EMRO Regional Database on HIV/AIDS)
	4.9% (FSWs; Štulhofer and Božicevic 2008)

MENA and are common among priority populations. It is estimated that the general prevalence of
syphilis in MENA is at 1%.[116] In Afghanistan, a
15-fold increase in syphilis prevalence was
reported among blood donors from 2002 to 2003,
apparently due to a massive influx of refugees
returning to the country.[117] In the Islamic Republic
of Iran, almost all FSWs reported a previous history of STDs and 60% reported frequent STD
infections.[118] Among truck drivers and youth,
31.9% and 27.9% reported a previous history
of STDs, respectively.[119] In Lebanon, a large
study of general population women reported a

---

[116] WHO/EMRO Regional Database on HIV/AIDS.

[117] Todd et al., "Prevalence of and Barriers to Testing."

[118] Tehrani and Malek-Afzalip, "Knowledge, Attitudes and Practices."

[119] Ibid.

Table 10.7 Gonorrhea Prevalence in Different Population Groups

Country	Gonorrhea prevalence
Djibouti	32.4% (promiscuous males; Fox et al. 1989)
Egypt, Arab Republic of	2.8% (family planning attendees; El-Sayed et al. 2002) 2.0% (ANC attendees; El-Sayed et al. 2002) 2.7% (IDUs; El-Sayed et al. 2002) 7.7% (FSWs; El-Sayed et al. 2002) 8.8% (MSM; El-Sayed et al. 2002)
Iran, Islamic Republic of	0.4% (a group of pregnant and nonpregnant women; Dezfulimanesh and Tehranian 2005) 1.0% (female prison inmates; Zangeneh 1999) 6.4% (obstetrics and gynecology clinics attendees; Chamani-Tabriz et al. 2007)
Jordan	0.7% (symptomatic hospital attendees; Jordan Ministry of Health 2004) 0.5% (asymptomatic hospital attendees; Jordan Ministry of Health 2004) 1.2% (symptomatic hospital attendees; As'ad 2004) 0.0% (asymptomatic hospital attendees; As'ad 2004) 0.6% (symptomatic hospital attendees; Mahafzah et al. 2008) 0.9% (asymptomatic hospital attendees; Mahafzah et al. 2008)
Kuwait	31.5% (STD clinic attendees; Al-Mutairi et al. 2007)
Lebanon	0.0% (rural population; Deeb et al. 2003)
Morocco	3.2% (family planning center attendees; Ryan et al. 1998) 5.4% (symptomatic primary health care center attendees; Ryan et al. 1998) 0.9% (ANC attendees; WHO/EMRO Regional Database on HIV/AIDS) 1.74% (female STD clinic attendees; Heikel et al. 1999) 0.8% (female STD clinic attendees; WHO/EMRO Regional Database on HIV/AIDS) 7.07% (male STD clinic attendees; Heikel et al. 1999) 10.0% (STD clinic attendees; Ryan et al. 1998) 42.0% (STD clinic attendees; WHO/EMRO Regional Database on HIV/AIDS) 52.4% (STD clinic attendees; Alami et al. 2002) 3.5% (FSWs; WHO/EMRO Regional Database on HIV/AIDS)
Pakistan	1%–4% (truck drivers; Pakistan National AIDS Control Program 2005a) 1%–2% (IDUs; Pakistan National AIDS Control Program 2005a) 1.3% (IDUs; Platt et al. 2009) 0.0% (IDUs; Platt et al. 2009) 10%–12% (FSWs; Pakistan National AIDS Control Program 2005a) 0%–18% (anal; MSWs; Pakistan National AIDS Control Program 2005a) 3%–6% (genital; MSWs; Pakistan National AIDS Control Program 2005a) 3%–4% (anal; *hijras;* Pakistan National AIDS Control Program 2005a) 15.0% (anal; *hijras;* Khan et al. 2008) 4.0% (urethral; *hijras;* Khan et al. 2008) 12.6% (anal; MSWs; *banthas;* Hawkes et al. 2009) 11.1% (anal; MSWs; *banthas;* Hawkes et al. 2009) 4.7% (anal; MSWs; *khotkis;* Hawkes et al. 2009) 0.0% (anal; MSWs; *khotkis;* Hawkes et al. 2009) 20.2% (anal; MSWs; *khusras;* Hawkes et al. 2009) 6.3% (anal; MSWs; *khusras;* Hawkes et al. 2009)
Somalia	0.8% (ANC attendees; WHO 2004) 0.5% (STD clinic attendees; WHO 2004) 6.7% (STD clinic attendees; Burans et al. 1990) 11.2% (FSWs; Burans et al. 1990)
Turkey	0.0% (family planning clinic attendees; Ortayli, Bulut, and Nalbant 2001; Ortayli et al. 2001)

Table 10.8 Chlamydia Prevalence in Different Population Groups

Country	Chlamydia prevalence
Algeria	100% (antichlamydia antibodies; obstetric clinic attendees; Kadi et al. 1989) 100% (antichlamydia antibodies; FSWs; Kadi et al. 1989)
Djibouti	5.7% (promiscuous males; Fox 1989)
Egypt, Arab Republic of	2.8% (family planning attendees; El-Sayed et al. 2002) 1.3% (ANC attendees; El-Sayed et al. 2002) 2.7% (IDUs; El-Sayed et al. 2002) 7.7% (FSWs; El-Sayed et al. 2002) 8.8% (MSM; El-Sayed et al. 2002)
Iran, Islamic Republic of	8.8% (male STI clinic attendees; Darougar et al. 1982) 9.3% (male patients with urethritis; Ghanaat et al. 2008) 6.9% (FSWs; Darougar et al. 1983)
Jordan	1.3% (symptomatic hospital attendees; Jordan Ministry of Health 2004) 0.5% (asymptomatic hospital attendees; Jordan Ministry of Health 2004) 0.8% (symptomatic hospital attendees; As'ad 2004) 0.0% (asymptomatic hospital attendees; As'ad 2004) 0.9% (symptomatic hospital attendees; Mahafzah et al. 2008) 2.2% (asymptomatic hospital attendees; Mahafzah et al. 2008) 3.9% (women attending infertility clinic; Al-Ramahi et al. 2008) 0.7% (hospital attendees; Al-Ramahi et al. 2008) 4.6% (symptomatic patients with urethritis; Awwad, Al-Amarat, and Shehabi 2003) 3.9% (symptomatic patients with urethritis; Al Ramahi et al. 2008)
Kuwait	4.1% (STD clinic attendees; Al-Mutairi et al. 2007)
Lebanon	0.0% (rural population; Deeb et al. 2003)
Morocco	2.6% (family planning center attendees; Ryan et al. 1998) 6.3% (symptomatic primary health care center attendees; Ryan et al. 1998) 4.2% (ANC attendees; WHO/EMRO Regional Database on HIV/AIDS) 5.6% (female STD clinic attendees; WHO/EMRO Regional Database on HIV/AIDS) 51.5% (STD clinic attendees; Heikel et al. 1991) 6.0% (STD clinic attendees; WHO/EMRO Regional Database on HIV/AIDS) 17.1% (STD clinic attendees; Alami et al. 2002) 5.0% (STD clinic attendees; Ryan et al. 1998) 19.1% (FSWs; WHO/EMRO Regional Database on HIV/AIDS)
Pakistan	1.0% (truck drivers; Pakistan National AIDS Control Program 2005a) 0%–1% (IDUs; Pakistan National AIDS Control Program 2005a) 0.7% (IDUs; Platt et al. 2009) 0.0% (IDUs; Platt et al. 2009) 5%–11% (FSWs; Pakistan National AIDS Control Program 2005a) 10.0% (anal; MSWs; Pakistan National AIDS Control Program 2005a) 1%–2% (genital; MSWs; Pakistan National AIDS Control Program 2005a) 29.0% (anal; *hijras;* Pakistan National AIDS Control Program 2005a) 0%–2% (genital; *hijras;* Pakistan National AIDS Control Program 2005a) 9.0% (anal; *hijras;* Khan et al. 2008) 1.0% (urethral; *hijras;* Khan et al. 2008) 4.7% (anal; MSWs; *banthas;* Hawkes et al. 2009) 4.9% (anal; MSWs; *banthas;* Hawkes et al. 2009) 3.6% (anal; MSWs; *khotkis;* Hawkes et al. 2009) 0.0% (anal; MSWs; *khotkis;* Hawkes et al. 2009) 9.9% (anal; MSWs; *khusras;* Hawkes et al. 2009) 6.3% (anal; MSWs; *khusras;* Hawkes et al. 2009)
Saudi Arabia	0.0% (asymptomatic females attending genitourinary or gynecological clinics; Massoud et al. 1991) 2.0% (asymptomatic males attending genitourinary or gynecological clinics; Massoud et al. 1991) 35.0% (symptomatic females attending genitourinary or gynecological clinics; Massoud et al. 1991) 46.0% (symptomatic males attending genitourinary or gynecological clinics; Massoud et al. 1991)

(continued)

Table 10.8 *(Continued)*

Country	Chlamydia prevalence
Somalia	1.1% (ANC attendees; WHO 2004) 0.8% (STD clinic attendees; WHO 2004) 14.0% (STD clinic attendees; Ismail et al. 1990)
Sudan	1.2% (randomly sampled women in a suburban community; Kafi, Mohamed, and Musa 2000)
Turkey	1.9% (family planning clinic attendees; Ortayli et al. 2001) 1.9% (family planning clinic attendees; Ortayli, Bulut, and Nalbant 2001) 12.0% (registered FSWs; Agacfidan et al. 1997) 14.4% (unregistered FSWs; Agacfidan et al. 1997) 12.9% (FSWs; Agacfidan et al. 1997)
United Arab Emirates	2.6% (female primary and secondary care attendees; Ghazal-Aswad et al. 2004)
West Bank and Gaza	8.0% (pregnant women; Lubbad and Al-Hindi 2007)

trichomonas prevalence of 0.53%.[120] In Pakistan, 15%–45% of different risk groups, including IDUs, FSWs, MSWs, and *hijras*, reported having an STI in the past six months.[121] Also in Pakistan, 3.2% of migrant workers had etiologically confirmed STI prevalence.[122] In Sudan, 7.3% of ANC attendees were found to have multiple STIs.[123] It appears that gonorrhea and chlamydia are the most common bacterial STIs among MSM in MENA.[124]

A few studies have also documented chancroid in MENA, a bacterial STI characteristic of very high levels of risky behavior.[125] This infection reappeared in Algeria in 1988 and was consistently associated with contacts with FSWs.[126] The infection was also common among STD clinic attendees in Kuwait.[127]

The magnitude of the burden of STIs is not well known in most countries of MENA due to the limited STI surveillance. In 2002, HIV and STIs together became the second leading cause of mortality among all infectious (and parasitic) diseases among people 15–44 years old in the region.[128] It is estimated that there are 3.5 million curable (mainly bacterial) STIs every year

among adults in MENA.[129] The yearly incidence of the four leading curable STIs (gonorrhea, chlamydia, syphilis, and trichomonas) is estimated at 7% per person, per year.[130] This is the second lowest incidence rate of all regions. In Djibouti, it is estimated that there are 25,000 reported STD cases every year.[131] In the Islamic Republic of Iran, 850,000 STDs are registered annually.[132] In Morocco, between 180,000 and 240,000 new STDs used to be reported annually in the late 1990s,[133] but in recent years the number of reported cases has increased considerably (370,000 in 2005).[134] Figure 10.5 shows the trend in STI notified cases in Morocco from 1992 to 2006.[135] In Saudi Arabia, gonorrhea incidence was estimated at 4.9 per 100,000 persons per year,[136] compared to 131.4 per 100,000 persons per year in the United States.[137] In the Republic of Yemen, it is estimated that there are 150,000 to 170,000 new STDs per year.[138]

Reproductive tract infections include, in addition to STIs, infections arising from overgrowth of natural organisms in the genital tract and infections acquired during improperly performed medical procedures such as unsafe

[120] Karam et al., "Prevalence of Sexually Transmitted Infections."
[121] Pakistan National AIDS Control Program, "Report of the Pilot Study in Karachi & Rawalpindi."
[122] Faisel and Cleland, "Migrant Men"
[123] Ortashi, El Khidir, and Herieka, "Prevalence of HIV."
[124] WHO/EMRO, *Strengthening Health Sector Response.*
[125] Brunham and Plummer, "A General Model"; Glasier et al., "Sexual and Reproductive Health."
[126] Boudghene-Stambouli and Merad-Boudia, "Chancroid in Algeria."
[127] Brunham and Plummer, "A General Model"; Al-Mutairi et al., "Clinical Patterns."
[128] WHO, *Shaping the Future.*

[129] WHO, "Global Prevalence and Incidence."
[130] Glasier et al., "Sexual and Reproductive Health."
[131] WHO/EMRO, "Prevention and Control."
[132] Iran Center for Disease Management, Three Month Statistics.
[133] Heikel et al., "The Prevalence of Sexually Transmitted Pathogens."
[134] Morocco MOH, "Situation épidémiologique actuelle du VIH/SIDA au Maroc."
[135] WHO/EMRO data reported to the WHO office of the Eastern Mediterranean Region.
[136] Madani, "Sexually Transmitted Infections in Saudi Arabia."
[137] CDC, "Tracking the Hidden Epidemics."
[138] Lambert, "HIV and Development Challenges in Yemen."

abortions.[139] Hence, caution needs to be exercised when interpreting STD data with no confirmed etiology. In a rural community in eastern Lebanon, STD prevalence was 1.2%, but there were no etiologically confirmed cases of syphilis, gonorrhea, or chlamydia.[140] Among general population women in Egypt, 19.7% of women self-reported STI symptoms in the previous 12 months,[141] but given the epidemiological context of sexual risk behavior highlighted in this synthesis, it seems unlikely that the majority of these symptoms are STI related. Facilities with etiologic diagnostic methods are not widely available in MENA.[142]

Figure 10.5 Trend in STI Notified Cases in Morocco, 1992–2006

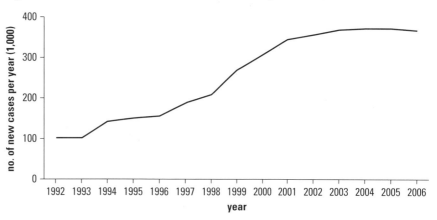

Source: WHO/EMRO data reported to the WHO office of the Eastern Mediterranean Region.

Analytical summary

Prevalence levels of bacterial STIs among the general population in MENA are low compared to other regions, but prevalence levels among priority populations are considerable, suggesting higher levels of sexual risk behavior. HIV infection is unlikely to have major inroads into the general population in MENA, confirming the results of HIV prevalence and behavioral measures (chapter 6). The considerable prevalence levels in priority groups suggest that there is potential for HIV spread among these groups.

UNSAFE ABORTIONS AS MARKERS OF SEXUAL RISK BEHAVIOR

Levels of unsafe abortions can be used as proxies of sexual risk behavior and may reflect levels of unprotected sexual intercourse in nonspousal partnerships. Figure 10.5 displays the rates of unsafe abortion in MENA compared to the rest of the regions.[143] Apart from Djibouti and Somalia, MENA has one of the lowest rates of unsafe abortions in the developing world. The rates are higher in the Maghreb than in the Mashriq parts of MENA, consistent with the results of STI measures.

It is estimated that about 1.5 million unsafe abortions occurred in MENA in 2003,[144] out of a world total of about 19 million.[145] Unsafe abortions account for 11% of maternal deaths in MENA,[146] compared to 30% of all maternal deaths globally.[147]

Analytical summary

The fact that MENA has one of the lowest rates of unsafe abortions in the developing world suggests that levels of risk behavior are lower than those in other regions. HIV infection is unlikely to have major inroads into the general population in MENA, confirming the results of HIV prevalence and behavioral measures (chapter 6).

Nevertheless, there is substantial heterogeneity in unsafe abortion rates across MENA. Countries closest to sub-Saharan Africa have the highest levels followed by the Maghreb countries. Lower levels are found in the rest of MENA.

BIOLOGICAL EVIDENCE ON PROXY MEASURES OF SEXUAL RISK BEHAVIORS: ANALYTICAL SUMMARY

The above sections presented data on several proxy biomarkers for sexual risk behavior in different population groups in MENA. The

---

[139] Roudi-Fahimi and Ashford, "Sexual & Reproductive Health."
[140] Deeb et al., "Prevalence of Reproductive Tract Infections."
[141] Measure DHS, "Egypt: Demographic and Health Survey 2005."
[142] Ibid.
[143] WHO, *Unsafe Abortion.*

[144] Roudi-Fahimi and Ashford, "Sexual & Reproductive Health."
[145] WHO, *Unsafe Abortion;* Ahman and Shah, "Unsafe Abortion."
[146] Roudi-Fahimi and Ashford, "Sexual & Reproductive Health."
[147] Glasier et al., "Sexual and Reproductive Health."

Figure 10.6 Estimated Annual Incidence of Unsafe Abortions per 1,000 Women Aged 15–44 Years, by United Nations Subregions in 2000

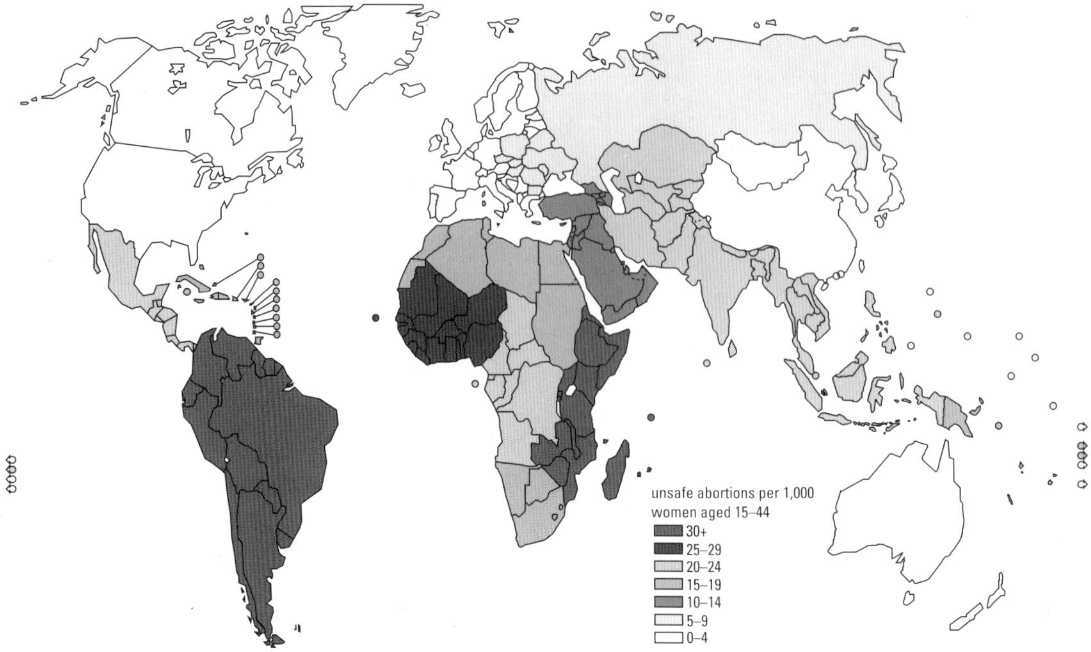

unsafe abortions per 1,000
women aged 15–44

- 30+
- 25–29
- 20–24
- 15–19
- 10–14
- 5–9
- 0–4

The designations employed and the presentation of material on this map do not imply the expression of any opinion whatsoever on the part of the World Health Organization concerning the legal status of any country, territory, city or area or of its authorities, or concerning the delimitation of its frontiers or boundaries. Dashed lines represent approximate border lines for which there may not yet be full agreement.

Source: Reproduced with permission from WHO (2004).

data derived from these different proxy biomarkers converge to the same conclusion: sexual risk behaviors are present in MENA; there are existing local sexual risk networks where STIs are propagating; and levels of sexual risk behavior appear to be considerable among priority groups. However, levels of risky behavior are low among the general population and overall they are among the lowest of all regions.

Sexual risk behaviors vary across MENA, with the highest levels found in countries closest to sub-Saharan Africa, followed by the Maghreb countries in the western part of MENA. The lowest levels appear to be in the Mashriq countries in the eastern part of MENA.

The evidence on the different proxy biomarkers suggests that it is unlikely that HIV infection will make major inroads into the general population in MENA, confirming the results of HIV prevalence and behavioral measures (chapter 7). However, the data on priority populations suggest that there is potential for HIV spread among these populations.

BIBLIOGRAPHY

Abdel, Aziz M. T., M. Z. Abdel Aziz, H. M. Atta, O. G. Shaker, M. M. Abdel Fattah, G. A. Mohsen, H. H. Ahmed, and D. A. El Derwi. 2006. "Screening for Human Papillomavirus (HPV) in Egyptian Women by the Second-Generation Hybrid Capture (HC II) Test." *Med Sci Monit* 12: MT43–49.

Abuharfeil, N., and M. M. Meqdam. 2000. "Seroepide-miologic Study of Herpes Simplex Virus Type 2 and Cytomegalovirus among Young Adults in Northern Jordan." *New Microbiol* 23: 235–39.

Abu-Raddad, L. J., A. S. Magaret, C. Celum, A. Wald, I. M. Longini, S. G. Self, and L. Corey. 2008. "Genital Herpes Has Played a More Important Role Than Any Other Sexually Transmitted Infection in Driving HIV Prevalence in Africa." *PLoS ONE* 3: e2230.

Abu-Raddad, L. J., J. T Schiffer, R. Ashley, R. A. Alsallaq, F. A. Akala, I. Semini, G. Riedner, and D. Wilson. Forthcoming. "HSV-2 Serology Can Be Predictive of HIV Epidemic Potential and Hidden Sexual Risk Behavior in the Middle East and North Africa."

Afghanistan Central Blood Bank. 2006. *Report of Testing of Blood Donors from March–December, 2006.* Ministry of Public Health, Kabul, Afghanistan.

Agacfidan, A., J. M. Chow, H. Pashazade, G. Ozarmagan, and S. Badur. 1997. "Screening of Sex Workers in Turkey for Chlamydia Trachomatis." *Sex Transm Dis* 24: 573–75.

Ahman, E., and I. Shah. 2002. "Unsafe Abortion: Worldwide Estimates for 2000." *Reprod Health Matters* 10: 13–17.

Ahmed, H. J., J. Mbwana, E. Gunnarsson, K. Ahlman, C. Guerino, L. A. Svensson, F. Mhalu, and T. Lagergard. 2003. "Etiology of Genital Ulcer Disease and Association with Human Immunodeficiency Virus Infection in Two Tanzanian Cities." *Sex Transm Dis* 30: 114–19.

Ahmed, H. J., K. Omar, S. Y. Adan, A. M. Guled, L. Grillner, and S. Bygdeman. 1991. "Syphilis and Human Immunodeficiency Virus Seroconversion during a 6-Month Follow-Up of Female Prostitutes in Mogadishu, Somalia." *Int J STD AIDS* 2: 119–23.

Aidaoui, M., S. Bouzbid, and M. Laouar. 2008. "Seroprevalence of HIV Infection in Pregnant Women in the Annaba Region (Algeria)." *Rev Epidemiol Sante Publique* 56: 261–66.

Al Sairafi, M., and F. A. Mohamed. 2009. "Knowledge, Attitudes, and Practice Related to Cervical Cancer Screening among Kuwaiti Women." *Med Princ Pract* 18: 35–42.

Alami, K. 2009. "Tendances récentes de l'épidémie à VIH/SIDA en Afrique du nord." Presentation, Research and AIDS Workshop in North Africa, Marrakech, Morocco.

Alami, K., N. Ait Mbarek, M. Akrim, B. Bellaji, A. Hansali, H. Khattabi, A. Sekkat, R. El Aouad, and J. Mahjour. 2002. "Urethral Discharge in Morocco: Prevalence of Microorganisms and Susceptibility of Gonococcos." *East Mediterr Health J* 8: 794–804.

Alim, A., M. O. Artan, Z. Baykan, and B. A. Alim. 2009. "Seroprevalence of Hepatitis B and C Viruses, HIV, and Syphilis Infections among Engaged Couples." *Saudi Med J* 30: 541–45.

Allahverdipour, H., and A. Emami. 2008. "Perceptions of Cervical Cancer Threat, Benefits, and Barriers of Papanicolaou Smear Screening Programs for Women in Iran." *Women Health* 47: 23–37.

Al-Muammar, T., M. N. Al-Ahdal, A. Hassan, G. Kessie, D. M. Dela Cruz, and G. E. Mohamed. 2007. "Human Papilloma Virus-16/18 Cervical Infection among Women Attending a Family Medical Clinic in Riyadh." *Ann Saudi Med* 27: 1–5.

Al-Mutairi, N., A. Joshi, O. Nour-Eldin, A. K. Sharma, I. El-Adawy, and M. Rijhwani. 2007. "Clinical Patterns of Sexually Transmitted Diseases, Associated Sociodemographic Characteristics, and Sexual Practices in the Farwaniya Region of Kuwait." *Int J Dermatol* 46: 594–99.

Al-Ramahi, M., A. Mahafzah, S. Saleh, and K. Fram. 2008. "Prevalence of Chlamydia Trachomatis Infection in Infertile Women at a University Hospital in Jordan." *East Mediterr Health J* 14: 1148–54.

Altaf, F. J. 2001. "Pattern of Cervical Smear Cytology in the Western Region of Saudi Arabia." *Ann Saudi Med* 21: 92–96.

———. 2006. "Cervical Cancer Screening with Pattern of Pap Smear: Review of Multicenter Studies." *Saudi Med J* 27: 1498–502.

Anwar, K., M. Inuzuka, T. Shiraishi, and K. Nakakuki. 1991. "Detection of HPV DNA in Neoplastic and Non-Neoplastic Cervical Specimens from Pakistan and Japan by Non-Isotopic in situ Hybridization." *Int J Cancer* 47: 675–80.

As'ad, A. 2004. "Final Report: Sexually Transmitted Infections (STI) Prevalence Study." National AIDS Program, Jordan.

Ashley, R., A. Cent, V. Maggs, A. Nahmias, and L. Corey. 1991. "Inability of Enzyme Immunoassays to Discriminate between Infections with Herpes Simplex Virus Types 1 and 2." *Ann Intern Med* 115: 520–26.

Ashley, R. L., and A. Wald. 1999. "Genital Herpes: Review of the Epidemic and Potential Use of Type-Specific Serology." *Clin Microbiol Rev* 12: 1–8.

Awwad, Z. M., A. A. Al-Amarat, and A. A. Shehabi. 2003. "Prevalence of Genital Chlamydial Infection in Symptomatic and Asymptomatic Jordanian Patients." *Int J Infect Dis* 7: 206–9.

Azaiza, F., and M. Cohen. 2008. "Between Traditional and Modern Perceptions of Breast and Cervical Cancer Screenings: A Qualitative Study of Arab Women in Israel." *Psychooncology* 17: 34–41.

Bailey, R. 2007. "Scaling Up Circumcision Programmes: The Road from Evidence to Practice." PowerPoint presentation at the 4th IAS Conference on HIV Pathogenesis, Treatment & Prevention, Sydney, Australia, July 22–25, 2007.

Baseman, J. G., and L. A. Koutsky. 2005. "The Epidemiology of Human Papillomavirus Infections." *J Clin Virol* 32 Suppl 1: S16–24.

Baqi, S. 1995. "HIV Seroprevalence and Risk Factors in Drug Abusers in Karachi." Second National Symposium, the Aga Khan University.

Baykal, C., A. Al, M. G. Ugur, N. Cetinkaya, R. Attar, and P. Arioglu. 2008. "Knowledge and Interest of Turkish Women about Cervical Cancer and HPV Vaccine." *Eur J Gynaecol Oncol* 29: 76–79.

Bener, A., S. Denic, and R. Alwash. 2001. "Screening for Cervical Cancer among Arab Women." *Int J Gynaecol Obstet* 74: 305–7.

Bennani, A., and K. Alami. 2006. "Surveillance sentinelle VIH, résultats 2005 et tendances de la séroprévalence du VIH." Morocco Ministry of Health, UNAIDS.

Bennis, S., S. Meniar, A. Amarti, and A. Bijou. 2007. "Role of Cervical Smear in the Diagnosis of Cervical Cancer in Fes-Boulemane Region of Morocco." *East Mediterr Health J* 13: 1153–59.

Bogaerts, J., J. Ahmed, N. Akhter, N. Begum, M. Rahman, S. Nahar, M. Van Ranst, and J. Verhaegen. 2001. "Sexually Transmitted Infections among Married Women in Dhaka, Bangladesh: Unexpected High Prevalence of Herpes Simplex Type 2 Infection." *Sex Transm Infect* 77: 114–19.

Bosch, F. X., M. M. Manos, N. Munoz, M. Sherman, A. M. Jansen, J. Peto, M. H. Schiffman, V. Moreno, R. Kurman, and K. V. Shah. 1995. "Prevalence of Human Papillomavirus in Cervical Cancer: A Worldwide Perspective." International Biological Study on Cervical Cancer (IBSCC) Study Group. *J Natl Cancer Inst* 87: 796–802.

Bosch, F. X., N. Munoz, S. de Sanjose, E. Guerrerro, A. M. Ghaffari, J. Kaldor, X. Castellsague, and K. V. Shah. 1994. "Importance of Human Papillomavirus

Endemicity in the Incidence of Cervical Cancer: An Extension of the Hypothesis on Sexual Behavior." *Cancer Epidemiol Biomarkers* Prev 3: 375–79.

Boudghene-Stambouli, O., and A. Merad-Boudia. 1997. "Chancroid in Algeria: The Status of This Sexually Transmitted Disease in 1995." *Bull Soc Pathol Exot* 90: 78–80.

Brown, Z. A., S. Selke, J. Zeh, J. Kopelman, A. Maslow, R. L. Ashley, D. H. Watts, S. Berry, M. Herd, and L. Corey. 1997. "The Acquisition of Herpes Simplex Virus during Pregnancy." *N Engl J Med* 337: 509–15.

Brunham, R. C., and F. A. Plummer. 1990. "A General Model of Sexually Transmitted Disease Epidemiology and Its Implications for Control." *Med Clin North Am* 74: 1339–52.

Burans, J. P., M. McCarthy, S. M. el Tayeb, A. el Tigani, J. George, R. Abu-Elyazeed, and J. N. Woody. 1990. "Serosurvey of Prevalence of Human Immunodeficiency Virus amongst High Risk Groups in Port Sudan, Sudan." *East Afr Med J* 67: 650–55.

Burchell, A. N., H. Richardson, S. M. Mahmud, H. Trottier, P. P. Tellier, J. Hanley, F. Coutlee, and E. L. Franco. 2006. "Modeling the Sexual Transmissibility of Human Papillomavirus Infection Using Stochastic Computer Simulation and Empirical Data from a Cohort Study of Young Women in Montreal, Canada." *Am J Epidemiol* 163: 534–43.

Burchell, A. N., R. L. Winer, S. de Sanjose, and E. L. Franco. 2006. "Chapter 6: Epidemiology and Transmission Dynamics of Genital HPV Infection." *Vaccine* 24 Suppl 3: S52–61.

Caldwell, C., and P. Quiggin. 1989. "The Social Context of AIDS in Sub-Saharan Africa." *Population and Development Review* 15: 185–234.

Castellsague, X., F. X. Bosch, N. Munoz, C. J. Meijer, K. V. Shah, S. de Sanjose, J. Eluf-Neto, C. A. Ngelangel, S. Chichareon, J. S. Smith, R. Herrero, V. Moreno, and S. Franceschi. 2002. "Male Circumcision, Penile Human Papillomavirus Infection, and Cervical Cancer in Female Partners." *N Engl J Med* 346: 1105–12.

Catania, J. A., D. R. Gibson, D. D. Chitwood, and T. J. Coates. 1990. "Methodological Problems in AIDS Behavioral Research: Influences on Measurement Error and Participation Bias in Studies of Sexual Behavior." *Psychol Bull* 108: 339–62.

CDC (Centers for Disease Control and Prevention). 2000. "Tracking the Hidden Epidemics." Trends in STDs in the United States, Atlanta, Georgia.

Cengiz, A. T., O. Kendi, M. Kiyan, Y. Bilge, S. Ugurel, and A. R. Tumer. 1992. "Detection of Herpes Simplex Virus 2 (HSV) IgG and IgM Using ELISA in Transsexuals and Homosexuals." *Mikrobiyol Bul* 26: 41–49.

———. 1993. "Demonstration of Herpes Simplex Virus (HSV)-2 IgG and IgM Using ELISA in Transsexuals and Homosexuals." *Mikrobiyol Bul* 27: 46–51.

Cengiz, L., M. Kiyan, A. T. Cengiz, F. Kara, and M. S. Ugurel. 1993. "Detection of Herpes Simplex Virus 1 and 2 (HSV-1 And HSV-2) Igg and Igm by ELISA in Cord Blood and Sera of Mothers with Pregnancy Complications." *Mikrobiyol Bul* 27: 299–307.

Chamani-Tabriz, L., M. J. Tehrani, M. M. Akhondi, A. Mosavi-Jarrahi, H. Zeraati, J. Ghasemi, S. Asgari, A. Kokab, and A. R. Eley. 2007. "Chlamydia Trachomatis Prevalence in Iranian Women Attending Obstetrics and Gynaecology Clinics." *Pak J Biol Sci* 10: 4490–94.

Chaouki, N., F. X. Bosch, N. Munoz, C. J. Meijer, B. El Gueddari, A. El Ghazi, J. Deacon, X. Castellsague, and J. M. Walboomers. 1998. "The Viral Origin of Cervical Cancer in Rabat, Morocco." *Int J Cancer* 75: 546–54.

Chuang, T. Y., H. O. Perry, L. T. Kurland, and D. M. Ilstrup. 1984. "Condyloma Acuminatum in Rochester, Minn., 1950–78: I. Epidemiology and Clinical Features." *Arch Dermatol* 120: 469–75.

Cirpan, T., A. Guliyeva, G. Onder, M. C. Terek, A. Ozsaran, Y. Kabasakal, O. Zekioglu, and S. Yucebilgin. 2007. "Comparison of Human Papillomavirus Testing and Cervical Cytology with Colposcopic Examination and Biopsy in Cervical Cancer Screening in a Cohort of Patients with Sjogren's Syndrome." *Eur J Gynaecol Oncol* 28: 302–6.

Cleland, J., J. T. Boerma, M. Carael, and S. S. Weir. 2004. "Measurement of Sexual Behaviour." *Sexually Transmitted Infections* 80: ii1–i90.

Collins, S. I., S. Mazloomzadeh, H. Winter, T. P. Rollason, P. Blomfield, L. S. Young, and C. B. Woodman. 2005. "Proximity of First Intercourse to Menarche and the Risk of Human Papillomavirus Infection: A Longitudinal Study." *Int J Cancer* 114: 498–500.

Corey, L., and H. H. Handsfield. 2000. "Genital Herpes and Public Health: Addressing a Global Problem." *JAMA* 283: 791–94.

Corey, L., A. Wald, C. L. Celum, and T. C. Quinn. 2004. "The Effects of Herpes Simplex Virus-2 on HIV-1 Acquisition and Transmission: A Review of Two Overlapping Epidemics." *J Acquir Immune Defic Syndr* 35: 435–45.

Corwin, A. L., J. G. Olson, M. A. Omar, A. Razaki, and D. M. Watts. 1991. "HIV-1 in Somalia: Prevalence and Knowledge among Prostitutes." *AIDS* 5: 902–4.

Coskun, O., C. Gul, H. Erdem, O. Bedir, and C. P. Eyigun. 2008. "Prevalence of HIV and Syphilis among Turkish Blood Donors." *Ann Saudi Med* 28: 470.

Cowan, F. M., R. S. French, P. Mayaud, R. Gopal, N. J. Robinson, S. A. de Oliveira, T. Faillace, A. Uuskula, M. Nygard-Kibur, S. Ramalingam, G. Sridharan, R. El Aouad, K. Alami, M. Rbai, N. P. Sunil-Chandra, and D. W. Brown. 2003. "Seroepidemiological Study of Herpes Simplex Virus Types 1 and 2 in Brazil, Estonia, India, Morocco, and Sri Lanka." *Sex Transm Infect* 79: 286–90.

Cowan, F. M., A. M. Johnson, R. Ashley, L. Corey, and A. Mindel. 1994. "Antibody to Herpes Simplex Virus Type 2 as Serological Marker of Sexual Lifestyle in Populations." *BMJ* 309: 1325–29.

Cunningham, A. L., F. K. Lee, D. W. Ho, P. R. Field, C. L. Law, D. R. Packham, I. D. McCrossin, E. Sjogren-Jansson, S. Jeansson, and A. J. Nahmias. 1993. "Herpes Simplex Virus Type 2 Antibody in Patients Attending Antenatal or STD Clinics." *Med J Aust* 158: 525–28.

Curado, M. P., B. Edwards, H. R. Shin, H. Storm, J. Ferlay, et al., eds. 2007. *Cancer Incidence in Five Continents*, Vol. IX. IARC Scientific Publications No. 160, International Agency for Research on Cancer.

Dan, M., O. Sadan, M. Glezerman, D. Raveh, and Z. Samra. 2003. "Prevalence and Risk Factors for Herpes Simplex Virus Type 2 Infection among Pregnant Women in Israel." *Sex Transm Dis* 30: 835–38.

Darougar, S., B. Aramesh, J. A. Gibson, J. D. Treharne, and B. R. Jones. 1983. "Chlamydial Genital Infection in Prostitutes in Iran." *Br J Vener Dis* 59: 53–55.

Darougar, S., B. R. Jones, L. Cornell, J. D. Treharne, R. S. Dwyer, and B. Aramesh. 1982. "Chlamydial Urethral Infection in Teheran: A Study of Male Patients Attending an STD Clinic." *Br J Vener Dis* 58: 374–76.

Deeb, M. E., J. Awwad, J. S. Yeretzian, and H. G. Kaspar. 2003. "Prevalence of Reproductive Tract Infections, Genital Prolapse, and Obesity in a Rural Community in Lebanon." *Bull World Health Organ* 81: 639–45.

Dezfulimanesh, M., and N. Tehranian. 2005. "Endocervical Gonorrhea in Pregnant and Non-Pregnant Women and Follow Up of the Infected Cases in Kermanshah, Iran, 2004." *Pak J Med Sci* July–September 21: 313–17.

Dolar, N., S. Serdaroglu, G. Yilmaz, and S. Ergin. 2006. "Seroprevalence of Herpes Simplex Virus Type 1 and Type 2 in Turkey." *J Eur Acad Dermatol Venereol* 20: 1232–36.

Drain, P. K., K. K. Holmes, J. P. Hughes, and L. A. Koutsky. 2002. "Determinants of Cervical Cancer Rates in Developing Countries." *Int J Cancer* 100: 199–205.

Duran, N., F. Yarkin, C. Evruke, and F. Koksal. 2004. "Asymptomatic Herpes Simplex Virus Type 2 (HSV-2) Infection among Pregnant Women in Turkey." *Indian J Med Res* 120: 106–10.

El-All, H. S., A. Refaat, and K. Dandash. 2007. "Prevalence of Cervical Neoplastic Lesions and Human Papilloma Virus Infection in Egypt: National Cervical Cancer Screening Project." *Infect Agent Cancer* 2: 12.

Elattar, I. A. A. 2004. "Cancer in the Arab World: Magnitude of the Problem." The 132nd Annual Meeting.

El-Gilany, A. H., and S. El-Fedawy. 2006. "Bloodborne Infections among Student Voluntary Blood Donors in Mansoura University, Egypt." *East Mediterr Health J* 12: 742–48.

El Ghrari, K., Z. Terrab, H. Benchikhi, H. Lakhdar, I. Jroundi, and M. Bennani. 2007. "Prevalence of Syphilis and HIV Infection in Female Prison Population in Morocco." *East Mediterr Health J* 13: 774–79.

El-Sayed, N., M. Abdallah, A. Abdel Mobdy, A. Abdel Sattar, E. Aoun, F. Beths, G. Dallabetta, M. Rakha, C. Soliman, and N. Wasef. 2002. "Evaluation of Selected Reproductive Health Infections in Various Egyptian Population Groups in Greater Cairo." Ministry of Health and Population (MOHP), Implementing AIDS Prevention and Care (IMPACT), Family Health International (FHI), and the United States Agency for International Development (USAID).

El-Sayed, N. M., P. J. Gomatos, G. R. Rodier, T. F. Wierzba, A. Darwish, S. Khashaba, and R. R. Arthur. 1996. "Seroprevalence Survey of Egyptian Tourism Workers for Hepatitis B Virus, Hepatitis C Virus, Human Immunodeficiency Virus, and Treponema Pallidum Infections: Association of Hepatitis C Virus Infections with Specific Regions of Egypt." *Am J Trop Med Hyg* 55: 179–84.

El-Sayed, M. Zaki, and H. Goda. 2007. "Relevance of Parvovirus B19, Herpes Simplex Virus 2, and Cytomegalovirus Virologic Markers in Maternal Serum for Diagnosis of Unexplained Recurrent Abortions." *Arch Pathol Lab Med* 131: 956–60.

Faisel, A., and J. Cleland. 2006. "Migrant Men: A Priority for HIV Control in Pakistan?" *Sex Transm Infect* 82: 307–10.

Farhadi, M., Z. Tahmasebi, S. Merat, F. Kamangar, D. Nasrollahzadeh, and R. Malekzadeh. 2005. "Human Papillomavirus in Squamous Cell Carcinoma of Esophagus in a High-Risk Population." *World J Gastroenterol* 11: 1200–203.

Feldman, P. A., J. Steinberg, R. Madeb, G. Bar, O. Nativ, J. Tal, and I. Srugo. 2003. "Herpes Simplex Virus Type 2 Seropositivity in a Sexually Transmitted Disease Clinic in Israel." *Isr Med Assoc J* 5: 626–28.

Ferlay, J., F. Bray, P. Pisani, and D. M. Parkin. 2004. "GLOBOCAN 2002: Cancer Incidence, Mortality and Prevalence Worldwide." IARC CancerBase 5.

Fleming, D. T., G. M. McQuillan, R. E. Johnson, A. J. Nahmias, S. O. Aral, F. K. Lee, and M. E. St. Louis. 1997. "Herpes Simplex Virus Type 2 in the United States, 1976 to 1994." *N Engl J Med* 337: 1105–11.

Fox, E., R. L. Haberberger, E. A. Abbatte, S. Said, D. Polycarpe, and N. T. Constantine. 1989. "Observations on Sexually Transmitted Diseases in Promiscuous Males in Djibouti." *J Egypt Public Health Assoc* 64: 561–69.

Freeman, E. E., H. A. Weiss, J. R. Glynn, P. L. Cross, J. A. Whitworth, and R. J. Hayes. 2006. "Herpes Simplex Virus 2 Infection Increases HIV Acquisition in Men and Women: Systematic Review and Meta-Analysis of Longitudinal Studies." *AIDS* 20: 73–83.

Ghaffari, S. R., T. Sabokbar, H. Mollahajian, J. Dastan, F. Ramezanzadeh, F. Ensani, F. Yarandi, A. Mousavi-Jarrahi, M. A. Mohagheghi, and A. Moradi. 2006. "Prevalence of Human Papillomavirus Genotypes in Women with Normal and Abnormal Cervical Cytology in Iran." *Asian Pac J Cancer Prev* 7: 529–32.

Ghanaat, J., J. T. Afshari, K. Ghazvini, and M. Malvandi. 2008. "Prevalence of Genital Chlamydia in Iranian Males with Urethritis Attending Clinics in Mashhad." *East Mediterr Health J* 14: 1333–37.

Ghani, A. C., J. Swinton, and G. P. Garnett. 1997. "The Role of Sexual Partnership Networks in the Epidemiology of Gonorrhea." *Sex Transm Dis* 24: 45–56.

Ghazal-Aswad, S., P. Badrinath, A. Osman, S. Abdul-Khaliq, S. Mc Ilvenny, and I. Sidky. 2004. "Prevalence of Chlamydia Trachomatis Infection among Women in a Middle Eastern Community." *BMC Womens Health* 4: 3.

Ghazi, H. O., A. M. Telmesani, and M. F. Mahomed. 2002. "TORCH Agents in Pregnant Saudi Women." *Med Princ Pract* 11: 180–82.

Ginsberg, G. M., M. Fisher, I. Ben-Shahar, and J. Bornstein. 2007. "Cost-Utility Analysis of Vaccination against HPV in Israel." *Vaccine* 25: 6677–91.

Glasier, A., A. M. Gulmezoglu, G. P. Schmid, C. G. Moreno, and P. F. Van Look. 2006. "Sexual and Reproductive Health: A Matter of Life and Death." *Lancet* 368: 1595–607.

Goldie, S. J., L. Kuhn, L. Denny, A. Pollack, and T. C. Wright. 2001. "Policy Analysis of Cervical Cancer Screening Strategies in Low-Resource Settings: Clinical Benefits and Cost-Effectiveness." *JAMA* 285: 3107–15.

Gul, U., A. Kilic, B. Sakizligil, S. Aksaray, S. Bilgili, O. Demirel, and C. Erinckan. 2008. "Magnitude of Sexually Transmitted Infections among Female Sex Workers in Turkey." *J Eur Acad Dermatol Venereol* 22: 1123–24.

Hajiabdolbaghi, M., N. Razani, N. Karami, P. Kheirandish, M. Mohraz, M. Rasoolinejad, K. Arefnia, Z. Kourorian, G. Rutherford, and W. McFarland. 2007. "Insights from a Survey of Sexual Behavior among a Group of At-Risk Women in Tehran, Iran, 2006." *AIDS Educ Prev* 19: 519–30.

Hajjaj, A. A., A. C. Senok, A. E. Al-Mahmeed, A. A. Issa, A. R. Arzese, and G. A. Botta. 2006. "Human Papillomavirus Infection among Women Attending Health Facilities in the Kingdom of Bahrain." *Saudi Med J* 27: 487–91.

Hamkar, R., T. M. Azad, M. Mahmoodi, S. Seyedirashti, A. Severini, and R. Nategh. 2002. "Prevalence of Human Papillomavirus in Mazandaran Province, Islamic Republic of Iran." *East Mediterr Health J* 8: 805–11.

Hammad, M. M., H. W. Jones, and M. Zayed. 1987. "Low Prevalence of Cervical Intraepithelial Neoplasia among Egyptian Females." *Gynecol Oncol* 28: 300–4.

Hammouda, D., N. Munoz, R. Herrero, A. Arslan, A. Bouhadef, M. Oublil, B. Djedeat, B. Fontaniere, P. Snijders, C. Meijer, and S. Franceschi. 2005. "Cervical Carcinoma in Algiers, Algeria: Human Papillomavirus and Lifestyle Risk Factors." *Int J Cancer* 113: 483–89.

Hassen, E., A. Chaieb, M. Letaief, H. Khairi, A. Zakhama, S. Remadi, and L. Chouchane. 2003. "Cervical Human Papillomavirus Infection in Tunisian Women." *Infection* 31: 143–48.

Hassen, E., S. Remadi, and L. Chouchane. 1999. "Detection and Molecular Typing of Human Papillomaviruses: Prevalence of Cervical Infection in the Tunisian Central Region." *Tunis Med* 77: 497–502.

Hawkes, S., M. Collumbien, L. Platt, N. Lalji, N. Rizvi, A. Andreasen, J. Chow, R. Muzaffar, H. ur-Rehman, N. Siddiqui, S. Hasan, and A. Bokhari. 2009. "HIV and Other Sexually Transmitted Infections among Men, Transgenders and Women Selling Sex in Two Cities in Pakistan: A Cross-Sectional Prevalence Survey." *Sex Transm Infect* 85 Suppl 2: ii8–16.

Heikel, J., S. Sekkat, F. Bouqdir, H. Rich, B. Takourt, F. Radouani, N. Hda, S. Ibrahimy, and A. Benslimane. 1999. "The Prevalence of Sexually Transmitted Pathogens in Patients Presenting to a Casablanca STD Clinic." *Eur J Epidemiol* 15: 711–15.

Holt, B. Y., P. Effler, W. Brady, J. Friday, E. Belay, K. Parker, and M. Toole. 2003. "Planning STI/HIV Prevention among Refugees and Mobile Populations: Situation Assessment of Sudanese Refugees." *Disasters* 27: 1–15.

IARC (International Agency for Research on Cancer). WHO http://www.iarc.fr/.

Ibrahim, A. I., K. M. Kouwatli, and M. T. Obeid. 2000. "Frequency of Herpes Simplex Virus in Syria Based on Type-Specific Serological Assay." *Saudi Med J* 21: 355–60.

Imam, S. Z., F. Rehman, M. M. Zeeshan, B. Maqsood, S. Asrar, N. Fatima, F. Aslam, and M. R. Khawaja. 2008. "Perceptions and Practices of a Pakistani Population regarding Cervical Cancer Screening." *Asian Pac J Cancer Prev* 9: 42–44.

Inal, M. M., S. Kose, Y. Yildirim, Y. Ozdemir, E. Toz, K. Ertopcu, I. Ozelmas, and S. Tinar. 2007. "The Relationship between Human Papillomavirus Infection and Cervical Intraepithelial Neoplasia in Turkish Women." *Int J Gynecol Cancer* 17: 1266–70.

Iran Center for Disease Management. 2005. Three Month Statistics of the MoH AIDS Office. Unpublished.

Ismail, S. O., H. J. Ahmed, L. Grillner, B. Hederstedt, A. Issa, and S. M. Bygdeman. 1990. "Sexually Transmitted Diseases in Men in Mogadishu, Somalia." *Int J STD AIDS* 1: 102–6.

Jamal, A., and J. A. Al-Maghrabi. 2003. "Profile of Pap Smear Cytology in the Western Region of Saudi Arabia." *Saudi Med J* 24: 1225–29.

Jordan Ministry of Health. 2004. "Prevalence of Reproductive Tract Infections in Women Attending Selected Urban OB/GYN Clinics in Jordan." Amman, Jordan.

Jordan National Cancer Registry. 2008. *Cancer Incidence in Jordan*. Annual reports, 2000–2004. Cancer Prevention Directorate, National Cancer Registry, Ministry of Health, Amman, Jordan.

Kadi, Z., A. Bouguermouh, N. Ait-Mokhtar, A. Allouache, A. Ziat, and J. Orfilla. 1989. "Genital Chlamydia Infections: A Seroepidemiologic Study in Algiers." *Arch Inst Pasteur Alger* 57: 73–82.

Kafi, S. K., A. O. Mohamed, and H. A. Musa. 2000. "Prevalence of Sexually Transmitted Diseases (STD) among Women in a Suburban Sudanese Community." *Ups J Med Sci* 105: 249–53.

Kaiser, R., T. Kedamo, J. Lane, G. Kessia, R. Downing, T. Handzel, E. Marum, P. Salama, J. Mermin, W. Brady, and P. Spiegel. 2006. "HIV, Syphilis, Herpes Simplex Virus 2, and Behavioral Surveillance among Conflict-Affected Populations in Yei and Rumbek, Southern Sudan." *AIDS* 20: 942–44.

Kapila, K., S. S. George, A. Al-Shaheen, M. S. Al-Ottibi, S. K. Pathan, Z. A. Sheikh, B. E. Haji, M. K. Mallik, D. K. Das, and I. M. Francis. 2006. "Changing Spectrum of Squamous Cell Abnormalities Observed on Papanicolaou Smears in Mubarak Al-Kabeer Hospital, Kuwait, over a 13-Year Period." *Med Princ Pract* 15: 253–59.

Karam, W., G. Aftimos, A. Jurjus, S. Khairallah, and N. Bedrossian. 2007. "Prevalence of Sexually Transmitted Infections in Lebanese Women as Revealed by Pap Smear Cytology: A Cross Sectional Study from 2002–2006." WHO/EMRO.

Kasraeian, M., M. Movaseghii, and A. F. Ghiam. 2004. "Seroepidemiological Study of Herpes Simplex Virus Type 2 (HSV-2) Antibody in Shiraz, Iran." *Iranian Journal of Immunology* 1: 3 (autumn).

Khair, M. M., M. E. Mzibri, R. A. Mhand, A. Benider, N. Benchekroun, E. M. Fahime, M. N. Benchekroun, and M. M. Ennaji. 2009. "Molecular Detection and Genotyping of Human Papillomavirus in Cervical Carcinoma Biopsies in an Area of High Incidence of Cancer from Moroccan Women." *J Med Virol* 81: 678–84.

Khan, A. A., N. Rehan, K. Qayyum, and A. Khan. 2008. "Correlates and Prevalence of HIV and Sexually Transmitted Infections among Hijras (Male Transgenders) in Pakistan." *Int J STD AIDS* 19: 817–20.

Khattabi, H., and K. Alami. 2005. "Surveillance sentinelle du VIH, résultats 2004 et tendance de la séroprévalence du VIH." Morocco Ministry of Health, UNAIDS.

Khedmat, H., F. Fallahian, H. Abolghasemi, S. M. Alavian, B. Hajibeigi, S. M. Miri, and A. M. Jafari. 2007. "Seroepidemiologic Study of Hepatitis B Virus, Hepatitis C Virus, Human Immunodeficiency Virus and Syphilis Infections in Iranian Blood Donors." *Pak J Biol Sci* 10: 4461–66.

Komoditi, C. 2005. "Cervical and Corpus Uterine Cancer." In *Cancer Incidence in Four Member Countries (Cyprus, Egypt, Israel, and Jordan) of the Middle East Cancer Consortium (MECC) Compared with US SEER*, eds. L. S. Freedman, B. K. Edwards, L. A. Ries, and J. L. Young, 83–90. Bethesda, MD: National Cancer Institute, NIH Pub. No. 06–5873.

Kretzschmar, M., and M. Morris. 1996. "Measures of Concurrency in Networks and the Spread of Infectious Disease." *Mathematical Biosciences* 133: 165–95.

Lacey, C. J., C. M. Lowndes, and K. V. Shah. 2006. "Chapter 4: Burden and Management of Non-Cancerous HPV-Related Conditions: HPV-6/11 Disease." *Vaccine* 24 Suppl 3: S35–41.

Lalaoui, K., M. El Mzibri, M. Amrani, M. A. Belabbas, and P. A. Lazo. 2003. "Human Papillomavirus DNA in Cervical Lesions from Morocco and Its Implications for Cancer Control." *Clin Microbiol Infect* 9: 144–48.

Lambert, L. 2007. "HIV and Development Challenges in Yemen: Which Grows Fastest?" *Health Policy and Planning* 22: 60.

Langenberg, A. G., L. Corey, R. L. Ashley, W. P. Leong, and S. E. Straus. 1999. "A Prospective Study of New Infections with Herpes Simplex Virus Type 1 and Type 2." Chiron HSV Vaccine Study Group. *N Engl J Med* 341: 1432–38.

Lee, R. M., and C. M. Renzetti. 1990. "The Problems of Researching Sensitive Topics." *American Behavioral Scientist* 33: 510–28.

Looker, K. J., G. P. Garnett, and G. P. Schmid. 2008. "An Estimate of the Global Prevalence and Incidence of Herpes Simplex Virus Type 2 Infections." *Bulletin of the World Health Organization* 86: 805–12, A.

Lu, B., Y. Wu, C. M. Nielson, R. Flores, M. Abrahamsen, M. Papenfuss, R. B. Harris, and A. R. Giuliano. 2009. "Factors Associated with Acquisition and Clearance of Human Papillomavirus Infection in a Cohort of U.S. Men: A Prospective Study." *J Infect Dis* 199: 362–71.

Lubbad, A. M., and A. I. Al-Hindi. 2007. "Bacterial, Viral and Fungal Genital Tract Infections in Palestinian Pregnant Women in Gaza, Palestine." *West Afr J Med* 26: 138–42.

Madani, T. A. 2006. "Sexually Transmitted Infections in Saudi Arabia." *BMC Infect Dis* 6: 3.

Mahafzah, A. M., M. Q. Al-Ramahi, A. M. Asa'd, and M. S. El-Khateeb. 2008. "Prevalence of Sexually Transmitted Infections among Sexually Active Jordanian Females." *Sex Transm Dis* 35: 607–10.

Malkawi, S. R., R. M. Abu Hazeem, B. M. Hajjat, and F. K. Hajjiri. 2004. "Evaluation of Cervical Smears at King Hussein Medical Centre, Jordan, over Three and a Half Years." *East Mediterr Health J* 10: 676–79.

Maral, I., A. Biri, U. Korucuoglu, C. Bakar, M. Cirak, and M. Ali Bumin. 2009. "Seroprevalences of Herpes Simplex Virus Type 2 and Chlamydia Trachomatis in Turkey." *Arch Gynecol Obstet* 280: 739–43.

Marcelin, A. G., M. Grandadam, P. Flandre, J. L. Koeck, M. Philippon, E. Nicand, R. Teyssou, H. Agut, J. M. Huraux, and N. Dupin. 2001. "Comparative Study of Heterosexual Transmission of HIV-1, HSV-2 and KSHV in Djibouti." *8th Retrovir Oppor Infect* (abstract no. 585).

Massenet, D., and A. Bouh. 1997. "Aspects of Blood Transfusion in Djibouti." *Med Trop (Mars)* 57: 202–5.

Massoud, M., A. Noweir, M. Salah, and W. A. Saleh. 1991. "Chlamydial Infection in Riyadh, Saudi Arabia." *J Egypt Public Health Assoc* 66: 411–19.

Matin, M., and S. LeBaron. 2004. "Attitudes toward Cervical Cancer Screening among Muslim Women: A Pilot Study." *Women Health* 39: 63–77.

McCaffery, K., S. Forrest, J. Waller, M. Desai, A. Szarewski, and J. Wardle. 2003. "Attitudes towards HPV Testing: A Qualitative Study of Beliefs among Indian, Pakistani, African-Caribbean and White British Women in the UK." *Br J Cancer* 88: 42–46.

McCarthy, M. C., J. P. Burans, N. T. Constantine, A. A. el-Hag, M. E. el-Tayeb, M. A. el-Dabi, J. G. Fahkry, J. N. Woody, and K. C. Hyams. 1989. "Hepatitis B and HIV in Sudan: A Serosurvey for Hepatitis B and Human Immunodeficiency Virus Antibodies among Sexually Active Heterosexuals." *Am J Trop Med Hyg* 41: 726–31.

Measure DHS. 2006. "Egypt: Demographic and Health Survey 2005."

Mertz, G. J., O. Schmidt, J. L. Jourden, M. E. Guinan, M. L. Remington, A. Fahnlander, C. Winter, K. K. Holmes, and L. Corey. 1985. "Frequency of Acquisition of First-Episode Genital Infection with Herpes Simplex Virus from Symptomatic and Asymptomatic Source Contacts." *Sex Transm Dis* 12: 33–39.

Mertz, K. J., D. Trees, W. C. Levine, J. S. Lewis, B. Litchfield, K. S. Pettus, S. A. Morse, M. E. St. Louis, J. B. Weiss, J. Schwebke, J. Dickes, R. Kee, J. Reynolds, D. Hutcheson, D. Green, I. Dyer, G. A. Richwald, J. Novotny, I. Weisfuse, M. Goldberg, J. A. O'Donnell, and R. Knaup. 1998. "Etiology of Genital Ulcers and Prevalence of Human Immunodeficiency Virus Coinfection in 10 US Cities." The Genital Ulcer Disease Surveillance Group. *J Infect Dis* 178: 1795–98.

Morocco MOH (Ministry of Health). Unknown. "Situation épidémiologique actuelle du VIH/SIDA au Maroc."

Morris, M. 1993. "Telling Tails Explain the Discrepancy in Sexual Partner Reports." *Nature* 365: 437–40.

———. 1997. "Sexual Networks and HIV." *AIDS* 11: S209–16.

———. 2004. *Network Epidemiology: A Handbook for Survey Design and Data Collection*. Oxford University Press.

Morse, S. A. 1999. "Etiology of Genital Ulcer Disease and Its Relationship to HIV Infection." *Sex Transm Dis* 26: 63–65.

Mroueh, A. M., M. A. Seoud, H. G. Kaspar, and P. A. Zalloua. 2002. "Prevalence of Genital Human Papillomavirus among Lebanese Women." *Eur J Gynaecol Oncol* 23: 429–32.

Munoz, N., X. Castellsague, A. B. de Gonzalez, and L. Gissmann. 2006. "Chapter 1: HPV in the Etiology of Human Cancer." *Vaccine* 24S3: S1–S10.

Nagelkerke, N. J., R. M. Bernsen, S. K. Sgaier, and P. Jha. 2006. "Body Mass Index, Sexual Behaviour, and Sexually Transmitted Infections: An Analysis Using the NHANES 1999–2000 Data." *BMC Public Health* 6: 199.

Nahmias, A. J., F. K. Lee, and S. Beckman-Nahmias. 1990. "Sero-Epidemiological and Sociological Patterns of Herpes Simplex Virus Infection in the World." *Scand J Infect Dis* Suppl 69: 19–36.

Obasi, A., F. Mosha, M. Quigley, Z. Sekirassa, T. Gibbs, K. Munguti, J. Todd, H. Grosskurth, P. Mayaud, J. Changalucha, D. Brown, D. Mabey, and R. Hayes. 1999. "Antibody to Herpes Simplex Virus Type 2 as a Marker of Sexual Risk Behavior in Rural Tanzania." *J Infect Dis* 179: 16–24.

O'Farrell, N. 1999. "Increasing Prevalence of Genital Herpes in Developing Countries: Implications for Heterosexual HIV Transmission and STI Control Programmes." *Sex Transm Infect* 75: 377–84.

Ortashi, O. M., I. El Khidir, and E. Herieka. 2004. "Prevalence of HIV, Syphilis, Chlamydia Trachomatis, Neisseria Gonorrhoea, Trichomonas Vaginalis and Candidiasis among Pregnant Women Attending an Antenatal Clinic in Khartoum, Sudan." *J Obstet Gynaecol* 24: 513–15.

Ortayli, N., A. Bulut, and H. Nalbant. 2001. "The Effectiveness of Preabortion Contraception Counseling." *Int J Gynaecol Obstet* 74: 281–85.

Ortayli, N., Y. Sahip, B. Amca, L. Say, N. Sahip, and D. Aydin. 2001. "Curable Sexually Transmitted Infections among the Clientele of a Family Planning Clinic in Istanbul, Turkey." *Sex Transm Dis* 28: 58–61.

Ozcelik, B., I. S. Serin, S. Gokahmetoglu, M. Basbug, and R. Erez. 2003. "Human Papillomavirus Frequency of Women at Low Risk of Developing Cervical Cancer: A Preliminary Study from a Turkish University Hospital." *Eur J Gynaecol Oncol* 24: 157–59.

Pakistan National AIDS Control Program. 2005a. *National Study of Reproductive Tract and Sexually Transmitted Infections. Survey of High Risk Groups in Lahore and Karachi*. Ministry of Health, Pakistan.

———. 2005b. "Report of the Pilot Study in Karachi & Rawalpindi." Ministry of Health Canada-Pakistan HIV/AIDS Surveillance Project, Integrated Biological & Behavioral Surveillance 2004–5.

Parkin, D. M., S. L. Whelan, J. Ferlay, L. Teppo, and D. B. Thomas, eds. 2002. *Cancer Incidence in Five Continents* Vol. VIII, IARC Scientific Publications No. 155, International Agency for Research on Cancer.

Partridge, J. M., J. P. Hughes, Q. Feng, R. L. Winer, B. A. Weaver, L. F. Xi, M. E. Stern, S. K. Lee, S. F. O'Reilly, S. E. Hawes, N. B. Kiviat, and L. A. Koutsky. 2007. "Genital Human Papillomavirus Infection in Men: Incidence and Risk Factors in a Cohort of University Students." *J Infect Dis* 196: 1128–36.

Patnaik, P., R. Herrero, R. A. Morrow, N. Munoz, F. X. Bosch, S. Bayo, B. El Gueddari, E. Caceres, S. B. Chicharoen, X. Castellsague, C. J. Meijer, P. J. Snijders, and J. S. Smith. 2007. "Type-Specific Seroprevalence of Herpes Simplex Virus Type 2 and Associated Risk Factors in Middle-Aged Women from 6 Countries: The IARC Multicentric Study." *Sex Transm Dis* 34: 1019–24.

Paz-Bailey, G., M. Ramaswamy, S. J. Hawkes, and A. M. Geretti. 2007. "Herpes Simplex Virus Type 2: Epidemiology and Management Options in Developing Countries." *Sex Transm Infect* 83: 16–22.

Pebody, R. G., N. Andrews, D. Brown, R. Gopal, H. De Melker, G. Francois, N. Gatcheva, W. Hellenbrand, S. Jokinen, I. Klavs, M. Kojouharova, T. Kortbeek, B. Kriz, K. Prosenc, K. Roubalova, P. Teocharov, W. Thierfelder, M. Valle, P. Van Damme, and R. Vranckx. 2004. "The Seroepidemiology of Herpes Simplex Virus Type 1 and 2 in Europe." *Sex Transm Infect* 80: 185–91.

Pisani, E., S. Lazzari, N. Walker, and B. Schwartlander. 2003. "HIV Surveillance: A Global Perspective." *J Acquir Immune Defic Syndr* 32 Suppl 1: S3–11.

Platt, L., P. Vickerman, M. Collumbien, S. Hasan, N. Lalji, S. Mayhew, R. Muzaffar, A. Andreasen, and S. Hawkes. 2009. "Prevalence of HIV, HCV and Sexually Transmitted Infections among Injecting Drug Users in Rawalpindi and Abbottabad, Pakistan: Evidence for an Emerging Injection-Related HIV Epidemic." *Sex Transm Infect* 85 Suppl 2: ii17–22.

Rodier, G. R., J. J. Morand, J. S. Olson, D. M. Watts, S. Said. 1993. "HIV Infection among Secondary School Students in Djibouti, Horn of Africa: Knowledge, Exposure, and Prevalence." *East Afr Med J* 70: 414–17.

Roudi-Fahimi, F., and L. Ashford. 2008. "Sexual & Reproductive Health in the Middle East and North Africa: A Guide for Reporters." Population Reference Bureau, Washington, DC.

Rowe, W. 2007. "Cultural Competence in HIV Prevention and Care: Different Histories, Shared Future." *Soc Work Health Care* 44: 45–54.

Ryan, C. A., A. Zidouh, L. E. Manhart, R. Selka, M. Xia, M. Moloney-Kitts, J. Mahjour, M. Krone, B. N. Courtois, G. Dallabetta, and K. K. Holmes. 1998. "Reproductive Tract Infections in Primary Healthcare, Family Planning, and Dermatovenereology Clinics: Evaluation of Syndromic Management in Morocco." *Sex Transm Infect* 74 Suppl 1: S95–105.

Sadjadi, A., R. Malekzadeh, M. H. Derakhshan, A. Sepehr, M. Nouraie, M. Sotoudeh, A. Yazdanbod, B. Shokoohi, A. Mashayekhi, S. Arshi, A. Majidpour, M. Babaei, A. Mosavi, M. A. Mohagheghi, and M. Alimohammadian. 2003. "Cancer Occurrence in Ardabil: Results of a Population-Based Cancer Registry from Iran." *Int J Cancer* 107: 113–18.

Saleh, E., W. McFarland, G. Rutherford, J. Mandel, M. El-Shazaly, and T. Coates. 2000. "Sentinel Surveillance for HIV and Markers for High Risk Behaviors among STD Clinic Attendees in Alexandria, Egypt." XIII International AIDS Conference, Durban, South Africa, Poster MoPeC2398.

Samra, Z., E. Scherf, and M. Dan. 2003. "Herpes Simplex Virus Type 1 Is the Prevailing Cause of Genital Herpes in the Tel Aviv Area, Israel." *Sex Transm Dis* 30: 794–96.

Schiffman, M., and P. E. Castle. 2005. "The Promise of Global Cervical-Cancer Prevention." *N Engl J Med* 353: 2101–4.

Scott, D. A., A. L. Corwin, N. T. Constantine, M. A. Omar, A. Guled, M. Yusef, C. R. Roberts, and D. M. Watts. 1991. "Low Prevalence of Human Immunodeficiency Virus-1 (HIV-1), HIV-2, and Human T Cell Lymphotropic Virus-1 Infection in Somalia." *American Journal of Tropical Medicine and Hygiene* 45: 653.

Shafiq, M., and S. H. Ali. 2006. "Sexually Transmitted Infections in Pakistan." *Lancet Infect Dis* 6: 321–22.

Skegg, D. C., P. A. Corwin, C. Paul, and R. Doll. 1982. "Importance of the Male Factor in Cancer of the Cervix." *Lancet* 2: 581–83.

Slomka, M. J. 1996. "Seroepidemiology and Control of Genital Herpes: The Value of Type Specific Antibodies to Herpes Simplex Virus." *Commun Dis Rep* CDR Rev 6: R41–45.

Smith, J. S., and N. J. Robinson. 2002. "Age-Specific Prevalence of Infection with Herpes Simplex Virus Types 2 and 1: A Global Review." *J Infect Dis* 186 Suppl 1: S3–28.

Somaliland Ministry of Health and Labour. 2007. *Somaliland 2007 HIV/Syphilis Seroprevalence Survey, A Technical Report.* Ministry of Health and Labour in collaboration with WHO, UNAIDS, UNICEF/GFATM, and SOLNAC.

Southern Sudan AIDS Commission. 2007. Southern Sudan ANC Sentinel Surveillance Data. Database, U.S. Centers for Disease Control and Prevention (CDC), Sudan, and Southern Sudan AIDS Commission.

Štulhofer, A., and I. Božicevic. 2008. "HIV Bio-Behavioural Survey among FSWs in Aden, Yemen."

Sudan National AIDS Program. 2008. "Update on the HIV Situation in Sudan." PowerPoint presenation.

Sudan National AIDS/STIs Program. 2008. "2007 ANC HIV Sentinel Sero-Survey, Technical Report." Federal Ministry of Health, Preventive Medicine Directorate, draft.

Sultan, F., T. Mehmood, and M. T. Mahmood. 2007. "Infectious Pathogens in Volunteer and Replacement Blood Donors in Pakistan: A Ten-Year Experience." *Int J Infect Dis* 11: 407–12.

Tehrani, F. R., and H. Malek-Afzalip. 2008. "Knowledge, Attitudes and Practices concerning HIV/AIDS among Iranian At-Risk Sub-Populations." *Eastern Mediterranean Health Journal* 14.

Testa, A. C., and K. Kriitmaa. 2009. "HIV and Syphilis Bio-Behavioural Surveillance Survey (BSS+) among Female Transactional Sex Workers in Hargeisa, Somaliland." International Organization for Migration, World Health Organization.

Todd, C. S., A. M. Abed, S. A. Strathdee, P. T. Scott, B. A. Botros, N. Safi, and K. C. Earhart. 2007. "HIV, Hepatitis C, and Hepatitis B Infections and Associated Risk Behavior in Injection Drug Users, Kabul, Afghanistan." *Emerg Infect Dis* 13: 1327–31.

Todd, C. S., M. Ahmadzai, F. Atiqzai, S. Miller, J. M. Smith, S. A. Ghazanfar, and S. A. Strathdee. 2008. "Seroprevalence and Correlates of HIV, Syphilis, and Hepatitis B and C Virus among Intrapartum Patients in Kabul, Afghanistan." *BMC Infect Dis* 8: 119.

Todd, C. S., M. Ahmadzai, F. Atiqzai, H. Siddiqui, P. Azfar, S. Miller, J. M. Smith, S. A. S. Ghazanfar, and S. A. Strathdee. 2007. "Seroprevalence and Correlates of HIV, Syphilis, and Hepatitis B and C Infection among Antenatal Patients and Testing Practices and Knowledge among Obstetric Care Providers in Kabul." PowerPoint presentation.

Todd, C. S., S. Strathdee, F. Atiqzai, M. Ahmadzai, M. Appelbaum, S. Miller, J. A. McCutchan, J. Smith, and K. Earhart. 2006. "Prevalence of and Barriers to Testing for Blood-Borne Infections in an Afghan Antenatal Population." Study proposal.

Trottier, H., and E. L. Franco. 2006. "The Epidemiology of Genital Human Papillomavirus Infection." *Vaccine* 24 Suppl 1: S1–15.

UNHCR (United Nations High Commissioner for Refugees). 2006–07. *HIV Sentinel Surveillance among Antenatal Clients and STI Patients.* Dadaab Refugee Camps, Kenya.

Unknown. "Statut de la réponse nationale: Caractéristiques de l'épidémie des IST/VIH/SIDA." Algeria.

Unknown. 2002. "Surveillance des infections à VIH et de la syphilis chez les femmes enceintes vues dans 8 centres de consultations prénatales dans le district de Djibouti." Grey Report.

Vahdani, P., S. M. Hosseini-Moghaddam, L. Gachkar, and K. Sharafi. 2006. "Prevalence of Hepatitis B, Hepatitis C, Human Immunodeficiency Virus, and Syphilis among Street Children Residing in Southern Tehran, Iran." *Arch Iran Med* 9: 153–55.

van de Laar, M. J. W., F. Termorshuizen, M. J. Slomka, G. J. J. van Doornum, J. M. Ossewaarde, D. W. G. Brown, R. A. Coutinho, and J. A. R. van den Hoek. 2001. "Prevalence and Correlates of Herpes Simplex Virus Type 2 Infection: Evaluation of Behavioural Risk Factors." *International Journal of Epidemiology* 27: 127–34.

Wadsworth, J., J. Field, A. M. Johnson, S. Bradshaw, and K. Wellings. 1993. "Methodology of the National Survey of Sexual Attitudes and Lifestyles." *J R Stat Soc Ser A Stat Soc* 156: 407–21.

Walboomers, J. M., M. V. Jacobs, M. M. Manos, F. X. Bosch, J. A. Kummer, K. V. Shah, P. J. Snijders, J. Peto, C. J. Meijer, and N. Munoz. 1999. "Human Papillomavirus Is a Necessary Cause of Invasive Cervical Cancer Worldwide." *J Pathol* 189: 12–19.

Watts, C. H., and R. M. May. 1992. "The Influence of Concurrent Partnerships on the Dynamics of HIV/AIDS." *Math Biosci* 108: 89–104.

Watts, D. M., A. L. Corwin, M. A. Omar, and K. C. Hyams. 1994. "Low Risk of Sexual Transmission of Hepatitis C Virus in Somalia." *Trans R Soc Trop Med Hyg* 88: 55–56.

Weiss, H. 2004. "Epidemiology of Herpes Simplex Virus Type 2 Infection in the Developing World." *Herpes* 11 Suppl 1: 24A–35A.

Weiss, H. A., S. L. Thomas, S. K. Munabi, and R. J. Hayes. 2006. "Male Circumcision and Risk of Syphilis, Chancroid, and Genital Herpes: A Systematic Review and Meta-Analysis." *Sex Transm Infect* 82: 101–9; discussion 110.

WHO (World Health Organization). 2001. "Global Prevalence and Incidence of Selected Curable Sexually Transmitted Infections, Overview and Estimates." Geneva, Switzerland.

———. 2003. *Shaping the Future*. World Health Report 2003. Geneva: World Health Organization.

———. 2004. *Unsafe Abortion, Global and Regional Estimates of the Incidence of Unsafe Abortion and Associated Mortality in 2000, 4th Edition*. Geneva: World Health Organization.

———. 2007. "Human Papillomavirus and HPV Vaccination: Technical Information for Policy-Makers and Health Professionals." Department of Immunization, Vaccines, and Biologicals, Geneva, Switzerland.

WHO/EMRO (Eastern Mediterranean Region Office). 1998. *Report on the Intercountry Workshop on STD Prevalence Study*. Amman, Jordan.

———. 2006. *Strengthening Health Sector Response to HIV/AIDS and Sexually Transmitted Infections in the Eastern Mediterranean Region 2006–2010*. Cairo: WHO/EMRO.

———. 2007. "Prevention and Control of Sexually Transmitted Infections in the WHO Eastern Mediterranean Region." Intercountry meeting, PowerPoint presentation.

Winer, R. L., S. K. Lee, J. P. Hughes, D. E. Adam, N. B. Kiviat, and L. A. Koutsky. 2003. "Genital Human Papillomavirus Infection: Incidence and Risk Factors in a Cohort of Female University Students." *Am J Epidemiol* 157: 218–26.

Yildirim, Y., M. M. Inal, and S. Tinar. 2005. "Reproductive and Obstetric Characteristics of Adolescent Pregnancies in Turkish Women." *J Pediatr Adolesc Gynecol* 18: 249–53.

Zangeneh, M. 1999. "Epidemiology of the Gonococcal Infection in Women Kermanshah." West Iran.

Ziyaeyan, M., A. Japoni, M. H. Roostaee, S. Salehi, and H. Soleimanjahi. 2007. "A Serological Survey of Herpes Simplex Virus Type 1 and 2 Immunity in Pregnant Women at Labor Stage in Tehran, Iran." *Pak J Biol Sci* 10: 148–51.

Chapter 11

Analytical Insights into HIV Transmission Dynamics and Epidemic Potential in MENA

Understanding the current status and future potential of the human immunodeficiency virus (HIV) epidemic is central to designing appropriate epidemic responses because surveillance efforts and the effectiveness and cost-effectiveness of interventions depend on the epidemiological context in which they are implemented.[1] This chapter discusses the analytical insights reached based on the conceptual framework described in chapter 1 and the data synthesis presented in the following chapters.

EVOLUTION OF THE HIV EPIDEMIC IN MENA

HIV found its way to the Middle East and North Africa (MENA) countries by the 1980s at the latest. Virtually all countries had reported their first HIV or AIDS (acquired immunodeficiency syndrome) case by 1990.[2] The majority of cases were linked to blood or blood products or exposures abroad. Transfusions of blood or blood

products were behind a large fraction of reported cases such as in the Arab Republic of Egypt,[3] the Islamic Republic of Iran,[4] Saudi Arabia,[5] and the West Bank and Gaza.[6] Quite often the blood or the blood products were imported.[7]

A high prevalence of blood-borne diseases was found at the time among people in need of blood or blood products. In Bahrain in the early 1990s, the prevalence of HIV among children with hereditary hemolytic anemias was 1.6%, 40% for people with hepatitis C virus (HCV), and 20.5% for people with hepatitis B virus (HBV).[8] In Egypt, recipients of blood or blood products had an HIV prevalence of 4.8% in the period from 1986 to 1990.[9] In Lebanon, multi-transfused patients had an HIV prevalence of 6%.[10] In Qatar, more than 75% of reported HIV infections up to 1989 were acquired via transfusion of imported blood,[11] and 38.5% of

---

[1] Grassly et al., "The Effectiveness of HIV Prevention."

[2] Shah et al., "An Outbreak of HIV"; Ryan, "Travel Report Summary"; Jenkins and Robalino, "HIV in the Middle East and North Africa"; Al-Fouzan and Al-Mutairi, "Overview of Incidence of Sexually Transmitted Diseases in Kuwait"; Elharti et al., "Some Characteristics of the HIV Epidemic in Morocco"; Kalaajieh, "Epidemiology of Human Immunodeficiency Virus"; Iran Center for Disease Management, *HIV/AIDS and STIs Surveillance Report*; Woodruff et al., "A Study of Viral and Rickettsial Exposure"; Khanani et al., "Human Immunodeficiency Virus-Associated Disorders in Pakistan"; Toukan and Schable, "Human Immunodeficiency Virus (HIV) Infection in Jordan"; Rodier et al., "Infection by the Human Immunodeficiency Virus."

[3] Faris and Shouman, "Study of the Knowledge, Attitude of Egyptian Health Care Workers."

[4] Rao, *Strengthening of AIDS/HIV Surveillance.*

[5] El-Hazmi and Ramia, "Frequencies of Hepatitis B"; Alrajhi, "Human Immunodeficiency Virus in Saudi Arabia"; Al-Nozha et al., "Horizontal versus Vertical Transmission."

[6] Maayan et al., "HIV/AIDS among Palestinian Arabs"; Moses et al., "HIV Infection and AIDS in Jerusalem."

[7] Mokhbat et al., "Clinical and Serological Study"; Novelli et al., "High Prevalence of Human Immunodeficiency Virus"; Harfi and Fakhry, "Acquired Immunodeficiency Syndrome in Saudi Arabia"; Kingston et al., "Acquired Immune Deficiency Syndrome."

[8] Al-Mahroos and Ebrahim, "Prevalence of Hepatitis B."

[9] Watts et al. "Prevalence of HIV Infection and AIDS."

[10] Mokhbat et al., "Clinical and Serological Study."

[11] Milder and Novelli, "Clinical, Social and Ethical Aspects of HIV-1."

children with thalassemia were found to be HIV positive.[12] In Saudi Arabia, 1.3% of multitransfused thalassemic and sickle cell disease patients tested positive for HIV,[13] and 34.5% of HIV-positive children became infected through blood or blood products.[14]

Organ transplants have also contributed to a number of HIV infections in this early phase of the epidemic. HIV infections were diagnosed among kidney transplant patients in Oman, Saudi Arabia, and the United Arab Emirates who bought kidneys from donors in Egypt and India.[15] HIV prevalence was 4.3% among 540 Saudi hemodialysis patients who received a commercial kidney transplant in India.[16]

Although blood safety measures were not implemented satisfactorily until the late 1990s, the region nonetheless made substantial progress in reducing HIV infections due to contaminated blood, from 12.1% in 1993 to 0.4% in 2003.[17] This progress, however, was not universal and some countries, such as Afghanistan and the Republic of Yemen, continued to lag behind in the screening of blood products.[18] It is believed that currently only 30% of all donated blood is screened in Afghanistan.[19]

The majority of reported infections acquired by a mode other than blood or blood products were either related to sexual or injecting drug exposures abroad[20] or acquired by sexual partners of those who worked or lived abroad.[21] This trend is not dissimilar to other regions such as in Western Europe, where the first AIDS cases were among travelers and expatriates who worked abroad.[22] However, the pattern of a large share of HIV acquisitions related to exposures abroad appears to persist in several countries. In Jordan, 450 out of 501 notified HIV/AIDS cases by 2006 were acquired abroad.[23] In Lebanon, 45.36% of notified HIV/AIDS cases up to 2004 were linked to travel abroad.[24] Half of reported AIDS cases in the Republic of Yemen were linked to traveling abroad.[25]

The travel-related exposures were from multiple destinations. In Lebanon, a considerable number of HIV/AIDS cases were found among returning migrants who resided in western and Central Africa.[26] In the West Bank and Gaza, HIV cases appeared among migrant workers working legally or illegally in Israel.[27] In Oman, a number of HIV cases were related to Omani historical links to East Africa.[28] In Pakistan, the majority of cases were acquired through contacts with female sex workers (FSWs) while working in the Persian Gulf region.[29] In Tunisia, HIV infections were found among Tunisian injecting drug users (IDUs) deported from France.[30] Generally, HIV infections in Maghreb countries were linked to exposures in Western Europe.[31]

A number of HIV sero-prevalence studies that were conducted in MENA in the 1980s and early 1990s included Djibouti,[32] Egypt,[33] the Islamic Republic of Iran,[34] Jordan,[35] Lebanon,[36]

[12] Novelli et al., "High Prevalence of Human Immunodeficiency Virus."

[13] El-Hazmi and Ramia, "Frequencies of Hepatitis B."

[14] Kordy et al., "Human Immunodeficiency Virus Infection."

[15] Alrajhi, Halim, and Al-Abdely, "Mode of Transmission of HIV-1"; Salahudeen et al., "High Mortality among Recipients"; Aghanashinikar et al., "Prevalence of Hepatitis B."

[16] Anonymous, "Commercially Motivated Renal Transplantation."

[17] UNAIDS, "Notes on AIDS in the Middle East and North Africa."

[18] WHO/EMRO, "Progress Report on HIV/AIDS and '3 by 5.'"

[19] Global Fund, Afghanistan Proposal, www.theglobalfund.org/search/docs/4AFGT_764_0_full.pdf.

[20] Iqbal and Rehan, "Sero-Prevalence of HIV"; Ryan, "Travel Report Summary"; Kayani et al., "A View of HIV-I Infection in Karachi"; Toukan and Schable, "Human Immunodeficiency Virus (HIV) Infection in Jordan"; Faris and Shouman, "Study of the Knowledge"; Maayan et al., "HIV/AIDS among Palestinian Arabs"; Naman et al., "Seroepidemiology of the Human Immunodeficiency Virus"; Dan, Rock, and Bar-Shany, "Prevalence of Antibodies"; Jemni et al., "AIDS and Tuberculosis in Central Tunisia."

[21] Tiouiri et al., "Study of Psychosocial Factors"; "Global Update: Morocco."

[22] Hawkes et al., "Risk Behaviour."

[23] Jordan National AIDS Program, personal communication.

[24] Jurjus et al., "Knowledge, Attitudes, Beliefs, and Practices."

[25] WHO, UNICEF, and UNAIDS, "Yemen, Epidemiological Facts Sheets."

[26] Jenkins and Robalino, "HIV in the Middle East and North Africa."

[27] UNAIDS, "Key Findings on HIV Status in the West Bank and Gaza."

[28] Tawilah and Tawil, Visit to Sultane of Oman.

[29] Shah et al., "HIV-Infected Workers Deported"; Baqi, Kayani, and Khan, "Epidemiology and Clinical Profile"; Khan et al., "HIV-1 Subtype A Infection."

[30] Jenkins and Robalino, "HIV in the Middle East and North Africa."

[31] "Global Update: Morocco."

[32] Rodier et al., "HIV Infection among Secondary School Students."

[33] Watts et al. "Prevalence of HIV Infection and AIDS"; El-Ghazzawi, Hunsmann, and Schneider, "Low Prevalence of Antibodies"; Constantine et al., "HIV Infection in Egypt"; Kandela, "Arab Nations: Attitudes to AIDS."

[34] Arbesser, Bashiribod, and Sixl, "Serological Examinations of HIV-I in Iran."

[35] Al Katheeb, Tarawneh, and Awidi, "Antibodies to HIV."

[36] Naman et al., "Seroepidemiology of the Human Immunodeficiency Virus."

Libya,[37] Mauritania,[38] Pakistan,[39] Saudi Arabia,[40] Somalia,[41] Sudan,[42] Turkey,[43] the West Bank and Gaza,[44] and the Republic of Yemen.[45] These studies included tens of thousands of blood samples from populations including pregnant women, healthy women, healthy men, neonates, drug users, IDUs, FSWs, sexually transmitted disease (STD) patients, prisoners, truck drivers, soldiers, refugees, leprous patients, outpatients, hospital patients, and blood or blood product donors and recipients.

In almost all of these surveys, few HIV infections were identified, if any. HIV prevalence was consistently at very low levels even in priority groups. The vast majority of diagnosed cases were linked to HIV exposures abroad, blood or blood products, or organ transplants. Nevertheless, a new pattern of HIV infectious spread started to appear in MENA by the early 1990s. HIV found its way to some of the high-risk networks in a few countries. Growing HIV prevalence was identified among a number of priority populations.

A classic example highlighting this emerging pattern is the epidemic in Djibouti. The first reported AIDS case was in 1986.[46] Although HIV prevalence was still nil in general population groups, such as high school students,[47] it was growing rapidly along the complex network of commercial sex. HIV prevalence among street-based FSWs, the most vulnerable of sex workers, increased tenfold from 4.6% in 1987 to 41.7% in 1990.[48] By the early 1990s, HIV prevalence among these sex workers appeared to be at levels as high as 70%.[49] The epidemic among bar-based FSWs was also growing rapidly;[50] over this period, it was documented by individual studies to be 1.4%,[51] 2.7%,[52] 5%,[53] 7%,[54] 14.2%,[55] 15.3%,[56] 21.7%,[57] and 25.6%.[58]

While HIV prevalence was stabilizing among FSWs by about 1990,[59] it was rising rapidly among their clients. The HIV prevalence among STD clinic attendees increased fivefold between 1990 and 1991 and reached 10.4%.[60] HIV infection then found its way to spouses of clients of FSWs and their children through mother-to-child transmission. HIV prevalence was rising among the spouses, but at a slower rate, and reached levels of about 5% by the late 1990s and has remained stable at about this level since then.[61]

Women from the general population in Djibouti were the dam at which the tide of HIV spread was absorbed and then stopped. Being at the receiving end, they carried a higher overall HIV prevalence than men (3.6% versus 3.1% in Djibouti-ville and 1.7% versus 0.3% in the rest of the country[62]). However, it does not appear that they engaged in much risk behavior and it seems that they rarely spread the infection further. This limited further inroads of HIV into the population. HIV prevalence appears to have leveled off at about 3% nationally since the late 1990s.[63] Although Djibouti was predicted to have a sky-rocketing epidemic a decade ago, this has not materialized.[64] HIV may have already traveled along the contours of risk and vulnerability in this country and saturated its potential.

[37] Giasuddin et al., "Failure to Find Antibody."
[38] Lepers et al., "Sero-Epidemiological Study in Mauritania."
[39] Mujeeb and Hafeez, "Prevalence and Pattern of HIV "; Mujeeb et al., "Prevalence of HIV-Infection among Blood Donors."
[40] Al Rasheed et al., "Screening for HIV Antibodies."
[41] Jama et al., "Sexually Transmitted Viral Infections"; Burans et al., "HIV Infection Surveillance in Mogadishu"; Ismail et al., "Sexually Transmitted Diseases in Men"; Fox et al., "AIDS."
[42] Burans et al., "Serosurvey of Prevalence"; McCarthy et al., "Hepatitis B and HIV in Sudan"; Hashim et al., "AIDS and HIV Infection in Sudanese Children."
[43] Rota et al., "HIV Antibody Screening"; Demiroz et al., "HIV Infections among Turkish Citizens."
[44] Maayan et al., "HIV-1 Prevalence."
[45] Leonard et al., "Prevalence of HIV Infection."
[46] Rodier et al., "Infection by the Human Immunodeficiency Virus."
[47] Rodier et al., "HIV Infection among Secondary School Students."
[48] Rodier et al., "Trends of Human Immunodeficiency Virus"; Rodier et al., "Infection by the Human Immunodeficiency Virus."
[49] Etchepare, "Programme National de Lutte"; Rodier et al., "Trends of Human Immunodeficiency Virus"; Marcelin et al., "Comparative Study."
[50] Couzineau et al., "Prevalence of Infection."
[51] Etchepare, "Programme National de Lutte."
[52] Ibid.
[53] Ibid.
[54] Marcelin et al., "Comparative Study."
[55] Etchepare, "Programme National de Lutte."
[56] Rodier et al., "Trends of Human Immunodeficiency Virus"; Rodier et al., "Infection by the Human Immunodeficiency Virus."
[57] Etchepare, "Programme National de Lutte."
[58] Ibid.
[59] Rodier et al., "Infection by the Human Immunodeficiency Virus."
[60] Rodier et al., "Trends of Human Immunodeficiency Virus"; Rodier et al., "Infection by the Human Immunodeficiency Virus."
[61] Marcelin et al., "Kaposi's Sarcoma Herpesvirus."
[62] WHO, "Summary Country Profile."
[63] UNAIDS, "Notes on AIDS in the Middle East and North Africa"; Djibouti (Ministère de La Santé de) and Association Internationale de Développement, Tome I; Maslin et al., "Epidemiology and Genetic Characterization."
[64] O'Grady, "WFP Consultant Visit to Djibouti Report."

In the Islamic Republic of Iran, the first HIV/AIDS case among IDUs was reported in 1992.[65] Only a few cases were reported per year in the three following years.[66] However, starting from 1996, the number of reported cases suddenly rose by thirtyfold.[67] The first reported outbreak was in 1996 in the prisons of Kerman and Kermanshah.[68] By 2000, the prevalence remained under 1%–2% in most studies.[69] In 2003, the prevalence started growing rapidly and was consistently above 5% in most point-prevalence surveys among IDUs.[70] Through overlapping risk behaviors,[71] HIV infection appears to have crossed into the sexual networks of men who have sex with men (MSM),[72] and, to a lesser extent, FSWs.[73] Then HIV infection moved to spouses of IDUs, whose contribution to the number of HIV/AIDS cases increased fourfold from 0.5% of all cases in 2001 to 2% of all cases in 2004.[74] Seventy-six percent of HIV-positive women in the Islamic Republic of Iran acquired the infection from their husbands, who were predominantly IDUs.[75]

More than two decades since the introduction of HIV into MENA populations, the epidemiological landscape continues to be dominated by two patterns. The first is that of exogenous HIV infections related to sexual and injecting drug exposures abroad among the nationals of MENA countries, followed by HIV transmissions to their sexual partners upon their return. The second is that of concentrated or low-intensity HIV epidemics among priority populations.

CONCEPTUAL FRAMEWORK: DYNAMICS OF HIV INFECTIOUS SPREAD IN MENA

There is substantial heterogeneity in HIV spread across MENA and different risk contexts are present throughout the region. However, we can grossly classify the HIV epidemic in MENA, in terms of the extent of HIV spread, into two groups. The first group, which has a considerable HIV prevalence and includes Djibouti, Somalia, and Southern Sudan, is labeled here as **Subregion with Considerable Prevalence**. The second group has a more modest HIV prevalence and includes the rest of MENA countries and is labeled here as the **Core MENA Region**. Because the latter group consists of most MENA countries, HIV epidemiology here represents the main patterns found in MENA.

HIV epidemic typology in the Core MENA Region

Two patterns describe HIV epidemiology in this group of MENA countries. The first is the pattern of exogenous HIV exposures among the nationals of these countries, and HIV transmissions to their sexual partners upon their return. This pattern exists in all MENA countries at some level or another, but also appears to be the dominant pattern in several MENA countries. The weak surveillance systems of priority populations prevent us from definitively concluding whether this is indeed the dominant epidemiologic pattern in these countries. HIV could be spreading among some of the priority groups, or within pockets of these populations, without current awareness of this endemic spread. However, there is no evidence to date that such considerable endemic transmission exists in these MENA countries.

The second pattern in several MENA countries is that of concentrated or low-intensity HIV epidemics among priority populations, particularly IDUs and MSM. Concentrated epidemics are defined as HIV epidemics in subpopulations at higher risk of HIV infection, such as IDUs, MSM, and FSWs; and HIV prevalence is consistently above 5% in at least one priority group, but remains below 1% in pregnant women in the general population.[76] There is already

[65] Iran Center for Disease Management, *Country Report on UNGASS.*
[66] Ibid.
[67] Ministry of Health and Medical Education of Iran, "Treatment and Medical Education"; Iran Center for Disease Management, *Country Report on UNGASS.*
[68] Afshar, "Health and Prison."
[69] Ministry of Health and Medical Education of Iran, "Treatment and Medical Education."
[70] Ibid.
[71] Tehrani and Malek-Afzalip, "Knowledge, Attitudes and Practices"; Farhoudi et al., "Human Immunodeficiency Virus"; Razzaghi, Rahimi, and Hosseini, *Rapid Situation Assessment (RSA) of Drug Abuse*; Narenjiha et al., "Rapid Situation Assessment"; Eftekhar et al., "Bio-Behavioural Survey on HIV"; Ministry of Health and Medical Education of Iran, "Treatment and Medical Education"; Mostashari, UNODC, and Darabi, "Summary of the Iranian Situation on HIV Epidemic"; Jahani et al., "Distribution and Risk Factors."
[72] Eftekhar et al., "Bio-Behavioural Survey on HIV."
[73] WHO/EMRO Regional Database on HIV/AIDS; Jahani et al., "Distribution and Risk Factors"; Tassie, "Assignment Report."
[74] Ministry of Health and Medical Education of Iran, "Treatment and Medical Education."
[75] Ramezani, Mohraz, and Gachkar, "Epidemiologic Situation"; Burrows, Wodak, and WHO, *Harm Reduction in Iran.*

[76] Pisani et al., "HIV Surveillance."

documented evidence for concentrated epidemics among priority groups in several MENA countries, such as the HIV epidemics among IDUs in the Islamic Republic of Iran and Pakistan, which are established concentrated epidemics.[77] There is evidence that suggests that this could also be the case in Afghanistan (in Kabul),[78] Bahrain,[79] Libya,[80] North Sudan,[81] and Oman.[82]

There is no definitive evidence of the existence of concentrated epidemics among MSM, the most hidden of all risk groups, in any of the MENA countries. However, there is evidence that suggests that this could be the case in Egypt,[83] North Sudan,[84] and Pakistan.[85] Though the evidence is not strong, there is an indication of an epidemic among MSM in Lebanon; however, it is not yet at the level to be categorized as a concentrated epidemic.[86]

There is no evidence of the existence of concentrated epidemics among FSWs in this group of MENA countries. HIV prevalence among FSWs has been found on occasions to be substantially higher than that of the general population, but not to the level of concentrated HIV epidemics (greater than 5%). Concentrated epidemics may exist, though, among subgroups of FSWs, such as in southern Algeria.[87]

HIV epidemic typology in the Subregion with Considerable Prevalence

Djibouti,[88] parts of Somalia,[89] and Southern Sudan[90] are in a state of generalized HIV epidemic,

defined as an epidemic with an HIV prevalence consistently exceeding 1% among pregnant women.[91] However, it appears that the epidemics in Djibouti and Somalia, and possibly Southern Sudan, are dynamically similar to those in West Africa where most HIV infections are concentrated in priority groups and bridging populations. The high HIV prevalence among FSWs in Djibouti[92] and Southern Sudan[93] suggests that commercial sex networks are playing the central role in these epidemics, just as in West Africa.[94]

There is no evidence of sustainable general population HIV epidemics in this group of MENA countries. The prevailing epidemics are best understood as concentrated epidemics focused around the commercial sex networks in settings where the size of the commercial sex network is large enough to support an epidemic with a prevalence exceeding 1% in the whole population.

Southern Sudan is of particular concern. There are no sufficient data to characterize satisfactorily HIV epidemiology in this part of Sudan. Southern Sudan is the only part of MENA where limited male circumcision coverage is found. It could already be in a state of general population epidemic. With the recent peace treaty, the resettlement of refugees and internally displaced persons (IDPs), demobilization of soldiers, influx of peacekeepers, and mushrooming of commercial centers, there is a concern as to whether there is fertile ground for further HIV expansion in Southern Sudan.[95]

The two key epidemiologic characteristics that distinguish this subregion of MENA from the Core MENA Region are the concentrated epidemics among FSWs, implying higher levels of risk behavior in commercial sex networks, and the sizes of commercial sex networks, which appear to be significantly larger than those in the rest of MENA.

[77] Pakistan National AIDS Control Program, *HIV Second Generation Surveillance* (Rounds I, II, and III); Ministry of Health and Medical Education of Iran, "Treatment and Medical Education."

[78] Todd et al., "HIV, Hepatitis C, and Hepatitis B Infections"; Sanders-Buell et al., "A Nascent HIV Type 1 Epidemic."

[79] Al-Haddad et al., "HIV Antibodies among Intravenous Drug Users."

[80] UNAIDS, and WHO, *AIDS Epidemic Update 2003;* Groterah, "Drug Abuse and HIV/AIDS."

[81] Bayoumi, *Baseline Survey of Intravenous Drug Users.*

[82] Aceijas et al., "Global Overview"; Tawilah and Tawil, *Visit to Sultane of Oman;* Oman MOH, "HIV Risk among Heroin and Injecting Drug Users."

[83] Egypt Ministry of Health and Population, and National AIDS Program, *HIV/AIDS Biological and Behavioral Surveillance Survey.*

[84] Elrashied, "Prevalence."

[85] Pakistan National AIDS Control Program, *HIV Second Generation Surveillance* (Rounds I, II, and III).

[86] Mishwar, "An Integrated Bio-Behavioral Surveillance Study" (final report).

[87] Fares et al., *Rapport sur l'enquête nationale.*

[88] UNAIDS, "Notes on AIDS in the Middle East and North Africa."

[89] WHO, *The 2004 First National Second Generation HIV/AIDS/STI Sentinel Surveillance Survey.*

[90] Ibid.

[91] Pisani et al., "HIV Surveillance."

[92] Etchepare, "Programme National de Lutte."

[93] McCarthy, Khalid, and El Tigani, "HIV-1 Infection in Juba, Southern Sudan."

[94] Cote et al., "Transactional Sex"; Alary and Lowndes, "The Central Role of Clients."

[95] NSNAC and UNAIDS, *HIV/AIDS Integrated Report South Sudan.*

Status of the HIV epidemic

Table 11.1 summarizes what is known of the current status of the HIV epidemic in MENA countries from the data collected through this synthesis and the epidemiological context. The limitations of the surveillance systems in MENA are manifest in this table. There are only a few examples where there are sufficient data to conclusively determine the status of the epidemic in the different risk groups in a given MENA country.

Table 11.1 Status of the HIV Epidemic in MENA Countries

Country	Concentrated epidemic among IDUs	Concentrated epidemic among MSM	Concentrated epidemic among FSWs	Generalized epidemic
Afghanistan	Possibly (in Kabul) Unknown (out of Kabul)	Unknown	Apparently not	Unlikely
Algeria	Possibly	Unknown	Possibly (southern part of Algeria) Apparently not (rest of country)	Unlikely
Bahrain	Possibly	Unknown	Unknown	Unlikely
Djibouti	Unknown	Unknown	Established	Established
Egypt, Arab Rep. of	Apparently not	Possibly	Apparently not	Unlikely
Iran, Islamic Rep of.	Established	Possibly	Apparently not	Unlikely
Iraq	Apparently not	Unknown	Unknown	Unlikely
Jordan	Apparently not	Unknown	Unknown	Unlikely
Kuwait	Unknown	Unknown	Apparently not	Unlikely
Lebanon	Apparently not	Apparently not	Apparently not	Unlikely
Libya	Possibly	Unknown	Unknown	Unlikely
Morocco	Unknown	Unknown	Apparently not	Unlikely
Oman	Possibly	Unknown	Unknown	Unlikely
Pakistan	Established	Possibly	Apparently not	Unlikely
Qatar	Unknown	Unknown	Unknown	Unlikely
Saudi Arabia	Unknown	Unknown	Unknown	Unlikely
Somalia	Unknown	Unknown	Likely	Possibly in some parts
Sudan	Possibly (North Sudan) Unknown (Southern Sudan)	Possibly (North Sudan) Unknown (Southern Sudan)	Apparently not (North Sudan) Likely (Southern Sudan)	Unlikely (North Sudan) Likely (Southern Sudan)
Syrian Arab Republic	Apparently not	Unknown	Apparently not	Unlikely
Tunisia	Apparently not	Unknown	Apparently not	Unlikely
United Arab Emirates	Unknown	Unknown	Unknown	Unlikely
West Bank and Gaza	Unknown	Unknown	Unknown	Unlikely
Yemen, Rep. of	Unknown	Unknown	Apparently not	Unlikely

Source: Authors.
Note: Established: direct empirical data support this conclusion; Likely: evidence suggests strongly the possibility, but no conclusive, direct, empirical evidence to date; Possibly: fragmented evidence suggests the possibility, but no direct empirical evidence; Apparently not: fragmented evidence suggests that this is not the case; Unlikely: evidence suggests that this is a very remote possibility; Unknown: evidence not available.

Essence of HIV dynamics in MENA

The essence of the HIV dynamics in MENA, with regard to the conceptual framework delineated in chapter 1, is illustrated in figure 11.1. The levels of HIV prevalence, risk behaviors, and biomarkers of risk all indicate that the HIV dynamics are focused in the circle containing priority and bridging populations. The groups of potential sustainable HIV transmission for each MENA country include the priority populations of IDUs, MSM, and possibly FSWs in a few countries. Concentrated epidemics among these groups either have occurred or have the potential to occur as described earlier in figure 1.3b. HIV is not sustainable in the general population in any MENA country, except possibly for Southern Sudan.

In addition to this epidemiologic profile, there is an epidemiologic pattern of randomly distributed exogenous HIV exposures among the nationals of MENA countries, and HIV infections among their sexual partners upon their return. This pattern appears to be dominant in a number of MENA countries where considerable HIV epidemics among priority populations have not occurred.

The conceptual framework describes HIV epidemiology in MENA, but there are still heterogeneities in scale and types of priority groups that drive HIV dynamics across the region. In Djibouti, parts of Somalia, and Southern Sudan, there are concentrated epidemics in commercial sex networks that continue to drive HIV transmission in these localities. The levels of sexual risk behaviors in the commercial sex networks are substantial and the sizes of these networks are significant, leading to a considerable HIV prevalence in the population of as much as a few percentage points. In the rest of the MENA countries, there do not appear to be concentrated HIV epidemics in commercial sex networks and the sizes of these networks appear to be considerably smaller.

Similar heterogeneities apply to the rest of the priority groups. While IDU is large in scale in the Islamic Republic of Iran and Pakistan and continues to be the major driver of the HIV epidemics in these countries, it is likely to be relatively smaller in scale and have a minor role in the HIV epidemics in Djibouti, Somalia, and Sudan. The nature and levels of HIV spread among MSM are the least understood in MENA.

GENERAL FEATURES OF HIV SPREAD IN MENA

HIV infection has already reached all corners of MENA and the vast majority of HIV infections

Figure 11.1 Analytical View of HIV Epidemiology in MENA

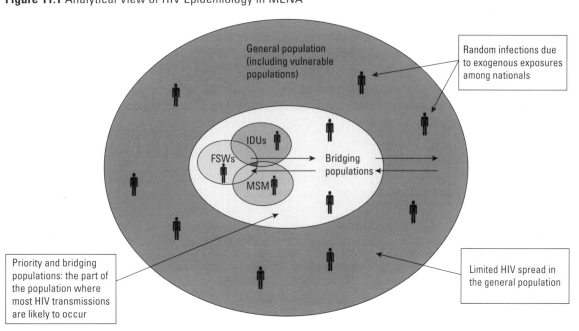

Source: Authors.
Note: The majority of infections are focused in the circle containing priority and bridging populations.

are coming from within the already existing sexual and injecting drug risk networks. MENA countries have made enormous progress in controlling parenteral HIV transmissions due to contaminated blood and poor safety measures. Nonetheless, the region as a whole is failing to control HIV spread along the contours of risk and vulnerability, despite promising recent efforts, such as in the Islamic Republic of Iran and Morocco. Priority populations, including IDUs, MSM, and FSWs, are documented to exist in every country of MENA. With the volume of evidence collected in this synthesis, there is no more room for denial that risk behaviors do exist and indeed are common in MENA.

Number of HIV infections

It is estimated that Sudan has the largest number of HIV infections, about 320,000 to 350,000, which account for roughly 60% of all HIV infections in the broad definition of the MENA region used in this report (chapter 1).[96] The majority of infections in this country appear to be concentrated in Southern Sudan, where the limitations in terms of public health are most severe.[97] HIV prevalence in Southern Sudan is estimated to be up to eight times higher than that in the capital, Khartoum.[98] For the rest of the MENA countries, the estimated number of HIV infections ranges between a few hundred in the small countries to tens of thousands in the larger countries.[99] It is important to note that these estimates have wide confidence margins and are based on limited data. Given the evidence collected in this synthesis, there might be room to conduct a more precise quantitative assessment of the number of HIV infections.

Reported numbers of HIV cases remain small and most HIV infections appear to be occurring in men and in urban areas.[100] However, the number of case notifications has been increasing

in recent years.[101] The large fraction of AIDS cases among newly discovered HIV infections and the short interval from HIV notification to AIDS diagnosis[102] suggest that HIV diagnosis and testing rates are low, and that a large fraction of HIV infections are being missed. The inertia in diagnosing HIV infections may be preventing a prompt response to ongoing or emerging HIV epidemics.

HIV prevalence

HIV prevalence overall continues to be at low levels compared to other regions. The overarching pattern is that of very limited HIV spread in the general population but growing epidemics in priority populations, including IDUs and MSM and, to a lesser extent, FSWs. Although there is a considerable fraction of HIV infections that are being characterized as unknown,[103] these infections possibly reflect the under-reporting of risky behavior due to the perceived adverse consequences that might come with admitting to culturally unacceptable behavior. The epidemic has reached the stages of a generalized epidemic, prevalence greater than 1% among pregnant women, in three countries, and the stages of a concentrated epidemic, prevalence greater than 5% in at least one priority group, in several other countries. The levels of reported sexual and injecting drug risk behaviors are substantial among the majority of the priority populations and are comparable to levels reported in other regions. The levels of proxy biomarkers including sexually transmitted infections (STIs) and HCV are also substantial in these groups. These facts confirm the potential for HIV infection to spread among at least some of the priority populations.

HIV is spreading at different rates among priority populations. Consistent with global patterns,[104] IDU epidemics are the fastest in terms of speed of growth. In Pakistan, HIV prevalence was 0.63% at the end of 2003 at a

[96] UNAIDS, *AIDS Epidemic Update 2007;* SNAP, "Update on the HIV Situation in Sudan;" UNAIDS Country Database 2007, http://www.unaids.org/en/CountryResponses/Countries/default.asp.

[97] Del Viso, "UNDP Supports HIV/AIDS/STD Project"; Mandal, Purdin, and McGinn "A Study of Health Facilities."

[98] SNAP, *HIV/AIDS/STIs Prevalence.*

[99] UNAIDS, *AIDS Epidemic Update 2007;* UNAIDS Country Database 2007, http://www.unaids.org/en/CountryResponses/Countries/default.asp.

[100] WHO/EMRO Regional Database on HIV/AIDS.

[101] WHO/EMRO Regional Database on HIV/AIDS; Madani et al., "Epidemiology of the Human Immunodeficiency Virus."

[102] WHO/EMRO Regional Database on HIV/AIDS; Chemtob and Srour, "Epidemiology of HIV Infection among Israeli Arabs."

[103] UNAIDS and WHO, *AIDS Epidemic Update 2006.*

[104] Piyasirisilp et al., "A Recent Outbreak"; Nguyen et al., "Genetic Analysis."

site in Karachi,[105] but the prevalence increased to 23% at this site by mid-2004.[106] This pattern has been witnessed in a few other MENA countries. However, it is also possible for HIV epidemics among MSM to grow rapidly as well. There are multiple indications that the epidemic among MSM is growing in the region. In a number of MENA countries, HIV prevalence among MSM could already be at considerable levels despite limited HIV prevalence among IDUs. MSM, however, are the most hidden and the hardest-to-reach priority group through surveillance and interventions.

Apart from the notable exceptions of Djibouti, Somalia, and Southern Sudan, HIV prevalence is at relatively low levels among commercial sex networks. The prevalence among FSWs appears to grow slowly in MENA and may not reach the high levels it reached in other regions. Given the prominent role of commercial sex networks in the epidemics of Djibouti, Somalia, and Sudan, interventions with FSWs and their clients might be the best method to control HIV spread in this part of MENA.[107]

No general population HIV epidemic in MENA

There is no evidence of an HIV epidemic in the general population in any of the MENA countries. Available HIV prevalence and behavioral data suggest that HIV infectious spread is not self-sustainable in the general population of MENA countries, except possibly for Southern Sudan. Low levels of STI prevalence including human papillomavirus (HPV) and herpes simplex virus 2 (HSV-2) in the general population support this inference. The fact that HIV is more likely to be sustainable and focused in priority populations does not imply that the general population is immune against HIV spread. HIV will find its way into the general population through transmission chains originating at the high-risk cores, although these chains are not self-sustainable and will eventually die out.

Protective factors

Several protective factors have slowed and limited HIV transmissions in MENA relative to other regions. Male circumcision is almost universally practiced in MENA and is associated with a 60% efficacy against HIV infection for men.[108] Male circumcision can also substantially slow the expansion of HIV in a population, thereby providing a window of opportunity to intervene against an epidemic before it reaches higher levels.[109]

The cultural traditions in MENA are influenced by Islamic teachings. Islam promotes a line of behavior that is consonant with several themes of HIV/AIDS prevention including prohibitions against premarital and extramarital sex[110]; prohibitions against alcohol consumption because of alcohol's strong association with higher risk behavior, paying for sex, and misuse of protective measures such as condoms[111]; closed sexual networks of monogamous or polygamous marriages[112]; prohibition against intercourse during menstruation[113]; and possibly ritual washing and penile and vaginal hygiene following intercourse.[114] Being a Muslim has been repeatedly associated with lower risk behavior,[115] and lower HIV prevalence,[116] in Muslim-majority countries as well as in Muslim minorities in predominantly non-Muslim nations.[117] Islamic religiosity was found in one study not to be associated with lower use of condoms for

[105] Altaf et al., "Harm Reduction among Injection Drug Users."
[106] Bokhari et al., "HIV Risk in Karachi and Lahore, Pakistan."
[107] Boily, Lowndes, and Alary, "The Impact of HIV Epidemic Phases"; Lowndes et al., "Interventions among Male Clients."

[108] Auvert et al., "Randomized, Controlled Intervention Trial"; Bailey et al., "Male Circumcision"; Gray et al., "Male Circumcision."
[109] Alsallaq et al., "Quantitative Assessment."
[110] Pickthall, The Meaning of the Glorious Qur'an.
[111] Mbulaiteye et al., "Alcohol and HIV"; Kaljee et al., "Alcohol Use and HIV Risk Behaviors"; Fisher, Bang, and Kapiga, "The Association between HIV Infection and Alcohol Use."
[112] Huff, "Male Circumcision: Cutting the Risk?"
[113] Elharti et al., "Some Characteristics."
[114] Lerman and Liao, "Neonatal Circumcision."
[115] Bailey, Neema, and Othieno, "Sexual Behaviors"; Shirazi and Morowatisharifabad, "Religiosity and Determinants of Safe Sex"; Rakwar et al., "Cofactors for the Acquisition of HIV-1"; Isiugo-Abanihe, "Extramarital Relations"; Biaya, "Les plaisirs de la ville"; Gilbert, "The Influence of Islam on AIDS."
[116] Gray, "HIV and Islam"; Mbulaiteye et al., "Alcohol and HIV"; Rakwar et al., "Cofactors for the Acquisition of HIV-1"; Kengeya-Kayondo et al., "Incidence of HIV-1 Infection in Adults"; Malamba et al., "Risk Factors for HIV-1 Infection in Adults"; Gray et al., "Male Circumcision and HIV"; Bwayo et al., "Human Immunodeficiency Virus Infection"; Nunn et al., "Risk Factors for HIV-1 Infection"; Abebe et al., "HIV Prevalence"; Drain et al., "Correlates of National HIV Seroprevalence"; Meda et al., "Low and Stable HIV Infection Rates."
[117] Gray, "HIV and Islam"; Kagee et al., "HIV Prevalence."

those who are sexually active.[118] Islamic cultural traditions have been cited as a protective factor even after adjustment for male circumcision.[119]

While Islamic values provide protection against HIV/AIDS,[120] several studies suggest that adherence to Islamic codes of conduct is not perfect and that Muslims do engage in sexual and injecting drug activities not sanctioned in Islam.[121] What is promoted religiously is not necessarily what is put into practice.[122] Though the social fabric of MENA societies is heavily influenced by Islamic traditions, the region is also experiencing a sociocultural transition that is leading to more tolerance and acceptance of behaviors such as premarital sex and extramarital sex.[123] The evidence for recent increases in risky behavior points to this direction (see youth section in chapter 9). Counting only on the "cultural immunity" of religious and traditional mores[124] is not enough to prevent the worst of the HIV epidemic.

Overlap of risky behaviors

A hallmark of risky behavior in MENA is the intersection of priority groups, with abundant evidence of overlapping risk factors.[125] The social, sexual, and injecting drug networks of priority groups overlap and intersect, allowing HIV to easily propagate between different priority populations (figure 11.2). HIV is spreading from one priority group to another. In the Islamic Republic of Iran and Pakistan, the epidemic among MSM appears to have been sparked by ample overlap with injecting drug practices.[126] If HIV establishes itself in one priority population, it can easily find ways to spread through the overlapping risks to other priority populations.

[118] Gilbert, "The Influence of Islam."

[119] Hargrove, "Migration, Mines and Mores."

[120] Ridanovic, "AIDS and Islam."

[121] Gilbert, "The Influence of Islam"; Gibney et al., "Behavioural Risk Factors"; Kagimu et al., "Evaluation of the Effectiveness."

[122] Ridanovic, "AIDS and Islam."

[123] Busulwa, "HIV/AIDS Situation Analysis Study."

[124] Khawaja et al., "HIV/AIDS and Its Risk Factors in Pakistan."

[125] UNAIDS, "Fact Sheet on Drug Use."

[126] Pakistan National AIDS Control Program, *HIV Second Generation Surveillance* (Rounds I, II, and III); Eftekhar et al., "Bio-Behavioural Survey on HIV."

Figure 11.2 A Schematic Diagram of the Overlap between Priority Populations in MENA

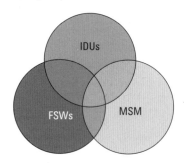

Source: Authors.

Risk network structures are not well understood

Network structures among priority populations, and even the general population, appear to be complex and intricate and are not yet well understood. Some of the injecting drug and sexual networks appear to be sparse, consisting of many subcomponents that are loosely connected to each other. Each of these components is small and tightly knit, such as possibly among IDUs in Lebanon.[127] Figure 10.3a illustrates this kind of network. Networks of this nature are not conducive to substantial HIV spread because the infection finds many obstacles in propagating from one subcomponent to another. It is not yet determined whether the sparse nature of some network structures has contributed to the limited HIV prevalence in MENA.

Vulnerability of spouses and other regular sexual partners

Ample evidence documents men acquiring the infection through high-risk practices including IDU and sexual contacts with FSWs or other males, and then passing the infection to their wives. Matrimony, rather than sexual or injecting risk behavior, is the leading risk factor for HIV infection among women in MENA. Sexual partners of priority populations form a key group at risk of exposure to HIV, but they appear to rarely engage in risky behavior or pass the infection further. Ninety-seven percent of HIV-positive women in Saudi Arabia, who

[127] Mishwar, "An Integrated Bio-Behavioral Surveillance Study" (midterm and final report).

acquired the infection sexually, acquired the infection from their husbands.[128] Seventy-six percent of HIV-positive women in the Islamic Republic of Iran acquired the infection from their husbands, who were predominantly IDUs.[129] HIV infections are repeatedly found among pregnant women with no identifiable risk behaviors, suggesting that the risk factor is heterosexual sex with the spouse.[130] Prevention efforts in the region need to address this vulnerability.

Settings of vulnerability

A large fraction of the MENA population belongs to one or another of several vulnerable groups including prisoners, youth, and mobile populations. The socioeconomic context that is leading to risky behavior includes poverty, unemployment, social disruption, gender roles and expectations, sexual exploitation, and inadequate social and health resources.[131] Socioeconomic disparities, large-scale population mobility, and political instability are contributing to increased vulnerability. Complex emergencies are prevalent in the region, such as in Afghanistan, Iraq, Lebanon, Somalia, Sudan, and the West Bank and Gaza.[132] Marginalization of priority groups is contributing to the vulnerability of these groups to HIV infection.[133]

HIV knowledge, attitudes, and practices

Though basic knowledge of HIV/AIDS is high in MENA, low levels of comprehensive knowledge of HIV/AIDS, and high levels of misconceptions, stigma, and discrimination, continue to plague MENA populations. Use of protective measures such as condoms is limited and condoms are not always widely or easily accessible. Most MENA populations perceive themselves not at risk of HIV infection even when they practice high-risk behaviors. There is a perception that minimizing apparent risk behaviors is the best protection against HIV, but at a cost of ignoring

safe sex practices. The majority of at-risk heterosexual and homosexual sex acts in MENA are unprotected against HIV. The concept that every sex act with any partner can carry some risk of HIV infection still eludes the majority of the population. The fact that a large fraction of HIV infections are being transmitted within socially acceptable partnerships, such as from a husband to his wife, is still beyond public comprehension.

FUTURE HIV EXPANSION IN MENA

The levels of risky behavior and biomarkers of risk among many priority populations are high and are conducive to substantial HIV epidemics. The fact that HIV prevalence continues to be at zero or low prevalence levels in many priority populations should not be mistaken for a lack of HIV epidemic potential. HIV may simply not yet have had the opportunity to be introduced into some of these groups. Some of the priority groups in MENA tend to be quite isolated, limiting the probability of virus introduction.

Even when the virus is introduced into a priority population at higher risk of HIV, it may take many years before HIV starts to appreciably expand. Figure 11.3 displays a simulated epidemic among an MSM community of 1,000 persons. Though the virus was introduced into the population in the year 2000, it did not start appreciable growth until a decade later. The low HIV transmission probability per coital act,[134] long duration of latent infection, and slow disease progression[135] limit the expansion of HIV spread initially, but once HIV prevalence becomes appreciable, HIV incidence and therefore prevalence can increase rapidly.

Indeed, this pattern of emerging epidemics in priority populations appears to be occurring at the moment in at least a few MENA countries. The best recent example to this end is Pakistan, where exogenous exposures dominated the epidemiological profile for two decades, but then rapidly rising epidemics emerged among IDUs and, to some extent, among MSM.[136]

[128] Alrajhi, Halim, and Al-Abdely, "Mode of Transmission of HIV-1."

[129] Ramezani, Mohraz, and Gachkar, "Epidemiologic Situation"; Burrows, Wodak, and WHO, *Harm Reduction in Iran.*

[130] Aidaoui, Bouzbid, and Laouar, "Seroprevalence of HIV Infection."

[131] World Bank, "Mapping and Situation Assessment."

[132] Salama and Dondero, "HIV Surveillance in Complex Emergencies."

[133] Tiouiri et al., "Study of Psychosocial Factors."

[134] Wawer et al., "Rates of HIV-1 Transmission per Coital Act."

[135] Mellors et al., "Prognosis in HIV-1 Infection."

[136] Pakistan National AIDS Control Program, *HIV Second Generation Surveillance (Rounds I, II, and III)..*

Figure 11.3 Simulation of a Typical HIV Epidemic among an MSM Population

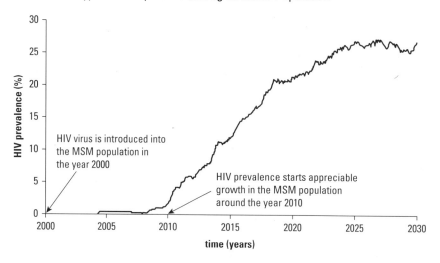

Source: Abu-Raddad 2009.
Note: Simulation produced using a stochastic compartmental model.

HIV prevalence among some IDU groups continues to be at low levels despite reported high-risk behaviors and high HCV prevalence. Therefore, it is likely that we will see further HIV spread and possibly explosive epidemics among IDUs in at least a few MENA countries. HIV epidemic expansion among MSM is a real possibility over the next few years in MENA considering the high levels of risky behavior. Although it does not appear that there is substantial HIV epidemic potential among FSWs in most MENA countries, commercial sex networks are much larger than IDU and MSM networks,[137] and there could be a considerable rise in the number of HIV infections if HIV establishes itself in some commercial sex networks or in subgroups of FSWs, such as those who inject drugs.

It is unlikely that MENA will experience a sustainable or a substantial HIV epidemic in the general population in the next decade, if ever. However, the region could be poised to see a rise in the number women in the general population who are infected with HIV largely due to the wave of HIV transmissions moving from priority populations and bridging populations to spouses of partners involved in these networks. Considering the relatively high probability of vertical and breastfeeding HIV transmission

from a mother to her child in the absence of HIV treatment,[138] the region may also be destined to see a rise in easily preventable HIV infections among children, as the HIV disease burden moves further to women.

Though the prevalence of drug injection is in the intermediate to high range at 0.2%,[139] it seems not as likely that drug injection alone will be the major driver of a substantial HIV epidemic at the level of the whole population in any MENA country. The prevalence of male same-sex practices, at a few percentage points, is consistent with global levels.[140] Therefore, it also seems unlikely that male same-sex contacts alone, within MSM networks as well as beyond these networks, will be the major driver of a large epidemic at the whole population level in a manner that is distinct from other regions.

Prevalence of sex work among women and the fraction of men who visit sex workers appear to be on the lower side of the global range.[141] Furthermore, the near universal coverage of male circumcision and the apparently lower risk behaviors in commercial sex networks

[137] Blanchard, Khan, and Bokhari, "Variations in the Population."

[138] Coutsoudis et al., "Late Postnatal Transmission"; Connor et al., "Reduction of Maternal-Infant Transmission."

[139] Aceijas et al., "Global Overview"; Aceijas et al., "Estimates of Injecting Drug Users."

[140] McFarland and Caceres, "HIV Surveillance"; W. McFarland, personal communication; UNAIDS, Epidemiological Software and Tools.

[141] Vandepitte et al., "Estimates of the Number of Female Sex Workers."

may prevent concentrated HIV epidemics among FSWs from materializing for at least a decade, if ever (apart from Djibouti, Somalia, and Sudan). Hence, it seems also unlikely that commercial sex networks alone will be the major driver of a large epidemic at the whole population level, except again for Djibouti, Somalia, and Sudan.

Considering all of the above, it is unlikely that the HIV epidemic in MENA will take a course similar to that in sub-Saharan Africa if the existing social and epidemiological context in the region remains largely the same. At most, the region may face up to few percentage points prevalence in several of its countries. This would still imply an immense disease burden and subsequent economic burden in a region that is mostly unprepared for such an epidemic.

A key unknown in the understanding of the epidemiology of HIV in MENA is that of the levels of recent increases, and future trends, in risky behavior. If the increases in risky behavior are substantial, this could put some aspects of this analytical view of the dynamics in question. The trajectory of the HIV epidemic may be different and we may observe somewhat considerable HIV epidemics in some MENA populations. Studying the levels of risky behavior and STI incidence among youth, such as using multicenter cohort studies, should be considered by scientific researchers in MENA.

The analytical insights drawn here from a synthesis of thousands of studies and data sources indicate that there is no escape from the necessity of developing robust surveillance systems to monitor HIV spread among priority populations. Effective and repeated surveillance of priority populations, particularly among IDUs and MSM, is key in MENA countries to definitively conclude whether HIV spread is indeed limited in priority populations, and to detect emerging epidemics among these groups at an early stage. This would offer a window of opportunity for targeted prevention at an early phase of an epidemic. Monitoring recent infections and examining the nature of exposures could also be useful in detecting emerging epidemic chains of transmission within MENA populations.

BIBLIOGRAPHY

Abebe, Y., A. Schaap, G. Mamo, A. Negussie, B. Darimo, D. Wolday, and E. J. Sanders. 2003. "HIV Prevalence in 72,000 Urban and Rural Male Army Recruits, Ethiopia." *AIDS* 17: 1835–40.

Abu-Raddad, L. J. 2009. "A Model for HIV Infectious Spread in an MSM Population in the Middle East and North Africa." Ongoing modeling work, Weill Cornell Medical College, Doha, Qatar.

Aceijas, C., S. R. Friedman, H. L. Cooper, L. Wiessing, G. V. Stimson, and M. Hickman. 2006. "Estimates of Injecting Drug Users at the National and Local Level in Developing and Transitional Countries, and Gender and Age Distribution." *Sex Transm Infect* 82 Suppl 3: iii10–17.

Aceijas, C., G. V. Stimson, M. Hickman, and T. Rhodes. 2004. "Global Overview of Injecting Drug Use and HIV Infection among Injecting Drug Users." *AIDS* 18: 2295–303.

Afshar, P. Unknown. "Health and Prison." Director General of Health, Office of Iran Prisons Organization.

Aghanashinikar, P. N., S. H. al-Dhahry, H. A. al-Marhuby, M. R. Buhl, A. S. Daar, and M. K. Al-Hasani. 1992. "Prevalence of Hepatitis B, Hepatitis Delta, and Human Immunodeficiency Virus Infections in Omani Patients with Renal Diseases." *Transplant Proc* 24: 1913–14.

Aidaoui, M., S. Bouzbid, and M. Laouar. 2008. "Seroprevalence of HIV Infection in Pregnant Women in the Annaba Region (Algeria)." *Rev Epidemiol Sante Publique* 56: 261–66.

Al Katheeb, M. S., M. S. Tarawneh, and A. S. Awidi. 1988. "Antibodies to HIV in Jordanian Blood Donors and Patients with Congenital Bleeding Disorders." IV International Conference on AIDS, Stockholm, abstract 5003.

Al Rasheed, A. M., D. Fairclough, Abu Al Sand, and A. O. Osoba. 1988. "Screening for HIV Antibodies among Blood Donors at Riadh Armed Forces Hospital." VI International Conference on AIDS, Stockholm, abstract 5001.

Alary, M., and C. M. Lowndes. 2004. "The Central Role of Clients of Female Sex Workers in the Dynamics of Heterosexual HIV Transmission in Sub-Saharan Africa." *AIDS* 18: 945–47.

Al-Fouzan, A., and N. Al-Mutairi. 2004. "Overview of Incidence of Sexually Transmitted Diseases in Kuwait." *Clin Dermatol* 22: 509–12.

Al-Haddad, M. K., A. S. Khashaba, B. Z. Baig, and S. Khalfan. 1994. "HIV Antibodies among Intravenous Drug Users in Bahrain." *J Commun Dis* 26: 127–32.

Al-Mahroos, F. T., and A. Ebrahim. 1995. "Prevalence of Hepatitis B, Hepatitis C and Human Immune Deficiency Virus Markers among Patients with Hereditary Haemolytic Anaemias." *Ann Trop Paediatr* 15: 121–28.

Al-Nozha, M. M., A. R. Al-Frayh, M. Al-Nasser, and S. Ramia. 1995. "Horizontal versus Vertical Transmission of Human Immunodeficiency Virus Type 1 (HIV-1): Experience from Southwestern Saudi Arabia." *Trop Geogr Med* 47: 293–95.

Alrajhi, A. A. 2004. "Human Immunodeficiency Virus in Saudi Arabia." *Saudi Med J 25*: 1559–63.

Alrajhi, A. A., M. A. Halim, and H. M. Al-Abdely. 2004. "Mode of Transmission of HIV-1 in Saudi Arabia." *AIDS* 18: 1478–80.

Alsallaq, R. A., B. Cash, H. A. Weiss, I. M. Longini, S. B. Omer, M. J. Wawer, R. H. Gray, and L. J. Abu-Raddad. 2008. "Quantitative Assessment of the Role of Male Circumcision in HIV Epidemiology at the Population Level." *Epidemics*.

Altaf, A., A. Memon, N. Rehman, and S. Shah. 2004. "Harm Reduction among Injection Drug Users in Karachi, Pakistan." International AIDS Conference 2004, Bangkok, abstract WePeC5992.

Anonymous. 1997. "Commercially Motivated Renal Transplantation: Results in 540 Patients Transplanted in India: The Living Non-Related Renal Transplant Study Group." *Clin Transplant* 11: 536–44.

Arbesser, C., H. Bashiribod, and W. Sixl. 1987. "Serological Examinations of HIV-I in Iran." *J Hyg Epidemiol Microbiol Immunol* 31: 504–5.

Auvert, B., D. Taljaard, E. Lagarde, J. Sobngwi-Tambekou, R. Sitta, and A. Puren. 2005. "Randomized, Controlled Intervention Trial of Male Circumcision for Reduction of HIV Infection Risk: The ANRS 1265 Trial." *PLoS Med* 2: e298.

Baidy, Lo B., M. Adimorty, C. Fatimata, and S. Amadou. 1993. "Surveillance of HIV Seroprevalence in Mauritania." *Bull Soc Pathol Exot* 86: 133–35.

Bailey, R. C., S. Moses, C. B. Parker, K. Agot, I. Maclean, J. N. Krieger, C. F. M. Williams, R. T. Campbell, and J. O. Ndinya-Achola. 2007. "Male Circumcision for HIV Prevention in Young Men in Kisumu, Kenya: A Randomised Controlled Trial." *Lancet* 369: 643–56.

Bailey, R. C., S. Neema, and R. Othieno. 1999. "Sexual Behaviors and Other HIV Risk Factors in Circumcised and Uncircumcised Men in Uganda." *J Acquir Immune Defic Syndr* 22: 294–301.

Baqi, S., N. Kayani, and J. A. Khan. 1999. "Epidemiology and Clinical Profile of HIV/AIDS in Pakistan." *Trop Doct 29*: 144–48.

Bayoumi, A. 2005. *Baseline Survey of Intravenous Drug Users (IDUs) in Karthoum State (KS): Cross-Sectional and Case-Control Study*. Assignment Report, Inter Agency Technical Committee, Sudan National AIDS Programme, Federal Ministry of Health, Khartoum, Sudan.

Biaya, T. K. 2001. "Les plaisirs de la ville: Masculinité, sexualité et féminité à Dakar (1997–2000)." *African Studies Review*: 71–85.

Blanchard, J. F., A. Khan, and A. Bokhari. 2008. "Variations in the Population Size, Distribution and Client Volume among Female Sex Workers in Seven Cities of Pakistan." *Sex Transm Infect* 84 Suppl 2: ii24–27.

Boily, M. C., C. Lowndes, and M. Alary. 2002. "The Impact of HIV Epidemic Phases on the Effectiveness of Core Group Interventions: Insights from Mathematical Models." *Sex Transm Infect* 78 Suppl 1: i78–90.

Bokhari, A., N. M. Nizamani, D. J. Jackson, N. E. Rehan, M. Rahman, R. Muzaffar, S. Mansoor, H. Raza,

K. Qayum, P. Girault, E. Pisani, and I. Thaver. 2007. "HIV Risk in Karachi and Lahore, Pakistan: An Emerging Epidemic in Injecting and Commercial Sex Networks." *Int J STD AIDS* 18: 486–92.

Burans, J. P., E. Fox, M. A. Omar, A. H. Farah, S. Abbass, S. Yusef, A. Guled, M. Mansour, R. Abu-Elyazeed, and J. N. Woody. 1990. "HIV Infection Surveillance in Mogadishu, Somalia." *East Afr Med J* 67: 466–72.

Burans, J. P., M. McCarthy, S. M. el Tayeb, A. el Tigani, J. George, R. Abu-Elyazeed, and J. N. Woody. 1990. "Serosurvey of Prevalence of Human Immuno-deficiency Virus amongst High Risk Groups in Port Sudan, Sudan." *East Afr Med J* 67: 650–55.

Burrows, D., A. Wodak, and WHO (World Health Organization). 2005. *Harm Reduction in Iran: Issues in National Scale-Up*.

Busulwa, R. 2003. "HIV/AIDS Situation Analysis Study." Conducted in Hodeidah, Taiz and Hadhramut, Republic of Yemen.

Bwayo, J., F. Plummer, M. Omari, A. Mutere, S. Moses, J. Ndinya-Achola, P. Velentgas, and J. Kreiss. 1994. "Human Immunodeficiency Virus Infection in Long-Distance Truck Drivers in East Africa." *Arch Intern Med* 154: 1391–96.

Chemtob, D., and S. F. Srour. 2005. "Epidemiology of HIV Infection among Israeli Arabs." *Public Health* 119: 138–43.

Connor, E. M., R. S. Sperling, R. Gelber, P. Kiselev, G. Scott, M. J. O'Sullivan, R. VanDyke, M. Bey, W. Shearer, R. L. Jacobson, et al. 1994. "Reduction of Maternal-Infant Transmission of Human Immuno-deficiency Virus Type 1 with Zidovudine Treatment." Pediatric AIDS Clinical Trials Group Protocol 076 Study Group. *N Engl J Med* 331: 1173–80.

Constantine, N. T., M. F. Sheba, D. M. Watts, Z. Farid, and M. Kamal. 1990. "HIV Infection in Egypt: A Two and a Half Year Surveillance." *J Trop Med Hyg* 93: 146–50.

Cote, A. M., F. Sobela, A. Dzokoto, K. Nzambi, C. Asamoah-Adu, A. C. Labbe, B. Masse, J. Mensah, E. Frost, and J. Pepin. 2004. "Transactional Sex Is the Driving Force in the Dynamics of HIV in Accra, Ghana." *AIDS* 18: 917–25.

Coutsoudis, A., F. Dabis, W. Fawzi, P. Gaillard, G. Haverkamp, D. R. Harris, J. B. Jackson, V. Leroy, N. Meda, P. Msellati, M. L. Newell, R. Nsuati, J. S. Read, and S. Wiktor. 2004. "Late Postnatal Transmission of HIV-1 in Breast-Fed Children: An Individual Patient Data Meta-Analysis." *J Infect Dis* 189: 2154–66.

Couzineau, B., J. Bouloumie, P. Hovette, and R. Laroche. 1991. "Prevalence of Infection by the Human Immunodeficiency Virus (HIV) in a Target Population in the Republic of Djibouti." *Med Trop* (Mars) 51: 485–86.

Dan, M., M. Rock, and S. Bar-Shany. 1989. "Prevalence of Antibodies to Human Immunodeficiency Virus among Intravenous Drug Users in Israel—Association with Travel Abroad." *Int J Epidemiol* 18: 239–41.

Del Viso, N. 1997. "UNDP Supports HIV/AIDS/STD Project for War-Torn South Sudan—A Special Report." *UNDP News* 21.

Demiroz, P., H. Irmak, A. Sengul, H. A. Ceviz, and F. Kocabalkan. 1989. "HIV Infections among Turkish Citizens Who Have Lived in Foreign Countries." *Mikrobiyol Bul* 23: 203–9.

Djibouti Ministère de La Santé, and Association Internationale de Développement. 2002. *Epidémie a VIH/SIDA/IST en République de Djibouti; Tome I: Analyse de la Situation et Analyse de la Réponse Nationale.* Décembre.

Drain, P. K., J. S. Smith, J. P. Hughes, D. T. Halperin, and K. K. Holmes. 2004. "Correlates of National HIV Seroprevalence: An Ecologic Analysis of 122 Developing Countries." *J Acquir Immune Defic Syndr* 35: 407–20.

Egypt Ministry of Health and Population, and National AIDS Program. 2006. *HIV/AIDS Biological and Behavioral Surveillance Survey.* Summary report.

El-Ghazzawi, E., G. Hunsmann, and J. Schneider. 1987. "Low Prevalence of Antibodies to HIV-1 and HTLV-I in Alexandria, Egypt." *AIDS Forsch* 2: 639.

Elharti, E., M. Alami, H. Khattabi, A. Bennani, A. Zidouh, A. Benjouad, and R. El Aouad. 2002. "Some Characteristics of the HIV Epidemic in Morocco." *East Mediterr Health J* 8: 819–25.

El-Hazmi, M. A., and S. Ramia. 1989. "Frequencies of Hepatitis B, Delta and Human Immune Deficiency Virus Markers in Multitransfused Saudi Patients with Thalassaemia and Sickle-Cell Disease." *J Trop Med Hyg* 92: 1–5.

Elrashied, S. 2006. "Prevalence, Knowledge and Related Risky Sexual Behaviours of HIV/AIDS among Receptive Men Who Have Sex with Men (MSM) in Khartoum State, Sudan, 2005." XVI International AIDS Conference, Toronto, August 13–18, abstract TUPE0509.

Etchepare, M. 2001. "Programme National de Lutte contre le SIDA et les MST." Draft report, World Bank Mission for Health Project Strategy Development, Djibouti.

Fares, G., et al. 2004. *Rapport sur l'enquête nationale de sero-surveillance sentinelle du VIH et de la syphilis en Algérie en 2004.* Ministère de la Santé de la population et de la reforme hospitalière, Alger, Décembre.

Farhoudi, B., A. Montevalian, M. Motamedi, M. M. Khameneh, M. Mohraz, M. Rassolinejad, S. Jafari, P. Afshar, I. Esmaili, and L. Mohseni. 2003. "Human Immunodeficiency Virus and HIV-Associated Tuberculosis Infection and Their Risk Factors in Injecting Drug Users in Prison in Iran."

Faris, R., and A. Shouman. 1994. "Study of the Knowledge, Attitude of Egyptian Health Care Workers towards Occupational HIV Infection." *J Egypt Public Health Assoc* 69: 115–28.

Fisher, J. C., H. Bang, and S. H. Kapiga. 2007. "The Association between HIV Infection and Alcohol Use: A Systematic Review and Meta-Analysis of African Studies." *Sex Transm Dis* 34: 856–63.

Fox, E., J. P. Burans, M. A. Omar, A. H. Farah, A. Guled, S. Yusef, J. C. Morrill, and J. N. Woody. 1989. "AIDS: The Situation in Mogadishu during Spring 1987." *J Egypt Public Health Assoc* 64: 135–43.

Giasuddin, A. S., M. M. Ziu, A. Abusadra, and A. Gamati. 1988. "Failure to Find Antibody to Human Immunodeficiency Virus Type I in Libya." *J Infect* 17: 192–93.

Gibney, L., P. Choudhury, Z. Khawaja, M. Sarker, and S. H. Vermund. 1999. "Behavioural Risk Factors for HIV/AIDS in a Low-HIV Prevalence Muslim Nation: Bangladesh." *Int J STD AIDS* 10: 186–94.

Gilbert, S. S. 2008. "The Influence of Islam on AIDS Prevention among Senegalese University Students." *AIDS Educ Prev* 20: 399–407.

"Global Update: Morocco." 1993. *AIDSlink* (23): 14.

Grassly, N. C., G. P. Garnett, B. Schwartlander, S. Gregson, and R. M. Anderson. 2001. "The Effectiveness of HIV Prevention and the Epidemiological Context." *Bull World Health Organ* 79: 1121–32.

Gray, P. B. 2004. "HIV and Islam: Is HIV Prevalence Lower among Muslims?" *Soc Sci Med* 58: 1751–56.

Gray, R. H., N. Kiwanuka, T. C. Quinn, N. K. Sewankambo, D. Serwadda, F. W. Mangen, T. Lutalo, F. Nalugoda, R. Kelly, M. Meehan, M. Z. Chen, C. Li, and M. J. Wawer. 2000. "Male Circumcision and HIV Acquisition and Transmission: Cohort Studies in Rakai, Uganda. Rakai Project Team." *AIDS* 14: 2371–81.

Groterah, A. 2002. "Drug Abuse and HIV/AIDS in the Middle East and North Africa: A Situation Assessment." UNODC, internal document.

Harfi, H. A., and B. M. Fakhry. 1986. "Acquired Immunodeficiency Syndrome in Saudi Arabia: The American-Saudi Connection." *JAMA* 255: 383–84.

Hargrove, J. 2007. "Migration, Mines and Mores: The HIV Epidemic in Southern Africa." Inaugural Address, Stellenbosch University.

Hashim, M. S., M. A. Salih, A. A. el Hag, Z. A. Karrar, E. M. Osman, F. S. el-Shiekh, I. A. el Tilib, and N. E. Attala. 1997. "AIDS and HIV Infection in Sudanese Children: A Clinical and Epidemiological Study." *AIDS Patient Care STDS* 11: 331–37.

Hawkes, S., G. J. Hart, A. M. Johnson, C. Shergold, E. Ross, K. M. Herbert, P. Mortimer, J. V. Parry, and D. Mabey. 1994. "Risk Behaviour and HIV Prevalence in International Travellers." *AIDS* 8: 247–52.

Huff, B. 2000. "Male Circumcision: Cutting the Risk?" American Foundation for AIDS Research, August.

Iqbal, J., and N. Rehan. 1996. "Sero-Prevalence of HIV: Six Years' Experience at Shaikh Zayed Hospital, Lahore." *J Pak Med Assoc* 46: 255–58.

Iran Center for Disease Management. Unknown. *Country Report on UNGASS Declaration of Commitment.* Office of Deputy Minister of Health in Health Affairs, Islamic Republic of Iran, in cooperation with UNAIDS Iran and the Iranian Center for AIDS Research.

———. 2004. *HIV/AIDS and STIs Surveillance Report.* Ministry of Health and Medical Education, Tehran.

Isiugo-Abanihe, U. C. 1994. "Extramarital Relations and Perceptions of HIV/AIDS in Nigeria." *Health Transit Rev* 4: 111–25.

Ismail, S. O., H. J. Ahmed, L. Grillner, B. Hederstedt, A. Issa, and S. M. Bygdeman. 1990. "Sexually Transmitted Diseases in Men in Mogadishu, Somalia." *Int J STD AIDS* 1: 102–6.

Jahani, M. R., S. M. Alavian, H. Shirzad, A. Kabir, and B. Hajarizadeh. 2005. "Distribution and Risk Factors of Hepatitis B, Hepatitis C, and HIV Infection in a Female Population with 'Illegal Social Behaviour.'" *Sex Transm Infect* 81: 185.

Jama, H., L. Grillner, G. Biberfeld, S. Osman, A. Isse, M. Abdirahman, and S. Bygdeman. 1987. "Sexually Transmitted Viral Infections in Various Population Groups in Mogadishu, Somalia." *Genitourin Med* 63: 329–32.

Jemni, L., S. Bahri, M. Saadi, A. Letaif, M. Dhidah, H. Lahdhiri, and S. Bouchoucha. 1991. "AIDS and Tuberculosis in Central Tunisia." *Tunis Med* 69: 349–52.

Jenkins, C., and D. A. Robalino. 2003. "HIV in the Middle East and North Africa: The Cost of Inaction." Orientations in Development Series, World Bank.

Jurjus, A. R., J. Kahhaleh, National AIDS Program, and WHO/EMRO (World Health Organization/Eastern Mediterranean Regional Office). 2004. "Knowledge, Attitudes, Beliefs, and Practices of the Lebanese concerning HIV/AIDS." Beirut, Lebanon.

Kagee, A., Y. Toefy, L. Simbayi, and S. Kalichman. 2005. "HIV Prevalence in Three Predominantly Muslim Residential Areas in the Cape Town Metropole." *S Afr Med J* 95: 512–16.

Kagimu, M., E. Marum, F. Wabwire-Mangen, N. Nakyanjo, Y. Walakira, and J. Hogle. 1998. "Evaluation of the Effectiveness of AIDS Health Education Interventions in the Muslim Community in Uganda." *AIDS Educ Prev* 10: 215–28.

Kalaajieh, W. K. 2000. "Epidemiology of Human Immunodeficiency Virus and Acquired Immuno-deficiency Syndrome in Lebanon from 1984 through 1998." *Int J Infect Dis* 4: 209–13.

Kaljee, L. M., B. L. Genberg, T. T. Minh, L. H. Tho, L. T. Thoa, and B. Stanton. 2005. "Alcohol Use and HIV Risk Behaviors among Rural Adolescents in Khanh Hoa Province Viet Nam." *Health Educ Res* 20: 71–80.

Kandela, P. 1993. "Arab Nations: Attitudes to AIDS." *Lancet* 341: 884–85.

Kayani, N., A. Sheikh, A. Khan, C. Mithani, and M. Khurshid. 1994. "A View of HIV-I Infection in Karachi." *J Pak Med Assoc* 44: 8–11.

Kengeya-Kayondo, J. F., A. Kamali, A. J. Nunn, A. Ruberantwari, H. U. Wagner, and D. W. Mulder. 1996. "Incidence of HIV-I Infection in Adults and Socio-Demographic Characteristics of Seroconverters in a Rural Population in Uganda: 1990–1994." *Int J Epidemiol* 25: 1077–82.

Khan, S., M. A. Rai, M. R. Khanani, M. N. Khan, and S. H. Ali. 2006. "HIV-1 Subtype A Infection in a Community of Intravenous Drug Users in Pakistan." *BMC Infect Dis* 6: 164.

Khanani, R. M., A. Hafeez, S. M. Rab, and S. Rasheed. 1988. "Human Immunodeficiency Virus-Associated Disorders in Pakistan." *AIDS Res Hum Retroviruses* 4: 149–54.

Khawaja, Z. A., L. Gibney, A. J. Ahmed, and S. H. Vermund. 1997. "HIV/AIDS and Its Risk Factors in Pakistan." *AIDS* 11: 843–48.

Kingston, M. E., E. J. Harder, M. M. Al-Jaberi, T. M. Bailey, G. T. Roberts, and K. V. Sheth. 1985. "Acquired Immune Deficiency Syndrome in the Middle East from Imported Blood." *Transfusion* 25: 317–18.

Kordy, F., S. Al-Hajjar, H. H. Frayha, R. Al-Khlaif, D. Al-Shahrani, and J. Akthar. 2006. "Human Immunodeficiency Virus Infection in Saudi Arabian Children: Transmission, Clinical Manifestations and Outcome." *Ann Saudi Med* 26: 92–99.

Leonard, G., A. Sangare, M. Verdier, E. Sassou-Guesseau, G. Petit, J. Milan, S. M'Boup, J. L. Rey, J. L. Dumas, J. Hugon, et al. 1990. "Prevalence of HIV Infection among Patients with Leprosy in African Countries and Yemen." *J Acquir Immune Defic Syndr* 3: 1109–13.

Lepers, J. P., C. Billon, J. L. Pesce, P. E. Rollin, and J. De Saint-Martin. 1988. "Sero-Epidemiological Study in Mauritania (1985–1986): Incidence of Treponema-tosis, Hepatitis B Virus, HIV Virus and Viral Hemorrhagic Fevers." *Bull Soc Pathol Exot Filiales* 81: 24–31.

Lerman, S. E., and J. C. Liao. 2001. "Neonatal Circumcision." *Pediatr Clin North Am* 48: 1539–57.

Lowndes, C. M., M. Alary, A. C. Labbe, C. Gnintoungbe, M. Belleau, L. Mukenge, H. Meda, M. Ndour, S. Anagonou, and A. Gbaguidi. 2007. "Interventions among Male Clients of Female Sex Workers in Benin, West Africa: An Essential Component of Targeted HIV Preventive Interventions." *Sex Transm Infect* 83: 577–81.

Maayan, S., E. Shinar, M. Aefani, M. Soughayer, R. Alkhoudary, S. Barshany, and N. Manny. 1994. "HIV-1 Prevalence among Israeli and Palestinian Blood Donors." *AIDS* 8: 133–34.

Maayan, S., E. Shinar, M. Aefani, M. Soughayer, R. el Khoudary, G. Rahav, and N. Manny. 1993. "HIV/AIDS among Palestinian Arabs." *Isr J Med Sci* 29: 7–10.

Madani, T. A., Y. Y. Al-Mazrou, M. H. Al-Jeffri, and N. S. Al Huzaim. 2004. "Epidemiology of the Human Immunodeficiency Virus in Saudi Arabia: 18-Year Surveillance Results and Prevention from an Islamic Perspective." *BMC Infect Dis* 4: 25.

Malamba, S. S., H. U. Wagner, G. Maude, M. Okongo, A. J. Nunn, J. F. Kengeya-Kayondo, and D. W. Mulder. 1994. "Risk Factors for HIV-1 Infection in Adults in a Rural Ugandan Community: A Case-Control Study." *AIDS* 8: 253–57.

Mandal, M., S. Purdin, and T. McGinn. 2005. "A Study of Health Facilities: Implications for Reproductive Health and HIV/AIDS Programs in Southern Sudan." *Int Q Community Health Educ* 24: 175–90.

Marcelin, A. G., M. Grandadam, P. Flandre, J. L. Koeck, M. Philippon, E. Nicand, R. Teyssou, H. Agut, J. M. Huraux, and N. Dupin. 2001. "Comparative Study of Heterosexual Transmission of HIV-1, HSV-2 and KSHV in Djibouti." *8th Retrovir Oppor Infect* (abstract no. 585).

Marcelin, A. G., M. Grandadam, P. Flandre, E. Nicand, C. Milliancourt, J. L. Koeck, M. Philippon, R. Teyssou, H. Agut, N. Dupin, and V. Calvez. 2002. "Kaposi's Sarcoma Herpesvirus and HIV-1 Seroprevalences in Prostitutes in Djibouti." *J Med Virol* 68: 164–67.

Maslin, J., C. Rogier, F. Berger, M. A. Khamil, D. Mattera, M. Grandadam, M. Caron, and E. Nicand. 2005. "Epidemiology and Genetic Characterization of HIV-1 Isolates in the General Population of Djibouti (Horn of Africa)." *J Acquir Immune Defic Syndr* 39: 129–32.

Mbulaiteye, S. M., A. Ruberantwari, J. S. Nakiyingi, L. M. Carpenter, A. Kamali, and J. A. Whitworth. 2000. "Alcohol and HIV: A Study among Sexually Active Adults in Rural Southwest Uganda." *Int J Epidemiol* 29: 911–15.

McCarthy, M. C., J. P. Burans, N. T. Constantine, A. A. el-Hag, M. E. el-Tayeb, M. A. el-Dabi, J. G. Fahkry, J. N. Woody, and K. C. Hyams. 1989. "Hepatitis B and HIV in Sudan: A Serosurvey for Hepatitis B and Human Immunodeficiency Virus Antibodies among Sexually Active Heterosexuals." *Am J Trop Med Hyg* 41: 726–31.

McCarthy, M. C., I. O. Khalid, and A. El Tigani. 1995. "HIV-1 Infection in Juba, Southern Sudan." *J Med Virol* 46: 18–20.

McFarland, W., and C. F. Caceres. 2001. "HIV Surveillance among Men Who Have Sex with Men." *AIDS* 15 Suppl 3: S23–32.

Meda, N., I. Ndoye, S. M'Boup, A. Wade, S. Ndiaye, C. Niang, F. Sarr, I. Diop, and M. Carael. 1999. "Low and Stable HIV Infection Rates in Senegal: Natural Course of the Epidemic or Evidence for Success of Prevention?" *AIDS* 13: 1397–405.

Mellors, J. W., C. R. Rinaldo, P. Gupta, R. M. White, J. A. Todd, and L. A. Kingsley. 1996. "Prognosis in HIV-1 Infection Predicted by the Quantity of Virus in Plasma." *Science* 272: 1167–70.

Milder, J. E., and V. M. Novelli. 1992. "Clinical, Social and Ethical Aspects of HIV-1 Infections in an Arab Gulf State." *J Trop Med Hyg* 95: 128–31.

Ministry of Health and Medical Education of Iran. 2006. "Treatment and Medical Education." Islamic Republic of Iran HIV/AIDS situation and response analysis.

Mishwar. 2008a. "An Integrated Bio-Behavioral Surveillance Study among Four Vulnerable Groups in Lebanon: Men Who Have Sex with Men; Prisoners; Commercial Sex Workers and Intravenous Drug Users." Mid-term report.

————. 2008b. "An Integrated Bio-Behavioral Surveillance Study among Four Vulnerable Groups in Lebanon: Men Who Have Sex with Men; Prisoners; Commercial Sex Workers and Intravenous Drug Users." Final report.

Mokhbat, J. E., R. E. Naman, F. S. Rahme, A. E. Farah, K. L. Zahar, and A. Maalouf. 1989. "Clinical and Serological Study of the Human Immunodeficiency Virus Infection in a Cohort of Multitransfused Persons." *J Med Liban* 38: 9–14.

Moses, A. E., S. Maayan, G. Rahav, M. Weinberger, D. Engelhard, M. Schlesinger, B. Knishkowy, A. Morag, and M. Shapiro. 1996. "HIV Infection and AIDS in Jerusalem: A Microcosm of Illness in Israel." *Isr J Med Sci* 32: 716–21.

Mostashari, G., UNODC (United Nations Office on Drugs and Crime), and M. Darabi. 2006. "Summary of the Iranian Situation on HIV Epidemic." NSP Situation Analysis.

Mujeeb, S. A., and A. Hafeez. 1993. "Prevalence and Pattern of HIV Infection in Karachi." *J Pak Med Assoc* 43: 2–4.

Mujeeb, S. A., M. R. Khanani, T. Khursheed, and A. Siddiqui. 1991. "Prevalence of HIV-Infection among Blood Donors." *J Pak Med Assoc* 41: 253–54.

Naman, R. E., J. E. Mokhbat, A. E. Farah, K. L. Zahar, and F. S. Ghorra. 1989. "Seroepidemiology of the Human Immunodeficiency Virus in Lebanon: Preliminary Evaluation." *J Med Liban* 38: 5–8.

Narenjiha, H., H. Rafiey, A. Baghestani, et al. 2005. "Rapid Situation Assessment of Drug Abuse and Drug Dependence in Iran, DARIUS Institute" (draft version, in Persian).

Nguyen, L., D. J. Hu, K. Choopanya, S. Vanichseni, D. Kitayaporn, F. van Griensven, P. A. Mock, W. Kittikraisak, N. L. Young, T. D. Mastro, and S. Subbarao. 2002. "Genetic Analysis of Incident HIV-1 Strains among Injection Drug Users in Bangkok: Evidence for Multiple Transmission Clusters during a Period of High Incidence." *J Acquir Immune Defic Syndr* 30: 248–56.

Novelli, V. M., H. Mostafavipour, M. Abulaban, F. Ekteish, J. Milder, and B. Azadeh. 1987. "High Prevalence of Human Immunodeficiency Virus Infection in Children with Thalassemia Exposed to Blood Imported from the United States." *Pediatr Infect Dis J* 6: 765–66.

NSNAC (New Sudan AIDS Council), and UNAIDS (Joint United Nations Programme on HIV/AIDS). 2006. *HIV/AIDS Integrated Report South Sudan, 2004–2005.* With United Nations General Assembly Special Session on HIV/AIDS Declaration of Commitment.

Nunn, A. J., J. F. Kengeya-Kayondo, S. S. Malamba, J. A. Seeley, and D. W. Mulder. 1994. "Risk Factors for HIV-1 Infection in Adults in a Rural Ugandan Community: A Population Study." *AIDS* 8: 81–86.

O'Grady, M. 2004. "WFP Consultant Visit to Djibouti Report." July 30.

Oman MOH (Ministry of Health). 2006. "HIV Risk among Heroin and Injecting Drug Users in Muscat, Oman." Quantitative survey, preliminary data.

Pakistan National AIDS Control Program. 2005. *HIV Second Generation Surveillance in Pakistan.* National Report Round 1. Ministry of Health, Pakistan, and Canada-Pakistan HIV/AIDS Surveillance Project.

————. 2006–7. *HIV Second Generation Surveillance in Pakistan.* National Report Round II. Ministry of Health, Pakistan, and Canada-Pakistan HIV/AIDS Surveillance Project.

————. 2008. *HIV Second Generation Surveillance in Pakistan.* National Report Round III. Ministry of Health, Pakistan, Canada-Pakistan HIV/AIDS Surveillance Project.

Pickthall, M. 1930. *The Meaning of the Glorious Qur'an.* Hyderabad, India. *Chapters and Verses* 17:32, 26:165–166, 5:90.

Pisani, E., S. Lazzari, N. Walker, and B. Schwartlander. 2003. "HIV Surveillance: A Global Perspective." *J Acquir Immune Defic Syndr* 32 Suppl 1: S3–11.

Piyasirisilp, S., F. E. McCutchan, J. K. Carr, E. Sanders-Buell, W. Liu, J. Chen, R. Wagner, H. Wolf, Y. Shao, S. Lai, C. Beyrer, and X. F. Yu. 2000. "A Recent Outbreak of Human Immunodeficiency Virus Type 1 Infection in Southern China Was Initiated by Two Highly Homogeneous, Geographically Separated Strains, Circulating Recombinant Form AE and a Novel BC Recombinant." *J Virol* 74: 11286–95.

Rakwar, J., L. Lavreys, M. L. Thompson, D. Jackson, J. Bwayo, S. Hassanali, K. Mandaliya, J. Ndinya-Achola, and J. Kreiss. 1999. "Cofactors for the Acquisition of HIV-1 among Heterosexual Men: Prospective Cohort Study of Trucking Company Workers in Kenya." *AIDS* 13: 607–14.

Ramezani, A., M. Mohraz, and L. Gachkar. 2006. "Epidemiologic Situation of Human Immuno-deficiency Virus (HIV/AIDS Patients) in a Private Clinic in Tehran, Iran." *Arch Iran Med* 9: 315–18.

Rao, C. K. 1993. *Strengthening of AIDS/HIV Surveillance in the Islamic Republic of Iran.* An Assignment Report, WHO/EMRO.

Razzaghi, E., A. Rahimi, and M. Hosseini. 1999. *Rapid Situation Assessment (RSA) of Drug Abuse in Iran.* Tehran: Prevention Department, State Welfare Organization, Ministry of Health, and United Nations International Drug Control Program.

Ridanovic, Z. 1997. "AIDS and Islam." *Med Arh* 51: 45–46.

Rodier, G. R., B. Couzineau, G. C. Gray, C. S. Omar, E. Fox, J. Bouloumie, and D. Watts. 1993. "Trends of Human Immunodeficiency Virus Type-1 Infection in Female Prostitutes and Males Diagnosed with a Sexually Transmitted Disease in Djibouti, East Africa." *Am J Trop Med Hyg* 48: 682–86.

Rodier, G., B. Couzineau, S. Salah, J. Bouloumie, J. P. Parra, E. Fox, N. Constantine, and D. Watts. 1993. "Infection by the Human Immunodeficiency Virus in the Republic of Djibouti: Literature Review and Regional Data." *Med Trop* (Mars) 53: 61–67.

Rodier, G. R., J. J. Morand, J. S. Olson, D. M. Watts, and S. Said. 1993. "HIV Infection among Secondary School Students in Djibouti, Horn of Africa: Knowledge, Exposure and Prevalence." *East Afr Med J* 70: 414–17.

Rota, S., A. Yildiz, H. Guner, and M. Erdem. 1989. "HIV Antibody Screening in a Gynecology and Obstetrics Clinic, Ankara, Turkey." *Int J Gynaecol Obstet* 30: 395–96.

Ryan, S. 2006. "Travel Report Summary." Kabul, Afghanistan, Joint United Nations Programme on HIV/AIDS, February 27 through March 7, 2006.

Salahudeen, A. K., H. F. Woods, A. Pingle, M. Nur-El-Huda Suleyman, K. Shakuntala, M. Nandakumar, T. M. Yahya, and A. S. Daar. 1990. "High Mortality among Recipients of Bought Living-Unrelated Donor Kidneys." *Lancet* 336: 725–28.

Salama, P., and T. J. Dondero. 2001. "HIV Surveillance in Complex Emergencies." *AIDS* 15 Suppl 3: S4–12.

Sanders-Buell, E., M. D. Saad, A. M. Abed, M. Bose, C. S. Todd, S. A. Strathdee, B. A. Botros, N. Safi, K. C. Earhart, P. T. Scott, N. Michael, and F. E. McCutchan. 2007. "A Nascent HIV Type 1 Epidemic among Injecting Drug Users in Kabul, Afghanistan Is Dominated by Complex AD Recombinant Strain, CRF35_AD." *AIDS Res Hum Retroviruses* 23: 834–39.

Shah, S. A., A. Altaf, S. A. Mujeeb, and A. Memon. 2004. "An Outbreak of HIV Infection among Injection Drug Users in a Small Town in Pakistan: Potential for National Implications." *Int J STD AIDS* 15: 209.

Shah, S. A., O. A. Khan, S. Kristensen, and S. H. Vermund. 1999. "HIV-Infected Workers Deported from the Gulf States: Impact on Southern Pakistan." *Int J STD AIDS* 10: 812–14.

Shirazi, K. K., and M. A. Morowatisharifabad. 2009. "Religiosity and Determinants of Safe Sex in Iranian Non-Medical Male Students." *J Relig Health* 48: 29–36.

SNAP (Sudan National HIV/AIDS Control Program). 2004. *HIV/AIDS/STIs Prevalence, Knowledge, Attitude, Practices and Risk Factors among University Students and Military Personnel.* Federal Ministry of Health, Khartoum.

———. 2008. "Update on the HIV Situation in Sudan." PowerPoint presentation.

Tassie, J.-M. Unknown. "Assignment Report HIV/AIDS/ STD Surveillance in I.R. of Iran." UNAIDS, Mission Internal Report.

Tawilah, J., and O. Tawil. 2001. *Visit to Sultane of Oman.* Travel report summary, National AIDS Programme at the Ministry of Health in Muscat and Salalah, and WHO Representative Office and EMRO.

Tehrani, F. R., and H. Malek-Afzalip. 2008. "Knowledge, Attitudes and Practices concerning HIV/AIDS among Iranian At-Risk Sub-Populations." *Eastern Mediter-ranean Health Journal* 14.

Tiouiri, H., B. Naddari, G. Khiari, S. Hajjem, and A. Zribi. 1999. "Study of Psychosocial Factors in HIV Infected Patients in Tunisia." *East Mediterr Health J* 5: 903–11.

Todd, C. S., A. M. Abed, S. A. Strathdee, P. T. Scott, B. A. Botros, N. Safi, and K. C. Earhart. 2007. "HIV, Hepatitis C, and Hepatitis B Infections and Associated Risk Behavior in Injection Drug Users, Kabul, Afghanistan." *Emerg Infect Dis* 13: 1327–31.

Toukan, A. U., and C. A. Schable. 1987. "Human Immunodeficiency Virus (HIV) Infection in Jordan: A Seroprevalence Study." *Int J Epidemiol* 16: 462–65.

UNAIDS (Joint United Nations Programme on HIV/ AIDS). 2006. "Fact Sheet on Drug Use and HIV in the Middle East and North Africa." MENA RST.

———. 2007a. *AIDS Epidemic Update 2007.* Geneva.

———. 2007b. Country Database, http://www.unaids .org/en/CountryResponses/Countries/default.asp.

———. 2007c. "Key Findings on HIV Status in the West Bank and Gaza." Working document, UNAIDS Regional Support Team for the Middle East and North Africa.

———. 2008. "Notes on AIDS in the Middle East and North Africa." RST MENA.

UNAIDS, and WHO (World Health Organization). 2003. *AIDS Epidemic Update 2003.* Geneva.

———. 2006. *AIDS Epidemic Update 2006.* Geneva.

Vandepitte, J., R. Lyerla, G. Dallabetta, F. Crabbe, M. Alary, and A. Buve. 2006. "Estimates of the Number of Female Sex Workers in Different Regions of the World." *Sex Transm Infect* 82 Suppl 3: iii18–25.

Watts, D. M., N. T. Constantine, M. F. Sheba, M. Kamal, J. D. Callahan, and M. E. Kilpatrick. 1993. "Prevalence of HIV Infection and AIDS in Egypt over Four Years of Surveillance (1986–1990)." *J Trop Med Hyg* 96: 113–17.

Wawer, M. J., R. H. Gray, N. K. Sewankambo, D. Serwadda, X. Li, O. Laeyendecker, N. Kiwanuka, G. Kigozi, M. Kiddugavu, T. Lutalo, F. Nalugoda, F. Wabwire-Mangen, M. P. Meehan, and T. C. Quinn. 2005. "Rates of HIV-1 Transmission per Coital Act, by Stage of HIV-1 Infection, in Rakai, Uganda." *J Infect Dis* 191: 1403–9.

WHO (World Health Organization). 2004. *The 2004 First National Second Generation HIV/AIDS/STI Sentinel Surveillance Survey, Somalia, A Technical Report.*

———. 2005. "Summary Country Profile for HIV/AIDS Treatment Scale-Up." Djibouti.

WHO/EMRO (Eastern Mediterranean Regional Office). 2005. "Progress Report on HIV/AIDS and '3 by 5.'" Cairo, July.

WHO, UNICEF (United Nations Children's Fund), and UNAIDS. 2006. "Yemen, Epidemiological Facts Sheets on HIV/AIDS and Sexually Transmitted Infections."

Woodruff, P. W., J. C. Morrill, J. P. Burans, K. C. Hyams, and J. N. Woody. 1988. "A Study of Viral and Rickettsial Exposure and Causes of Fever in Juba, Southern Sudan." *Trans R Soc Trop Med Hyg* 82: 761–66.

World Bank. 2008. "Mapping and Situation Assessment of Key Populations at High Risk of HIV in Three Cities of Afghanistan." Human Development Sector, South Asia Region (SAR) AIDS Team, World Bank.

Chapter 12

Snapshot on Response to HIV Epidemic in MENA: Linking Evidence with Policy and Programmatic Action to Avert the Epidemic

The epidemiological assessment detailed in the previous chapters highlights that the human immunodeficiency virus (HIV) disease burden in the Middle East and North Africa (MENA) is concentrated in priority populations, including injecting drug users (IDUs), men who have sex with men (MSM), and commercial sex networks, as well as the partners of these populations. There is very limited HIV spread in the general population. While HIV is likely to expand its spread in priority populations over the next decade, it is unlikely that MENA will experience substantial HIV epidemics in the general population such as those found in sub-Saharan Africa.

For any HIV response to be successful and cost-effective, it must be tailored to the epidemiological reality of HIV transmission patterns. The analytical synthesis in this report provides the strategic evidence necessary for determining the effectiveness of the HIV response in MENA, and the appropriateness of current resource allocation to control HIV spread.

This chapter provides a snapshot of HIV efforts in the region from the perspective of assessing the extent to which the response is in alignment with HIV epidemiology. This chapter is not an attempt to provide a comprehensive or exhaustive review of HIV efforts in MENA. A detailed analysis of response and resource allocation is beyond the scope of this report. HIV efforts are highly heterogeneous and cover a

wide spectrum of interventions across MENA. This chapter discusses mainly the HIV response through the lens of the epidemiological findings of this research work.

HIV PREVENTION IN MENA

Scaling up HIV prevention for people most at risk is the key to averting further spread of the HIV epidemic in MENA. As documented in the previous chapters, the relatively limited magnitude and current potential for HIV transmission across the region continue to provide a window of opportunity for containing the epidemic.[1] Timing, however, is critical, and effective HIV prevention should be pursued with great vigor and unyielding intensity.

While HIV prevention remains limited in scope and scale in MENA, based on a review of national strategic plans (NSPs), a few countries have made some advances, such as prevention efforts designed to engage female sex workers (FSWs), MSM, and IDUs in Morocco, and IDUs in the Islamic Republic of Iran. Prevention efforts in the region are impeded by generic and routine planning, competing priorities, limited human capital, and lack of monitoring and evaluation,

---

[1] Jenkins and Robalino, "HIV in the Middle East and North Africa"; World Bank, "Preventing HIV/AIDS in the Middle East and North Africa."

while national policies remain inadequate and do not sufficiently reflect evidence-informed approaches. Although there are noteworthy and recent examples, still very few prevention programs in MENA have adopted a comprehensive approach encompassing policy dimensions, strategic information, and an optimal mix of interventions developed with and implemented by members of the concerned populations.

FOCUSED HIV PREVENTION PROGRAMS FOR PEOPLE EXPOSED TO RISK

Priority populations in MENA are either disproportionately affected or more vulnerable to contracting HIV compared to other populations. As in all low prevalence and concentrated epidemic settings in the world, it is expected that MENA countries strategically focus their response on key populations at risk, namely, IDUs, MSM, and FSWs. However, a review of national strategic plans revealed that only those of Lebanon, Morocco, and Pakistan aim to engage each of the three priority populations.[2] Other countries have either included strategies for one or two key populations only, or mentioned a lump of key populations at risk without including specific strategies to address their specific needs and risks.

It is worth noting that countries that have clearly stated objectives or strategies addressing priority populations have been more successful in directing their response to effective interventions. Morocco, for example, is the only country in the region that was able to implement and rapidly scale up comprehensive services for MSM and FSWs, in spite of the cultural sensitivity. Similarly, the Islamic Republic of Iran and Pakistan have introduced harm reduction services for IDUs (but these need to be at a larger scale), and Djibouti could introduce targeted interventions for FSWs. Promising programs are currently developing in Afghanistan for IDUs and in Lebanon and Tunisia for the three key populations at risk.

The role of civil society and nongovernmental organizations (NGOs) in implementing activities addressing priority populations has been pivotal.

It can be noted that where NGOs are strong, the response is strong (for example, Algeria, the Islamic Republic of Iran, Lebanon, Morocco, and Pakistan).

While there is wider recognition in MENA countries of the importance of implementing targeted interventions for priority populations, there is concern over the coverage and the quality of those services and whether the services have the potential to avert the epidemic. Program monitoring data are scarce and thus cannot confirm the appropriateness of the response in terms of service coverage or specific services.

Injecting drug users

With the emergence of IDU as an important driver of the epidemic in MENA, and with the wealth of evidence accumulated around the world regarding the effectiveness of harm reduction interventions in preventing, slowing, or even reversing HIV epidemics among IDUs,[3] harm reduction is increasingly appropriate in MENA.

MENA countries, however, are at different stages of introducing the different components of the harm reduction package. The Islamic Republic of Iran is a model country in its response to HIV among IDUs, with a rapidly scaled-up plan to make available needles and syringes, opioid substitution therapy (OST), HIV testing and counseling, and sexually transmitted infection (STI) services. Once stabilized on OST, eligible HIV-positive IDUs are provided with antiretroviral therapy (ART).

After conducting an assessment of risk behaviors among IDUs, Morocco developed its harm reduction policies and integrated them into its national AIDS strategic plan. Currently, pilot drop-in centers performing needle and syringe exchange are in place, while preparations for introducing OST are underway.[4] Similarly, the Lebanese Minister of Health has publicly announced his commitment to introducing OST into the public health system as a national response, after a successful buprenorphine substitution program was introduced by the NGO

[2] UNAIDS and ASAP, "Review of National AIDS Strategic Plan."

[3] Des Jarlais et al., "HIV Incidence"; Metzger et al., Human Immunodeficiency Virus Seroconversion"; van Ameijden et al., "Interventions among Injecting Drug Users."

[4] G. Riedner, personal communication (2008), and site visits to drop-in centers in Tangier and Tetouane.

Skoun.[5] Lebanon's National AIDS Program is currently putting in place measures to expand OST. Needle and syringe programs are also being implemented by NGOs through outreach workers. Over the last few years Pakistan has scaled up its outreach, needle and syringe exchange, testing, and counseling services for IDUs.[6] Multisectoral national consultation is currently being held to initiate OST. Afghanistan has initiated drop-in centers providing harm reduction services, except for OST, which is expected to start in the near future.[7] A few NGOs in the Arab Republic of Egypt are providing sterile needles and syringes to IDUs through outreach.[8] Oman is reviewing its national policies and regulations to assess the need for and feasibility of OST.[9]

A regional civil society movement has formed and is called the Middle East and North Africa Harm Reduction Association (MENAHRA).[10] MENHARA's objective is to build the capacity of civil society organizations for harm reduction through training, sharing information, networking, and providing direct support to NGOs to initiate or scale up harm reduction services. MENAHRA includes three subregional knowledge hubs: Lebanon's hub is hosted by an NGO (SIDC [*Soins Infirmiers et Developpement Communautaire*]), the Islamic Republic of Iran's hub is hosted by the Iranian National Center for Addiction Studies (INCAS), and Morocco's hub is hosted by the Ar-Razi psychiatric hospital. The MENAHRA network connects over 350 professionals in the field of drug use and HIV through its Web site, bimonthly newsletter, and ad hoc announcements.

Men who have sex with men

Data on MSM have been the most difficult to obtain, but have begun to emerge over the last five years and are indicating the need for immediate action. Limited adoption of safe sexual practices and low access to services are heightened by marginalizing sociocultural attitudes, as a study of MSM suggests in Lebanon.[11] The majority of MSM in the study indicated that they face exclusion from their communities and families.[12] As far as their own practices are concerned, they often engage in unprotected sex, with 74% of those surveyed identifying unprotected sex as the main reason for seeking voluntary counseling and testing (VCT).

In a study in Sudan, more than half (55.6%) of MSM study participants had exchanged sex for money.[13] Close to half of those who had commercial sexual partners did not use a condom in the last sexual contact, and 85.3% indicated nonavailability of condoms at the time of the sexual act as the reason for lack of use. High-risk practices coupled with a significant HIV prevalence rate (9.3%) for this group emphasize the need for immediate prevention services for MSM.

In Tunisia, the qualitative and quantitative survey conducted among MSM documented substantive risk behaviors, limited access to services, and that more than 92.2% of those surveyed had both male and female partners.[14]

Customary claims that stringent legal and social context deters implementation of prevention programs should not be a reason to shy away from adapting programs and denying services to MSM. A number of countries are now addressing this population directly, although this remains particularly sensitive with the general public, community leaders, and law enforcement agencies. Examples include Lebanon, where NGOs such as Helem and SIDC, along with the National AIDS Program, have implemented outreach and HIV prevention for MSM. In Algeria, the first outreach HIV prevention program for people most at risk has reached out to male sex workers (MSWs) with services and condoms. In Tunisia and Morocco, MSM are the outreach workers informing their peers on HIV prevention services, accompanying them to VCT, and providing condoms and lubricants (when available). The assessment undertaken in Sudan on better understanding the needs of MSM and their vulnerabilities is

[5] Skoun, "New Perspectives."
[6] Punjab Provincial AIDS Control Programme, "The Lethal Overdose";
    Nai Zindagi quarterly reports 2007 (www.naizindagi.com/Reports).
[7] WHO/EMRO, unpublished country information.
[8] Aziz et al., "The Impact of Harm Reduction."
[9] WHO/EMRO, unpublished country information.
[10] MENAHRA, http://www.menahra.org/.

[11] Dewachi, "HIV/AIDS Prevention."
[12] Ibid.
[13] Elrashied, "Prevalence, Knowledge and Related Risky Sexual Behaviours."
[14] Hsairi and Ben Abdallah, "Analyse de la situation de vulnérabilité."

a stepping stone to establishing trust with the communities and tailoring HIV prevention programs to their needs. In Pakistan, a special program is set for MSM, MSWs, and *hijras*.[15] Through NGOs, outreach peer education and condom distribution are expected to reach over 56,000 members of these priority groups by 2013.

Commercial sex

As demonstrated in the previous chapters, men and women involved in sex work face an increased risk of HIV infection. In addition to the illegal status of FSWs in the majority of MENA countries, social taboos and lack of means to protect FSWs from exploitation cause clandestine prostitution to thrive in all countries, as well as in Tunisia, where sex work is regulated by law. Consequently, those involved are secluded and often reluctant to seek health, social, or legal services or to disclose their risk of HIV exposure.[16]

This is compounded by social exclusion and the negative attitudes of communities and service providers, attitudes mainly due to sociocultural conservative attitudes on sexual behavior.

Despite overall reluctance and the stringent context, HIV prevention programs started in Morocco in the 1990s and have provided male and female sex workers with prevention information and prevention, condoms, testing, counseling, and STI services. In Lebanon, one NGO, Dar el Amal (the *House of Hope*), which has provided health, social, and vocational services for female FSWs since the 1970s, has mainstreamed HIV services into its activities. The first outreach peer-educator FSWs were recruited from this NGO.

Similarly, an NGO in Tunisia (ATL MST/sida-section de Tunis [Association Tunisienne de Lutte contre les MST et le sida-Section de Tunis]), through outreach work implemented by FSWs and MSM, provides HIV information and prevention kits (including condoms and lubricants) and conducts awareness-raising services and referral for VCT or treatment services. A qualitative survey of FSWs[17] in Algeria resulted

in programs for those people most at risk. Subsequently, in 2008, AIDS Algerie provided more than 1,500 males and females involved in sex work in Oran and Alger with condoms and HIV prevention information and materials.

The first project for women in vulnerable situations, established in Cairo in 2006 and implemented through Shehab NGOs, resulted in awareness-raising services mainly for FSWs, reaching more than 900 FSWs in the first two years of implementation.[18] The project, through outreach work and a drop-in center, established trust with the concerned communities; ensured access to STI treatment, legal services, and training on negotiation skills and condom use; and generated crucial information on the structural vulnerabilities of those involved in sex work.

In the Islamic Republic of Iran, a promising experience is currently unfolding. It includes the provision of services to FSWs through the establishment of drop-in centers for women in risky situations. Interventions include HIV testing and counseling, harm reduction services for women using drugs, condom distribution, and STI services. This is believed to be an adapted approach to engaging FSWs given sociocultural sensitivity and their illegal status.

Starting in 2003, in Djibouti, programs designed to engage FSWs were implemented; they included awareness raising, STI services, HIV testing and counseling, and condom promotion and distribution. Other countries such as Afghanistan, Jordan, Pakistan, and Sudan are reportedly conducting awareness raising for FSWs through outreach. The results generated and trust built with the communities in some of these examples have led to expansion of the programs through NGOs and community organizations. It has also led to initiating partnerships with police and community leaders to facilitate implementation of programs and to protect the well-being of concerned communities. Support mobilized from the Joint United Nations Programme on HIV/AIDS (UNAIDS), the Global Fund to Fight AIDS, Tuberculosis and Malaria (GFATM), HIV International Alliance, and others has been instrumental in expanding efforts in several countries.

[15] Pakistan National AIDS Control Program, *HIV Second Generation Surveillance* (Rounds II and III).

[16] Karouaoui, "Report of Mission on HIV and Sex Work in Oman."

[17] AIDS Algérie, UNAIDS, and UNFPA, *Travail du Sexe et VIH/SIDA en Algérie.*

[18] ONUSIDA, *Rapport de fin de Mission Appui aux Programmes de Prévention SIDA.*

Young people

Peer influence can encourage risky behavior, but it can also be used to spread knowledge through peer educators.[19] The Islamic Republic of Iran has spearheaded a peer education program in schools that has trained thousands of students to educate peers on HIV.[20] A special course on AIDS was developed as an appendix to biology books and 13,000 teachers and school physicians have been trained to educate 1.5 million students in high schools.[21] Tunisia had a program to reach out to youth through appropriate education, counseling and testing, condoms, and STI services that reached 10% of the youth.[22] In Sudan, an intervention for youth has provided over 300,000 young people with health education sessions covering various topics.[23]

Progress in HIV prevention

Progress made over the last four years in terms of generating crucial information on HIV prevalence, risks, and vulnerabilities for priority populations and settings has been a breakthrough in informing advocacy efforts and programmatic choices, contributing to policy change, and creating an enabling environment.

With just a few exceptions, HIV prevention programs have recently taken a qualitative step forward by combining several communication and service-delivery approaches and focusing on behavior change in the form of risk and harm reduction. Enhancing the quality of interventions, expanding coverage, and intensifying implementation remain key challenges for HIV prevention programs that engage high-risk populations in the region.

One of the main obstacles that prevention efforts had to overcome was the limited knowledge on, contacts with, and participation of the concerned populations. To overcome these obstacles, peer education and outreach strategies were introduced and are now essential components in evolving HIV prevention efforts, encouraging and facilitating the engagement of civil society and national AIDS programs with the concerned populations and communities.

HIV prevention efforts raise awareness and provide information, materials, and services (for example, condoms; interpersonal communication; referrals to VCT; and STI, ART, and other health care and social support programs) including risk or harm reduction. Prevention efforts focus on changing risky or maintaining safe behaviors through channels such as interpersonal communication, peer education, and outreach.

ACCESS TO MEANS OF PREVENTION

While this shift over time from HIV prevention based mainly on health promotion to a more focused approach on behavior change is notable, the coverage and quality of services and means of prevention in the region are still far from adequate. Access to HIV-related prevention means and services remains sporadic, with very limited coverage, and is therefore unlikely to lead to significant behavior change.

With regard to condom availability, some progress has been made with some countries (such as in Algeria, Jordan, Morocco, and Sudan) reporting an increase in condom availability and distribution, mainly as part of indicators to monitor progress of GFATM-supported projects. These data are an important leap toward making means of prevention available; however, little is known about whether condom distribution is part of a behavior change approach reaching people most at risk. However, stigma related to the very nature of HIV transmission, compounded by the social marginalization of those exposed, hampers efforts to include condoms and other means of prevention as part of prevention programs in many countries. It is also noted that in specific programs for people most at risk, the messages delivered and means of prevention have not been adapted to their needs; therefore, they have little impact on behaviors, especially while negotiation skills with their sexual partners are limited.

Information, education, and communication (IEC) materials for refugees and mobile

[19] Busulwa, "HIV/AIDS Situation Analysis Study"; Kocken et al., "Effects of Peer-Led AIDS Education."
[20] Gheiratmand et al., "A Country Study."
[21] Gheiratmand et al., "A Country Study"; Mohebbi and Navipour, "Preventive Education."
[22] Jenkins and Robalino, "HIV in the Middle East and North Africa."
[23] SNAP and UNAIDS, "HIV/AIDS Integrated Report North Sudan, 2004–5."

populations in the Republic of Yemen, for example, were not adapted to the languages of those concerned, nor were the messages explicit in terms of transmission modes and prevention methods. Condoms were not included as part of prevention activities, and referrals to VCT were lacking. The situation is compounded by the limited capacities and resources of implementing partners to provide prevention materials, such as condoms and lubricants, and make them accessible as part of outreach activities.[24]

In a review of programs for IDUs in Egypt, provision of needles, syringes, condoms, and other HIV prevention commodities appeared to be inconsistent at the three sites reviewed.[25] The outreach program for MSM in Tunisia is in desperate need of a robust and sustainable procurement system for water-based lubricants for distribution with the prevention kit.

The use of condoms in HIV prevention protective strategies is reported to be generally low in the region (chapter 8). Condom use is also low and irregular among people who need them the most, including those reporting multiple and casual unprotected sexual contacts, although utilization rates among such groups are still considerably higher than in the general population (chapter 8). Despite the above evidence, condom promotion, access, and distribution are still conspicuously missing from many HIV prevention programs being implemented in the region. Even when programs have included condoms, access has remained difficult and limited to certain distribution points.

Continuing to ignore the sensitive but essential issue of condom accessibility and neglecting the promotion of its protective role for everyone, particularly for people most at risk, are undoubtedly crippling effective HIV prevention efforts, as is the case in many countries of the region.

HIV TESTING AND COUNSELING

Initially, most VCT centers across the region were located only in the capital cities as part of governmental health facilities, discouraging those fearing stigma from checking their HIV status. There was substantial delay in the establishment of VCT services at a community level across the region.

Morocco is one of the first countries to establish VCT centers with broad, national coverage. Today, Algeria has expanded its VCT network across the country and more than 75 centers have been established in Sudan. In Lebanon, the innovative model of establishing and managing VCTs through NGOs was adopted by the National AIDS Program and partners.[26]

However, the recent increase in VCT services has not translated into enhanced prevention efforts or an increased number of those who know their HIV status. A recent review revealed that VCT services are either not available or limited to major cities in most countries.[27] Where they exist, these VCT services are underused. Different reasons may account for this, including the absence or low coverage of HIV prevention programs among priority groups and vulnerable and other populations, as well as weak message quality and lack of referrals to the VCT. Other factors could be the general concern that confidentiality may not be maintained and the negative attitudes of service providers in the VCT centers, which have been documented in some countries.

The same review has demonstrated that HIV rapid tests have not been fully adopted in MENA. Where they are used, laboratory confirmation of reactive tests requires the use of ELISA (enzyme-linked immunosorbent assay), and, in many cases, Western blot assay. The resulting waiting time and cumbersome procedure for the clients to get their HIV test results increase the risk of losing the client before he or she is informed of the test result.

Moreover, the review has shown that the majority of people in MENA learn their HIV status through mandatory testing. Out of tens of millions of HIV tests conducted in the region since 1995, only a little over 400,000 were administered through VCT. All countries of the region (except Djibouti and Morocco, which do mandatory testing only on military recruits to establish physical fitness) have mandated HIV testing for different purposes including preoperative, pre-employment, in-migration, and

---

[24] Semini, Njogou, and Mortagy, *UNHCR/UNAIDS Joint Mission.*
[25] UNAIDS/APMG, *Recommendations for Interventions.*

[26] Lebanon National AIDS Control Program, "A Case Study."
[27] WHO/EMRO, "Regional Review of HIV Testing."

high-risk populations upon arrest or admission to health care. The consequences of positive HIV test results can be deportation of migrant workers, denial of visa, or denial of health care services.

Provider-initiated testing and counseling (PITC) is rarely adopted. Where it is reportedly undertaken in health care settings (for example, in tuberculosis clinics, antenatal clinic services, surgical units, STI clinics, and others), PITC is often confused with mandatory screening, where the requirement for consent is not respected.

EXPANDING COVERAGE

Currently, scaled-up and decentralized HIV prevention programs are the exception to the rule in MENA. Partially due to the fact that the current HIV prevention programs for priority populations are nascent in the region, current efforts are mainly patchy projects providing access to populations in selected areas of urban cities. The programs that have expanded in various regions of Morocco demonstrate the feasibility of scaled-up programs for those involved in sex work, even in a stringent context. In Morocco in 2007, 51.8% of FSWs were tested in VCT centers and received the result. Of the above, 53.2% declared using a condom during the last sexual contact compared to 37.5% in 2003.

Massive efforts are needed to address the challenges impeding coverage expansion and the implementation of quality and focused HIV prevention programs. One of the challenges of scaling up programs for HIV prevention is the variety of contexts where risk behaviors take place. People involved in sex work are not a homogeneous group, existing networks relate to subpopulations (those working in the streets, hotels, and so forth), and various motivations and several underlying factors determine involvement in sex work. The variations among existing networks make it even more challenging to inform an effective programmatic approach. In the MENA context, current programs reach only a few subpopulations of FSWs, drug users, and MSM, mainly determined by the initial entry point of how these populations were reached.

Information generated by situation assessments in terms of underlying vulnerability factors and context variety needs to be effectively used to adapt programs to the needs of people most at risk and expand coverage and intensity to reach all of those in need. Adapted programmatic approaches are necessary to provide services to those in bars, residences, streets, and other high-risk areas. Biobehavior information disaggregated on settings and specific geographical locations at higher risk needs to take into account the geographical variations to determine the priority settings and focus of expanded HIV prevention. As an example, in Morocco, HIV prevalence among sex workers is substantively higher in Marrakesh and Agadir, while IDU is prevalent in Tangier and Tetouan, and this information should be used in planning prevention programs in each setting. In Algeria, Tamanrasset and Tiaret are characterized by a considerably higher HIV prevalence rate among FSWs compared to other regions (9% in Tamanrasset, 3%–8% in some regions in 2004–07, and 11% in Tiaret[28]), and the NSP for 2008–12 places a priority focus on programs for sex work in these selected areas.

CIVIL SOCIETY AND PEOPLE LIVING WITH HIV AS IMPLEMENTATION PARTNERS

A wider proliferation of NGOs and community-based organizations to help implement HIV prevention programs will improve HIV prevention services and programs and help focus these programs on priority populations that are harder to reach. There is a limited presence of NGOs and community organizations implementing HIV prevention, particularly for people most at risk, and this significantly hinders the decentralization and expansion of service coverage. Pioneering NGOs have initiated breakthrough projects on HIV prevention; however, their scope and coverage remain limited.

Thus, it is essential that other NGOs and community-based organizations are identified in the priority areas and are trained to deliver HIV prevention services and information to people most in need. These NGOs can be developmental partners working on thematics other than AIDS that have community access and the trust of the populations, but not necessarily the required competence on HIV-related services.

---

[28] Algeria National AIDS Council, "Algeria National Strategy."

Despite an environment of limited awareness, apprehension, and stigma associated with HIV/AIDS, associations of people living with HIV (PLHIV) have now emerged as partners in more than 10 countries of the region. Civil society organizations and, in some cases, the national AIDS programs have contributed to establishing support groups and associations for PLHIV in recent years. In countries such as Algeria, Djibouti, Morocco, and Sudan, socioeconomic support mechanisms have also been put in place through joint government and civil society initiatives, including for a sizable number of orphaned children in Djibouti. The role of people living with HIV and their association as equal partners is essential to ensure access to HIV prevention, treatment, care, and support services.

From evidence to programs

Translating evidence generated through research, biobehavior surveys, and surveillance into adapted programming is essential to devise an optimal combination of interventions tailored to the needs of concerned populations.

Overlapping risks have been documented (chapters 2–4); however, few programs include a comprehensive package of interventions and referral to services to address the needs of people who are exposed to multiple risks. Such packages need to be an integral part of prevention programs and are crucial to averting an epidemic. Specific programming and focus are necessary to address the needs of these subpopulations.

Strikingly, there appears to be considerable multiplicity and overlap of risk factors in urban settings in MENA, including injecting drug use and unprotected sexual contacts (chapter 2). The overlap of sexual and drug injecting risks, which was featured in nearly all of the behavioral surveys among drug users,[29] and was also documented among FSWs and MSM, could spark more serious HIV outbreaks across populations at a time when consistent condom use is strikingly low. Over 40% of drug users in Algeria, 36% in Cairo, and 33% in Lebanon had engaged in sex work contacts in the month preceding the interview, with the reported use of condoms

being inconsistent or nonexistent among the vast majority. In Afghanistan, more than 70% of IDUs surveyed in Kabul had paid women for sex, while condom use is exceptionally low in the country.[30] Conversely, in the Syrian Arab Republic, 10% FSWs reported drug injection.[31]

A study in Alexandria, Egypt, showed that 10.9% of MSM had injected drugs in the previous 12 months.[32] High-risk sexual practices were also prevalent, with 53% of drug users interviewed in Syria having engaged in sex work, and 40% of the sexually experienced had never used a condom, while only 20% had done so consistently.[33] Likewise, among a sample of IDUs in treatment in the Islamic Republic of Iran, most were sexually active and exchanging money for sex was not uncommon, yet almost half of them had never used a condom.[34] However, few programs integrate adapted approaches to address the multiple and overlapping risks. The NGOs providing HIV prevention services to FSWs in Egypt, despite the holistic approach adopted and the willingness to address the needs of women who also inject drugs, do not provide drug injection–related HIV prevention information and material as part of the prevention package, nor have they the capacity to do so. A few programs on drug use and HIV have included a focus on sexual risks, with limited integration of education about sexual risks or condom provision.

This lack of integration in adapted approaches is also due to the focus and capacities of the NGOs implementing the HIV prevention programs. Involving the concerned communities in planning the prevention services and management of implementation will help to redeem the programming shortfalls.

In almost all of the MENA countries, an impediment to measuring progress and determining the priorities for prevention programs is the absence of monitoring and evaluation (M&E) systems to assess program impact over time. Integrating data collection from the inception of the program, using the data to inform the program and national M&E system,

[29] UNAIDS, UNODC, and WHO, "Fact Sheet on Drug Use."

[30] Todd et al., "Prevalence of Human Immunodeficiency Virus."
[31] Syria National AIDS Programme, "HIV/AIDS Female Sex Workers."
[32] Egypt Ministry of Health and Population, and National AIDS Program, *HIV/AIDS Biological and Behavioral Surveillance Survey*.
[33] Syria Ministry of Health, UNODC, and UNAIDS, "Assessment on Drug Use and HIV in Syria."
[34] Zamani et al., "Prevalence."

and the participation of concerned populations will yield much-needed information on service delivery and prevention progress.

Scope, quality, and outreach are essential for sustainable HIV prevention programs

Because HIV prevention efforts need to focus on the people who are likely to be reluctant to approach facility-based services, outreach and peer education are the keys to providing these hard-to-reach people with information and services.

Experience confirms that it is essential that outreach workers come from the concerned communities; this helps to ensure behavior change and empowers the communities themselves. Health and social workers, and NGO volunteers face increasing challenges to establish regular contacts and deliver HIV prevention messages to IDUs in Egypt, while ex- and active IDUs have proven to be very efficient and trusted by the communities, leading to increased adoption of safe methods.

Outreach is an efficient technique for getting information and services to people who need them most. However, high rotation and change of personnel over time hampers effective and quality behavior change interventions, because there is limited incremental experience in the implementing partner institutions. The complexities and challenges are magnified as the programs try to expand coverage. In addition to management challenges, maintaining a core mass of outreach workers with adequate, updated skills is proving difficult.

Education and referral for large HIV prevention programs demand significant resources, and continuous training quality may be affected over time. While recognizing the necessity of ensuring that outreach workers are peers of the populations being engaged, programs in MENA should try to institutionalize outreach work to ensure their sustainability and long-term impact on HIV prevention.

BLOOD SAFETY AND UNIVERSAL PRECAUTIONS

Infections as a result of blood products, blood transfusion, and lack of infection control measures in health care settings are generally on the decline, although this mode of transmission continues to be present in a small number of countries. Overall, the percentage of reported HIV and AIDS cases attributed to contaminated blood has fallen from 12.1% in 1993 to 0.4% for the entire MENA region in 2003.[35]

According to countries' universal access indicator reports for 2007, the screening of donated blood was fully operational at 100% in all facilities in Djibouti, the Islamic Republic of Iran, Iraq, Jordan, Lebanon, Oman, Saudi Arabia, Somalia, Sudan, Syria, Tunisia, and the United Arab Emirates.[36] Afghanistan and Pakistan report that 39% and 87%, respectively, of donated blood units were screened for HIV in a quality assured manner.[37] No data were available for Sudan, the West Bank and Gaza, and the Republic of Yemen.[38]

HIV CARE AND TREATMENT

By 2005, in the majority of MENA countries, ART was available at least at one central health facility. During the following years, access to ART was expanded to include low-income countries that had succeeded in mobilizing donor support through the GFATM.

The introduction of ART had an almost immediate and visible impact on the quality of life of PLHIV, which was also evident in the reduced mortality rates. In Tunisia, the mortality of AIDS patients fell from 45% to 7.8% between 2000 and 2003. However, the gap between PLHIV receiving treatment and the overall estimated need for treatment has remained substantial.

Based on the most recent UNAIDS and World Health Organization (WHO) estimates, at the end of 2008, approximately 151,000 PLHIV were in need of ART in MENA[39]; two-thirds of them are living in Pakistan and Sudan. Only 9,622 PLHIV in need of ART were reportedly receiving treatment.[40] Accordingly, in 2007, the

[35] UNAIDS, "Notes on AIDS in the Middle East and North Africa."
[36] WHO/EMRO, "Progress towards Universal Access" (2007).
[37] Ibid.
[38] WHO/EMRO, Progress towards Universal Access" (2006); WHO and EMRO, "Progress towards Universal Access" (2007).
[39] WHO, UNAIDS, and UNICEF, "Towards Universal Access."
[40] WHO/EMRO, "Progress towards Universal Access" (2007).

Figure 12.1 ART Scale Up in Somalia and Southern Sudan between 2005 and 2008

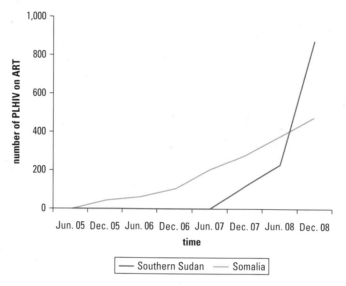

Source: WHO/EMRO. Country data reported to the WHO Office of the Eastern Mediterranean Region.

Table 12.1 Number of PLHIV on ART in Selected Countries, 2006–08

Country	2006	2007	2008
Djibouti	578	705	816
Iran, Islamic Rep. of	522	827	921
Morocco	1,370	1,648	2,207
Pakistan	164	523	907
Somalia	111	211	413
Sudan	986	1,198	2,317
Yemen, Republic of	0	107	189

Source: WHO/EMRO Regional Database on HIV/AIDS; WHO/EMRO 2008a.

regional ART coverage of the estimated need was 6%, the lowest among all regions. By 2008, all countries in MENA, except for Afghanistan, Iraq, and the West Bank and Gaza, had established HIV care and treatment services and were steadily expanding access to ART (table 12.1).[41]

Experience with establishing and expanding access to HIV care and treatment in Southern Sudan and Somalia shows that providing ART is possible, even in very difficult contexts. Southern Sudan initiated its HIV care and treatment program by mid-2007, and by December 2008, almost 1,000 of the PLHIV received ART.[42]

Somalia started in June 2005, and by the end of 2008, more than 500 of the PLHIV were receiving ART (figure 12.1).[43]

A main reason for the low ART coverage in MENA is that a very small proportion of PLHIV know their HIV status, and approximately 80% of PLHIV known to the health care system to be in need of ART are actually receiving treatment.[44] At local and regional meetings of support groups, PLHIV frequently voice their fear of nonconfidentiality if they disclose their HIV status to health service providers and the resulting stigma and discrimination they could face within the health system, their workplaces, and communities. Accordingly, there is reason to assume that a considerable proportion of PLHIV who know their HIV status try to avoid contact with the public health system and attempt to find access to treatment in the private sector or outside their countries. The limited ability of most countries to implement interventions for reaching high-risk populations is likely to considerably affect access to and use of HIV VCT, and therefore impact treatment.

Large gaps in geographical coverage of ART services are another reason for the low treatment coverage in MENA countries with the highest burden of HIV. In 2007, per 1,000 PLHIV in need of ART, 1.5 health facilities

---

[41] WHO/EMRO Regional Database on HIV/AIDS.
[42] WHO/EMRO, data reported to the WHO Office of the Eastern Mediterranean Region.

[43] Ibid.
[44] WHO/EMRO, "Survey on Status."

offered ART in Pakistan, 0.9 in Somalia, 0.4 in Sudan, and 0.6 in the Republic of Yemen.[45]

Treatment outcomes reported by country ART programs in low-income countries in the region are comparable to globally reported outcomes. In 2008, the reported survival rate of PLHIV on ART during one year was 92% in Pakistan and ranged between 72% and 91% in Djibouti, the Islamic Republic of Iran, Morocco, Somalia, and the Republic of Yemen.[46]

Despite rather newly established national ART programs and low ART coverage, some countries, such as the Islamic Republic of Iran and Pakistan, already report a high proportion (greater than 10%) of patients receiving second line ART, indicating the emergence of HIV drug resistance.

Good adherence to ART has been observed in Morocco,[47] though noncompliance and treatment interruptions have been observed, for example, in Oman.[48] Some of the identified challenges to adherence are the difficulty in following the administration schedule, long distances between home and ART services, or the presence of adverse effects.[49] This suggests the need for education and counseling programs to ensure that patients understand ART and thereby improve adherence.[50] There is also evidence of obtaining drugs with no prescription and no clinical and psychosocial support.[51] Some countries report problems such as drug stock outs, lack of second line drugs, over-centralization of services, and lack of comprehensive care and psychosocial support.[52]

Few countries are implementing HIV drug resistance monitoring and surveillance activities, according to the WHO global strategy. In 2008, only Djibouti published an annual report on HIV drug resistance early warning indicators.[53]

HIV MOTHER-TO-CHILD TRANSMISSION

In 2008, half of the MENA countries had established national programs for prevention of mother-to-child transmission (PMTCT), compared to one-third in 2006.[54] However, major challenges remain to ensure the effectiveness of PMTCT programs, including low antenatal care attendance rates in some countries, geographical availability of PMTCT services, provision of HIV testing and counseling in antenatal care clinics (opt-out approach), antiretroviral (ARV) prophylaxis regimen efficacy, and retention of women and children in PMTCT services. According to reports on universal access indicators in 2008 from Jordan, Morocco, Somalia, Sudan, and the Republic of Yemen, less than 1% of the estimated total number of pregnant women underwent an HIV test. Based on the same reports, between less than 1% and 24% of the estimated number of HIV-positive pregnant women received antiretroviral prophylaxis to reduce the risk of mother-to-child HIV transmission in the Islamic Republic of Iran (23.6%), Morocco (14.3%), North Sudan (0.2%), Pakistan (0.02%), Somalia (0.3%), and the Republic of Yemen (0.4%).[55]

PREVENTION AND CONTROL OF STIs: CURRENT RESPONSE AND CHALLENGES

According to information on the status of STI surveillance and control obtained from focal points in the ministries of health, surveillance is limited or not established in most MENA countries. Only one country (Morocco) reported establishing a surveillance system that makes it possible to chart trends, quantify the situation, guide program planning, and assess the impact of interventions (chapter 10). Thus, reliable data on STIs are not often available in the region.

The degree to which MENA countries have already established STI control programs and their ability to implement recommended STI prevention and control interventions, in terms of available political support, resources, and systems, vary widely. Most STI programs are not appropriately equipped with human and financial resources. According to an unpublished review of the STI response conducted by the World Health Organization Eastern Mediterranean Regional Office (WHO/EMRO), 12 countries (Afghanistan, Bahrain, Djibouti, Egypt, the

[45] WHO/EMRO, "Progress towards Universal Access" (2007).
[46] WHO/EMRO, "Progress towards Universal Access" (2007); WHO/EMRO, "Progress towards Universal Access" (2008).
[47] Benjaber, Rey, and Himmich, "A Study on Antiretroviral Treatment."
[48] Al Dhahry et al., "Human Immunodeficiency Virus."
[49] Benjaber, Rey, and Himmich, "A Study on Antiretroviral Treatment."
[50] Ibid.
[51] Shah et al., "Antiretroviral Drugs."
[52] UNAIDS, "Notes on AIDS in the Middle East and North Africa."
[53] Djibouti National AIDS Programme, "Programme de lutte contre le sida."
[54] WHO/EMRO, "Progress towards Universal Access" (2007).
[55] WHO/EMRO, "Progress towards Universal Access" (2008).

Islamic Republic of Iran, Iraq, Morocco, Oman, Pakistan, Saudi Arabia, Somalia, and the West Bank and Gaza) reported having a national strategy for STIs. Only five countries (Bahrain, the Islamic Republic of Iran, Morocco, Pakistan, and Saudi Arabia) have a national action plan to implement these strategies and have allocated more than 50% of the funds required for the response from the national health budget.

STI interventions currently being implemented in several countries often do not build on evidence-based, effective public health approaches, as recommended in the global strategy for the prevention and control of STIs. According to a survey carried out by WHO/EMRO in 2008, 13 countries have implemented the syndromic approach for STI case management, but only 6 (Djibouti, Egypt, Jordan, Morocco, Pakistan, and Somalia) have carried out etiological studies to validate the WHO flowcharts relating to the syndromic approach.[56]

The same survey found that most countries in the region do not provide any special STI services for priority populations. Only six countries (Djibouti, Egypt, Jordan, Morocco, Pakistan, and Sudan) have implemented an outreach peer education program among sex workers. Egypt, Morocco, and Pakistan also provide special consultation and treatment services for this group. Any response that does not address priority populations, such as FSWs, MSM, and IDUs, will fall short of having any significant impact on the spread of STIs in MENA. As in other regions, STI and HIV transmission are concentrated among groups that have higher rates of partner change and higher-risk behaviors than the general population. Although these groups are socially marginalized, the infection spreads to the general public via other population subgroups, known as bridging populations, which connect the higher-risk groups (such as clients of sex workers) and the general population.

CONCLUDING REMARKS AND SUMMARY OF FINDINGS

HIV prevention and treatment efforts in MENA continue to be rather limited despite recent improvements. Ample efforts continue to be focused on the general population despite the limited HIV prevalence in this population. Coverage of and access to HIV prevention services among priority populations continue to be far below the needs. Access to HIV treatment varies and is among the lowest globally.

A key structural problem in MENA is the poor mapping of risk, vulnerabilities, and HIV infection in the population. Most HIV infections are not diagnosed until years after infection. There is an urgent need for all MENA countries to develop robust surveillance systems for HIV and STIs and to base their policies on the epidemiological outcome of this surveillance. Due to the absence of such surveillance, resources are not being allocated according to need.

Essential to transforming social attitudes in MENA is the growing participation of PLHIV in the national response. Prevailing stigma and discrimination in relation to HIV/AIDS have been a serious impediment to the proliferation and visibility of the HIV engagement of civil society and other nongovernmental partners. However, MENA has witnessed a growing movement of PLHIV over the past few years.

Walking the fine line between law enforcement and public health will necessitate strong political commitment and a solid and effective partnership between different sectors, such as the police, national AIDS programs, NGOs, and communities. Without a multisectoral approach and partnerships with civil society, key populations, and PLHIV, the HIV response in MENA will be severely limited in its ability to control HIV spread.

BIBLIOGRAPHY

AIDS Algérie/UNAIDS/UNFPA. 2005. *Travail du Sexe et VIH/SIDA en Algérie; Enquête qualitative sur le travail du sexe et le VIH/SIDA.* AIDS Algeria/UNAIDS/UNFPA. 2005.

Al Dhahry, S. H., E. M. Scrimgeour, A. R. Al Suwaid, M. R. Al Lawati, H. S. El Khatim, M. F. Al Kobaisi, and T. C. Merigan. 2004. "Human Immunodeficiency Virus Type 1 Infection in Oman: Antiretroviral Therapy and Frequencies of Drug Resistance Mutations." *AIDS Res Hum Retroviruses* 20: 1166–72.

Algeria National AIDS Council. 2009. "Algeria National Strategy of the HIV/AIDS Response for 2009–2012."

Aziz, A., A. Malek, S. Kozman, D. Rezk, A. Sawy, and Y. Shafei. 2007. "The Impact of Harm Reduction Program on IDUs Knowledge and Preventive Practice:

---

[56] WHO/EMRO, "Technical Paper."

A Pilot Experience." International Conference on the Reduction of Drug Related Harm, Warsaw, abstract.

Benjaber, K., J. L. Rey, and H. Himmich. 2005. "A Study on Antiretroviral Treatment Compliance in Casablanca (Morocco)." *Med Mal Infect* 35: 390–95.

Busulwa, R. 2003. "HIV/AIDS Situation Analysis Study." Conducted in Hodeidah, Taiz and Hadhramut, Republic of Yemen.

Des Jarlais, D. C., M. Marmor, D. Paone, S. Titus, Q. Shi, T. Perlis, B. Jose, and S. R. Friedman. 1996. "HIV Incidence among Injecting Drug Users in New York City Syringe—Exchange Programmes." *Lancet* 348: 987–91.

Dewachi, O. 2001. "HIV/AIDS Prevention through Outreach to Vulnerable Populations in Beirut, Lebanon: Men Who Have Sex with Other Men and HIV AIDS; A Situation Analysis in Beirut, Lebanon." Final report, April 29.

Djibouti National AIDS Programme. 2008. "Programme de lutte contre le sida: Suivi des indicateurs d'alerte rapide à la résistance aux médicaments antirétroviraux en République de Djibouti." République de Djibouti, Ministère de la Sante, document de référence.

Egypt Ministry of Health and Population, and National AIDS Program. 2006. *HIV/AIDS Biological and Behavioral Surveillance Survey*. Summary report, Cairo, Egypt.

Elrashied, S. 2006. "Prevalence, Knowledge and Related Risky Sexual Behaviours of HIV/AIDS among Receptive Men Who Have Sex with Men (MSM) in Khartoum State, Sudan, 2005." XVI International AIDS Conference, Toronto, August 13–18, abstract TUPE0509.

Gheiratmand, R., R. Navipour, M. Mohebbi, K. Hosseini, M. Motaghian-Monazzam, A. Mallik, et al. 2004. "A Country Study to Review Existing Capacity Building and Management of the Training of Teachers on Preventive Education against HIV/AIDS in the Schools in I.R. Iran."

Hsairi, M., and S. Ben Abdallah. 2007. "Analyse de la situation de vulnérabilité vis-à-vis de l'infection à VIH des hommes ayant des relations sexuelles avec des hommes." For ATL MST sida NGO–Tunis Section, National AIDS Programme/DSSB, UNAIDS. Final report, abridged version.

Jenkins, C., and D. A. Robalino. 2003. "HIV in the Middle East and North Africa: The Cost of Inaction." Orientations in Development Series, World Bank.

Karouaoui, A. 2008. "Report of Mission on HIV and Sex Work in Oman." UNAIDS, RST, Cairo, Egypt.

Kocken, P., T. Voorham, J. Brandsma, and W. Swart. 2001. "Effects of Peer-Led AIDS Education Aimed at Turkish and Moroccan Male Immigrants in the Netherlands: A Randomised Controlled Evaluation Study." *Eur J Public Health* 11: 153–59.

Lebanon National AIDS Control Program. 2008. "A Case Study of the First Legal, Above-Ground LGBT Organization in the Mena Region." Helem, Beirut, Lebanon.

———. 2004. "AIDS/HIV National Strategic Plan: Lebanon 2004–2009." Ministry of Public Health, United Nations Theme Group on HIV/AIDS.

Metzger, D. S., G. E. Woody, A. T. McLellan, C. P. O'Brien, P. Druley, H. Navaline, D. DePhilippis, P. Stolley, and E. Abrutyn. 1993. "Human Immunodeficiency Virus Seroconversion among Intravenous Drug Users in- and out-of-Treatment: An 18-Month Prospective Follow-Up." *J Acquir Immune Defic Syndr* 6: 1049–56.

Mohebbi, M. R., and R. Navipour. 2004. "Preventive Education against HIV/AIDS in the Schools of Iran." *Indian Pediatr* 41: 966–67.

Morocco National STI/AIDS Programme. 2007. "National Strategic Plan to Fight AIDS 2007–2011." Ministry of Public Health/Department of Epidemiology and Disease Response, Kingdom of Morocco.

ONUSIDA/El Karaouaoui A. 2008. *Rapport de fin de Mission Appui aux Programmes de Prévention SIDA auprès des Professionnelles du Sexe*. Caire-Egypte-2008.

Pakistan National AIDS Control Program. 2006–7. *HIV Second Generation Surveillance in Pakistan*. National Report Round II. Ministry of Health, Pakistan, and Canada-Pakistan HIV/AIDS Surveillance Project.

———. 2008. *HIV Second Generation Surveillance in Pakistan*. National Report Round III. Ministry of Health, Pakistan, Canada-Pakistan HIV/AIDS Surveillance Project.

Punjab Provincial AIDS Control Programme. 2005. "The Lethal Overdose: Injecting Drug Use and HIV/AIDS."

Semini, I., P. Njogou, and I. Mortagy. 2004. *UNHCR/UNAIDS Joint Mission; HIV/AIDS Assessment Mission in Refugee Setting in Yemen*. September.

Shah, S. A., A. Altaf, R. Khanani, and S. H. Vermund. 2005. "Antiretroviral Drugs Obtained without Prescription for Treatment of HIV/AIDS in Pakistan: Patient Mismanagement as a Serious Threat for Drug Resistance." *J Coll Physicians Surg Pak* 15: 378.

Skoun. 2009. "New Perspectives for the Prevention and Treatment of Addictions." Conference proceedings, October 7–9, 2009.

SNAP (Sudan National AIDS Programme), and UNAIDS (Joint United Nations Programme on HIV/AIDS). 2006. "HIV/AIDS Integrated Report North Sudan, 2004–2005 (Draft)." With United Nations General Assembly Special Session on HIV/AIDS Declaration of Commitment.

Syria Ministry of Health, UNODC (United Nations Office on Drugs and Crime), and UNAIDS. 2007. "Assessment on Drug Use and HIV in Syria." Draft report, July.

Syria National AIDS Programme. 2004. "HIV/AIDS Female Sex Workers KABP Survey in Syria."

Todd, C. S., Y. Barbera-Lainez, S. C. Doocy, A. Ahmadzai, F. M. Delawar, and G. M. Burnham. 2007. "Prevalence of Human Immunodeficiency Virus Infection, Risk Behavior, and HIV Knowledge among Tuberculosis Patients in Afghanistan." *Sex Transm Dis* 34: 878–82.

UNAIDS (Joint United Nations Programme on HIV/AIDS). 2008. "Notes on AIDS in the Middle East and North Africa." RST MENA.

UNAIDS/AIDS Project Management Group (APMG) (2007). *Recommendations for Interventions Addressing Injecting Drug Use and Related HIV Infection in Egypt; Egypt HIV and Injecting Drug Use Supplementary Report*. UNAIDS. October 2007.

UNAIDS, and ASAP. 2008. "Review of National AIDS Strategic Plan in the Middle East and North Africa." RST MENA, December.

UNAIDS, UNODC (United Nations Office on Drugs and Crime), and WHO (World Health Organization). 2006. "Fact Sheet on Drug Use and HIV in MENA." November.

van Ameijden, E. J., J. K. Watters, J. A. van den Hoek, and R. A. Coutinho. 1995. "Interventions among Injecting Drug Users: Do They Work?" *AIDS* 9 Suppl A: S75–84.

WHO/EMRO (Eastern Mediterranean Regional Office). "Technical Paper on the Regional Strategy for STI Prevention and Control in the Eastern Mediterranean Region of WHO presented at the Regional Committee 55.

———. 2005. "Survey on Status of National AIDS Programme Implementation in the Health Sector."

——— . 2006 "Progress towards Universal Access to HIV Prevention, Treatment and Care in the Health Sector." Report on a baseline survey for the year 2005 in the WHO Eastern Mediterranean Region. Draft.

———. 2007. "Progress towards Universal Access to HIV Prevention, Treatment and Care in the Health Sector." Report on an indicator survey for the year 2007 in the WHO Eastern Mediterranean Region.

———. 2008a. "Progress towards Universal Access to HIV Prevention, Treatment and Care in the Health Sector. Report on an indicator survey for the year 2007 in the WHO Eastern Mediterranean Region."

———. 2008b. "Regional Review of HIV Testing and Counseling Policies and Practices in the EMR." WHO/EMRO, FHI, unpublished.

WHO, UNAIDS, and UNICEF (United Nations Children's Fund). 2008. "Towards Universal Access: Scaling Up Priority HIV/AIDS Interventions in the Health Sector." Progress report, WHO/UNAIDS/UNICEF, Geneva.

World Bank. 2005. "Preventing HIV/AIDS in the Middle East and North Africa: A Window of Opportunity to Act." Orientations in Development Series, World Bank.

Zamani, S., M. Kihara, M. M. Gouya, M. Vazirian, M. Ono-Kihara, E. M. Razzaghi, and S. Ichikawa. 2005. "Prevalence of and Factors Associated with HIV-1 Infection among Drug Users Visiting Treatment Centers in Tehran, Iran." *AIDS* 19: 709–16.

Chapter 13

Summary of Recommendations

This chapter focuses on key strategic recommendations related to the human immunodeficiency virus (HIV) epidemiology in the Middle East and North Africa (MENA) presented in this report. The following recommendations are based on the identification of the HIV epidemic status in MENA, through this synthesis, as a low HIV prevalence setting, but with rising concentrated epidemics among priority populations. General directions for prevention interventions as warranted by the outcome of this synthesis are also briefly discussed, but detailed recommendations are beyond the realm of this report. It is not part of the scope of this report to provide intervention recommendations for each MENA country.

RECOMMENDATION 1: INCREASE AND EXPAND BASELINE AND CONTINUED SURVEILLANCE

The data synthesis and HIV transmission concentration in priority populations, as described in this report, highlight the need for HIV surveillance of these at-risk groups. However, resistance to acknowledging the existence of priority populations including injecting drug users (IDUs), men who have sex with men (MSM), and female sex workers (FSWs) can still be found among stakeholders in MENA. The low HIV prevalence found in sporadic and nonrepresentative populations at low risk of infection, such as blood donors, is feeding a culture of complacency toward the epidemic that is blind to the reality of nascent HIV epidemics in hard-to-reach and stigmatized populations. The low HIV prevalence in the general population may mask a much higher prevalence in priority populations.

HIV is not spreading evenly among the different subpopulations within each MENA country. Finding the subpopulations where HIV is currently spreading is a key challenge.[1] Inadequate surveillance continues to be one of the most pervasive problems in the region.[2] Despite recent progress in several countries such as Morocco and Sudan, epidemiological and methodological surveillance remains limited.[3] Although surveillance has been expanded to include sentinel surveillance of pregnant women in a few countries, efforts need to be expanded and focused on surveillance of priority and vulnerable populations, including the mapping of risk and vulnerability factors, risk behavior measures, population size estimations, and, importantly, measurements of HIV prevalence and biomarkers of risk such as sexually transmitted infections (STIs) and hepatitis C virus (HCV) prevalence levels. Mapping of priority populations is a necessary prerequisite to prevention efforts among these groups. The

---

[1] El Feki, "Middle-Eastern AIDS Efforts."
[2] UNAIDS and WHO, *AIDS Epidemic Update 2006.*
[3] Obermeyer, "HIV in the Middle East."

surveillance system must be tailored to the epidemic state of each country.[4]

Integrated biobehavioral surveillance surveys (IBBSS) of representative priority populations should be the main component of surveillance efforts,[5] rather than relying on facility-based surveillance using convenient population samples. This is particularly true in settings of low prevalence or concentrated HIV epidemics, as is the case in MENA.[6] Resources should not be wasted on surveillance of low-risk populations while overlooking HIV spread in priority populations. Surveillance systems in the former Soviet republics focused on pregnant women and tested millions of them, but found very limited HIV spread.[7] At the time, HIV was raging among IDUs.[8]

Repeated IBBSS monitors trends over time by combining HIV sero-surveillance with biomarker surveillance and risk behavior surveillance.[9] This allows pinpointing of windows of opportunity for early intervention when necessary.[10] Biomarker surveillance, such as that of herpes simplex virus 2 (HSV-2) and HCV, is an indispensable component of HIV surveillance. This facilitates the collection and analysis of essential data needed for programming interventions and evaluating impact.

The surveillance should be appropriate for the phase of the epidemic and focus resources where they can provide the most useful data. Biological and behavioral data should be used to validate one another, and information from other sources as well should be integrated within the surveillance system. Programmatic data from voluntary counseling and testing (VCT) and antiretroviral therapy (ART) clinics can also inform epidemic patterns. This allows a deeper understanding of the factors involved in emerging epidemics. In other words, "know your epidemic," and at a local level.[11]

RECOMMENDATION 2: EXPAND SCIENTIFIC RESEARCH AND FORMULATE EVIDENCE-INFORMED POLICIES

This data synthesis highlights a large gap in methodological, scientific research in relation to HIV and other STI epidemiology in MENA. Although scientific research is often recognized in HIV national policies,[12] limited human and financial resources are key challenges. In turn, this is preventing the region from formulating effective and evidence-informed policies.[13]

MENA also has a poor record in utilizing existing sources of data. Valuable data sources are often ignored even though they can provide useful insights into HIV dynamics and trends. For instance, methodological analyses of the millions of HIV tests that are conducted yearly may provide hints about populations where HIV incidence is increasing. The depth and breadth of these analyses would significantly increase if HIV tests were supplemented with the collection of basic demographic and behavioral data and if additional serological tests, such as for HSV-2, were conducted on subsamples of these tests.

In terms of research priorities, the first priority is conducting repeated multicenter IBBSS studies of priority groups to monitor trends over time, combining HIV sero-surveillance with STI, HCV, and risk behavior surveillance: These studies also need to explore the network structures among these risk groups, including both sexual and injecting drug networks.

The second priority is research on mapping and size estimation of hard-to-reach priority populations because this will be essential for the quantitative assessments of HIV epidemiology and trends and would help in planning more effective prevention strategies and programs.

The third priority is conducting multicenter cohort or cross-sectional studies of the vulnerable populations, particularly the youth, to assess HIV and other STIs' incidence, other infectious disease incidence such as HCV, sexual and injecting drug use risk behaviors, and drivers of risky behavior. With the high rates of population mobility in MENA, it is also informative to assess the levels of risky behavior and infection

[4] Pisani et al., "HIV Surveillance."

[5] UNAIDS and WHO, Guidelines; Reider and Dehne, "HIV/AIDS Surveillance"; Sun et al., "The Development of HIV/AIDS Surveillance in China."

[6] Ghys, Jenkins, and Pisani, "HIV Surveillance."

[7] Pisani et al., "HIV Surveillance."

[8] Ibid.

[9] Reintjes and Wiessing, "2nd-Generation HIV Surveillance."

[10] Pisani et al., "HIV Surveillance."

[11] Wilson and Halperin, "Know Your Epidemic."

[12] SNAP, National Policy on HIV/AIDS.

[13] Khan and Hyder, "Responses to an Emerging Threat."

among migrants because data on this population remain rather limited, and the socioeconomic context of migration in this region may predispose this population to risk behavior practices.

The fourth priority is conducting mathematical modeling and cost-effectiveness studies to explore the full range of the complex HIV dynamics and intervention impacts in MENA. These studies would build inferences and suggest policy recommendations by utilizing the individual and population-level data that will become increasingly available over the next few years from surveillance studies on priority populations.[14]

RECOMMENDATION 3: FOCUS ON RISK AND VULNERABILITY, NOT ON LAW ENFORCEMENT

MENA has a history of approaching challenges through a "security" prism and often stakeholders believe that the HIV question is a question of law enforcement to prevent risk practices. This is at odds with the reality gleaned from this synthesis. HIV is merely a reflection of existing contours of risk and vulnerability in the societies in which it is spreading and cannot be addressed fundamentally except by addressing the underlying causes of these risks and vulnerabilities. Sex work, for example, is a reflection of demand and supply mechanisms where the existence of a massive bulge of single and often unemployed youth, and omnipresent pockets of wealth, are creating strong demand for sex work, and on the supply side, the large income disparity, poverty, and complex emergencies are fueling an ample supply of sex workers. Repressive measures on priority populations will only complicate efforts, increase hidden risky behaviors, and discourage the these populations from seeking aid and information. This would not change the vulnerability settings, but would deprive us of the ability to control the epidemic and administer prevention interventions as needed.

The failure of the "security" approach is manifest in the case of injecting drug use. For a long time the region depended on failed supply-reduction policies that focused on criminalizing drug use.[15] This only acted to exacerbate the problem. In Libya, restrictions imposed on the sale of needles and syringes at pharmacies in the late 1990s contributed to an increase in the use of nonsterile injecting equipment and led consequently to a rapid growth of HIV infections among IDUs since 2000.[16] Following this policy failure, Libya has made progress in moving to harm reduction policies.[17] The Islamic Republic of Iran passed through a similar path of policy failure only to become a world leader in a much celebrated harm reduction approach.[18] Use of nonsterile equipment decreased by half in the Islamic Republic of Iran after making needles and syringes easily available in pharmacies.[19]

Policy, programs, and resources continue to be diverted from where they are needed. The mandatory testing of many population groups at low risk of HIV infection is disconnected from the epidemiological reality of HIV infection in the region. Some of this testing may also violate basic human rights and is likely not effective from a public health perspective. Efforts need to be prioritized to the contours of risk and vulnerability and focus on priority groups. Recognizing the settings of risks and targeting them with effective interventions is the only available path for controlling HIV spread in MENA.

RECOMMENDATION 4: STRENGTHEN CIVIL SOCIETY CONTRIBUTIONS TO HIV EFFORTS

The contribution of civil society to HIV prevention efforts remains limited in MENA despite recent progress. One of the structural weaknesses of the HIV response is the meager contribution of nongovernmental organizations (NGOs), community organizations, and people living with HIV (PLHIV) groups in the formulation, planning, and implementation of the response. Strengthening civil society contributions to HIV efforts is essential due to the epidemiological reality of HIV transmission

[14] American University, "Reaching 'Hard to Reach' Population."
[15] Razzaghi et al., "HIV/AIDS Harm Reduction in Iran."
[16] Tawilah and Ball, "WHO/EMRO & WHO/HQ Mission."
[17] Razzaghi et al., "HIV/AIDS Harm Reduction in Iran"; Butler, "Libya Progresses on HIV."
[18] Zamani et al., "Prevalence"; Razzaghi et al., "HIV/AIDS Harm Reduction in Iran"; Ministry of Health and Medical Education of Iran, "Treatment and Medical Education"; Afshar, "From the Assessment to the Implementation"; Afshar and Kasraee, "HIV Prevention Experiences"; WHO/EMRO, "Best Practice."
[19] UNAIDS and WHO, *AIDS Epidemic Update 2004.*

being concentrated in priority groups, as delineated in this synthesis.

Despite this limitation, the region has seen the foundation of a number of effective NGOs working on HIV efforts in recent years. By the mid-1990s, there were at least 100 NGOs in MENA involved in HIV/AIDS prevention and education, although with limited capacity.[20] There are a growing number of NGOs and associations in countries such as Algeria, Djibouti, the Arab Republic of Egypt, the Islamic Republic of Iran, Jordan, Lebanon, Morocco, and Sudan. These organizations provide much needed support for HIV prevention and treatment, including outreach centers for IDUs, FSWs, and MSM.

Some of the NGOs have made impressive achievements, such as the comprehensive harm reduction approach by the Iranian NGO Persepolis that provides needle exchange, methadone maintenance, general medical care, VCT, and referral.[21] In the Islamic Republic of Iran, NGOs have played a leading role in the transformation to effective policies as well as the promotion of close cooperation between health authorities, prison departments, judiciary authorities, academic institutions, religious leaders, and other stakeholders.[22]

Another achievement is Helem in Lebanon, the first and only aboveground organization working with MSM in MENA.[23] Helem has made admirable contributions in addressing the health, legal, psychological, and social needs of MSM, by far the most culturally sensitive group of all priority groups.[24] Helem is also involved in scientific surveillance research work and VCT efforts with MSM.[25] In Djibouti, there have been a number of initiatives to address the high-risk behaviors among truck drivers and FSWs along the trade corridor, such as the High Risk Corridor Initiative.[26]

The attitude toward NGOs from outside the region can be negative among MENA populations.[27] There is no escaping the fact that grassroots NGOs need to be developed within MENA. Considering the cultural sensitivity of working with priority groups, a successful formula for HIV efforts may be government organized NGOs (GONGOs), where governments fund and support NGOs to discreetly provide services to priority groups, such as sex worker self-help groups.[28] NGOs may enable governments to deal with priority groups indirectly, thereby avoiding cultural sensitivities in explicit outreach efforts among stigmatized populations.[29] Discreet interventions for HIV prevention have been proven effective in Bangladesh,[30] Lebanon,[31] Morocco,[32] and Pakistan.[33]

RECOMMENDATION 5: AN OPPORTUNITY FOR PREVENTION

There is still an opportunity for prevention that should not be missed to avert a larger epidemic[34] and avoid the health and socioeconomic cost that the MENA region is largely unprepared to pay.[35] It appears that there is increasingly a political feasibility for implementing and scaling up interventions, including those involving priority populations.[36] Resources need to be allocated for interventions for the priority populations irrespective of whether these groups are "culturally safe" or not.[37] Developing mechanisms for working with priority populations, even if discreetly, need to be explored. Efforts in MENA continue to be focused on awareness-raising activities among the general population, which is the group at the lowest risk of infection.

[20] Wahdan, "The Middle East."

[21] Razzaghi et al., "HIV/AIDS Harm Reduction in Iran"; Vazirian et al., "Needle and Syringe Sharing."

[22] Razzaghi et al., "HIV/AIDS Harm Reduction in Iran"; Ohiri et al., "HIV/AIDS."

[23] Lebanon National AIDS Control Program, "A Case Study" (2008a).

[24] International HIV/AIDS Alliance, "Supporting Men Who Have Sex with Men in Lebanon," http://www.aidsalliance.org/sw51051.asp, accessed on January 12, 2007.

[25] Mishwar, "An Integrated Bio-Behavioral Surveillance Study"; Lebanon National AIDS Control Program, "A Case Study" (2008a); Lebanon National AIDS Control Program, "A Case Study" (2008b).

[26] O'Grady, "WFP Consultant Visit to Djibouti Report."

[27] Blowfield, "Fundamentalists Call the Shots."

[28] Jenkins, "Report on Sex Worker Consultation in Iran."

[29] Razzaghi et al., "HIV/AIDS Harm Reduction in Iran"; Vazirian et al., "Needle and Syringe Sharing."

[30] Jenkins et al., "Male Prostitutes."

[31] Jenkins and Robalino, "HIV in the Middle East and North Africa."

[32] Tawil et al., "HIV Prevention"; Boushaba et al., "Marginalization and Vulnerability."

[33] Jenkins et al., "Male Prostitutes."

[34] Khawaja et al., "HIV/AIDS and Its Risk Factors in Pakistan"; World Bank, "Preventing HIV/AIDS in the Middle East and North Africa"; Zaheer et al., "STIs and HIV in Pakistan."

[35] Jenkins and Robalino, "HIV in the Middle East and North Africa."

[36] Buse, "Political Feasibility of Scaling-Up."

[37] UNAIDS, "Notes on AIDS in the Middle East and North Africa"; Jordan National AIDS Program, "National HIV/AIDS Strategy for Jordan 2005–9."

There is a need to invest in comprehensive analysis of the current gaps of as well as intervention opportunities for the HIV response. This can be started by combining implementation of the transmission modes analysis for each country with the mapping of current interventions, including the taxonomy of prevention.

To maximize intervention impact, emphasis should be on using existing resources, such as integrating STI prevention into the reproductive health programs. Blood banks and facilities can also help in communicating blood-borne virus prevention messages.[38]

Interventions need to capitalize on the strengths represented by cultural traditions, and yet be culturally sensitive while fostering effective responses to the epidemic.[39] Interventions among IDUs, including those in prison, such as needle and syringe exchange, opioid substitution therapies, and HIV testing and counseling, have shown effectiveness against HIV infection[40] and need to be expanded. Lessons also need to be learned from other successful experiences in the control of sexually transmitted diseases, particularly from resource-limited settings.[41]

Intervention methodology should emphasize identifying places, rather than individuals, where high-risk sexual or injecting activities are present.[42] In this fashion, the central and key nodes of risk networks, instead of the peripheral ones, can be reached and used as a springboard for interventions such as condom distribution.[43] This would also help targeting the "cut points" and the "bridges" between subcomponents in sexual and injecting networks where interventions are most needed and effective.[44]

Access to testing, care, and treatment services should be expanded substantially. It is imperative to remove all barriers to HIV testing and diagnosis, particularly among priority groups, to impede the transmission chains driven by the short primary stage of infection following HIV infection.[45] Molecular epidemiology studies and quantitative assessments of priority populations have shown high levels of genetic clustering where at least 25% of HIV infections originate from HIV-positive persons in their primary infection.[46] It is believed that the large disparity in HIV testing and diagnosis between Caucasian and African American MSM in the United States is a key determinant of the striking difference in HIV incidence among these two racial groups.[47] Anonymous testing needs to be expanded, and it has already proved its utility in attracting hidden populations.[48]

Although countries need to address the structural factors that drive risk behavior practices, the priority in the public health sector should be on addressing the direct factors that put individuals at risk of HIV exposure, because tackling structural factors takes time and is beyond the control of the public health community.[49] Because almost all infections occur when an infected individual shares body fluids with an uninfected individual, prevention programs must focus on addressing the situations in which this is happening.[50] Careful analysis of the transmission patterns must be conducted to inform policy decisions.[51]

Beyond doubt, *harm reduction* should be at the core of intervention policy, and targeted prevention should go further than harm reduction. The concept of harm reduction should be applied not only to IDUs, but should also be considered for MSM and FSWs as well. Harm reduction is a direct and effective strategy to stem the tide of HIV, considering that addressing the root causes of risks and vulnerabilities might be a much more challenging task. The Islamic Republic of Iran has already paved the way by showing how harm reduction can be implemented within the cultural fabric of MENA and in consonance with religious values.

[38] Razzaghi et al., "Profiles of Risk."

[39] Obermeyer, "HIV in the Middle East"; Lazarus et al., "HIV/AIDS Knowledge and Condom Use"; Aden, Dahlgren, and Guerra, "Experiences against HIV/AIDS/STDS."

[40] Des Jarlais et al., "HIV Incidence"; Metzger et al., "Human Immunodeficiency Virus Seroconversion"; van Ameijden et al., "Interventions among Injecting Drug Users"; Jurgens, Ball, and Verster, "Interventions to Reduce HIV Transmission."

[41] Cohen et al., "Successful Eradication of Sexually Transmitted Diseases."

[42] Weir et al., "From People to Places."

[43] Doherty et al., "Determinants and Consequences of Sexual Networks."

[44] Wasserman and Faust, *Social Network Analysis.*

[45] Pilcher, et al., "Brief but Efficient."

[46] Abu-Raddad et al., "Genital Herpes"; Brenner et al., "High Rates of Forward Transmission"; Pao et al., "Transmission of HIV-1"; Yerly et al., "Acute HIV Infection"; Lewis et al., "Episodic Sexual Transmission."

[47] MacKellar et al., "Unrecognized HIV Infection."

[48] Levi et al., "Characteristics of Clients."

[49] Pisani et al., "Back to Basics in HIV Prevention."

[50] Pisani et al., "Back to Basics in HIV Prevention"; Ainsworth and Teokul, "Breaking the Silence."

[51] Ainsworth and Teokul, "Breaking the Silence."

BIBLIOGRAPHY

Abu-Raddad, L. J., A. S. Magaret, C. Celum, A. Wald, I. M. Longini, S. G. Self, and L. Corey. 2008. "Genital Herpes Has Played a More Important Role Than Any Other Sexually Transmitted Infection in Driving HIV Prevalence in Africa." *PLoS ONE* 3: e2230.

Aden, A. S., L. Dahlgren, and R. Guerra. 2004. "Experiences against HIV/AIDS/STDS of Somalis in Exile in Gothenburg, Sweden." *Ann Ig* 16: 141–55.

Afshar, P. Unknown. "From the Assessment to the Implementation of Services Available for Drug Abuse and HIV/AIDS Prevention and Care in Prison Setting: The Experience of Iran." PowerPoint presentation.

Afshar, P., and F. Kasraee. 2005. "HIV Prevention Experiences and Programs in Iranian Prisons" [MoPC0057]. Presented at the Seventh International Congress on AIDS in Asia and the Pacific, Kobe.

Ainsworth, M., and W. Teokul. 2000. "Breaking the Silence: Setting Realistic Priorities for AIDS Control in Less-Developed Countries." *Lancet* 356: 55–60.

American University of Beirut. "Reaching 'Hard to Reach' Population in HIV/AIDS Research in the Middle East: Methodological and Ethical Issues." Workshop held at the American University of Beirut, Lebanon, October 23–25, 2008.

Blowfield, M. 1994. "Fundamentalists Call the Shots." *WorldAIDS*: 3.

Boushaba, A., O. Tawil, L. Imane, and H. Himmich. 1999. "Marginalization and Vulnerability: Male Sex Work in Morocco." In *Men Who Sell Sex: International Perspectives on Males Sex Work and AIDS*, ed. Peter Angleton, 263–74. London: UCL Press.

Brenner, B. G., M. Roger, J. P. Routy, D. Moisi, M. Ntemgwa, C. Matte, J. G. Baril, R. Thomas, D. Rouleau, J. Bruneau, R. Leblanc, M. Legault, C. Tremblay, H. Charest, and M. A. Wainberg. 2007. "High Rates of Forward Transmission Events after Acute/Early HIV-1 Infection." *J Infect Dis* 195: 951–59.

Buse, K., N. Lalji, S. H. Mayhew, M. Imran, and S. J. Hawkes. 2009. "Political Feasibility of Scaling-Up Five Evidence-Informed HIV Interventions in Pakistan: A Policy Analysis." *Sex Transm Infect* 85 Suppl 2: ii37–42.

Butler, D. 2008. "Libya Progresses on HIV." *Nature* 452: 138.

Chen, L., P. Jha, B. Stirling, S. K. Sgaier, T. Daid, R. Kaul, and N. Nagelkerke. 2007. "Sexual Risk Factors for HIV Infection in Early and Advanced HIV Epidemics in Sub-Saharan Africa: Systematic Overview of 68 Epidemiological Studies." *PLoS ONE* 2: e1001.

Cohen, M. S., G. E. Henderson, P. Aiello, and H. Zheng. 1996. "Successful Eradication of Sexually Transmitted Diseases in the People's Republic of China: Implications for the 21st Century." *J Infect Dis* 174 Suppl 2: S223–29.

Des Jarlais, D. C., M. Marmor, D. Paone, S. Titus, Q. Shi, T. Perlis, B. Jose, and S. R. Friedman. 1996. "HIV Incidence among Injecting Drug Users in New York City Syringe-Exchange Programmes." *Lancet* 348: 987–91.

Doherty, I. A., N. S. Padian, C. Marlow, and S. O. Aral. 2005. "Determinants and Consequences of Sexual Networks as They Affect the Spread of Sexually Transmitted Infections." *J Infect Dis* 191 Suppl 1: S42–54.

El Feki, S. 2006. "Middle-Eastern AIDS Efforts Are Starting to Tackle Taboos." *Lancet* 367: 975–76.

Ghys, P. D., C. Jenkins, and E. Pisani. 2001. "HIV Surveillance among Female Sex Workers." *AIDS* 15 Suppl 3: S33–40.

Jenkins, C. 2006. "Report on Sex Worker Consultation in Iran." Sponsored by UNAIDS and UNFPA, Dec 2–18.

Jenkins, C., and D. A. Robalino. 2003. "HIV in the Middle East and North Africa: The Cost of Inaction." Orientations in Development Series, World Bank.

Jenkins, C., A. Shale, R. Habibur, and M. M. Faisal. 2001. "Male Prostitutes in Dhaka: Risk Reduction through Effective Intervention." Paper presented at the International Conference on AIDS in the Asia-Pacific, Melbourne, October.

Jordan National AIDS Program. 2005. "National HIV/AIDS Strategy for Jordan 2005–9." Draft.

Jurgens, R., A. Ball, and A. Verster. 2009. "Interventions to Reduce HIV Transmission Related to Injecting Drug Use in Prison." *Lancet Infect Dis* 9: 57–66.

Khan, O. A., and A. A. Hyder. 2001. "Responses to an Emerging Threat: HIV/AIDS Policy in Pakistan." *Health Policy Plan* 16: 214–18.

Khawaja, Z. A., L. Gibney, A. J. Ahmed, and S. H. Vermund. 1997. "HIV/AIDS and Its Risk Factors in Pakistan." *AIDS* 11: 843–48.

Lazarus, J. V., H. M. Himedan, L. R. Ostergaard, and J. Liljestrand. 2006. "HIV/AIDS Knowledge and Condom Use among Somali and Sudanese Immigrants in Denmark." *Scand J Public Health* 34: 92–99.

Lebanon National AIDS Control Program. 2008a. "A Case Study of the First Legal, Above-Ground LGBT Organization in the MENA Region." Helem.

———. 2008b. "A Case Study on Establishing and Building Capacities for VCT Centers for HIV/AIDS in Lebanon." Beirut, Lebanon.

Levi, I., B. Modan, T. Blumstein, O. Luxenburg, T. Yehuda-Cohen, B. Shasha, A. Lotan, A. Bundstein, A. Barzilai, and E. Rubinstein. 2001. "Characteristics of Clients Attending Confidential versus Anonymous Testing Clinics for Human Immunodeficiency Virus." *Isr Med Assoc J* 3: 184–87.

Lewis, F., G. J. Hughes, A. Rambaut, A. Pozniak, and A. J. Leigh Brown. 2008. "Episodic Sexual Transmission of HIV Revealed by Molecular Phylodynamics." *PLoS Med* 5: e50.

MacKellar, D. A., L. A. Valleroy, G. M. Secura, S. Behel, T. Bingham, D. D. Celentano, B. A. Koblin, M. Lalota, W. McFarland, D. Shehan, H. Thiede, L. V. Torian, and R. S. Janssen. 2005. "Unrecognized HIV Infection, Risk Behaviors, and Perceptions of Risk among Young Men Who Have Sex with Men: Opportunities for Advancing HIV Prevention in the Third Decade of HIV/AIDS." *J Acquir Immune Defic Syndr* 38: 603–14.

Metzger, D. S., G. E. Woody, A. T. McLellan, C. P. O'Brien, P. Druley, H. Navaline, D. DePhilippis, P. Stolley, and E. Abrutyn. 1993. "Human

Immunodeficiency Virus Seroconversion among Intravenous Drug Users in- and out-of-Treatment: An 18-Month Prospective Follow-Up." *J Acquir Immune Defic Syndr* 6: 1049–56.

Ministry of Health and Medical Education of Iran. 2006. "Treatment and Medical Education." Islamic Republic of Iran HIV/AIDS situation and response analysis.

Mishwar. 2008. "An Integrated Bio-Behavioral Surveillance Study among Four Vulnerable Groups in Lebanon: Men Who Have Sex with Men; Prisoners; Commercial Sex Workers and Intravenous Drug Users." Final report.

O'Grady, M. 2004. "WFP Consultant Visit to Djibouti Report." July 30.

Obermeyer, C. M. 2006. "HIV in the Middle East." *BMJ* 333: 851–54.

Ohiri, K., M. Claeson, E. Razzaghi, B. Nassirimanesh, P. Afshar, and R. Power. 2006. "HIV/AIDS Prevention among Injecting Drug Users Learning from Harm Reduction in Iran." Iranian National Center for Addiction Studies, Persepolis NGO, Iran Prison Organization, and the World Bank

Pao, D., M. Fisher, S. Hue, G. Dean, G. Murphy, P. A. Cane, C. A. Sabin, and D. Pillay. 2005. "Transmission of HIV-1 during Primary Infection: Relationship to Sexual Risk and Sexually Transmitted Infections." *AIDS* 19: 85–90.

Pilcher, C. D., H. C. Tien, J. J. Eron, Jr., P. L. Vernazza, S. Y. Leu, P. W. Stewart, L. E. Goh, and M. S. Cohen. 2004. "Brief but Efficient: Acute HIV Infection and the Sexual Transmission of HIV." *J Infect Dis* 189: 1785–92.

Pisani, E., G. P. Garnett, N. C. Grassly, T. Brown, J. Stover, C. Hankins, N. Walker, and P. D. Ghys. 2003. "Back to Basics in HIV Prevention: Focus on Exposure." *BMJ* 326: 1384–87.

Pisani, E., S. Lazzari, N. Walker, and B. Schwartlander. 2003. "HIV Surveillance: A Global Perspective." *J Acquir Immune Defic Syndr* 32 Suppl 1: S3–11.

Razzaghi, E. M., A. R. Movaghar, T. C. Green, and K. Khoshnood. 2006. "Profiles of Risk: A Qualitative Study of Injecting Drug Users in Tehran, Iran." *Harm Reduct J* 3: 12.

Razzaghi, E., B. Nassirimanesh, P. Afshar, K. Ohiri, M. Claeson, and R. Power. 2006. "HIV/AIDS Harm Reduction in Iran." *Lancet* 368: 434–35.

Reider, G., and K. L. Dehne. 1999. "HIV/AIDS Surveillance in Developing Countries: Experiences and Issues." Eschborn, Germany, Deutsche Gesellschaft für Technische Zusammenarbeit (GTZ).

Reintjes, R., and L. Wiessing. 2007. "2nd-generation HIV Surveillance and Injecting Drug Use: Uncovering the Epidemiological Ice-Berg." *Int J Public Health* 52: 166–72.

SNAP (Sudan National AIDS Control Programme). 2005. *National Policy on HIV/AIDS*. Ministry of Health.

Sun, X. N. Wang, D. Li, X. Zheng, S. Qu, L. Wang, F. Lu, and K. Poundstone. 2007. "The Development of HIV/AIDS Surveillance in China." *AIDS* 21 Suppl 8: S33–38.

Tawil, O., K. O'Reilly, I. M. Coulibaly, A. Tiemele, H. Himmich, A. Boushaba, K. Pradeep, and M. Carael.

1999. "HIV Prevention among Vulnerable Populations: Outreach in the Developing World." *AIDS* 13 Suppl A: S239–47.

Tawilah, J., and A. Ball. 2003. "WHO/EMRO & WHO/HQ Mission to Libyan Arab Jamahiriya to Undertake an Initial Assessment of the HIV/AIDS and STI Situation and National AIDS Programme." Tripoli, June 15–19.

UNAIDS (Joint United Nations Programme on HIV/AIDS). 2008. "Notes on AIDS in the Middle East and North Africa." RST MENA.

UNAIDS, and WHO (World Health Organization). 2000. *Guidelines for Second Generation HIV Surveillance: The Next Decade*. Geneva: WHO.

———. 2004. *AIDS Epidemic Update 2004*. Geneva.

———. 2006. *AIDS Epidemic Update 2006*. Geneva.

van Ameijden, E. J., J. K. Watters, J. A. van den Hoek, and R. A. Coutinho. 1995. "Interventions among Injecting Drug Users: Do They Work?" *AIDS* 9 Suppl A: S75–84.

Vazirian, M., B. Nassirimanesh, S. Zamani, M. Ono-Kihara, M. Kihara, S. M. Ravari, and M. M. Gouya. 2005. "Needle and Syringe Sharing Practices of Injecting Drug Users Participating in an Outreach HIV Prevention Program in Tehran, Iran: A Cross-Sectional Study." *Harm Reduct J* 2: 19.

Wahdan, M. H. 1995. "The Middle East: Past, Present, and Future." *AIDS Asia* 2: 21–23.

Wasserman, S., and K. Faust. 1994. *Social Network Analysis: Methods and Applications*. New York: Cambridge University Press.

Weir, S. S., C. Pailman, X. Mahlalela, N. Coetzee, F. Meidany, and J. T. Boerma. 2003. "From People to Places: Focusing AIDS Prevention Efforts Where It Matters Most." *AIDS* 17: 895–903.

WHO/EMRO (World Health Organization/Eastern Mediterranean Regional Office). 2004. "Best Practice in HIV/AIDS Prevention and Care for Injecting Drug Abusers: The Triangular Clinic in Kermanshah, Islamic Republic of Iran."

Wilson, D., and D. T. Halperin. 2008. "'Know Your Epidemic, Know Your Response': A Useful Approach, If We Get It Right." *Lancet* 372: 423–26.

World Bank. 2005. "Preventing HIV/AIDS in the Middle East and North Africa: A Window of Opportunity to Act." Orientations in Development Series, World Bank.

Yerly, S., S. Vora, P. Rizzardi, J. P. Chave, P. L. Vernazza, M. Flepp, A. Telenti, M. Battegay, A. L. Veuthey, J. P. Bru, M. Rickenbach, B. Hirschel, and L. Perrin. 2001. "Acute HIV Infection: Impact on the Spread of HIV and Transmission of Drug Resistance." *AIDS* 15: 2287–92.

Zaheer, H. A., S. Hawkes, K. Buse, and M. O'Dwyer. 2009. "STIs and HIV in Pakistan: From Analysis to Action." *Sex Transm Infect* 85 Suppl 2: ii1–2.

Zamani, S., M. Kihara, M. M. Gouya, M. Vazirian, M. Ono-Kihara, E. M. Razzaghi, and S. Ichikawa. 2005. "Prevalence of and Factors Associated with HIV-1 Infection among Drug Users Visiting Treatment Centers in Tehran, Iran." *AIDS* 19: 709–16.

Appendix A

Table A.1 Estimated Number of People Living with HIV in MENA Countries

Country	Number of PLHIV
Afghanistan	Not available
Algeria	21,000 (11,000–43,000)
Bahrain	Not available
Djibouti	16,000 (12,000–19,000)
Egypt, Arab Rep. of	9,200 (7,200–13,000)
Iran, Islamic Rep. of	86,000 (68,000–110,000)
Iraq	Not available
Jordan	Not available
Kuwait	Not available
Lebanon	3,000 (1,700–7,200)
Libya	Not available
Morocco	21,000 (15,000–31,000)
Oman	Not available
Pakistan	96,000 (69,000–150,000)
Qatar	Not available
Saudi Arabia	Not available
Somalia	24,000 (13,000–45,000)
Sudan	320,000 (220,000–440,000)
Syrian Arab Republic	Not available
Tunisia	3,700 (2,700–5,400)
United Arab Emirates	Not available
West Bank and Gaza	Not available
Yemen, Rep. of	Not available

Source: UNAIDS Country Database 2008, http://www.unaids.org/en/CountryResponses/Countries/default.asp.
Note: PLHIV = people living with HIV. Numbers within parentheses indicate the range within which the estimate could lie.

Appendix B

Table B.1 shows key differences in the epidemiologic characteristics of several sexually transmitted infections (STIs). These characteristics play a leading role in determining the nature of the infectious spread of these STIs. The effective sexual partner acquisition rate determines the size of the population where the STI transmission chains are sustainable (group of sustainable transmission, GST).[1] The size of the GST in any community determines the potential size of the STI epidemic. Different STIs have different GST sizes.

CRITERIA FOR SCIENTIFIC LITERATURE REVIEW

We used the following criteria for the scientific literature searches in peer-reviewed publications using the Medline (PubMed) database:

1. Studies of HIV infectious spread in its different transmission modes under the strategy of "HIV Seropositivity" OR "HIV" OR "HIV Infections" AND "Middle East" OR "Islam"

Table B.1 Threshold for Sustainable Transmission and Transmission Probability per Partnership for Key STIs

| STI | Duration of infectiousness in years | Transmission probability per partnership | | | Effective mean rate of new sexual partner acquisition per year for sustainable transmission |
		1-Year partnership	10-Year partnership	20-Year partnership	
Gonorrhea[a]	0.5	0.50	0.50	0.50	4
Chlamydia[b]	1.25	0.20	0.20	0.20	4
Syphilis[c]	0.5	0.30	0.30	0.30	7
Chancroid[d]	0.08	0.80	0.80	0.80	15
Herpes simplex virus type 2[e]	Chronic reactivations for lifetime	0.20	0.89	0.99	0.4
Human papillomavirus[f]	Chronic	~1.00	~1.00	~1.00	<0.1
human immunodeficiency virus–1[g]	10	0.16	0.83	0.83	1.4

[a] Brunham and Plummer 1990; Yorke, Hethcote, and Nold 1978.
[b] Brunham and Plummer 1990; Lycke et al. 1980.
[c] Brunham and Plummer 1990; Schroeter et al. 1971.
[d] Brunham and Plummer 1990; Plummer et al. 1983.
[e] Abu-Raddad et al. 2008.
[f] Winer et al. 2003.
[g] Abu-Raddad et al. 2008.

---

[1] Abu-Raddad et al., "Genital Herpes"; Boily and Masse, "Mathematical Models"; Brunham and Plummer, "A General Model."

OR "Arabs" OR "Arab World" OR "Africa, Northern" OR "Mauritania" OR "Sudan" OR "Somalia" OR "Djibouti" OR "Pakistan." As of July 30, 2009, 1,036 publications were identified, covering studies from the early days of the HIV epidemic in MENA up to today. The number of studies has increased substantially in the last few years.

2. Studies of sexual behavior and levels of risk behavior under the strategy of "Sexual Behavior" OR "Sexual Partners" OR "Sexual Abstinence" OR "Unsafe Sex" OR "Sexology" OR "Reproductive Behavior" OR "Safe Sex" OR "Condoms" OR "Sex" AND "Middle East" OR "Islam" OR "Arabs" OR "Arab World" OR "Africa, Northern" OR "Mauritania" OR "Sudan" OR "Somalia" OR "Djibouti" OR "Pakistan." As of July 30, 2009, 1,393 publications were identified, covering diverse issues in sexual and reproductive behavior. Most of these articles are focused on demographic and reproductive issues such as fertility, but still hundreds of articles study or discuss sexual behavior in MENA.

3. Studies of herpes simplex virus type 2 seroprevalence under the strategy of "Herpesvirus 2, Human" OR "Herpes Genitalis" AND "Middle East" OR "Islam" OR "Arabs" OR "Arab World" OR "Africa, Northern" OR "Mauritania" OR "Sudan" OR "Somalia" OR "Djibouti" OR "Pakistan." As of July 30, 2009, 27 publications were identified.

4. Studies of human papillomavirus and cervical cancer under the strategy of "HPV" OR "Human Papillomavirus" OR "Human Papilloma Virus" OR "Cervical Cancer" AND "Middle East" OR "Islam" OR "Arabs" OR "Arab World" OR "Africa, Northern" OR "Mauritania" OR "Sudan" OR "Somalia" OR "Djibouti" OR "Pakistan." As of July 30, 2009, 188 publications were identified.

5. Studies of bacterial STIs under the strategy of "Chlamydia" OR "Chlamydia Infections" OR "Chlamydia Trachomatis" OR "Gonorrhea" OR "Neisseria Gonorrhoeae" OR "Syphilis" OR "Vaginosis, Bacterial" OR "Pelvic Inflammatory Disease" AND "Middle East" OR "Arabs" OR "Islam" OR "Arab World" OR "Africa, Northern" OR "Mauritania" OR "Sudan" OR "Somalia" OR "Djibouti" OR "Pakistan". As of July 30, 2009, 523 publications were identified.

6. Studies of hepatitis C virus under the strategy of "Hepatitis C" OR "Hepatitis C Antibodies" OR "Hepatitis C Antigens" AND "Middle East" OR "Islam" OR "Iran" OR "Arabs" OR "Arab World" OR "Africa, Northern" OR "Mauritania" OR "Sudan" OR "Somalia" OR "Djibouti" OR "Pakistan". As of July 30, 2009, 788 publications were identified.

Appendix C

Table C.1 summarizes the results of HIV point-prevalence surveys in different population groups within the general population in MENA, in addition to the data shown in chapter 6.

Table C.1 HIV Prevalence of Different Population Groups in MENA

Country	HIV prevalence among different population groups
Bahrain	0.0% (outpatient pediatric clinic; Al-Mahroos and Ebrahim 1995)
Djibouti	0.0% (women; Marcelin et al. 2001) 5.0% (women; Marcelin et al. 2002) 5.0% (men; Marcelin et al. 2002)
Egypt, Arab Republic of	0.0% (different population groups; Constantine et al. 1990) 0.0% (tourism workers; El-Sayed et al. 1996) 0.18% (fever patients; Watts et al. 1993) 1.9% (sexual contacts of HIV patients; Watts et al. 1993) 0.07% (international travelers; Watts et al. 1993) 0.97% (non-Egyptian residents; Watts et al. 1993) 0.0% (hospital patients; El-Ghazzawi, Hunsmann, and Schneider 1987) 0.0% (control group in a study; El-Ghazzawi et al. 1995) 0.0% (fire brigade personnel; Quinti et al. 1995; Renganathan et al. 1995) 0.0% (university students; El-Gilany and El-Fedawy 2006)
Iran, Islamic Republic of	0.34% (healthy children; Karimi and Ghavanini 2001) 1.8% (gypsy population; Hosseini Asl, Avijgan, and Mohamadnejad 2004) 0.0% (runaways and other women seeking safe haven; Hajiabdolbaghi et al. 2007)
Jordan	0.0% (public employees; Zamani et al. 2005; Razzaghi et al. 2006; Ministry of Health and Medical Education of Iran 2006; Afshar [date unknown(a)]; Afshar and Kasrace 2005; WHO/EMRO 2004) 0.0% (military personnel; Jordan National AIDS Program, personal communication) 0.0% (prisoners; Jordan National AIDS Program, personal communication) 0.64% (at-risk populations; Anonymous 2006)
Mauritania	0.28% (general population; Baidy et al. 1993)
Morocco	0.0% (newly recruited employees; Morocco MOH 2007) 0.0% (people seeking a health insurance card; Morocco MOH 2007) 0.0% (traditional barbers and their customers; Zahraoui-Mehadji et al. 2004) 0.10% (STD clinic attendees, pregnant women, and patients with pulmonary tuberculosis; Elharti et al. 2002) 0.0% (women at family planning clinics; WHO/EMRO Regional Database on HIV/AIDS) 0.32% (seasonal female laborers; Khattabi and Alami 2005) 0.72% (seasonal female laborers; Bennani and Alami 2006) 0.75% (seasonal female laborers; Morocco MOH 2007) 5.26% (male laborers; Khattabi and Alami 2005) 0.0% (male laborers; Bennani and Alami 2006) 0.0% (hotel staff; Khattabi and Alami 2005) 0.16% (hotel staff; Bennani and Alami 2006) 0.12% (hotel staff; Morocco MOH 2007)

Table C.1 *(Continued)*

Country	HIV prevalence among different population groups
Pakistan	0.23% (15,000 individuals with various characteristics including people suspected of living with HIV; Kayani et al. 1994)
	0.06% (STD attendees, IDUs, hemodialysis patients, suspected people living with HIV, blood donors, ANC attendees, TB patients, travelers abroad, and multitransfused patients; Iqbal and Rehan 1996)
	0.064% (general population; Hyder and Khan 1998)
	5.4% (men reporting extramarital contacts; Hyder and Khan 1998)
	0.0% (health care workers; Aziz et al. 2002)
	0.97% (blood donors and recipients, IDUs, and suspected AIDS cases; Khanani et al. 1990)
	0.06% (blood donors and deported Pakistanis from Persian Gulf countries; Tariq et al. 1993)
	0.0% (IDUs in rehabilitation centers and drug-related arrestees; Khawaja et al. 1997)
	0.1% (high-risk and low-risk populations; Raziq, Alam, and Ali 1993)
	0.007% (general population; Khattak et al. 2002)
	0.0% (two surveys; earthquake victims; Khan et al. 2008)
Saudi Arabia	0% (controls in a study; Bakir et al. 1995)
Somalia	0.0% (military cadets; Corwin et al. 1991)
	0.0% (blood donors and hospitalized children and adults; Nur et al. 2000)
	0.0% (women and neonates; Jama et al. 1987)
	0.0% (hospitalized persons; Scott et al. 1991)
	1.0% (hospitalized persons; Kulane et al. 2000)
Sudan	1.1% (general population; Southern Sudan; Arbesser, Mose, and Sixl 1987)
	2.7% (general population; Southern Sudan; NSNAC and UNAIDS 2006)
	4.3% (women; Southern Sudan; NSNAC and UNAIDS 2006)
	1.0% (general population; Malakal, Southern Sudan; IGAD 2006)
	7.2% (general population; Yambio, Southern Sudan; IGAD 2006)
	12.0% (tea sellers; Southern Sudan; NSNAC and UNAIDS 2006)
	3.0% (female outpatients; Southern Sudan; McCarthy, Khalid, and El Tigani 1995)
	3.0% (outpatients; Juba; Southern Sudan; UNAIDS 2007b ; UNAIDS 2007a)
	4.0% (outpatients; Juba; Southern Sudan; UNAIDS 2007b; UNAIDS 2007a)
	0.8% (pregnant women and STI patients; Komo and Ardi Kanan; Southern Sudan; NSNAC and UNAIDS 2006)
	1.1% (university students; North Sudan; Ahmed 2004l),
	1.2% (women in a suburban community in Khartoum; North Sudan; Kafi, Mohamed, and Musa 2000)
	2.5% (tea sellers; North Sudan; UNAIDS 2008; Ahmed 2004j)
	0.4% (tea sellers; North Sudan; Anonymous 2007)
	0.2% (patients with various malignancies and normal subjects; North Sudan; Fahal et al. 1995)
	0.12% (hospital attendees; North Sudan; Ati 2005)
	1.0% (police officers in Khartoum; North Sudan; Abdelwahab 2006)
Turkey	0.1% (engaged couples; Alim et al. 2009)
Yemen, Republic of	0.0%, 0.17%, 1.26%, and 1.19% (travelers seeking visas to work abroad in different years, respectively; WHO, UNICEF, and UNAIDS 2006s)

Note: ANC = antenatal clinic; IDU = injecting drug use/user; STD = sexually transmitted disease; TB = tuberculosis.

Appendix D

Table D.1 HIV Prevalence among STD Clinic Attendees, VCT Attendees, and People Suspected of Living with HIV

Country	HIV prevalence among STD clinic attendees, VCT attendees, and people suspected of living with HIV
Algeria	2.0% (Institut de Formation Paramédicale de Parnet 2004) 1.24% (Unknown, "Statut de la réponse nationale") 1.26% (Unknown, "Statut de la réponse nationale") 0.25% (Alami 2009) 1.19% (Alami 2009) 2.4% (Alami 2009)
Djibouti	1.0% (Fox et al. 1989) 10.4% (Rodier et al. 1993)
Egypt, Arab Republic of	0.0% (Saleh et al. 2000) 0.23% (Watts et al. 1993) 8.4% (Ali et al. 1998)
Iran, Islamic Republic of	4.1% (Ghannad et al. 2009) 2.0% (Ghannad et al. 2009) 2.2% (Ghannad et al. 2009)
Kuwait	0.0% (Al-Owaish et al. 2000) 0.0% (Al-Fouzan and Al-Mutairi 2004) 0.0% (Al-Mutairi et al. 2007)
Morocco	0.15% (Khattabi and Alami 2005) 0.08% (Khattabi and Alami 2005) 0.25% (Khattabi and Alami 2005) 0.16% (Khattabi and Alami 2005) 0.1 (women; Ryan et al. 1998) 0.3% (women; Ryan et al. 1998) 2.9% (Ryan et al. 1998) 0.0% (men; WHO/EMRO Regional Database on HIV/AIDS) 0.2% (women; WHO/EMRO Regional Database on HIV/AIDS) 0.09% (Khattabi and Alami 2005) 0.23% (Khattabi and Alami 2005) 0.62% (Heikel et al. 1999) 5.0% (attendees with high risk and/or symptoms; Elmir et al. 2002) 0.10% (Khattabi and Alami 2005; Elharti et al. 2002) 0.25% (Elharti et al. 2002) 0.34% (Khattabi and Alami 2005) 0.26% (Khattabi and Alami 2005) 0.19% (Morocco MOH 2007)

Country	HIV prevalence among STD clinic attendees, VCT attendees, and people suspected of living with HIV
Pakistan	0.0% (Iqbal and Rehan 1996)
	0.0% (Mujeeb and Hafeez 1993)
	0.3% (Shrestha 1996)
	6.1% (Shrestha 1996)
	0.22% (Rehan 2006)
Somalia	0.0% (Corwin et al. 1991)
	0.0% (Burans et al. 1990)
	0.0% (Scott et al. 1991)
	0.9% (UNAIDS 2006)
	4.3% (WHO 2004)
	5.5% (UNAIDS 2006)
	6.3% (Somaliland Ministry of Health and Labour 2007)
	12.3% (Somaliland Ministry of Health and Labour 2007)
	7.4% (men; Somaliland Ministry of Health and Labour 2007)
	5.4% (women; Somaliland Ministry of Health and Labour 2007)
	1.7% (refugees; UNHCR 2006–07a)
	0.9% (refugees; UNHCR 2006–07a)
	2.0% (refugees; UNHCR 2006–07a)
	1.0% (refugees; UNHCR 2006–07a)
	2.0% (refugees; UNHCR 2006–07a)
	0.3% (refugees; UNHCR 2006–07a)
	0.0% (refugees; UNHCR 2006–07a)
	2.3% (refugees; UNHCR 2006–07a)
	1.9% (refugees; UNHCR 2006–07a)
Sudan	5.8% (Southern Sudan; NSNAC and UNAIDS 2006)
	5.8% (Yei town, Southern Sudan; SNAP, NSNAC, and UNAIDS 2006)
	17.0% (VCT; Southern Sudan; SNAP, NSNAC, and UNAIDS 2006)
	19.1% (VCT; Southern Sudan; NSNAC and UNAIDS 2006)
	16.1% (VCT; Southern Sudan; NSNAC and UNAIDS 2006)
	20.0% (VCT; Southern Sudan; UNHCR 2007)
	2.0% (VCT; Southern Sudan; UNHCR 2007)
	5.0% (VCT; Southern Sudan; UNHCR 2007)
	6.2% (VCT; Southern Sudan; UNHCR 2007)
	1.1% (North Sudan; Ahmed 2004g)
	1.94% (North Sudan; SNAP 2008)
	1.47% (North Sudan; SNAP 2008)
	2.0% (North Sudan; Sudan MOH 2005)
	1.86% (Red Sea; North Sudan; Sudan National AIDS Control Program 2005)
	2.0% (Khartoum; North Sudan; Sudan National AIDS Control Program 2005; Sudan MOH 2005)
	0%–4.4% (three Khartoum sites; North Sudan; SNAP and UNAIDS 2006)
	2.0% (Khartoum; North Sudan; SNAP and UNAIDS 2006)
	1.86% (Red Sea; North Sudan; SNAP and UNAIDS 2006)
	0.0% (Khartoum; North Sudan; SNAP and UNAIDS 2006)
	0.0% (Khartoum; North Sudan; SNAP and UNAIDS 2006)
	4.4% (Khartoum; North Sudan; SNAP and UNAIDS 2006)
	26.0% (suspected AIDS patients; North Sudan; Ahmed 2004a)
	3.1% (refugees; UNHCR 2006–07b)
Tunisia	1.8% (Sellami et al. 2003)
Yemen, Republic of	1.8% (Al-Serouri 2005; WHO, UNICEF, and UNAIDS 2006s)

Table D.2 HIV Prevalence of Tuberculosis (TB) Patients

Country	HIV prevalence among tuberculosis patients
Afghanistan	0.2% (Todd et al. 2007)
Algeria	0.2% (Unknown, "Rapport de l'enquête nationale de séro-surveillance") 0.3% (Unknown, "Rapport de l'enquête nationale de séro-surveillance")
Djibouti	5.7% (Rodier et al. 1993) 44.4% (estimate; WHO 2005) 10.1% (estimate; Djibouti National TB Programme 2006)
Iran, Islamic Republic of	1.8% (WHO/EMRO 2007) 3.0% (hospital attendees; Tabarsi et al. 2008)
Iraq	0.0% (Abdul-Abbas, al-Delami, and Yousif 2000) 0.0% (estimate; Iraq National TB Programme 2006)
Jordan	0.0% (Jordan National TB Programme 2006)
Kuwait	0.3% (Kuwait National TB Programme 2006)
Lebanon	0.5% (estimate; Lebanon National TB Programme 2006)
Mauritania	1.5% (WHO 2002)
Morocco	0.36% (WHO/EMRO 2007; Elharti et al. 2002) 0.12% (Khattabi and Alami 2005) 0.4% (Khattabi and Alami 2005) 0.94% (Khattabi and Alami 2005) 0.14% (Khattabi and Alami 2005) 0.5% (Khattabi and Alami 2005) 0.19% (Khattabi and Alami 2005) 0.34% (Khattabi and Alami 2005) 1.6% (Alami 2009) 0.39% (Bennani and Alami 2006) 0.76% (Morocco MOH 2007)
Oman	2.0 (WHO/EMRO 2007)
Pakistan	1.8% (Hussain et al. 2004)
Qatar	0.0% (Qatar National TB Programme 2006)
Saudi Arabia	1.1% (Alrajhi et al. 2002)
Somalia	0.0% (Corwin et al. 1991) 0.0% (Scott et al. 1991) 1.6% (Kulane et al. 2000) 6.0% (UNAIDS 2006)]] 2.4% (UNAIDS 2006) 4.5% (WHO 2004) 5.6% (UNAIDS 2006)
Sudan	1.6% (SNAP 2006) 7.2% (Sudan National AIDS Control Program 1999) 4.9% (settled population; El-Sony et al. 2002) 2.6% (IDPs; El-Sony et al. 2002) 4.0% (El-Sony et al. 2002) 2.0% (Ahmed 2004i) 1.85% (SNAP and UNAIDS 2006) 4.8% (Southern Sudan origin; El-Sony et al. 2002) 0.0% (Red Sea; North Sudan; Sudan National AIDS Control Program 2005) 3.0% (Algadarif; North Sudan; Sudan National AIDS Control Program 2005) 1.6% (White Nile; North Sudan; Sudan Government of National Unity 2007) 2.0% (White Nile; North Sudan; Sudan National AIDS Control Program 2005; SNAP and UNAIDS 2006) 1.3% (South Darfur; North Sudan; Sudan National AIDS Control Program 2005)

Table D.2 *(Continued)*

Country	HIV prevalence among tuberculosis patients
	3.6% (North Kurdofan; North Sudan; Sudan National AIDS Control Program 2005)
	5.1% (North Kurdofan; North Sudan; SNAP and UNAIDS 2006)
	0.33% (Kassala; North Sudan; SNAP and UNAIDS 2006)
	2.8% (Khartoum; North Sudan; Sudan National AIDS Control Program 2005)
	1.89%–5.65% (four Khartoum sites; North Sudan; SNAP and UNAIDS 2006)
	3.6% (North Sudan origin; El-Sony et al. 2002)
Tunisia	0.0% (Jemni et al. 1991)
Yemen, Republic of	3.3% (WHO/EMRO 2007)
	2.1% (Al-Serouri 2005; WHO, UNICEF, and UNAIDS 2006s)
	6.9% (Al-Serouri 2005; WHO, UNICEF, and UNAIDS 2006s)
	1.9% (Al-Serouri 2005; WHO, UNICEF, and UNAIDS 2006s)
	0.7% (Yemen National TB Programme 2006)

Table D.3 Point-Prevalence Surveys on Different Population Groups

Country	Injecting drug users	Men who have sex with men	Female sex workers	STI clinic patients	Tuberculosis patients	Pregnant women
Algeria[a]			3.0% (2000)	0.0% (1998) 0.4% (2000)	0.2% (2000)	1% (2000)
Bahrain[b]	21.1% (1991) 0.9% (1998) 1.4% (1993) 1.6% (1994) 0.0% (1995) 1.1% (1996) 0.0% (1997) 0.0% (1999)			0.0% (1998) 0.0% (1990) 0.0% (1993) 0.0% (1994) 0.2% (1995) 0.0% (1996) 0.0% (1997)	2.9% (1994) 0.0% (1995) 0.8% (1996) 0.7% (1997) 0.7% (1998)	0.2% (1998) 0.0% (1993) 0.0% (1994) 0.0% (1995) 0.2% (1996) 0.2% (1997)
Djibouti[c]			19.5% (1990) 26% (1991) 36.6% (1992) 37.7% (1993) 26.3% (1993) 25.5% (1994) 36.8% (1995) 32.6% (1996) 32.7% (1997) 27.5% (1998)	1.9% (1990) 10.4% (1991) 11.6% (1992) 14.4% (1993) 16.3% (1993) 19.9% (1994) 19.5% (1995) 22.2% (1996)	5.9% (1991) 6.2% (1992) 7.4% (1993) 15% (1996) 44% (2000) 8.7% (1994) 12.8% (1995) 14.9% (1996) 16.7% (1997) 17.2% (1998) 13% (1999) 24% (2000) 23% (2001)	0.5% (1991) 1.6% (1992) 4% (1993) 2.5% (2002) 3.4% (1993) 2.8% (1994) 9.3% (1995) 2.9% (1996) 1.9% (2000)
Egypt, Arab Republic of[d]	2.8% (1992) 3.8% (1994) 0.0% (1996) 0.0% (1993) 0.0% (1994) 0.0% (1995) 0.0% (1996) 0.0% (1997) 0.0% (1998)	0.0% (1991) 0.7% (1992) 0.0% (1993) 0.0% (1994) 0.0% (1995) 0.0% (1996) 0.0% (1997) 1.3% (1998) 1.4% (1999)	0.0% (1991) 0.0% (1993) 0.0% (1992) 0.0% (1993) 0.0% (1994) 0.0% (1995) 0.9% (1996) 1.1% (1997) 1.5% (1998)	0.8% (1990) 0.0% (1991) 0.0% (1992) 0.2% (1993) 0.0% (1994) 0.0% (1995) 0.0% (1996) 0.0% (1997) 0.0% (1998)	0.0% (1991) 0.0% (1992) 0.2% (1993) 0.3% (1994) 0.0% (1995) 0.1% (1996) 0.0% (1997) 0.3% (1998) 0.2% (1999)	0.0% (1991) 0.0% (1992) 0.0% (1993) 0.0% (1994) 0.0% (1992) 0.0% (1993) 0.0% (1994) 0.0% (1995) 0.0% (1996)

(continued)

Appendix D   **229**

Table D.3 *(Continued)*

Country	Injecting drug users	Men who have sex with men	Female sex workers	STI clinic patients	Tuberculosis patients	Pregnant women
	0.0% (1999) 0.0% (2004)	0.8% (2000) 1% (2001) 0.0% (2004)	1.1% (1999) 0.0% (2000) 0 % (2001) 0.0% (2004)	0.0% (1999) 0.0% (2000) 0.0% (2001) 0.0% (1992) 0.0% (1993) 0.0% (1994) 0.0% (1995) 0.0% (1996) 0.0% (1997) 0.0% (1998) 0.0% (1999) 0.0% (2002) 0.0% (2004)	0.3% (2000) 0.2% (2001) 0.0% (1991) 0.0% (1992) 0.0% (1993) 0.1% (1994) 0.0% (1995) 0.1% (1996) 0.0% (1997) 0.7% (1998) 0.5% (1999) 0.6% (2001) 0.1% (2004)	0.0% (2004)
Iran, Islamic Republic of[f]	5.7% (1996) 1.8% (1997) 0.5% (1998)		0.0% (1993) 0.0% (1994) 0.0% (1995) 0.0% (1996) 0.0% (1997) 0.0% (1998)	0.0% (1992) 0.1% (1993) 0.0% (1994) 0.0% (1992) 0.0% (1993) 0.0% (1994) 0.0% (1995) 0.0% (1996) 0.0% (1997) 0.0% (1998)	0.0% (1995) 0.0% (1997) 0.0% (1998) 6.5% (2000) 4.2% (2001)	0.0% (1993) 0.0% (1992) 0.0% (1994)
Iraq[e]	0.0% (1993) 0.0% (1994) 0.0% (1995) 0.0% (1996) 0.0% (1997) 0.0% (1998) 0.0% (1999)	0.0% (1993) 0.0% (1994) 0.0% (1995) 0.0% (1996) 0.0% (1997) 0.0% (1998)	0.0% (1993) 0.0% (1994) 0.0% (1995) 0.1% (1996) 0.0% (1997)	0.0% (1993) 0.0% (1994) 0.0% (1995) 0.0% (1996) 0.0% (1997) 0.0% (1998) 0.0% (1999)	0.0% (1997) 0.0% (1993) 0.0% (1994) 0.0% (1995) 0.0% (1996) 0.0% (1997) 0.0% (1998) 0.0% (1999)	0.0% (1993) 0.0% (1996) 0.0% (1997) 0.0% (1998) 0.0% (1999)
Jordan[g]			1.3% (1991)	1% (1992) 0.0% (1993) 0.0% (1994) 0.0% (1995)	0.0% (2001)	0.0% (1992) 0.0% (1993) 0.0% (1994) 0.0% (1999)
Kuwait[h]	1% (1993) 0.0% (1994) 0.0% (1995) 0.6% (1996) 0.0% (1997) 0.0% (1998) 0.0% (1999)			0.0% (1997) 0.0% (1993) 0.0% (1994) 0.0% (1995) 0.0% (1996) 0.0% (1997) 0.0% (1998) 0.0% (1999)		0.0% (1995) 0.0% (1996) 0.0% (1997) 0.0% (1998) 0.0% (1993) 0.0% (1994) 0.0% (1995) 0.0% (1996) 0.0% (1997) 0.0% (1998) 0.0% (1999)
Lebanon[i]			0.3% (1992) 0.1% (1993) 0.1% (1994) 0.0% (1995)	1.1% (1994)		0.1% (1994) 0.0% (1995)
Libya[j]	0.5% (1998)		1.1% (1993) 1.2% (1994)	0.0% (1990)	0.3% (1998)	0.0% (1998)

Characterizing the HIV/AIDS Epidemic in the Middle East and North Africa

Table D.3 *(Continued)*

Country	Injecting drug users	Men who have sex with men	Female sex workers	STI clinic patients	Tuberculosis patients	Pregnant women
Morocco[k]				0.0% (1993)	0.0% (1996)	0.0% (1994)
				0.0% (1994)	0.0% (1997)	0.0% (1996)
				0.0% (1996)	2% (1999)	0.0% (1997)
				0.9% (1997)	0.0% (1996)	0.1% (1999)
				0.4% (1999)	0.0% (1997)	0.0% (1996)
				0.0% (1996)	0.6% (1999)	0.0% (1997)
				0.0% (1997)		0.0% (1999)
				0.0% (1999)		
Oman[l]				0.0% (1999)	4.2% (1996)	
					2.3% (1997)	
					1.9% (1998)	
					1.4% (1999)	
Pakistan[m]	1.1% (1996)	1.6% (1993)	0.0% (1995)	6.1% (1994)	0.0% (1994)	0.0% (1993)
	0.0% (2000)	0.3% (1995)	1.2% (1993)	0.3% (1995)	2.8% (1995)	0.0% (1995)
	0.0% (2001)		0.7% (1995)	0.5% (2001)	0.0% (1992)	0.0% (2001)
	0.3% (1993)		0.0% (1996)	4.2% (1992)	0.0% (1993)	0.0% (1992)
	0.0% (1994)		0.5% (1997)	0.8% (1993)	0.1% (1994)	0.0% (1993)
	5.4% (1995)		1.7% (2001)	6.1% (1994)	0.8% (1995)	0.0% (1994)
				0.7% (1995)	1% (1997)	0.1% (1995)
				1.5% (1996)	0.2% (1998)	0.0% (1996)
				0.1% (1997)	0.0% (1999)	0.2% (1997)
				0.0% (1998)	2.1% (2001)	0.0% (1998)
				0.0% (1999)		0.0% (1999)
Qatar[n]				4.5% (1999)	0.0% (1993)	
					0.8% (1996)	
Somalia[o]			2.4% (1990)	0.0% (1990)	1.6% (1998)	0.0% (1998)
				4% (2004)	2.4% (2004)	0.9% (2004)
				4% (2005)	2% (2005)	1% (2005)
				0.9% (1999)	6% (1999)	2% (1997)
				4.3% (2002)	4.5% (2002)	0.6% (1997)
				5.5% (2004)	5.6% (2004)	0.8% (2004)
						0.0% (2005)
Sudan[p]			4.4% (2002)	1.8% (2004)	17% (1995)	4.5% (1996)
				6.8% (1991)	75% (1998)	0.5% (1998)
				2% (1993)	2.8% (2004)	0.3% (2004)
				3.6% (1994)	6.8% (1993)	0.0% (1994)
				3.2% (1997)	14.2% (1994)	1.8% (1995)
				1.1% (2002)	2.8% (1995)	1.7% (1996)
				1.9% (2004)	2.1% (1996)	2.9% (1997)
					9.9% (1997)	3.8% (1998)
					7.2% (1999)	0.9% (2002)
					1.4% (2004)	0.8% (2004)
Syrian Arab Republic[q]	0.1% (1992)	0.0% (1992)	0.0% (1990)	0.1% (1995)	0.0% (1995)	0.0% (1993)
	0.0% (1993)	0.6% (1994)	0.0% (1991)	0.3% (1996)		
	0.2% (1994)	3.6% (1995)	0.0% (1992)	0.2% (1997)		
	0.0% (1995)	0.9% (1996)	0.0% (1993)	0.1% (1998)		
	0.0% (1996)	0.0% (1997)	0.0% (1994)	0.0% (1990)		
	0.0% (1997)	0.6% (1998)	0.0% (1995)	0.2% (1993)		
	0.0% (1998)	0.0% (1999)	0.0% (1996)	1% (1994)		

(continued)

Table D.3 *(Continued)*

Country	Injecting drug users	Men who have sex with men	Female sex workers	STI clinic patients	Tuberculosis patients	Pregnant women
	0.0% (1999)		0.0% (1997) 0.1% (1998) 0.0% (1999)	0.2% (1995) 0.0% (1996) 0.0% (1997) 0.1% (1998) 0.0% (1999)		
Tunisia[r]	1.1% (1993) 0.9% (1994) 0.7% (1995) 1% (1996) 0.3% (1997)		0.0% (1990) 0.3% (1993) 0.1% (1994) 0.0% (1995) 0.4% (1996) 0.1% (1997) 0.0% (1998) 0.0% (1999)	0.0% (1995)	0.7% (1990) 0.4% (1993) 0.3% (1994) 0.0% (1995) 0.3% (1996) 0.0% (1998)	0.0% (1991) 0.2% (1996) 0.2% (1997) 0.2% (1998) 0.2% (1999) 0.2% (2000) 0.0% (1999)
Yemen, Republic of[s]			4.5% (1998)	1.7% (1993) 5.3% (1997) 2.9% (1998)	2.1% (1996) 0.5% (1998)	

Note: This table is a summary of all point–prevalence surveys as extracted from UNAIDS epidemiological facts sheets on each MENA country over the years. STI = sexually transmitted infection.

[a] WHO, UNICEF, and UNAIDS 2006a.
[b] WHO, UNICEF, and UNAIDS 2006b.
[c] WHO, UNICEF, and UNAIDS 2006c.
[d] WHO, UNICEF, and UNAIDS 2006d.
[e] WHO, UNICEF, and UNAIDS 2006e.
[f] WHO, UNICEF, and UNAIDS 2006f.
[g] WHO, UNICEF, and UNAIDS 2006g.
[h] WHO, UNICEF, and UNAIDS 2006h.
[i] WHO, UNICEF, and UNAIDS 2006i.
[j] WHO, UNICEF, and UNAIDS 2006j.

[k] WHO, UNICEF, and UNAIDS 2006k.
[l] WHO, UNICEF, and UNAIDS 2006l.
[m] WHO, UNICEF, and UNAIDS 2006m.
[n] WHO, UNICEF, and UNAIDS 2006n.
[o] WHO, UNICEF, and UNAIDS 2006o.
[p] WHO, UNICEF, and UNAIDS 2006p.
[q] WHO, UNICEF, and UNAIDS 2006q.
[r] WHO, UNICEF, and UNAIDS 2006r.
[s] WHO, UNICEF, and UNAIDS 2006s.

Table D.4 Hepatitis C Virus Prevalence in Different Population Groups

Country	Hepatitis C virus prevalence in different population groups
Afghanistan	0.31% (ANC attendees; Todd et al. 2008) 0.3% (blood donors; Dupire et al. 1999) 1.9% (blood donors; Afghanistan Central Blood Bank 2006) 36.6% (IDUs; Todd et al. 2007)
Algeria	0.18 % (blood donors; Ayed et al. 1995) 0.19% (pregnant women; Ayed et al. 1995) 0.63% (pregnant women; Aidaoui, Bouzbid, and Laouar 2008)
Bahrain	0.3% (blood donors including Saudi subjects; Almawi et al. 2004) 9.24% (dialysis patients including Saudi patients; Almawi et al. 2004) 40.0% (children with hemolytic anemias; Al-Mahroos and Ebrahim 1995)
Djibouti	0.3% (blood donors; Dray et al. 2005)
Egypt, Arab Republic of	13.9% (healthy populations; meta-analyses; Lehman and Wilson 2009), 78.5% (hepatocellular carcinoma patients; meta-analyses; Lehman and Wilson 2009) 13.6% (blood donors; Darwish et al. 1993) 26.6% (blood donors; Bassily et al. 1995)

Table D.4 *(Continued)*

Country	Hepatitis C virus prevalence in different population groups
	14.5% (blood donors; El Gohary et al. 1995)
	2.7% (blood donors; El-Gilany and El-Fedawy 2006)
	8.8% (blood donors; Tanaka et al. 2004)
	24.8% (blood donors; Arthur et al. 1997)
	20.8% (blood donors; Quinti et al. 1995)
	10.0% (general population; Shemer-Avni et al. 1998)
	27.5% (general population; El-Ghazzawi et al. 1995)
	24.0% (rural population; Mohamed et al. 2005)
	9.0% (rural population; Mohamed et al. 2005)
	14.8% (rural population; Marzouk et al. 2007)
	18.5% (rural population; Mohamed et al. 2006)
	2.7% (rural population; Arafa et al. 2005)
	19.0% (rural population; 10–19 years old; Darwish et al. 2001)
	60.0% (rural population; >30 years old; Darwish et al. 2001)
	8.7% (rural population; Nafeh et al. 2000)
	14.4% (rural population; El Gohary et al. 1995)
	15.5% (rural population; El Gohary et al. 1995)
	24.3% (rural population; Abdel-Aziz et al. 2000)
	10.3% (rural population; El-Sayed et al. 1997)
	18.1% (rural population; Abdel-Wahab et al. 1994)
	13.0% (healthy women; Kumar, Frossad, and Hughes 1997)
	15.7% (pregnant women; rural area; Shebl et al. 2009)
	19.0% (pregnant women; Kassem et al. 2000)
	15.8% (pregnant women; Stoszek et al. 2006)
	2.02% (children; El-Raziky et al. 2007)
	12.0% (children; Quinti et al. 1995; El-Nanawy et al. 1995)
	12.1% (children; Abdel-Wahab et al. 1994)
	31.5% (applicants for visa abroad; Mohamed et al. 1996a)
	39.0% (fire brigade personnel; Quinti et al. 1995)
	22.1% (army recruits; Abdel-Wahab et al. 1994)
	14.3% (tourism workers; El-Sayed et al. 1996)
	31.4% (prisoners; Quinti et al. 1995)
	7.7% (health care workers; El Gohary et al. 1995)
	1.4% (dentists; Hindy, Abdelhaleem, and Aly 1995)
	63.0% (IDUs; Saleh et al. 2000; El-Ghazzawi 1995)
	5.3% (STD patients; Ali et al. 1998)
	23.3% (kidney transplant recipients; Gheith et al. 2007)
	84.0% (hepatocellular carcinoma patients; Mabrouk 1997)
	27.3% (acute jaundice patients; Quinti et al. 1997)
	73.5% (chronic liver disease patients; Waked et al. 1995)
	46.2% (chronic liver disease patients; Abdel-Wahab et al. 1994)
	70.4% (hemodialysis patients; El Gohary et al. 1995)
	87.5% (hemodialysis patients; Gohar et al. 1995)
	46.2% (hemodialysis patients; Abdel-Wahab et al. 1994)
	81.25% (hemodialysis patients; Gohar et al. 1995)
	16.4% (children with hepatosplenomegaly; Abdel-Wahab et al. 1994)
	54.9% (hospitalized and multitransfused children; Abdel-Wahab et al. 1994)
	44.0% (thalassemic children; Quinti et al. 1995; El-Nanawy et al. 1995)
	75.6% (thalassemic children; El Gohary et al. 1995)
	14.0% (family members of HCV positive patients; spouses; Madwar et al. 1999)
	0.0% (family members of HCV positive patients; children; Madwar et al. 1999)
	5–50% (various populations; Mohamed et al. 1996b)

(continued)

Table D.4 *(Continued)*

Country	Hepatitis C virus prevalence in different population groups
Iran, Islamic Republic of	0.5% (blood donors; Ansar and Kooloobandi 2002) 0.59% (blood donors; Karimi and Ghavanini 2001; Ghavanini and Sabri 2000) 0.3% (blood donors; Rezvan et al. 1994) 0.1% (blood donors; Rahbar, Rooholamini, and Khoshnood 2004) 0.4% (blood donors; Pourshams et al. 2005) 0.4% (blood donors; Taziki and Espahbodi 2008) 0.8% (blood donors; Taziki and Espahbodi 2008) 2.07% (blood donors; Khedmat et al. 2007) 0.12% (general population; Alavian, Gholami and Masarrat 2002) 3.1% (general population; gypsy; Hosseini Asl, Avijgan, and Mohamadnejad 2004) 12.3% (adult population; Gholamreza et al. 2007) 0.0% (street children; Vahdani et al. 2006) 0.59% (healthy children; Karimi and Ghavanini 2001) 2.7% (FSWs; Jahani et al. 2005) 52.0% (IDUs; Zamani et al. 2007) 59.4% (IDUs; Rahbar, Rooholamini, and Khoshnood 2004) 78.0% (IDUs; local prison; Nassirimanesh 2002) 47.4% (IDUs; Khani and Vakili 2003) 45.3% (IDUs; Zali et al. 2001) 30.0% (injecting and noninjecting drug users; Alizadeh et al. 2005) 11.2% (IDUs; Imani et al. 2008) 80.0% (incarcerated IDUs; Kheirandish et al. 2009) 7.35% (injecting and noninjecting drug users; Mohammad Alizadeh et al. 2003) 14.4% (noninjecting drug users; Talaie et al. 2007) 30.0% (prisoners; Alizadeh et al. 2005) 45.4% (prisoners; Mutter, Grimes, and Labarthe 1994) 47.0% (prisoners; Khani and Vakili 2003) 78.0% (prisoners; Nassirimanesh 2002) 35.8% (prisoners; Javadi, Avijgan, and Hafizi 2006) 1.33% (household contacts of HCV positive patients; Hajiani et al. 2006) 12.3% (HBV positive patients; Semnani et al. 2007) 11.5% (HIV-infected patients; Sharifi-Mood et al. 2006) 5.5% (hemodialysis patients; Rais-Jalali and Khajehdehi 1999) 21.0% (hemodialysis patients; Nobakht, Zali, and Nowroozi 2001) 2.9% (hemodialysis patients; Khamispoor and Tahmasebi 1999) 13.2% (hemodialysis patients; Mohammad et al. 2003) 24.8% (hemodialysis patients; Amiri, Shakib, and Toorchi 2005) 55.9% (hemodialysis patients; Ansar and Kooloobandi 2002) 42.6% (hemodialysis patients; Hosseini-Moghaddam et al. 2006) 60.2% (hemophiliac patients; Alavian, Ardeshiri, and Hajarizadeh 2001) 16.0% (hemophiliac patients; Karimi, Yarmohammadi, and Ardeshiri 2002) 51.0% (hemophiliac patients; Torabi et al. 2006) 48.6% (hemophiliac patients; Javadzadeh, Attar, and Taher Yavari 2006) 41.9% (hemophiliac patients; Khamispoor and Tahmasebi 1999) 43.4% (hemophiliac patients; Samimi-Rad and Shahbaz 2007) 29.6% (hemophiliac patients; Sharifi-Mood et al. 2007) 71.3% (hemophiliac patients; Mansour-Ghanaei et al. 2002) 15.65% (hemophiliac patients; Karimi and Ghavanini 2001) 24.2% (thalassemia patients; Alavian, Gholami and Masarrat 2002) 9.4% (thalassemia patients; Javadzadeh, Attar, and Taher Yavari 2006) 13.0% (thalassemia patients; Khamispoor and Tahmasebi 1999) 24.0% (thalassemia patients; Nakhaie and Talachian 2003) 27.2% (thalassemia patients; Kadivar et al., 2001) 23.0% (thalassemia patients; Basiratnia, HosseiniAsl, and Avijegan 1999) 25.0% (thalassemia patients; Jafroodi and Asadi 2006) 21.0% (thalassemia patients; Rezvan, Abolghassemi, and Kafiabad 2007)

Table D.4 *(Continued)*

Country	Hepatitis C virus prevalence in different population groups
	63.8% (thalassemia patients; Ansar and Kooloobandi 2002)
	18.3% (thalassemia patients; Kashef et al. 2008)
	5.1% (thalassemia patients; Samimi-Rad and Shahbaz 2007)
	15.7% (thalassemia patients; children; Karimi and Ghavanini 2001)
	19.3% (thalassemia patients; Mirmomen et al. 2006)
	15.65% (multitransfused hemophiliac patients; Karimi and Ghavanini 2001)
Iraq	3.21% (pregnant women; Al-Kubaisy, Niazi, and Kubba 2002)
	66.0% (HIV-infected hemophilia patients; Al-Kubaisy, Al-Naib, and Habib 2006a)
	67.3% (children with thalassemia; Al-Kubaisy, Al-Naib, and Habib 2006b)
Jordan	0.65 to 6.25% (hospitalized populations; Quadan 2002)
	40.5% (multitransfused patients; Al-Sheyyab, Batieha, and El-Khateeb 2001)
Kuwait	33.0% (thalassemia patients; Al-Fuzae, Aboolbacker, and Al-Saleh 1998)
	0.8% (blood donors; Kuwaiti; Ameen et al. 2005)
	5.4% (blood donors; non-Kuwaiti; Ameen et al. 2005)
Lebanon	0.4% (blood donors; Tamim et al. 2001)
	0.6% (blood donors; Irani-Hakime et al. 2001b)
	0.40% (blood donors; Irani-Hakime et al. 2006)
	0.7% (blood donors; Araj et al. 1995)
	0.7% (general population; Baddoura, Haddad, and Germanos 2002)
	2.6% (health care workers; Irani-Hakime et al. 2001a)
	25.0% (HIV infected IDUs; Ramia et al. 2004)
Libya	1.19% (national survey; Libya National Center for the Prevention of and Control of Infectious Diseases 2005)
	7.9% (healthy subjects; Saleh et al. 1994)
Morocco	1.1% (blood donors; Benjelloun et al. 1996)
	1.0% (pregnant women; Benjelloun et al. 1996)
	0.5% (ANC attendees and family planning clinic; WHO/EMRO Regional Database on HIV/AIDS)
	5.0% (male barbers; Zahraoui-Mehadji et al. 2004)
	35.1% (hemodialysis patients; Benjelloun et al. 1996)
	76% (hemodialysis patients; Boulaajaj et al. 2005)
	68.3% (hemodialysis patients; Sekkat et al. 2008)
	42.4% (hemophiliacs; Benjelloun et al. 1996)
Oman	1.5% (blood donors; Alnaqy et al. 2006)
	0.9% (blood donors; Al-Dhahry et al. 1993)
	26.5% (hemodialysis patients; Al-Dhahry et al. 1993)
	13.4% (kidney transplant patients; Al-Dhahry et al. 1993)
	0.0% (medical students; Al-Dhahry et al. 1993)
	11%–53% (IDUs; Unknown 2006)
Pakistan	1.70% (youth; Butt and Amin 2008)
	16% (blood donors; Ahmad et al. 2007)
	3.6% (blood donors; Abdul Mujeeb et al. 2006)
	4.0% (blood donors; Khattak et al. 2002)
	0.5% (blood donors; Abdul Mujeeb, Aamir, and Mehmood 2000)
	3.01%–4.99% (blood donors; Sultan, Mehmood, and Mahmood 2007)
	1.8% (blood donors; Akhtar et al. 2004)
	1.18% (blood donors; Kakepoto et al. 1996)
	7.5% (blood donors; Mujeeb and Pearce 2008)
	4.1% (blood donors; Khattak et al. 2008)
	0.5% (blood donors; college students; Mujeeb, Aamir, and Mehmood 2006; Abdul Mujeeb, Aamir, and Mehmood 2000)
	2.8% (blood donors; weighted average in a review; Ali et al. 2009)
	6.7% (general population; women; Parker, Khan, and Cubitt 1999)

(continued)

Table D.4 *(Continued)*

Country	Hepatitis C virus prevalence in different population groups
	5.31% (general population; Khokhar, Gill, and Malik 2004)
	15.9% (general population; Aslam and Aslam 2001)
	4.6% (general population; Aslam et al. 2005)
	33.7% (general population; rural area; Abbas et al. 2008)
	5.4% (general population; weighted average in a review; Ali et al. 2009)
	1.3% (children; Parker, Khan, and Cubitt 1999)
	1.6 % (children; Jafri et al. 2006)
	0.44% (children; Agboatwalla et al. 1994)
	1.3% (children with HCV positive mothers; Parker, Khan, and Cubitt 1999),
	2.1% (children; weighted average in a review; Ali et al. 2009)
	21.0% (vaccinated population for smallpox; Aslam et al. 2005)
	5.6% (health care workers; Aziz et al. 2002)
	5.5% (health care workers; weighted average in a review; Ali et al. 2009)
	3.12% (hospital attendees; Khan et al. 2007)
	31.0% (operation room personnel; Mujeeb, Khatri, and Khanani 1998)
	88.0% (IDUs; Kuo et al. 2006)
	89.0% (IDUs; United Nations Office for Drug Control and Crime Prevention and UNAIDS 1999)
	60.0% (IDUs; Achakzai, Kassi, and Kasi 2007)
	87.0% (IDUs; Pakistan National AIDS Control Program 2005b)
	91.0% (IDUs; Pakistan National AIDS Control Program 2005b)
	22.0% (noninjecting drug users; Kuo et al. 2006)
	20.5% (household contacts of HCV positive thalassemic children; Akhtar et al. 2002)
	36.0% (type II diabetes patients; Ali et al. 2007)
	13.2% (transfusion patients; Rizvi and Fatima 2003)
	15.4% (transfusion patients; Rizvi and Fatima 2003)
	44.0% (patients who received frequent injections; Khan et al. 2000)
	33.0% (hepatocellular carcinoma cases; Abdul Mujeeb et al. 1997)
	60.0% (thalassemia patients; Bhatti, Amin, and Saleem 1995)
	34.8% (children with thalassemia; Akhtar and Moatter 2004)
	68.0% (hemodialysis patients; Gul and Iqbal 2003)
	23.7%–68.0% (hemodialysis patients; range in a review; Raja and Janjua 2008)
Saudi Arabia	4.3% (blood donors; Mahaba, el-Tayeb Ael, and Elbaz 1999)
	0.59% (blood donors; Bashawri et al. 2004)
	0.4% (blood donors; El-Hazmi 2004)
	1.7% (blood donors; Abdelaal et al. 1994)
	1.1% (blood donors; Shobokshi et al. 2003)
	3.6% (general population; males; Al Nasser 1992)
	3.1% (general population; females; Al Nasser 1992)
	1.7% (general population; males; Njoh and Zimmo 1997)
	3.2% (general population; non-Saudi persons; Njoh and Zimmo 1997)
	1.0% (children; Bakir et al. 1995)
	1.8% (children; Al-Faleh et al. 1991)
	0.1% (children; Shobokshi et al. 2003)
	0.7% (pregnant women; Shobokshi et al. 2003)
	2.2% (health care workers; Khan, Alkhalife, and Fathalla 2004)
	5.09% (different population groups; Mahaba, el-Tayeb Ael, and Elbaz 1999)
	74.6% (IDUs; Njoh and Zimmo 1997)
	10.5% (non-IDU drug dependent patients; Njoh and Zimmo 1997)
	5.87% (patients attending outpatient clinics; Saudis; Fakeeh and Zaki 1999)
	22.54% (patients attending outpatient clinics; Egyptians; Fakeeh and Zaki 1999)
	2.12% (patients attending outpatient clinics; Yemenis; Fakeeh and Zaki 1999)
	3.38% (patients attending outpatient clinics; other Middle Eastern origins; Fakeeh and Zaki 1999)
	4.98% (patients attending outpatient clinics; Asian countries origins; Fakeeh and Zaki 1999)
	41.9% (hemodialysis patients; Ayoola et al. 1991)
	9.24% (hemodialysis patients; including Bahraini patients; Qadi et al. 2004)

Table D.4 *(Continued)*

Country	Hepatitis C virus prevalence in different population groups
	15%–80% (hemodialysis patients; different dialysis units; Karkar 2007)
	6.9% (hemodialysis patients; Mahaba, el-Tayeb Ael, and Elbaz 1999)
	45.5% (hemodialysis patients; Al Nasser 1992)
	55.7% (hemodialysis patients; Shobokshi et al. 2003)
	43.4% (hemodialysis patients; Saxena and Panhotra 2004)
	17.9% (schistosomiasis patients; Khan, Alkhalife, and Fathalla 2004)
	21.0% (non-Hodgkin's lymphoma patients; Harakati, Abualkhair, and Al-Knawy 2000)
	63.6% (chronic liver disease patients; Ayoola et al. 1992)
	11.0% (children under cancer chemotherapy; Bakir et al. 1995)
	45.0% (multitransfused children; Al-Mugeiren et al. 1992)
Somalia	0.6% (blood donors; Nur et al. 2000)
	0.97% (healthy adults; Aceti et al. 1993)
	6.5% (healthy adults; Bile et al. 1993)
	0.0% (children; Bile et al. 1992)
	1.5% (children; Bile et al. 1992)
	0.0% (children; Aceti et al. 1993)
	1.8% (FSWs, STD clinic attendees, male soldiers, and tuberculosis patients; Watts et al. 1994)
	2.4% (blood donors, hospitalized children and adults; Nur et al. 2000)
	2.2% (hospitalized persons; Aceti et al. 1993)
	40.3% (chronic liver disease patients; Bile et al. 1993)
Sudan	0.6% (pregnant women; Elsheikh et al. 2007)
	0.36% (hospital attendees; Ati 2005)
	2.2% (an area with a high prevalence of schistosomiasis; Mudawi et al. 2007)
	34.0% (hemodialysis patients; El-Amin et al. 2007)
	19.0% (hemodialysis patients; Kose et al. 2009)
	3.0% (out-patient attendees; McCarthy et al. 1994)
Syrian Arab Republic	0.95% (blood donors; Othman and Monem 2002)
	1.96% (FSWs; Othman and Monem 2002)
	60.5% (IDUs; Othman and Monem 2002)
	3.0% (health care workers; Othman and Monem 2001)
	0.0% (laboratory workers; Othman and Monem 2001)
	54.4% (hemodialysis patients; Moukeh et al. 2009)
	6.0% (hemodialysis staff; Othman and Monem 2001)
	0.0% (dentistry workers; Othman and Monem 2001)
	0.0% (surgery workers; Othman and Monem 2001)
Tunisia	0.56% (blood donors; Hatira et al. 2000)
	1.09% (blood donors; Slama et al. 1991)
	1.7% (general population; Mejri et al. 2005)
	0.2% (general population; Mejri et al. 2005)
	0.71% (general population; Gorgi et al. 1998)
	0.4% (general population; Triki et al. 1997)
	39.7% (HIV patients; Kilani et al. 2007)
	20.0% (hemodialysis patients; Hmaied et al. 2006)
	32.6% (hemodialysis patients; Ben Othman et al. 2004)
	45.10% (hemodialysis patients; Hmida et al. 1995)
	42% (hemodialysis patients; Hachicha et al. 1995)
	42.0% (hemodialysis patients; Jemni et al. 1994)
	50.0% (hemophiliacs; Langar et al. 2005)
	50.5% (hemophiliacs; Djebbi et al. 2008)
Turkey	0.4% (blood donors; Ozsoy et al. 2003)
	0.38% (blood donors; Gurol et al. 2006)
	0.19% (blood donors; Sakarya et al. 2004)
	0.45% (blood donors; Altindis et al. 2006)

(continued)

Table D.4 *(Continued)*

Country	Hepatitis C virus prevalence in different population groups
	0.37% (blood donors; Mutlu, Meric, and Willke 2004)
	0.39% (blood donors; Afsar et al. 2008)
	0.28% (blood donors; Afsar et al. 2008)
	0.37% (blood donors; Afsar et al. 2008)
	1.0% (rural areas; general population; Akcam et al. 2009)
	2.3% (general population; men; Bozkurt et al. 2008)
	2.0% (general population; women; Bozkurt et al. 2008)
	2.1% (general population; Yildirim et al. 2009)
	0.6% (general population; Alim et al. 2009)
	0.1% (engaged couples; Alim et al. 2009)
	1.3% (study controls; Gulcan et al. 2008)
	2.8% (barbers; Candan et al. 2002)
	0.56% (soldiers; Altindis et al. 2006)
	0.45% (soldiers; Altindis et al. 2006)
	1.5% (health personnel; Koksal et al. 1991)
	0.3% (health care workers; Ozsoy et al. 2003)
	2.0% (spouses of chronic HCV patients; Tahan et al. 2005)
	0.77% (FSWs; Gul et al. 2008)
	2.8% (lymphoma patients; Sonmez et al. 2007)
	0.9% (gynecology and obstetrics patients; Tekay and Ozbek 2006)
	2.2% (outpatients; Demirturk et al. 2006)
	7.0% (predialytic chronic kidney disease patients; Sit et al. 2007)
	26.0% (hemodialysis patients; Selcuk et al. 2006)
	12.7% (hemodialysis patients; Ocak et al. 2006)
	43.6% (hemodialysis patients; Bozdayi et al. 2002)
	20.2% (hemodialysis patients; Selcuk et al. 2006)
	16.0% (hemodialysis patients; Selcuk et al. 2006)
	51.2% (hemodialysis patients; Koksal et al. 1991)
	0.0% (new hemodialysis patients; Koksal et al. 1991)
	24.4% (children with hemophilia; Kocabas et al. 1997b)
	4.0% (patients with multiple blood transfusions; Koksal et al. 1991)
	20.8% (diabetic patients; Ocak et al. 2006)
	3.2% (diabetic patients; Gulcan et al. 2008)
	5.8% (children with cancer; Kocabas et al. 1997a)
	2.0% at diagnosis and 14.0% at the end of cancer therapy (children with cancer; Kebudi et al. 2000)
West Bank and Gaza	2.2% (general population; Shemer-Avni et al. 1998)
Yemen, Republic of	1.1% (blood donors; Haidar 2002)
	2.1% (healthy persons; El Guneid et al. 1993)
	4.2% (healthy persons; Al-Moslih and Al-Huraibi 2001)
	0.5% (health care workers; Haidar 2002)
	3.5% (health care workers; Shidrawi et al. 2004)
	37.1% (patients with liver disease; Al-Moslih and Al-Huraibi 2001)
	21.5% (patients with liver disease; El Guneid et al. 1993)

Note: ANC = antenatal clinic; FSW = female sex worker; IDU = injecting drug user; STD = sexually transmitted disease.

Appendix E

Table E.1 Levels of HIV/AIDS Basic Knowledge in Different Population Groups

Country	High basic knowledge	Low basic knowledge
Afghanistan	University students (Mansoor et al. 2008) FSWs (World Bank 2008) HCWs (Todd et al. 2009)	General population women (Todd et al. 2007) General population women (van Egmond et al. 2004) Intrapartum patients (Todd et al. 2009) TB patients (Todd et al. 2007) High-risk groups (Action Aid Afghanistan 2006) IDUs (Zafar et al. 2003) FSWs (Action Aid Afghanistan 2006)
Djibouti	High school students (Rodier et al. 1993)	
Egypt, Arab Republic of	Nurses and university graduates (Mohsen 1998) General population women (Measure DHS 2004) General population women (*NEJM* 2008) Ever-married women (Measure DHS 2006) General population (Kabbash et al. 2007) Drug users (Salama et al. 1998) IDUs (Egypt MOH and Population National AIDS Program 2006) FSWs (Egypt MOH and Population National AIDS Program 2006) MSM (Egypt MOH and Population National AIDS Program 2006) MSM (El-Sayyed, Kabbash, and El-Gueniedy 2008)	Street children (Egypt MOH and Population National AIDS Program 2006) Squatter populations (Shama, Fiala, and Abbas 2002)
Iran, Islamic Republic of	Adolescents (Yazdi et al. 2006) Youth (Tehrani and Malek-Afzalip 2008) General population (Montazeri 2005) General population (Askarian, Mirzaei, and Assadian 2007) Truck drivers (Tehrani and Malek-Afzalip 2008) Teachers (Mazloomy and Baghianimoghadam 2008) Runaways and other women seeking safe haven (Hajiabdolbaghi et al. 2007) Prisoners (Nakhaee 2002) FSWs (Tehrani and Malek-Afzalip 2008) MSM (Eftekhar et al. 2008) Former prisoners (Ebrahim 2008)	
Iraq	General population women (*NEJM* 2008)	
Jordan	General population women (Measure DHS 1998) General population women (Measure DHS 2003) General population women (*NEJM* 2008)	
Kuwait	Different populations (Al-Owaish et al. 1999)	

(continued)

Table E.1 *(Continued)*

Country	High basic knowledge	Low basic knowledge
Lebanon	General population (Lebanon National AIDS Control Program 1996; Jurjus et al. 2004) Prisoners (Mishwar 2008) IDUs (Aaraj [unknown]; Hermez et al. [unknown]) IDUs (Mishwar 2008) FSWs (Mishwar 2008) FSWs (Hermez et al. [unknown]) FSWs (Rady 2005) MSM (Mishwar 2008) MSM (Hermez et al. [unknown]; Dewachi 2001)	
Morocco	General population women (*NEJM* 2008) General population women (Zidouh [unknown]) Blood donors (Boutayeb, Aamoum, and Benchemsi 2006)	
Oman	College students (Al-Jabri and Al-Abri 2003)	
Pakistan	Female college students (Khan et al. 2005) Medical students (Ali et al. 1996) School students (Shaikh and Assad 2001) Obstetrics and gynecology clinic attendees (Haider et al. 2009) General population (Raza et al. 1998) Migrant workers (Faisel and Cleland 2006) IDUs (Pakistan National AIDS Control Program 2005a) IDUs (Pakistan National AIDS Control Program 2006–07) IDUs (Pakistan National AIDS Control Program 2008) Clients of FSWs (Bokhari et al. 2007) Clients of MSWs (Bokhari et al. 2007) Different high-risk groups (Pakistan National AIDS Control Program 2005c) FSWs (Jamal, Khushk, and Naeem 2006) FSWs (Bokhari et al. 2007) FSWs (Pakistan National AIDS Control Program 2005a) FSWs (Pakistan National AIDS Control Program 2006–07) MSWs (Pakistan National AIDS Control Program 2005a) MSWs (Pakistan National AIDS Control Program 2006–07) 66.5% MSWs (Pakistan National AIDS Control Program 2008) HSWs (Pakistan National AIDS Control Program 2005a) HSWs (Pakistan National AIDS Control Program 2006–07) 66.5% HSWs (Pakistan National AIDS Control Program 2008) *Hijras* (Baqi et al. 1999) *Hijras* (Bokhari et al. 2007)	Rural adolescents (Raheel et al. 2007) Ever-married women (Measure DHS 2007) Paramedicals (Siddiqi, Majeed, and Saeed Khan 1995) Private health practitioners (Khan 1995) Pakistanis traveling abroad (Pakistan AIDS Prevention Society 1992–93) Fishermen (Sheikh et al. 2003) Male prisoners (Khawaja et al. 1997) IDUs (Haque et al. 2004) IDUs (Afghani refugees; Zafar et al. 2003) IDUs (Khawaja et al. 1997) Dancing girls, usually FSWs and their clients (Haroon 1994)
Saudi Arabia	Students (Abolfotouh 1995) Paramedical students (Al-Mazrou, Abouzeid, and Al-Jeffri 2005) Men in a management training institute (Badahdah 2005) HCWs (Al-Ghanim 2005)	General population women (IGAD 2006) HCWs (Mahfouz et al. 1995)
Somalia		Youth (WHO/EMRO 2000) General population (WHO/EMRO 2000) Traveling merchants/drivers (WHO/EMRO 2000)

Table E.1 *(Continued)*

Country	High basic knowledge	Low basic knowledge
Sudan	Street children (Ahmed 2004h) Youth (SNAP, UNICEF, and UNAIDS 2005) High school students (Elzubier, el Nour, and Ansari 1996) High school teachers and students (Elzubier, el Nour, and Ansari 1996) University students (Sudan National HIV/AIDS Control Program 2004) University students (Sudan National HIV/AIDS Control Program 2004; Ahmed 2004l) ANC women attendees (Mahmoud et al. 2007) ANC women attendees (Ahmed 2004b) Pregnant women (UNAIDS/WHO 2005) General population (Southern Sudan; NSNAC and UNAIDS 2006) General population (Southern Sudan; UNHCR 2007) Tea sellers (Gutbi and Eldin 2006) Tea sellers (Ati 2005) Tea sellers (Ahmed 2004j) Rural populations (SNAP, UNICEF, and UNAIDS 2005) Military personnel (Ahmed 2004d) Military personnel (Sudan National HIV/AIDS Control Program 2004) Prisoners (Assal 2006) Prisoners (Ahmed 2004e) Prisoners (Ati 2005) Truck drivers (Ahmed 2004k) Truck drivers (Farah and Hussein 2006) Internally displaced persons (Ahmed 2004c) Internally displaced persons (IGAD 2006) Sudanese refugees in Ethiopia (Holt et al. 2003) TB patients (Ahmed 2004i) STD clinic attendees (Ahmed 2004g) Suspected PLHIV (Ahmed 2004a) IDUs (Bayoumi 2005) FSWs (ACORD 2005) FSWs (Ati 2005) FSWs (ACORD 2006) FSWs (Yousif 2006) FSWs (Ahmed 2004f) MSM (Elrashied 2006)	
Syrian Arab Republic	FSWs (Syria National AIDS Programme 2004) IDUs (Syria Mental Health Directorate 2008)	
Tunisia	MSM (Hsairi and Ben Abdallah 2007)	
Turkey	High school students (Savaser 2003) General population (Ayranci 2005) Drug users and nondrug users (Soskolne and Maayan 1998) FSWs (Gul et al. 2008)	
United Arab Emirates	University students (Ganczak et al. 2007)	

(continued)

Table E.1 *(Continued)*

Country	High basic knowledge	Low basic knowledge
Yemen, Republic of	Youth (Al-Serouri 2005) Secondary school students (Gharamah and Baktayan 2006) Secondary school students (Raja and Farhan 2005) General population (Al-Serouri et al. 2002) General population (Busulwa 2003) Marginalized minority (Al-Akhdam) (Busulwa 2003) Returnee families from abroad (Busulwa 2003)	

Note: ANC = antenatal clinic; FSW = female sex worker; HCW = health care worker; HSW = *hrija* sex worker; IDU = injecting drug user; MSM = men who have sex with men; PLHIV = people living with HIV; STD = sexually transmitted disease; TB = tuberculosis.

Table E.2 MENA Populations with Low Levels of Comprehensive HIV/AIDS Knowledge

Country	Low comprehensive knowledge
Afghanistan	University students (Mansoor et al. 2008) Intrapartum patients (Todd et al. 2009) HCWs (Todd et al. 2007; Todd et al. 2009)
Egypt, Arab Republic of	Adolescents (El-Tawila et al. 1999) Students (Farghaly and Kamal 1991) Teachers (Farghaly and Kamal 1991) General population women (Measure DHS 2006) General population women (Measure DHS 2004) HCWs (Faris and Shouman 1994) Physicians (Sallam et al. 1995)
Iran, Islamic Republic of	Youth (Tehrani and Malek-Afzalip 2008) High school students (Tavoosi et al. 2004) Dentists (Askarian, Mirzaei, and Cookson 2007) Truck drivers (Tehrani and Malek-Afzalip 2008) Prisoners (Nakhaee 2002) FSWs (Tehrani and Malek-Afzalip 2008) MSM (Eftekhar et al. 2008)
Jordan	University students (Petro-Nustas, Kulwicki, and Zumout 2002; Petro-Nustas 2000) General population women (Measure DHS 1998) General population women (Measure DHS 2003)
Kuwait	Physicians (Fido and Al Kazemi 2002)
Lebanon	General population (Jurjus et al. 2004)
Morocco	General population women (Zidouh [unknown])
Pakistan	Adolescents (Ali, Bhatti, and Ushijima 2004) Medical students (Shaikh et al. 2007) General population (Raza et al. 1998) HCWs (Najmi 1998) IDUs (Khawaja et al. 1997) FSWs (Jamal, Khushk, and Naeem 2006) FSWs (Pakistan National AIDS Control Program 2005a) FSWs (Pakistan National AIDS Control Program 2006–07) *Hijras* (Baqi et al. 1999)
Saudi Arabia	Paramedical students (Al-Mazrou, Abouzeid, and Al-Jeffri 2005) Primary health care users (Al-Ghanim 2005) Men in a management training institute (Badahdah 2005) Bus drivers (Abdelmoneim et al. 2002)

Table E.2 *(Continued)*

Country	Low comprehensive knowledge
Somalia	Young women (Somaliland Ministry of Health and Labour 2007) General population (WHO 2004) Somali immigrants to Denmark (Lazarus et al. 2006)
Sudan	Street children (Ahmed 2004h) Youth (SNAP, UNICEF, and UNAIDS 2005) University students (Sudan National HIV/AIDS Control Program 2004) University students (Ahmed 2004l) ANC women attendees (Ahmed 2004b) General population (Southern Sudan; NSNAC and UNAIDS 2006) Tea sellers (Ahmed 2004j) Tea sellers (Ati 2005) Internally displaced persons (Ahmed 2004c) Sudanese immigrants to Denmark (Lazarus et al. 2006) Sudanese immigrant to the U.S.A. (Tompkins et al. 2006) Sudanese refugees in Ethiopia (Holt et al. 2003) Military personnel (Ahmed 2004d) Military personnel (Sudan National HIV/AIDS Control Program 2004) Prisoners (Ahmed 2004e) Prisoners (Assal 2006) Truck drivers (Farah and Hussein 2006) Truck drivers (Ahmed 2004k) TB patients (Ahmed 2004i) STD clinic attendees (Ahmed 2004g) Suspected AIDS patients (Ahmed 2004a) FSWs and tea sellers (Basha 2006) FSWs (ACORD 2005) FSWs (Ati 2005) FSWs (ACORD 2006) FSWs (Yousif 2006) FSWs (Ahmed 2004f) MSM (Elrashied 2006)
Syrian Arab Republic	IDUs (Syria Mental Health Directoràte 2008)
Turkey	Street children (Baybuga and Celik 2004) Youth (Baybuga and Celik 2004)
United Arab Emirates	University students (Ganczak et al. 2007)
West Bank and Gaza	Youth (PFPPA 2005)
Yemen, Republic of	Youth (Al-Serouri 2005) General population (Busulwa 2003) Marginalized minority (Al-Akhdam) (Busulwa 2003) Returnee families from abroad (Busulwa 2003)

Note: ANC = antenatal clinic; FSW = female sex worker; HCW = health care worker; IDU = injecting drug user; MSM = men who have sex with men; STD = sexually transmitted disease; TB = tuberculosis.

Table E.3 MENA Populations with High Levels of HIV/AIDS Misinformation

Country	High levels of misinformation
Djibouti	Truck drivers (O'Grady 2004)
Egypt, Arab Republic of	Squatter populations (Shama, Fiala, and Abbas 2002) Physicians (Sallam et al. 1995) HCWs (Faris and Shouman 1994) IDUs (Egypt MOH and Population National AIDS Program 2006) FSWs (Egypt MOH and Population National AIDS Program 2006) MSM (Egypt MOH and Population National AIDS Program 2006)
Iran, Islamic Republic of	Adolescents (Mohammadi et al. 2006) Adolescents (Yazdi et al. 2006) Youth (Tehrani and Malek-Afzalip 2008) Teachers (Mazloomy and Baghianimoghadam 2008) General population (Askarian, Mirzaei, and Assadian 2007) General population (Montazeri 2005) General population (Hedayati-Moghaddam 2008) Truck drivers (Tehrani and Malek-Afzalip 2008) FSWs (Tehrani and Malek-Afzalip 2008) MSM (Eftekhar et al. 2008)
Jordan	Youth (Jordan National AIDS Control Programme 2005)
Kuwait	Different populations (Al-Owaish et al. 1999)
Lebanon	Prisoners (Mishwar 2008)
Morocco	General population women (Zidouh [unknown])
Oman	College students (Al-Jabri and Al-Abri 2003)
Pakistan	Adolescents (Ali, Bhatti, and Ushijima 2004) Female college students (Farid and Choudhry 2003) School students (Shaikh and Assad 2001) Obstetrics and gynecology clinic attendees (Haider et al. 2009) General population (Raza et al. 1998) Pakistanis traveling abroad (Pakistan AIDS Prevention Society 1992–93) FSWs (Jamal, Khushk, and Naeem 2006)
Saudi Arabia	Paramedical students (Al-Mazrou, Abouzeid, and Al-Jeffri 2005)
Sudan	Street children (Ahmed 2004h) Street children (Kudrati et al. 2002; Kudrati, Plummer, and Yousif 2008) Youth (SNAP, UNICEF, and UNAIDS 2005) High school students (Elzubier, el Nour, and Ansari 1996) University students (Ahmed 2004l) University students (Sudan National HIV/AIDS Control Program 2004) Teachers (Elzubier, el Nour, and Ansari 1996) ANC women attendees (Ahmed 2004b) General population (Southern Sudan) (NSNAC and UNAIDS 2006) Tea sellers (Gutbi and Eldin 2006), Tea sellers (Ahmed 2004j) Internally displaced persons (Ahmed 2004c) Military personnel (Sudan National HIV/AIDS Control Program 2004) Military personnel (Ahmed 2004d) Prisoners (Ahmed 2004e) Prisoners (Assal 2006) Truck drivers (Ahmed 2004k) Truck drivers (Farah and Hussein 2006) TB patients (Ahmed 2004i) STD clinic attendees (Ahmed 2004g) Suspected PLHIV (Ahmed 2004a)

Table E.3 *(Continued)*

Country	High levels of misinformation
	FSWs and tea sellers (Basha 2006) FSWs (ACORD 2006) FSWs (Yousif 2006) FSWs (ACORD 2005) FSWs (Ahmed 2004f) MSM (Elrashied 2006)
Syrian Arab Republic	FSWs (Syria National AIDS Programme 2004) IDUs (Syria Mental Health Directorate 2008)
Tunisia	MSM (Hsairi and Ben Abdallah 2007)
Turkey	Street children (Baybuga and Celik 2004) Youth (Baybuga and Celik 2004) General population (Ayranci 2005) Drug users and nondrug users (Soskolne and Maayan 1998)
United Arab Emirates	University students (Ganczak et al. 2007)
West Bank and Gaza	Youth (PFPPA 2005)
Yemen, Republic of	Youth (Al-Serouri 2005) Secondary school students (Gharamah and Baktayan 2006) General population (Al-Serouri et al. 2002)

Note: ANC = antenatal clinic; FSW = female sex worker; IDU = injecting drug user; MSM = men who have sex with men; PLHIV = people living with HIV; STD = sexually transmitted disease; TB = tuberculosis.

Table E.4 Nature of Attitudes toward People Living with HIV/AIDS by Different Population Groups

Country	Negative attitudes toward people living with HIV/AIDS	Positive attitudes toward people living with HIV/AIDS
Djibouti	Dockers and truck drivers (O'Grady 2004)	
Egypt, Arab Republic of	General population women (Measure DHS 2006) Tourism workers (El-Sayyed, Kabbash, and El-Gueniedy 2008) Industrial workers (El-Sayyed, Kabbash, and El-Gueniedy 2008) Drug users (Salama et al. 1998)	
Iran, Islamic Republic of	Adolescents (Yazdi et al. 2006) High school students (Tavoosi et al. 2004) Teachers (Mazloomy and Baghianimoghadam 2008) PLHIV (Sherafat-Kazemzadeh et al. 2003) MSM (Eftekhar et al. 2008)	General population (Montazeri 2005) General population (IRIB 2006) Former prisoners (Ebrahim 2008)
Jordan	College students (Petro-Nustas, Kulwicki, and Zumout 2002) General population women (Measure DHS 2003) General population women (Measure DHS 2003) Dentists (El-Maaytah et al. 2005)	

(continued)

Table E.4 *(Continued)*

Country	Negative attitudes toward people living with HIV/AIDS	Positive attitudes toward people living with HIV/AIDS
Lebanon	General population (Othman and Monem 2002; Lebanon National AIDS Control Program 1996) General population (Lebanon National AIDS Control Program 2003)	General population (Jurjus et al. 2004) General population (Lebanon National AIDS Control Program 2003)
Libya	High school students (El-Gadi, Abudher, and Sammud 2008)	High school students (El-Gadi, Abudher, and Sammud 2008)
Morocco		General population (Zidouh [unknown])
Saudi Arabia	Paramedical students (Al-Mazrou, Abouzeid, and Al-Jeffri 2005)	
Somalia		Youth (WHO/EMRO 2000) General population (WHO 2004) General population (WHO/EMRO 2000) Traveling merchants/drivers (WHO/EMRO 2000)
Sudan	Street children (Ahmed 2004h) Youth (SNAP, UNICEF, and UNAIDS 2005) University students (Sudan National HIV/AIDS Control Program 2004) University students (Ahmed 2004l) ANC women attendees (Ahmed 2004b) General population (Southern Sudan; UNHCR 2007) Tea sellers (Ahmed 2004j) Internally displaced persons (Ahmed 2004c) Military personnel (Ahmed 2004d) Military personnel (Sudan National HIV/AIDS Control Program 2004) Prisoners (Assal 2006) Prisoners (Ahmed 2004e) Truck drivers (Farah and Hussein 2006) Truck drivers (Ahmed 2004k) TB patients (Ahmed 2004i) STD clinic attendees (Ahmed 2004g) Suspected AIDS patients (Ahmed 2004a) FSWs (Yousif 2006) FSWs (Ahmed 2004f) MSM (Elrashied 2006)	University students (Sudan National HIV/AIDS Control Program 2004) General population (Southern Sudan; UNHCR 2007)
Syrian Arab Republic	FSWs (Syria National AIDS Programme 2004)	
Turkey		General population (Ayranci 2005)
United Arab Emirates	University students (Ganczak et al. 2007)	
West Bank and Gaza	General population (UNAIDS 2007c) General population women (UNAIDS 2007c)	

Table E.4 *(Continued)*

Country	Negative attitudes toward people living with HIV/AIDS	Positive attitudes toward people living with HIV/AIDS
Yemen, Republic of	Youth (Al-Serouri 2005) Secondary school students (Gharamah and Baktayan 2006) General population (Busulwa 2003) Marginalized minority (Al-Akhdam; Busulwa 2003) Returnee families from abroad (Busulwa 2003)	Secondary school students (Gharamah and Baktayan 2006) General population (Al-Serouri et al. 2002)

Note: ANC = antenatal clinic; FSW = female sex worker; MSM = men who have sex with men; STD = sexually transmitted disease; TB = tuberculosis.

Table E.5 Television as the Main Source of HIV/AIDS Knowledge, by MENA Population Groups

Country	Populations that identified television as the main source of HIV/AIDS knowledge
Egypt, Arab Republic of	Street children (Egypt MOH and Population National AIDS Program 2006) University students (Refaat 2004) General population women (Measure DHS 2004) General population women (Measure DHS 2006) Squatter populations (Shama, Fiala, and Abbas 2002) HCWs (Faris and Shouman 1994) IDUs (Egypt MOH and Population National AIDS Program 2006) FSWs (Egypt MOH and Population National AIDS Program 2006) MSM (Egypt MOH and Population National AIDS Program 2006)
Iran, Islamic Republic of	Adolescents (Yazdi et al. 2006) Youth (Tehrani and Malek-Afzalip 2008) High school students (Tavoosi et al. 2004) High school students (Karimi and Ataei 2007) Teachers (Mazloomy and Baghianimoghadam 2008) General population (Montazeri 2005) General population (Ministry of Health and Medical Education of Iran 2006) Truck drivers (Tehrani and Malek-Afzalip 2008) FSWs (Tehrani and Malek-Afzalip 2008)
Pakistan	Female college students (Khan et al. 2005) Male prisoners (Khawaja et al. 1997) IDUs (Khawaja et al. 1997) FSWs (Jamal, Khushk, and Naeem 2006)
Sudan	Youth (SNAP, UNICEF, and UNAIDS.2005) University students (Ahmed 2004l) University students (Sudan National HIV/AIDS Control Program 2004) Military personnel (Sudan National HIV/AIDS Control Program 2004)
Turkey	High school students (Savaser 2003) College students (Ungan and Yaman 2003)
West Bank and Gaza	General population women (Husseini and Abu-Rmeileh 2007)
Yemen, Republic of	Youth (Al-Serouri 2005) High school students (Raja and Farhan 2005) General population (Al-Serouri et al. 2002) General population (Busulwa 2003) Marginalized minority (Al-Akhdam) (Busulwa 2003) Returnee families from abroad (Busulwa 2003)

Note: FSW = female sex worker; HCW = health care worker; IDU = injecting drug user; MSM = men who have sex with men.

BIBLIOGRAPHY FOR APPENDIXES A–E

Aaraj, E. Unknown. "Report on the Situation Analysis on Vulnerable Groups in Beirut, Lebanon." IVDU Group.

Abbas, Z., N. L. Jeswani, G. N. Kakepoto, M. Islam, K. Mehdi, and W. Jafri. 2008. "Prevalence and Mode of Spread of Hepatitis B and C in Rural Sindh, Pakistan." *Trop Gastroenterol* 29: 210–16.

Abdelaal, M., D. Rowbottom, T. Zawawi, T. Scott, and C. Gilpin. 1994. "Epidemiology of Hepatitis C Virus: A Study of Male Blood Donors in Saudi Arabia." *Transfusion* 34: 135–37.

Abdel-Aziz, F., M. Habib, M. K. Mohamed, M. Abdel-Hamid, F. Gamil, S. Madkour, N. N. Mikhail, D. Thomas, A. D. Fix, G. T. Strickland, W. Anwar, and I. Sallam. 2000. "Hepatitis C Virus (HCV) Infection in a Community in the Nile Delta: Population Description and HCV Prevalence." *Hepatology* 32: 111–15.

Abdelmoneim, I., M. Y. Khan, A. Daffalla, S. Al-Ghamdi, and M. Al-Gamal. 2002. "Knowledge and Attitudes towards AIDS among Saudi and Non-Saudi Bus Drivers." *East Mediterr Health J* 8: 716–24.

Abdel-Wahab, M. F., S. Zakaria, M. Kamel, M. K. Abdel-Khaliq, M. A. Mabrouk, H. Salama, G. Esmat, D. L. Thomas, and G. T. Strickland. 1994. "High Seroprevalence of Hepatitis C Infection among Risk Groups in Egypt." *Am J Trop Med Hyg* 51: 563–67.

Abdelwahab, O. 2006. "Prevalence, Knowledge of AIDS and HIV Risk-Related Sexual Behaviour among Police Personnel in Khartoum State, Sudan 2005." XVI International AIDS Conference, Toronto, August 13–18, abstract CDC0792.

Abdul Mujeeb, S., K. Aamir, and K. Mehmood. 2000. "Seroprevalence of HBV, HCV and HIV Infections among College Going First Time Voluntary Blood Donors." *J Pak Med Assoc* 50: 269–70.

Abdul Mujeeb, S., Q. Jamal, R. Khanani, N. Iqbal, and S. Kaher. 1997. "Prevalence of Hepatitis B Surface Antigen and HCV Antibodies in Hepatocellular Carcinoma Cases in Karachi, Pakistan." *Trop Doct* 27: 45–46.

Abdul Mujeeb, S., D. Nanan, S. Sabir, A. Altaf, and M. Kadir. 2006. "Hepatitis B and C Infection in First-Time Blood Donors in Karachi—A Possible Subgroup for Sentinel Surveillance." *East Mediterr Health J* 12: 735–41.

Abdul-Abbas, A. J., A. M. al-Delami, and T. K. Yousif. 2000. "HIV Infection in Patients with Tuberculosis in Baghdad (1996–98)." *East Mediterr Health J* 6: 1103–6.

Abolfotouh, M. A. 1995. "The Impact of a Lecture on AIDS on Knowledge, Attitudes and Beliefs of Male School-Age Adolescents in the Asir Region of Southwestern Saudi Arabia." *J Community Health* 20: 271–81.

Abu-Raddad, L. J., A. S. Magaret, C. Celum, A. Wald, I. M. Longini, S. G. Self, and L. Corey. 2008. "Genital Herpes Has Played a More Important Role Than Any Other Sexually Transmitted Infection in Driving HIV Prevalence in Africa." *PLoS ONE* 3: e2230.

ACORD (Agency for Co-operation and Research Development). 2005. "Socio Economic Research on HIV/AIDS Prevention among Informal Sex Workers." Agency for Co-operation and Research in Development, Federal Ministry of Health, Sudan National AIDS Control Program, and the World Health Organization.

———. 2006. "Qualitative Socio Economic Research on Female Sex Workers and Their Vulnerability to HIV/AIDS in Khartoum State." Agency for Co-operation and Research in Development.

Aceti, A., G. Taliani, R. Bruni, O. S. Sharif, K. A. Moallin, D. Celestino, G. Quaranta, and A. Sebastiani. 1993. "Hepatitis C Virus Infection in Chronic Liver Disease in Somalia." *Am J Trop Med Hyg* 48: 581–84.

Achakzai, M., M. Kassi, and P. M. Kasi. 2007. "Seroprevalences and Co-Infections of HIV, Hepatitis C Virus and Hepatitis B Virus in Injecting Drug Users in Quetta, Pakistan." *Trop Doct* 37: 43–45.

Action Aid Afghanistan. 2006. "HIV AIDS in Afghanistan: A Study on Knowledge, Attitude, Behavior, and Practice in High Risk and Vulnerable Groups in Afghanistan."

Afghanistan Central Blood Bank. 2006. *Report of Testing of Blood Donors from March–December, 2006.* Ministry of Public Health, Kabul, Afghanistan.

Afsar, I., S. Gungor, A. G. Sener, and S. G. Yurtsever. 2008. "The Prevalence of HBV, HCV and HIV Infections among Blood Donors in Izmir, Turkey." *Indian J Med Microbiol* 26: 288–89.

Afshar, P., and F. Kasrace. 2005. "HIV Prevention Experiences and Programs in Iranian Prisons" [MoPC0057]. Presented at the Seventh International Congress on AIDS in Asia and the Pacific, July 1–5, Kobe, Japan.

Afshar, P. Unknown (a). "From the Assessment to the Implementation of Services Available for Drug Abuse and HIV/AIDS Prevention and Care in Prison Setting: The Experience of Iran." PowerPoint presentation

———. Unknown (b). "Health and Prison." Director General of Health, Office of Iran Prisons Organization.

Agboatwalla, M., S. Isomura, K. Miyake, T. Yamashita, T. Morishita, and D. S. Akram. 1994. "Hepatitis A, B and C Seroprevalence in Pakistan." *Indian J Pediatr* 61: 545–49.

Ahmad, N., M. Asgher, M. Shafique, and J. A. Qureshi. 2007. "An Evidence of High Prevalence of Hepatitis C Virus in Faisalabad, Pakistan." *Saudi Med J* 28: 390–95.

Ahmed, S. M. 2004a. *AIDS Patients: Situation Analysis-Behavioral Survey Results & Discussions.* Report, Sudan National AIDS Control Program.

———. 2004b. *Antenatal: Situation Analysis-Behavioral Survey Results & Discussions.* Report. Sudan National AIDS Control Program.

———. 2004c. *Internally Displaced People: Situation Analysis-Behavioral Survey Results & Discussions.* Report, Sudan National AIDS Control Program.

———. 2004d. *Military Situation: Analysis-Behavioral Survey Results & Discussions.* Report. Sudan National AIDS Control Program.

————. 2004e. *Prisoners: Situation Analysis-Behavioral Survey Results & Discussions*. Report. Sudan National AIDS Control Program.

————. 2004f. *Sex Sellers: Situation Analysis-Behavioral Survey Results & Discussions Report*. Sudan National AIDS Control Program.

————. 2004g. *STDs: Situation Analysis-Behavioral Survey Results & Discussions*. Report, Sudan National AIDS Control Program.

————. 2004h. *Street Children: Situation Analysis-Behavioral Survey Results & Discussions*. Report, Sudan National AIDS Control Program.

————. 2004i. *TB Patients: Situation Analysis-Behavioral Survey Results & Discussions*. Report. Sudan National AIDS Control Program.

————. 2004j. *Tea Sellers: Situation Analysis-Behavioral Survey Results & Discussions*. Report. Sudan National AIDS Control Program.

————. 2004k. *Truck Drivers: Situation Analysis-Behavioral Survey Results & Discussions*. Report. Sudan National AIDS Control Program.

————. 2004l. *University Students: Situation Analysis-Behavioral Survey, Results & Discussions*. Report, Sudan National AIDS Control Program.

Aidaoui, M., S. Bouzbid, and M. Laouar. 2008. "Seroprevalence of HIV Infection in Pregnant Women in the Annaba Region (Algeria)." *Rev Epidemiol Sante Publique* 56: 261–66.

Akcam, F. Z., E. Uskun, K. Avsar, and Y. Songur. 2009. "Hepatitis B Virus and Hepatitis C Virus Seroprevalence in Rural Areas of the Southwestern Region of Turkey." *Int J Infect Dis* 13: 274–84.

Akhtar, S., and T. Moatter. 2004. "Hepatitis C Virus Infection in Polytransfused Thalassemic Children in Pakistan." *Indian Pediatr* 41: 1072–73.

Akhtar, S., T. Moatter, S. I. Azam, M. H. Rahbar, and S. Adil. 2002. "Prevalence and Risk Factors for Intrafamilial Transmission of Hepatitis C Virus in Karachi, Pakistan." *J Viral Hepat* 9: 309–14.

Akhtar, S., M. Younus, S. Adil, S. H. Jafri, and F. Hassan. 2004. "Hepatitis C Virus Infection in Asymptomatic Male Volunteer Blood Donors in Karachi, Pakistan." *J Viral Hepat* 11: 527–35.

Al Nasser, M. N. 1992. "Intrafamilial Transmission of Hepatitis C Virus (HCV): A Major Mode of Spread in the Saudi Arabia Population." *Ann Trop Paediatr* 12: 211–15.

Alami, K. 2009. "Tendances récentes de l'épidémie à VIH/SIDA en Afrique du nord." Presentation, Research and AIDS Workshop in North Africa/Marrakech, Morocco.

Alavian, S. M., A. Ardeshiri, and B. Hajarizadeh. 2001. "Prevalence of HCV, HBV and HIV Infections among Hemophiliacs." *Transfusion Today* 49: 4–5.

Alavian, S. M., B. Gholami, and S. Masarrat. 2002. "Hepatitis C Risk Factors in Iranian Volunteer Blood Donors: A Case-Control Study." *J Gastroenterol Hepatol* 17: 1092–97.

Al-Dhahry, S. H. S., M. R. Buhl, A. S. Daar, P. N. Aganashinikar, and M. K. Al-Hasani. 1993. "Prevalence of Antibodies to Hepatitis C Virus among Omani Patients with Renal Disease." *Infection* 21: 164–67.

Al-Faleh, F. Z., E. A. Ayoola, M. Al-Jeffry, R. Al-Rashed, M. Al-Mofarreh, M. Arif, S. Ramia, M. Al-Karawi, and M. Al-Shabrawy. 1991. "Prevalence of Antibody to Hepatitis C Virus among Saudi Arabian Children: A Community-Based Study." *Hepatology* 14: 215–18.

Al-Fouzan, A., and N. Al-Mutairi. 2004. "Overview of Incidence of Sexually Transmitted Diseases in Kuwait." *Clin Dermatol* 22: 509–12.

Al-Fuzae, L., K. C. Aboolbacker, and Q. Al-Saleh. 1998. "Beta-Thalassaemia Major in Kuwait." *J Trop Pediatr* 44: 311–12.

Al-Ghanim, S. A. 2005. "Exploring Public Knowledge and Attitudes towards HIV/AIDS in Saudi Arabia: A Survey of Primary Health Care Users." *Saudi Med J* 26: 812–18.

Ali, F., A. Abdel-Aziz, M. F. Helmy, A. Abdel-Mobdy, and M. Darwish. 1998. "Prevalence of Certain Sexually Transmitted Viruses in Egypt." *J Egypt Public Health Assoc* 73: 181–92.

Ali, G., R. Khanani, M. A. Shaikh, A. R. Memon, and H. N. Naqvi. 1996. "Knowledge and Attitudes of Medical Students to People with HIV and AIDS." *J Coll Physicians Surg Pak* 6: 58–61.

Ali, M., M. A. Bhatti, and H. Ushijima. 2004. "Reproductive Health Needs of Adolescent Males in Rural Pakistan: An Exploratory Study." *Tohoku J Exp Med* 204: 17–25.

Ali, S. A., R. M. Donahue, H. Qureshi, and S. H. Vermund. 2009. "Hepatitis B and Hepatitis C in Pakistan: Prevalence and Risk Factors." *Int J Infect Dis* 13: 9–19.

Ali, S. S., I. S. Ali, A. H. Aamir, Z. Jadoon, and S. Inayatullah. 2007. "Frequency of Hepatitis C Infection in Diabetic Patients." *J Ayub Med Coll Abbottabad* 19: 46–49.

Alim, A., M. O. Artan, Z. Baykan, and B. A. Alim. 2009. "Seroprevalence of Hepatitis B and C Viruses, HIV, and Syphilis Infections among Engaged Couples." *Saudi Med J* 30: 541–45.

Alizadeh, A. H., S. M. Alavian, K. Jafari, and N. Yazdi. 2005. "Prevalence of Hepatitis C Virus Infection and Its Related Risk Factors in Drug Abuser Prisoners in Hamedan—Iran." *World J Gastroenterol* 11: 4085–89.

Al-Jabri, A. A., and J. H. Al-Abri. 2003. "Knowledge and Attitudes of Undergraduate Medical and Non-Medical Students in Sultan Qaboos University toward Acquired Immune Deficiency Syndrome." *Saudi Med J* 24: 273–77.

Al-Kubaisy, W. A., K. T. Al-Naib, and M. A. Habib. 2006a. "Prevalence of HCV/HIV Co-Infection among Haemophilia Patients in Baghdad." *East Mediterr Health J* 12: 264–69.

————. 2006b. "Seroprevalence of Hepatitis C Virus Specific Antibodies among Iraqi Children with Thalassaemia." *East Mediterr Health J* 12: 204–10.

Al-Kubaisy, W. A., A. D. Niazi, and K. Kubba. 2002. "History of Miscarriage as a Risk Factor for Hepatitis C Virus Infection in Pregnant Iraqi Women." *East Mediterr Health J* 8: 239–44.

Al-Mahroos, F. T., and A. Ebrahim. 1995. "Prevalence of Hepatitis B, Hepatitis C and Human Immune Deficiency Virus Markers among Patients with Hereditary Haemolytic Anaemias." *Ann Trop Paediatr* 15: 121–28.

Almawi, W. Y., A. A. Qadi, H. Tamim, G. Ameen, A. Bu-Ali, S. Arrayid, and M. M. Abou Jaoude. 2004. "Seroprevalence of Hepatitis C Virus and Hepatitis B Virus among Dialysis Patients in Bahrain and Saudi Arabia." *Transplant Proc* 36: 1824–26.

Al-Mazrou, Y. Y., M. S. Abouzeid, and M. H. Al-Jeffri. 2005. "Knowledge and Attitudes of Paramedical Students in Saudi Arabia toward HIV/AIDS." *Saudi Med J* 26: 1183–89.

Al-Moslih, M. I., and M. A. Al-Huraibi. 2001. "Prevalence of Hepatitis C Virus among Patients with Liver Disease in the Republic of Yemen." *East Mediterr Health J* 7: 771–78.

Al-Mugeiren, M., F. Z. Al-Faleh, S. Ramia, S. al-Rasheed, M. A. Mahmoud, and M. Al-Nasser. 1992. "Seropositivity to Hepatitis C Virus (HCV) in Saudi Children with Chronic Renal Failure Maintained on Haemodialysis." *Ann Trop Paediatr* 12: 217–19.

Al-Mutairi, N., A. Joshi, O. Nour-Eldin, A. K. Sharma, I. El-Adawy, and M. Rijhwani. 2007. "Clinical Patterns of Sexually Transmitted Diseases, Associated Sociodemographic Characteristics, and Sexual Practices in the Farwaniya Region of Kuwait." *Int J Dermatol* 46: 594–99.

Alnaqy, A., S. Al-Harthy, G. Kaminski, and S. Al-Dhahry. 2006. "Detection of Serum Antibodies to Hepatitis C Virus in 'False-Seronegative' Blood Donors in Oman." *Med Princ Pract* 15: 111–13.

Al-Owaish, R. A., S. Anwar, P. Sharma, and S. F. Shah. 2000. "HIV/AIDS Prevalence among Male Patients in Kuwait." *Saudi Med J* 21: 852–59.

Al-Owaish, R., M. A. Moussa, S. Anwar, H. Al-Shoumer, and P. Sharma. 1999. "Knowledge, Attitudes, Beliefs, and Practices about HIV/AIDS in Kuwait." *AIDS Educ Prev* 11: 163–73.

Alrajhi, A. A., A. Nematallah, S. Abdulwahab, and Z. Bukhary. 2002. "Human Immunodeficiency Virus and Tuberculosis Co-Infection in Saudi Arabia." *East Mediterr Health J* 8: 749–53.

Al-Serouri, A. W. 2005. "Assessment of Knowledge, Attitudes and Beliefs about HIV/AIDS among Young People Residing in High Risk Communities in Aden Governatore, Republic of Yemen." Society for the Development of Women & Children (SOUL), Education, Health, Welfare, and United Nations Children's Fund, Yemen Country Office, HIV/AIDS Project.

Al-Serouri, A. W., M. Takioldin, H. Oshish, A. Aldobaibi, and A. Abdelmajed. 2002. "Knowledge, Attitudes and Beliefs about HIV/AIDS in Sana'a, Yemen." *East Mediterr Health J* 8: 706–15.

Al-Sheyyab, M., A. Batieha, and M. El-Khateeb. 2001. "The Prevalence of Hepatitis B, Hepatitis C and Human Immune Deficiency Virus Markers in Multi-Transfused Patients." *J Trop Pediatr* 47: 239–42.

Altindis, M., S. Yilmaz, T. Dikengil, H. Acemoglu, and S. Hosoglu. 2006. "Seroprevalence and Genotyping of Hepatitis B, Hepatitis C and HIV among Healthy Population and Turkish Soldiers in Northern Cyprus." *World J Gastroenterol* 12: 6792–96.

Ameen, R., N. Sanad, S. Al-Shemmari, I. Siddique, R. I. Chowdhury, S. Al-Hamdan, and A. Al-Bashir. 2005. "Prevalence of Viral Markers among First-Time Arab Blood Donors in Kuwait." *Transfusion* 45: 1973–80.

Amiri, Z. M., A. J. Shakib, and M. Toorchi. 2005. "Seroprevalence of Hepatitis C and Risk Factors in Haemodialysis Patients in Guilan, Islamic Republic of Iran." *East Mediterr Health J* 11: 372–76.

Anonymous. 2006. *Scaling Up the HIV Response toward Universal Access to Prevention, Treatment, Care and Support in Jordan.* Summary report of the national consultation.

Anonymous. 2007. "Improving HIV/AIDS Response among Most at Risk Population in Sudan." Orientation Workshop, 16 April 2007.

Ansar, M. M., and A. Kooloobandi. 2002. "Prevalence of Hepatitis C Virus Infection in Thalassemia and Haemodialysis Patients in North Iran-Rasht." *J Viral Hepat* 9: 390–92.

Arafa, N., M. El Hoseiny, C. Rekacewicz, I. Bakr, S. El-Kafrawy, M. El Daly, S. Aoun, D. Marzouk, M. K. Mohamed, and A. Fontanet. 2005. "Changing Pattern of Hepatitis C Virus Spread in Rural Areas of Egypt." *J Hepatol* 43: 418–24.

Araj, G. F., E. E. Kfoury-Baz, K. A. Barada, R. E. Nassif, and S. Y. Alami. 1995. "Hepatitis C Virus: Prevalence in Lebanese Blood Donors and Brief Overview of the Disease." *J Med Liban* 43(1): 11–6.

Arbesser, C., J. R. Mose, and W. Sixl. 1987. "Serological Examinations of HIV-I Virus in Sudan." *J Hyg Epidemiol Microbiol Immunol* 31: 480–82.

Arthur, R. R., N. F. Hassan, M. Y. Abdallah, M. S. el-Sharkawy, M. D. Saad, B. G. Hackbart, and I. Z. Imam. 1997. "Hepatitis C Antibody Prevalence in Blood Donors in Different Governorates in Egypt." *Trans R Soc Trop Med Hyg* 91: 271–74.

Askarian, M., K. Mirzaei, and B. Cookson. 2007. "Knowledge, Attitudes, and Practice of Iranian Dentists with regard to HIV-Related Disease." *Infect Control Hosp Epidemiol* 28: 83–87.

Askarian, M., K. Mirzaei, and O. Assadian. 2007. "Iranians' Attitudes about Possible Human Immunodeficiency Virus Transmission in Dental Settings." *Infect Control Hosp Epidemiol* 28: 234–37.

Aslam, M., and J. Aslam. 2001. "Seroprevalence of the Antibody to Hepatitis C in Select Groups in the Punjab Region of Pakistan." *J Clin Gastroenterol* 33: 407–11.

Aslam, M., J. Aslam, B. D. Mitchell, and K. M. Munir. 2005. "Association between Smallpox Vaccination and Hepatitis C Antibody Positive Serology in Pakistani Volunteers." *J Clin Gastroenterol* 39: 243–46.

Assal, M. 2006. "HIV Prevalence, Knowledge, Attitude, Practices, and Risk Factors among Prisoners in Khartoum State, Sudan."

Ati, H. A. 2005. "HIV/AIDS/STIs Social and Geographical Mapping of Prisoners, Tea Sellers and Commercial Sex Workers in Port Sudan Town, Red Sea State." Draft 2, Ockenden International, Sudan.

Ayed, Z., D. Houinato, M. Hocine, S. Ranger-Rogez, and F. Denis. 1995. "Prevalence of Serum Markers of Hepatitis B and C in Blood Donors and Pregnant Women in Algeria." *Bull Soc Pathol Exot* 88: 225–28.

Ayoola, E. A., I. A. al-Mofleh, F. Z. al-Faleh, R. al-Rashed, M. A. Arif, S. Ramia, and I. Mayet. 1992. "Prevalence of Antibodies to Hepatitis C Virus among Saudi Patients with Chronic Liver Diseases." *Hepatogastroenterology* 39: 337–39.

Ayoola, E. A., S. Huraib, M. Arif, F. Z. al-Faleh, R. al-Rashed, S. Ramia, I. A. al-Mofleh, and H. Abu-Aisha. 1991. "Prevalence and Significance of Antibodies to Hepatitis C Virus among Saudi Haemodialysis Patients." *J Med Virol* 35: 155–59.

Ayranci, U. 2005. "AIDS Knowledge and Attitudes in a Turkish Population: An Epidemiological Study." *BMC Public Health* 5: 95.

Aziz, S., A. Memon, H. I. Tily, K. Rasheed, K. Jehangir, and M. S. Quraishy. 2002. "Prevalence of HIV, Hepatitis B and C amongst Health Workers of Civil Hospital Karachi." *J Pak Med Assoc* 52: 92–94.

Badahdah, A. 2005. "Saudi Attitudes towards People Living with HIV/AIDS." *Int J STD AIDS* 16: 837–38.

Baddoura, R., C. Haddad, and M. Germanos. 2002. "Hepatitis B and C Seroprevalence in the Lebanese Population." *East Mediterr Health J* 8: 150–56.

Baidy, Lo B., M. Adimorty, C. Fatimata, and S. Amadou. 1993. "Surveillance of HIV Seroprevalence in Mauritania." *Bull Soc Pathol Exot* 86: 133–35.

Bakir, T. M., K. M. Kurbaan, I. al Fawaz, and S. Ramia. 1995. "Infection with Hepatitis Viruses (B and C) and Human Retroviruses (HTLV-1 and HIV) in Saudi Children Receiving Cycled Cancer Chemotherapy." *J Trop Pediatr* 41: 206–9.

Baqi, S., S. A. Shah, M. A. Baig, S. A. Mujeeb, and A. Memon. 1999. "Seroprevalence of HIV, HBV, and Syphilis and Associated Risk Behaviours in Male Transvestites (Hijras) in Karachi, Pakistan." *Int J STD AIDS* 10: 300–4.

Basha, H. M. 2006. "Vulnerable Population Research in Darfur." Grey Report.

Bashawri, L. A., N. A. Fawaz, M. S. Ahmad, A. A. Qadi, and W. Y. Almawi. 2004. "Prevalence of Seromarkers of HBV and HCV among Blood Donors in Eastern Saudi Arabia, 1998–2001." *Clin Lab Haematol* 26: 225–28.

Basiratnia, M., S. M. K. HosseiniAsl, and M. Avijegan. 1999. "Hepatitis C Prevalence in Thalassemia Patients in Sharkord, Iran (Farsi)." *Shahrkord University Medical Science Journal* 4: 13–18.

Bassily, S., K. C. Hyams, R. A. Fouad, M. D. Samaan, and R. G. Hibbs. 1995. "A High Risk of Hepatitis C Infection among Egyptian Blood Donors: The Role of Parenteral Drug Abuse." *Am J Trop Med Hyg* 52: 503–5.

Baybuga, M. S., and S. S. Celik. 2004. "The Level of Knowledge and Views of the Street Children/Youth about AIDS in Turkey." *Int J Nurs Stud* 41: 591–97.

Bayoumi, A. 2005. *Baseline Survey of Intravenous Drug Users (IDUs) in Karthoum State (KS): Cross-Sectional and Case-Control Study*. Assignment Report, Inter Agency Technical Committee, Sudan National AIDS Programme, Federal Ministry of Health, Khartoum, Sudan.

Ben, Othman S., N. Bouzgarrou, A. Achour, T. Bourlet, B. Pozzetto, and A. Trabelsi. 2004. "High Prevalence and Incidence of Hepatitis C Virus Infections among Dialysis Patients in the East-Centre of Tunisia." *Pathol Biol* (Paris) 52: 323–27.

Benjelloun, S., B. Bahbouhi, S. Sekkat, A. Bennani, N. Hda, and A. Benslimane. 1996. "Anti-HCV Seroprevalence and Risk Factors of Hepatitis C Virus Infection in Moroccan Population Groups." *Res Virol* 147: 247–55.

Bennani, A., and K. Alami. 2006. "Surveillance sentinelle VIH, résultats 2005 et tendances de la séroprévalence du VIH." Morocco Ministry of Health, UNAIDS.

Bhatti, F. A., M. Amin, and M. Saleem. 1995. "Prevalence of Antibody to Hepatitis C Virus in Pakistani Thalassaemics by Particle Agglutination Test Utilizing C 200 and C 22-3 Viral Antigen Coated Particles." *J Pak Med Assoc* 45: 269–71.

Bile, K., C. Aden, H. Norder, L. Magnius, G. Lindberg, and L. Nilsson. 1993. "Important Role of Hepatitis C Virus Infection as a Cause of Chronic Liver Disease in Somalia." *Scand J Infect Dis* 25: 559–64.

Bile, K., O. Mohamud, C. Aden, A. Isse, H. Norder, L. Nilsson, and L. Magnius. 1992. "The Risk for Hepatitis A, B, and C at Two Institutions for Children in Somalia with Different Socioeconomic Conditions." *Am J Trop Med Hyg* 47: 357–64.

Boily, M. C., and B. Masse. 1997. "Mathematical Models of Disease Transmission: A Precious Tool for the Study of Sexually Transmitted Diseases." *Can J Public Health* 88: 255–65.

Bokhari, A., N. M. Nizamani, D. J. Jackson, N. E. Rehan, M. Rahman, R. Muzaffar, S. Mansoor, H. Raza, K. Qayum, P. Girault, E. Pisani, and I. Thaver. 2007. "HIV Risk in Karachi and Lahore, Pakistan: An Emerging Epidemic in Injecting and Commercial Sex Networks." *Int J STD AIDS* 18: 486–92.

Boulaajaj, K., Y. Elomari, B. Elmaliki, B. Madkouri, D. Zaid, and N. Benchemsi. 2005. "Prevalence of Hepatitis C, Hepatitis B and HIV Infection among Haemodialysis Patients in Ibn-Rochd University Hospital, Casablanca." *Nephrol Ther* 1: 274–84.

Boutayeb, H., A. Aamoum, and N. Benchemsi. 2006. "Knowledge about Hepatitis B and C Viruses and HIV among Blood Donors in Casablanca." *East Mediterr Health J* 12: 538–47.

Bozdayi, G., S. Rota, H. Verdi, U. Derici, S. Sindel, M. Bali, and T. Basay. 2002. "The Presence of Hepatitis C Virus (HCV) Infection in Hemodialysis Patients and Determination of HCV Genotype Distribution." *Mikrobiyol Bul* 36: 291–300.

Bozkurt, H., M. G. Kurtoglu, Y. Bayram, R. Kesli, and M. Berktas. 2008. "Distribution of Hepatitis C Prevalence in Individuals according to Their Age Level in Eastern Turkey." *Eur J Gastroenterol Hepatol* 20: 1249.

Brunham, R. C., and F. A. Plummer. 1990. "A General Model of Sexually Transmitted Disease Epidemiology and Its Implications for Control." *Med Clin North Am* 74: 1339–52.

Burans, J. P., M. McCarthy, S. M. el Tayeb, A. el Tigani, J. George, R. Abu-Elyazeed, and J. N. Woody. 1990. "Serosurvey of Prevalence of Human Immunodeficiency Virus amongst High Risk Groups in Port Sudan, Sudan." *East Afr Med J* 67: 650–55.

Busulwa, R. 2003. "HIV/AIDS Situation Analysis Study." Conducted in Hodeidah, Taiz and Hadhramut, Republic of Yemen.

Butt, T., and M. S. Amin. 2008. "Seroprevalence of Hepatitis B and C Infections among Young Adult Males in Pakistan. *East Mediterr Health J* 14: 791–97.

Candan, F., H. Alagozlu, O. Poyraz, and H. Sumer. 2002. "Prevalence of Hepatitis B and C Virus Infection in Barbers in the Sivas Region of Turkey." *Occup Med (Lond)* 52: 31–34.

Constantine, N. T., M. F. Sheba, D. M. Watts, Z. Farid, and M. Kamal. 1990. "HIV Infection in Egypt: A Two and a Half Year Surveillance." *J Trop Med Hyg* 93: 146–50.

Corwin, A. L., J. G. Olson, M. A. Omar, A. Razaki, and D. M. Watts. 1991. "HIV-1 in Somalia: Prevalence and Knowledge among Prostitutes." *AIDS* 5: 902–4.

Darwish, M. A., R. Faris, N. Darwish, A. Shouman, M. Gadallah, M. S. El-Sharkawy, R. Edelman, K. Grumbach, M. R. Rao, and J. D. Clemens. 2001. "Hepatitis C and Cirrhotic Liver Disease in the Nile Delta of Egypt: A Community-Based Study." *Am J Trop Med Hyg* 64: 147–53.

Darwish, M. A., T. A. Raouf, P. Rushdy, N. T. Constantine, M. R. Rao, and R. Edelman. 1993. "Risk Factors Associated with a High Seroprevalence of Hepatitis C Virus Infection in Egyptian Blood Donors." *Am J Trop Med Hyg* 49: 440–47.

Demirturk, N., T. Demirdal, D. Toprak, M. Altindis, and O. C. Aktepe. 2006. "Hepatitis B and C Virus in West-Central Turkey: Seroprevalence in Healthy Individuals Admitted to a University Hospital for Routine Health Checks." *Turk J Gastroenterol* 17: 267–72.

Dewachi, O. 2001. "HIV/AIDS Prevention through Outreach to Vulnerable Populations in Beirut, Lebanon: Men Who Have Sex with Other Men and HIV AIDS; A Situation Analysis in Beirut, Lebanon." Final report, April 29, 2001.

Djebbi, A., O. Bahri, H. Langar, A. Sadraoui, S. Mejri, and H. Triki. 2008. "Genetic Variability of Genotype 1 Hepatitis C Virus Isolates from Tunisian Haemophiliacs." *New Microbiol* 31: 473–80.

Djibouti National TB Programme. 2006. "TB Facts and Figures of Djibouti." Responsable du PNT, Ministere de la Santé, Republique de Djibouti.

Dray, X., R. Dray-Spira, J. A. Bronstein, and D. Mattera. 2005. "Prevalences of HIV, Hepatitis B and Hepatitis C in Blood Donors in the Republic of Djibouti." *Med Trop (Mars)* 65: 39–42.

Dupire, B., A. K. Abawi, C. Ganteaume, T. Lam, P. Truze, and G. Martet. 1999. "Establishment of a Blood Transfusion Center at Kabul (Afghanistan)." *Sante* 9: 18–22.

Ebrahim, H. 2008. "Iranian Epidemiological Training Programs for AIDS Prevention in Mazandaran Province." *Pak J Biol Sci* 11: 2109–15.

Eftekhar, M., M.-M. Gouya, A. Feizzadeh, N. Moshtagh, H. Setayesh, K. Azadmanesh, and A.-R. Vassigh. 2008. "Bio-Behavioural Survey on HIV and Its Risk Factors among Homeless Men Who Have Sex with Men in Teheran, 2006–07."

Egypt MOH (Ministry of Health), and Population National AIDS Program. 2006. *HIV/AIDS Biological and Behavioral Surveillance Survey*. Summary report.

El-Amin, H. H., E. M. Osman, M. O. Mekki, M. B. Abdelraheem, M. O. Ismail, M. E. Yousif, A. M. Abass, H. S. El-haj, and H. K. Ammar. 2007. "Hepatitis C Virus Infection in Hemodialysis Patients in Sudan: Two Centers' Report." *Saudi J Kidney Dis Transpl* 18: 101–6.

El-Gadi, S., A. Abudher, and M. Sammud. 2008. "HIV-Related Knowledge and Stigma among High School Students in Libya." *Int J STD AIDS* 19: 178–83.

El-Ghazzawi, E., L. Drew, L. Hamdy, E. El-Sherbini, Sel D. Sadek, and E. Saleh. 1995. "Intravenous Drug Addicts: A High Risk Group for Infection with Human Immunodeficiency Virus, Hepatitis Viruses, Cytomegalo Virus and Bacterial Infections in Alexandria Egypt." *J Egypt Public Health Assoc* 70: 127–50.

El-Ghazzawi, E., G. Hunsmann, and J. Schneider. 1987. "Low Prevalence of Antibodies to HIV-1 and HTLV-I in Alexandria, Egypt." *AIDS Forsch* 2: 639.

El-Gilany, A. H., and S. El-Fedawy. 2006. "Bloodborne Infections among Student Voluntary Blood Donors in Mansoura University, Egypt." *East Mediterr Health J* 12: 742–48.

El Gohary, A., A. Hassan, Z. Nooman, D. Lavanchy, C. Mayerat, A. El Ayat, N. Fawaz, F. Gobran, M. Ahmed, F. Kawano, et al. 1995. "High Prevalence of Hepatitis C Virus among Urban and Rural Population Groups in Egypt." *Acta Trop* 59: 155–61.

El Guneid, A. M., A. A. Gunaid, A. M. O'Neill, N. I. Zureikat, J. C. Coleman, and I. M. Murray-Lyon. 1993. "Prevalence of Hepatitis B, C, and D Virus Markers in Yemeni Patients with Chronic Liver Disease." *J Med Virol* 40: 330–33.

Elharti, E. E., Z. A. Zidouh, M. R. Mengad, B. O. Bennani, S. A. Siwani, K. H. Khattabi, A. M. Alami, and E. R. Elaouad. 2002. "Result of HIV Sentinel Surveillance Studies in Morocco during 2001." *Int Conf AIDS*: 14.

El-Hazmi, M. M. 2004. "Prevalence of HBV, HCV, HIV-1, 2 and HTLV-I/II Infections among Blood Donors in a Teaching Hospital in the Central Region of Saudi Arabia." *Saudi Med J* 25: 26–33.

El-Maaytah, M., A. Al Kayed, M. Al Qudah, H. Al Ahmad, K. Al-Dabbagh, W. Jerjes, M. Al Khawalde, O. Abu Hammad, N. Dar Odeh, K. El-Maaytah, Y. Al Shmailan, S. Porter, and C. Scully. 2005. "Willingness of Dentists in Jordan to Treat HIV-Infected Patients." *Oral Dis* 11: 318–22.

Elmir, E., S. Nadia, B. Ouafae, M. Rajae, S. Amina, and A. Rajae el. 2002. "HIV Epidemiology in Morocco: A Nine-Year Survey (1991–1999)." *Int J STD AIDS* 13: 839–42.

El-Nanawy, A. A., O. F. El Azzouni, A. T. Soliman, A. E. Amer, R. S. Demian, and H. M. El-Sayed. 1995.

"Prevalence of Hepatitis-C Antibody Seropositivity in Healthy Egyptian Children and Four High Risk Groups." *J Trop Pediatr* 41: 341–43.

Elrashied, S. M. 2006. "Generating Strategic Information and Assessing HIV/AIDS Knowledge, Attitude and Behaviour and Practices as well as Prevalence of HIV1 among MSM in Khartoum State, 2005." A draft report submitted to Sudan National AIDS Control Programme, Together Against AIDS Organization (TAG), Khartoum, Sudan.

El-Raziky, M. S., M. El-Hawary, G. Esmat, A. M. Abouzied, N. El-Koofy, N. Mohsen, S. Mansour, A. Shaheen, M. Abdel Hamid, and H. El-Karaksy. 2007. "Prevalence and Risk Factors of Asymptomatic Hepatitis C Virus Infection in Egyptian Children." *World J Gastroenterol* 13: 1828–32.

El-Sayed, H. F., S. M. Abaza, S. Mehanna, and P. J. Winch. 1997. "The Prevalence of Hepatitis B and C Infections among Immigrants to a Newly Reclaimed Area Endemic for Schistosoma Mansoni in Sinai, Egypt." *Acta Trop* 68: 229–37.

El-Sayed, N. M., P. J. Gomatos, G. R. Rodier, T. F. Wierzba, A. Darwish, S. Khashaba, and R. R. Arthur. 1996. "Seroprevalence Survey of Egyptian Tourism Workers for Hepatitis B Virus, Hepatitis C Virus, Human Immunodeficiency Virus, and Treponema Pallidum Infections: Association of Hepatitis C Virus Infections with Specific Regions of Egypt." *Am J Trop Med Hyg* 55: 179–84.

El-Sayyed, N., I. A. Kabbash, and M. El-Gueniedy. 2008. "Risk Behaviours for HIV/AIDS Infection among Men Who Have Sex with Men in Cairo, Egypt." *East Mediterr Health J* 14: 905–15.

Elsheikh, R. M., A. A. Daak, M. A. Elsheikh, M. S. Karsany, and I. Adam. 2007. "Hepatitis B Virus and Hepatitis C Virus in Pregnant Sudanese Women." *Virol J* 4: 104.

El-Sony, A. I., A. H. Khamis, D. A. Enarson, O. Baraka, S. A. Mustafa, and G. Bjune. 2002. "Treatment Results of DOTS in 1797 Sudanese Tuberculosis Patients with or without HIV Co-Infection." *Int J Tuberc Lung Dis* 6: 1058–66.

El-Tawila, S., O. El-Gibaly, B. Ibrahim, et al. 1999. *Transitions to Adulthood: A National Survey of Adolescents in Egypt.* Cairo, Egypt: Population Council.

Elzubier, A. G., M. H. el Nour, and E. H. Ansari. 1996. "AIDS-Related Knowledge and Misconceptions among High Secondary School Teachers and Students in Kassala, Sudan." *East Afr Med J* 73: 295–97.

Fahal, A. H., S. A. el Razig, S. H. Suliman, S. Z. Ibrahim, and A. E. Tigani. 1995. "Gastrointestinal Tract Cancer in Association with Hepatitis and HIV Infection." *East Afr Med J* 72: 424–26.

Faisel, A., and J. Cleland. 2006. "Study of the Sexual Behaviours and Prevalence of STIs among Migrant Men in Lahore, Pakistan." Arjumand and Associates, Centre for Population Studies, London School of Hygiene and Tropical Medicine.

Fakeeh, M., and A. M. Zaki. 1999. "Hepatitis C: Prevalence and Common Genotypes among Ethnic Groups in Jeddah, Saudi Arabia." *Am J Trop Med Hyg* 61: 889–92.

Farah, M. S., and S. Hussein. 2006. "HIV Prevalence, Knowledge, Attitude, Practices and Risk Factors among Truck Drivers in Karthoum State."

Farghaly, A. G., and M. M. Kamal. 1991. "Study of the Opinion and Level of Knowledge about AIDS Problem among Secondary School Students and Teachers in Alexandria." *J Egypt Public Health Assoc* 66: 209–25.

Farid, R., and A. J. Choudhry. 2003. "Knowledge about AIDS/HIV Infection among Female College Students." *J Coll Physicians Surg Pak* 13: 135–37.

Faris, R., and A. Shouman. 1994. "Study of the Knowledge, Attitude of Egyptian Health Care Workers towards Occupational HIV Infection." *J Egypt Public Health Assoc* 69: 115–28.

Fido, A., and R. Al Kazemi. 2002. "Survey of HIV/AIDS Knowledge and Attitudes of Kuwaiti Family Physicians." *Fam Pract* 19: 682–84.

Fox, E., R. L. Haberberger, E. A. Abbatte, S. Said, D. Polycarpe, and N. T. Constantine. 1989. "Observations on Sexually Transmitted Diseases in Promiscuous Males in Djibouti." *J Egypt Public Health Assoc* 64: 561–69.

Ganczak, M., P. Barss, F. Alfaresi, S. Almazrouei, A. Muraddad, and F. Al-Maskari. 2007. "Break the Silence: HIV/AIDS Knowledge, Attitudes, and Educational Needs among Arab University Students in United Arab Emirates." *J Adolesc Health* 40: 572 e571–78.

Ghannad, M. S., S. M. Arab, M. Mirzaei, and A. Moinipur. 2009. "Epidemiologic Study of Human Immunodeficiency Virus (HIV) Infection in the Patients Referred to Health Centers in Hamadan Province, Iran." *AIDS Res Hum Retroviruses* 25: 277–83.

Gharamah, F. A., and N. A. Baktayan. 2006. "Exploring HIV/AIDS Knowledge and Attitudes of Secondary School Students (10th &11th Grade) in Al-Tahreer District Sana'a City." Republic of Yemen, March–April.

Ghavanini, A. A., and M. R. Sabri. 2000. "Hepatitis B Surface Antigen and Anti-Hepatitis C Antibodies among Blood Donors in the Islamic Republic of Iran." *East Mediterr Health J* 6: 1114–16.

Gheith, O. A., M. A. Saad, A. A. Hassan, A. E. Agroudy, H. Sheashaa, and M. A. Ghoneim. 2007. "Hepatic Dysfunction in Kidney Transplant Recipients: Prevalence and Impact on Graft and Patient Survival." *Clin Exp Nephrol* 11: 309–15.

Gholamreza, R., S. Shahryar, K. Abbasali, J. Hamidreza, M. Abdolvahab, K. Khodaberdi, R. Danyal, and A. Nafiseh. 2007. "Seroprevalence of Hepatitis B Virus and Its Co-Infection with Hepatitis D Virus and Hepatitis C Virus in Iranian Adult Population." *Indian J Med Sci* 61: 263–68.

Gohar, S. A., R. Y. Khalil, N. M. Elaish, E. M. Khedr, and M. S. Ahmed. 1995. "Prevalence of Antibodies to Hepatitis C Virus in Hemodialysis Patients and Renal Transplant Recipients." *J Egypt Public Health Assoc* 70: 465–84.

Gorgi, Y., S. Yalaoui, H. L. Ben Nejma, M. M. Azzouz, M. Hsairi, H. Ben Khelifa, and K. Ayed. 1998. "Detection of Hepatitis C Virus in the General Population of Tunisia." *Bull Soc Pathol Exot* 91: 177.

Gul, A., and F. Iqbal. 2003. "Prevalence of Hepatitis C in Patients on Maintenance Haemodialysis." *J Coll Physicians Surg Pak* 13: 15–18.

Gul, U., A. Kilic, B. Sakizligil, S. Aksaray, S. Bilgili, O. Demirel, and C. Erinckan. 2008. "Magnitude of Sexually Transmitted Infections among Female Sex Workers in Turkey." *J Eur Acad Dermatol Venereol* 22: 1123–24.

Gulcan, A., E. Gulcan, A. Toker, I. Bulut, and Y. Akcan. 2008. "Evaluation of Risk Factors and Seroprevalence of Hepatitis B and C in Diabetic Patients in Kutahya, Turkey." *J Investig Med* 56: 858–63.

Gurol, E., C. Saban, O. Oral, A. Cigdem, and A. Armagan. 2006. "Trends in Hepatitis B and Hepatitis C Virus among Blood Donors over 16 Years in Turkey." *Eur J Epidemiol* 21: 299–305.

Gutbi, O. S.-A., and A. M. G. Eldin. 2006. "Women Tea-Sellers in Khartoum and HIV/AIDS: Surviving Against the Odds." Khartoum, Sudan.

Hachicha, J., A. Hammami, H. Masmoudi, M. Ben Hmida, H. Karray, M. Kharrat, F. Kammoun, and A. Jarraya. 1995. "Viral Hepatitis C in Chronic Hemodialyzed Patients in Southern Tunisia: Prevalence and Risk Factors." *Ann Med Interne* (Paris) 146: 295–98.

Haidar, N. A. 2002. "Prevalence of Hepatitis B and Hepatitis C in Blood Donors and High Risk Groups in Hajjah, Yemen Republic." *Saudi Med J* 23: 1090–94.

Haider, G., N. Zohra, N. Nisar, and A. A. Munir. 2009. "Knowledge about AIDS/HIV Infection among Women Attending Obstetrics and Gynaecology Clinic at a University Hospital." *J Pak Med Assoc* 59: 95–98.

Hajiabdolbaghi, M., N. Razani, N. Karami, P. Kheirandish, M. Mohraz, M. Rasoolinejad, K. Arefnia, Z. Kourorian, G. Rutherford, and W. McFarland. 2007. "Insights from a Survey of Sexual Behavior among a Group of At-Risk Women in Tehran, Iran, 2006." *AIDS Educ Prev* 19: 519–30.

Hajiani, E., J. Hashemi, R. Masjedizadeh, A. A. Shayesteh, E. Idani, and T. Rajabi. 2006. "Seroepidemiology of Hepatitis C and Its Risk Factors in Khuzestan Province, South-West of Iran: A Case-Control Study." *World J Gastroenterol* 12: 4884–87.

Haque, N., T. Zafar, H. Brahmbhatt, G. Imam, S. ul Hassan, and S. A. Strathdee. 2004. "High-Risk Sexual Behaviours among Drug Users in Pakistan: Implications for Prevention of STDs and HIV/AIDS." *Int J STD AIDS* 15: 601–7.

Harakati, M. S., O. A. Abualkhair, and B. A. Al-Knawy. 2000. "Hepatitis C Virus Infection in Saudi Arab Patients with B-Cell Non-Hodgkin's Lymphoma." *Saudi Med J* 21: 755–58.

Haroon, A. 1994. "Dancers of the Night." *World AIDS* 11.

Hatira, S. A., S. Yacoub-Jemni, B. Houissa, H. Kaabi, M. Zaeir, M. Kortas, and L. Ghachem. 2000. "Hepatitis C Virus Antibodies in 34,130 Blood Donors in Tunisian Sahel." *Tunis Med* 78: 101–5.

Hedayati-Moghaddam, M. R. 2008. "Knowledge of and Attitudes towards HIV/AIDS in Mashhad, Islamic Republic of Iran." *East Mediterr Health J* 14: 1321–32.

Heikel, J., S. Sekkat, F. Bouqdir, H. Rich, B. Takourt, F. Radouani, N. Hda, S. Ibrahimy, and A. Benslimane. 1999. "The Prevalence of Sexually Transmitted Pathogens in Patients Presenting to a Casablanca STD Clinic." *Eur J Epidemiol* 15: 711–15.

Hermez, J., E. Aaraj, O. Dewachi, and N. Chemaly. Unknown. "HIV/AIDS Prevention among Vulnerable Groups in Beirut, Lebanon." PowerPoint presentation.

Hindy, A. M., E. S. Abdelhaleem, and R. H. Aly. 1995. "Hepatitis B and C Viruses among Egyptian Dentists." *Egypt Dent J* 41: 1217–26.

Hmaied, F., M. Ben Mamou, K. Saune-Sandres, L. Rostaing, A. Slim, Z. Arrouji, S. Ben Redjeb, and J. Izopet. 2006. "Hepatitis C Virus Infection among Dialysis Patients in Tunisia: Incidence and Molecular Evidence for Nosocomial Transmission." *J Med Virol* 78: 185–91.

Hmida, S., N. Mojaat, E. Chaouchi, T. Mahjoub, B. Khlass, S. Abid, and K. Boukef. 1995. "HCV Antibodies in Hemodialyzed Patients in Tunisia." *Pathol Biol* (Paris) 43: 581–83.

Holt, B. Y., P. Effler, W. Brady, J. Friday, E. Belay, K. Parker, and M. Toole. 2003. "Planning STI/HIV Prevention among Refugees and Mobile Populations: Situation Assessment of Sudanese Refugees." *Disasters* 27: 1–15.

Hosseini Asl, S. K., M. Avijgan, and M. Mohamadnejad. 2004. "High Prevalence of HBV, HCV, and HIV Infections: In Gypsy Population Residing in Shar-e-kord." *Arch Iranian Med* 7: 22–24.

Hosseini-Moghaddam, S. M., H. Keyvani, H. Kasiri, S. M. Kazemeyni, A. Basiri, N. Aghel, and S. M. Alavian. 2006. "Distribution of Hepatitis C Virus Genotypes among Hemodialysis Patients in Tehran—A Multicenter Study." *J Med Virol* 78: 569–73.

Hsairi, M., and S. Ben Abdallah. 2007. "Analyse de la situation de vulnérabilité vis-à-vis de l'infection à VIH des hommes ayant des relations sexuelles avec des hommes." For ATL MST sida NGO–Tunis Section, National AIDS Programme/DSSB, UNAIDS. Final report, abridged version.

Hussain, S. F., M. Irfan, M. Abbasi, S. S. Anwer, S. Davidson, R. Haqqee, J. A. Khan, and M. Islam. 2004. "Clinical Characteristics of 110 Miliary Tuberculosis Patients from a Low HIV Prevalence Country." *Int J Tuberc Lung Dis* 8: 493–99.

Husseini, A., and N. M. Abu-Rmeileh. 2007. "HIV/AIDS-Related Knowledge and Attitudes of Palestinian Women in the Occupied Palestinian Territory." *Am J Health Behav* 31: 323–34.

Hyder, A. A., and O. A. Khan. 1998. "HIV/AIDS in Pakistan: The Context and Magnitude of an Emerging Threat." *J Epidemiol Community Health* 52: 579–85.

IGAD (Intergovernmental Authority on Development). 2006. "IGAD/World Bank Cross Border Mobile Population Mapping Exercise." Sudan, draft report.

Imani, R., A. Karimi, R. Rouzbahani, and A. Rouzbahani. 2008. "Seroprevalence of HBV, HCV and HIV Infection among Intravenous Drug Users in Shahr-e-Kord, Islamic Republic of Iran." *East Mediterr Health J* 14: 1136–41.

Institut de Formation Paramédicale de Parnet. 2004. *Rapport de la réunion d'évaluation a mis-parcours de l'enquête de sero-surveillance du VIH*. Juin.

Iqbal, J., and N. Rehan. 1996. "Sero-Prevalence of HIV: Six Years' Experience at Shaikh Zayed Hospital, Lahore." *J Pak Med Assoc* 46: 255–58.

Irani-Hakime, N., J. Aoun, S. Khoury, H. R. Samaha, H. Tamim, and W. Y. Almawi. 2001a. "Seroprevalence of Hepatitis C Infection among Health Care Personnel in Beirut, Lebanon." *Am J Infect Control* 29: 20–23.

Irani-Hakime, N., H. Tamim, H. Samaha, and W. Y. Almawi. 2001b. "Prevalence of Antibodies against Hepatitis C Virus among Blood Donors in Lebanon, 1997–2000." *Clin Lab Haematol* 23: 317–23.

Irani-Hakime, N., U. Musharrafieh, H. Samaha, and W. Y. Almawi. 2006. "Prevalence of Antibodies against Hepatitis B Virus and Hepatitis C Virus among Blood Donors in Lebanon, 1997–2003." *Am J Infect Control* 34: 241–43.

Iraq National TB Programme. 2006. "TB Facts and Figures of Iraq." Directorate of General Health & Primary Health Care. Ministry of Health.

IRIB (Islamic Republic of Iran Broadcasting). 2006. "Poll of Teheran Public on AIDS." Unpublished.

Jafri, W., N. Jafri, J. Yakoob, M. Islam, S. F. Tirmizi, T. Jafar, S. Akhtar, S. Hamid, H. A. Shah, and S. Q. Nizami. 2006. "Hepatitis B and C: Prevalence and Risk Factors Associated with Seropositivity among Children in Karachi, Pakistan." *BMC Infect Dis* 6: 101.

Jafroodi, M., and R. Asadi. 2006. "Prevalence of HCV in Thalassemia Major Patients in Guilan Province, Iran." The 4th Congress of Iranian Pediatric Hematology, Oncology Society. Kerman, Iran. September.

Jahani, M. R., S. M. Alavian, H. Shirzad, A. Kabir, and B. Hajarizadeh. 2005. "Distribution and Risk Factors of Hepatitis B, Hepatitis C, and HIV Infection in a Female Population with 'Illegal Social Behaviour.'" *Sex Transm Infect* 81: 185.

Jama, H., L. Grillner, G. Biberfeld, S. Osman, A. Isse, M. Abdirahman, and S. Bygdeman. 1987. "Sexually Transmitted Viral Infections in Various Population Groups in Mogadishu, Somalia." *Genitourin Med* 63: 329–32.

Jamal, N., I. A. Khushk, and Z. Naeem. 2006. "Knowledge and Attitudes regarding AIDS among Female Commercial Sex Workers at Hyderabad City, Pakistan. *J Coll Physicians Surg Pak* 16: 91–93.

Javadi, A. A., M. Avijgan, and M. Hafizi. 2006. "Prevalence of HBV and HCV Infections and Associated Risk Factors in Addict Prisoners." *Iranian J Publ Health* 35: 33–36.

Javadzadeh, H., M. Attar, and M. Taher Yavari. 2006. "Study of the Prevalence of HBV, HCV, and HIV Infection in Hemophilia and Thalassemia Population of Yazd (Farsi)." *Khoon (Blood)* 2: 315–22.

Jemni, L., S. Bahri, M. Saadi, A. Letaif, M. Dhidah, H. Lahdhiri, and S. Bouchoucha. 1991. "AIDS and Tuberculosis in Central Tunisia." *Tunis Med* 69: 349–52.

Jemni, S., K. Ikbel, M. Kortas, J. Mahjoub, L. Ghachem, J. M. Bidet, and K. Boukef. 1994. "Seropositivity to Hepatitis C Virus in Tunisian Haemodialysis Patients." *Nouv Rev Fr Hematol* 36: 349–51.

Jordan National AIDS Control Programme. 2005. *Report on the National KABP Survey on HIV/AIDS among Jordanian Youth*. NAP Jordan. Amman, Jordan: Ministry of Health.

Jordan National TB Programme. 2006. "TB Facts and Figures of Jordan." Directorate of Chest Diseases and Foreigner's Health, Ministry of Health.

Jurjus, A. R., J. Kahhaleh, National AIDS Program, and WHO/EMRO. 2004. "Knowledge, Attitudes, Beliefs, and Practices of the Lebanese concerning HIV/AIDS." Beirut, Lebanon.

Kabbash, I. A., N. M. El-Sayed, A. N. Al-Nawawy, I. K. Shady, and M. S. Abou Zeid. 2007. "Condom Use among Males (15–49 Years) in Lower Egypt: Knowledge, Attitudes and Patterns of Use." *East Mediterr Health J* 13: 1405–16.

Kadivar, M. R., A. R. Mirahmadizadeh, A. Karimi, and A. Hemmati. 2001. "The Prevalence of HCV and HIV in Thalassemia Patients in Shiraz, Iran." *Medical Journal of Iranian Hospital* 4: 18–20.

Kafi, S. K., A. O. Mohamed, and H. A. Musa. 2000. "Prevalence of Sexually Transmitted Diseases (STD) among Women in a Suburban Sudanese Community." *Ups J Med Sci* 105: 249–53.

Kakepoto, G. N., H. S. Bhally, G. Khaliq, N. Kayani, I. A. Burney, T. Siddiqui, and M. Khurshid. 1996. "Epidemiology of Blood-Borne Viruses: A Study of Healthy Blood Donors in Southern Pakistan." *Southeast Asian J Trop Med Public Health* 27: 703–6.

Karimi, I, and B. Ataei. 2007. "The Assessment of Knowledge about AIDS and Its Prevention on Isfahan High School Students." European Society of Clinical Microbiology and Infectious Diseases, Munich, Germany.

Karimi, M., and A. A. Ghavanini. 2001. "Seroprevalence of Hepatitis B, Hepatitis C and Human Immunodeficiency Virus Antibodies among Multitransfused Thalassaemic Children in Shiraz, Iran." *J Paediatr Child Health* 37: 564–66.

Karimi, M., H. Yarmohammadi, and R. Ardeshiri. 2002. "Inherited Coagulation Disorders in Southern Iran." *Haemophilia* 8: 740–44.

Karkar, A. 2007. "Hepatitis C in Dialysis Units: The Saudi Experience." *Hemodial Int* 11: 354–67.

Kashef, S., M. Karimi, Z. Amirghofran, M. Ayatollahi, M. Pasalar, M. M. Ghaedian, and M. A. Kashef. 2008. "Antiphospholipid Antibodies and Hepatitis C Virus Infection in Iranian Thalassemia Major Patients." *Int J Lab Hematol* 30: 11–16.

Kassem, A. S., A. A. el-Nawawy, M. N. Massoud, S. Y. el-Nazar, and E. M. Sobhi. 2000. "Prevalence of Hepatitis C Virus (HCV) Infection and Its Vertical Transmission in Egyptian Pregnant Women and Their Newborns." *J Trop Pediatr* 46: 231–33.

Kayani, N., A. Sheikh, A. Khan, C. Mithani, and M. Khurshid. 1994. "A View of HIV-I Infection in Karachi." *J Pak Med Assoc* 44: 8–11.

Kebudi, R., I. Ayan, G. Yilmaz, F. Akici, O. Gorgun, and S. Badur. 2000. "Seroprevalence of Hepatitis B, Hepatitis C, and Human Immunodeficiency Virus

Infections in Children with Cancer at Diagnosis and following Therapy in Turkey." *Med Pediatr Oncol* 34: 102–5.

Khamispoor, G., and R. Tahmasebi. 1999. "Prevalence of HIV, HBV, HCV and Syphilis in High Risk Groups of Bushehr Province (Farsi)." *Iranian South Medical Journal* 1: 59–53.

Khan, A. J., S. P. Luby, F. Fikree, A. Karim, S. Obaid, S. Dellawala, S. Mirza, T. Malik, S. Fisher-Hoch, and J. B. McCormick. 2000. "Unsafe Injections and the Transmission of Hepatitis B and C in a Periurban Community in Pakistan." *Bull World Health Organ* 78: 956–63.

Khan, M. S., M. Jamil, S. Jan, S. Zardad, S. Sultan, and A. S. Sahibzada. 2007. "Prevalence of Hepatitis 'B' and 'C' in Orthopaedics Patients at Ayub Teaching Hospital Abbottabad." *J Ayub Med Coll Abbottabad* 19: 82–84.

Khan, S. J., Q. Anjum, N. U. Khan, and F. G. Nabi. 2005. "Awareness about Common Diseases in Selected Female College Students of Karachi." *J Pak Med Assoc* 55: 195–98.

Khan, S., M. A. Rai, A. Khan, A. Farooqui, S. U. Kazmi, and S. H. Ali. 2008. "Prevalence of HCV and HIV Infections in 2005-Earthquake-Affected Areas of Pakistan." *BMC Infect Dis* 8: 147.

Khan, T. M. 1995. "Country Watch: Pakistan." *AIDS STD Health Promot Exch* 7–8.

Khan, Z. A., I. S. Alkhalife, and S. E. Fathalla. 2004. "Prevalence of Hepatitis C Virus among Bilharziasis Patients." *Saudi Med J* 25: 204–6.

Khanani, R. M., A. Hafeez, S. M. Rab, and S. Rasheed. 1990. "AIDS and HIV Associated Disorders in Karachi." *J Pak Med Assoc* 40: 82–85.

Khani, M., and M. M. Vakili. 2003. "Prevalence and Risk Factors of HIV, Hepatitis B Virus, and Hepatitis C Virus Infections in Drug Addicts among Zanjan Prisoners." *Arch Iranian Med* 6: 1–4.

Khattabi, H., and K. Alami. 2005. "Surveillance sentinelle du VIH, Résultats 2004 et tendance de la séroprévalence du VIH." Morocco Ministry of Health, UNAIDS.

Khattak, M. F., N. Salamat, F. A. Bhatti, and T. Z. Qureshi. 2002. "Seroprevalence of Hepatitis B, C and HIV in Blood Donors in Northern Pakistan." *J Pak Med Assoc* 52: 398–402.

Khattak, M. N., S. Akhtar, S. Mahmud, and T. M. Roshan. 2008. "Factors Influencing Hepatitis C Virus Sero-Prevalence among Blood Donors in North West Pakistan." *J Public Health Policy* 29: 207–25.

Khawaja, Z. A., L. Gibney, A. J. Ahmed, and S. H. Vermund. 1997. "HIV/AIDS and Its Risk Factors in Pakistan." *AIDS* 11: 843–48.

Khedmat, H., F. Fallahian, H. Abolghasemi, S. M. Alavian, B. Hajibeigi, S. M. Miri, and A. M. Jafari. 2007. "Seroepidemiologic Study of Hepatitis B Virus, Hepatitis C Virus, Human Immunodeficiency Virus and Syphilis Infections in Iranian Blood Donors." *Pak J Biol Sci* 10: 4461–66.

Kheirandish, P., S. SeyedAlinaghi, M. Hosseini, M. Jahani, H. Shirzad, M. Foroughi, M. Seyed Ahmadian, H. Jabbari, M. Mohraz, and W. McFarland. 2009. "Prevalence and Correlates of HIV Infection among Male Injection Drug Users in Detention, Tehran, Iran." Unpublished.

Khokhar, N., M. L. Gill, and G. J. Malik. 2004. "General Seroprevalence of Hepatitis C and Hepatitis B Virus Infections in Population." *J Coll Physicians Surg Pak* 14: 534–36.

Kilani, B., L. Ammari, C. Marrakchi, A. Letaief, M. Chakroun, M. Ben Jemaa, H. T. Ben Aissa, F. Kanoun, and T. Ben Chaabene. 2007. "Seroepidemiology of HCV-HIV Coinfection in Tunisia." *Tunis Med* 85: 121–23.

Kocabas, E., N. Aksaray, E. Alhan, A. Tanyeli, F. Koksal, and F. Yarkin. 1997a. "Hepatitis B and C Virus Infections in Turkish Children with Cancer." *Eur J Epidemiol* 13: 869–73.

Kocabas, E., N. Aksaray, E. Alhan, F. Yarkin, F. Koksal, and Y. Kilinc. 1997b. "Hepatitis B and C Virus Infections in Turkish Children with Haemophilia." *Acta Paediatr* 86: 1135–37.

Koksal, I., K. Biberoglu, S. Biberoglu, F. Koc, Y. Ayma, F. Aker, and H. Koksal. 1991. "Hepatitis C Virus Antibodies among Risk Groups in Turkey." *Infection* 19: 228–29.

Kose, S., A. Gurkan, F. Akman, M. Kelesoglu, and U. Uner. 2009. "Treatment of Hepatitis C in Hemodialysis Patients Using Pegylated Interferon Alpha-2a in Turkey." *J Gastroenterol* 44: 353–58.

Kudrati, M., M. L. Plummer, and N. D. Yousif. 2008. "Children of the Sug: A Study of the Daily Lives of Street Children in Khartoum, Sudan, with Intervention Recommendations." *Child Abuse Negl* 32: 439–48.

Kudrati, M., M. Plummer, N. Dafaalla El Hag Yousif, A. Mohamed Adam Adham, W. Mohamed Osman Khalifa, A. Khogali Eltayeb, J. Mohamed Jubara, V. Omujwok Apieker, S. Ali Yousif, and S. Mohamed Elnour. 2002. "Sexual Health and Risk Behaviour of Full-Time Street Children in Khartoum, Sudan." International Conference on AIDS, Barcelona, Spain, July 7–12; 14: Abstract no. LbOr04.

Kulane, A., A. A. Hilowle, A. A. Hassan, and R. Thorstensson. 2000. "Prevalence of HIV, HTLV I/II and HBV Infections during Long Lasting Civil Conflicts in Somalia." *Int Conf AIDS*: 13.

Kumar, R. M., P. M. Frossad, and P. F. Hughes. 1997. "Seroprevalence and Mother-to-Infant Transmission of Hepatitis C in Asymptomatic Egyptian Women." *Eur J Obstet Gynecol Reprod Biol* 75: 177–82.

Kuo, I., S. ul-Hasan, N. Galai, D. L. Thomas, T. Zafar, M. A. Ahmed, and S. A. Strathdee. 2006. "High HCV Seroprevalence and HIV Drug Use Risk Behaviors among Injection Drug Users in Pakistan." *Harm Reduct J* 3: 26.

Kuwait National TB Programme. 2006. "TB Facts and Figures of Kuwait." Kuwait, Department of Public Health, Ministry of Health.

Langar, H., H. Triki, E. Gouider, O. Bahri, A. Djebbi, A. Sadraoui, A. Hafsia, and R. Hafsia. 2005. "Blood-Transmitted Viral Infections among Haemophiliacs in Tunisia." *Transfusion clinique et biologique* 12: 301–5.

Lazarus, J. V., H. M. Himedan, L. R. Ostergaard, and J. Liljestrand. 2006. "HIV/AIDS Knowledge and Condom Use among Somali and Sudanese Immigrants in Denmark." *Scand J Public Health* 34: 92–99.

Lebanon National AIDS Control Program. 1996. "General Population Evaluation Survey Assessing Knowledge, Attitudes, Beliefs and Practices Related to HIV/AIDS in Lebanon." Ministry of Public Health.

———. 2003. "Soins Infirmiers et Développement Communautaire (SIDC) (2003) Rapid Appraisal Study on Stigma and Discrimination in Lebanon." Ministry of Public Health, Beirut, Lebanon.

Lebanon National TB Programme. 2006. "TB Facts and Figures of Lebanon." Ministry of Public Health, Karantina, Beirut, Lebanon.

Lehman, E. M., and M. L. Wilson. 2009. "Epidemiology of Hepatitis Viruses among Hepatocellular Carcinoma Cases and Healthy People in Egypt: A Systematic Review and Meta-Analysis." *Int J Cancer* 124: 690–97.

Libya National Center for the Prevention of and Control of Infectious Diseases. 2005. "Results of the National Seroprevalence Survey."

Lycke, E., G. B. Lowhagen, G. Hallhagen, G. Johannisson, and K. Ramstedt. 1980. "The Risk of Transmission of Genital Chlamydia Trachomatis Infection Is Less Than That of Genital Neisseria Gonorrhoeae Infection." *Sex Transm Dis* 7: 6–10.

Mabrouk, G. M. 1997. "Prevalence of Hepatitis C Infection and Schistosomiasis in Egyptian Patients with Hepatocellular Carcinoma." *Dis Markers* 13: 177–82.

Madwar, M. A., I. El-Gindy, H. M. Fahmy, N. M. Shoeb, and B. A. Massoud. 1999. "Hepatitis C Virus Transmission in Family Members of Egyptian Patients with HCV Related Chronic Liver Disease." *J Egypt Public Health Assoc* 74: 313–32.

Mahaba, H., K. el-Tayeb Ael, and H. Elbaz. 1999. "The Prevalence of Antibodies to Hepatitis C Virus in Hail Region, Saudi Arabia." *J Egypt Public Health Assoc* 74: 69–80.

Mahfouz, A. A., W. Alakija, A. A. al-Khozayem, and R. A. al-Erian. 1995. "Knowledge and Attitudes towards AIDS among Primary Health Care Physicians in the Asir Region, Saudi Arabia." *J R Soc Health* 115: 23–25.

Mahmoud, M. M., A. M. Nasr, D. E. Gassmelseed, M. A. Abdalelhafiz, M. A. Elsheikh, and I. Adam. 2007. "Knowledge and Attitude toward HIV Voluntary Counseling and Testing Services among Pregnant Women Attending an Antenatal Clinic in Sudan." *J Med Virol* 79: 469–73.

Mansoor, A. B., W. Fungladda, J. Kaewkungwal, and W. Wongwit. 2008. "Gender Differences in KAP Related to HIV/AIDS among Freshmen in Afghan Universities." *Southeast Asian J Trop Med Public Health* 39: 404–418.

Mansour-Ghanaei, F., M. S. Fallah, A. Shafaghi, M. Yousefi-Mashhoor, N. Ramezani, F. Farzaneh, and R. Nassiri. 2002. "Prevalence of Hepatitis B and C Seromarkers and Abnormal Liver Function Tests among Hemophiliacs in Guilan (Northern Province of Iran)." *Med Sci Monit* 8: CR797–800.

Marcelin, A. G., M. Grandadam, P. Flandre, E. Nicand, C. Milliancourt, J. L. Koeck, M. Philippon, R. Teyssou, H. Agut, N. Dupin, and V. Calvez. 2002. "Kaposi's Sarcoma Herpesvirus and HIV-1 Seroprevalences in Prostitutes in Djibouti." *J Med Virol* 68: 164–67.

Marcelin, A. G., M. Grandadam, P. Flandre, J. L. Koeck, M. Philippon, E. Nicand, R. Teyssou, H. Agut, J. M. Huraux, and N. Dupin. 2001. "Comparative Study of Heterosexual Transmission of HIV-1, HSV-2 and KSHV in Djibouti." *8th Retrovir Oppor Infect* (abstract no. 585).

Marzouk, D., J. Sass, I. Bakr, M. El Hosseiny, M. Abdel-Hamid, C. Rekacewicz, N. Chaturvedi, M. K. Mohamed, and A. Fontanet. 2007. "Metabolic and Cardiovascular Risk Profiles and Hepatitis C Virus Infection in Rural Egypt." *Gut* 56: 1105–10.

Mazloomy, S. S., and M. H. Baghianimoghadam. 2008. "Knowledge and Attitude about HIV/AIDS of Schoolteachers in Yazd, Islamic Republic of Iran." *East Mediterr Health J* 14: 292–97.

McCarthy, M. C., A. el-Tigani, I. O. Khalid, and K. C. Hyams. 1994. "Hepatitis B and C in Juba, Southern Sudan: Results of a Serosurvey." *Trans R Soc Trop Med Hyg* 88: 534–36.

McCarthy, M. C., I. O. Khalid, and A. El Tigani. 1995. "HIV-1 Infection in Juba, Southern Sudan." *J Med Virol* 46: 18–20.

Measure DHS. 1998. "Jordan: Demographic and Health Survey 1997."

———. 2003. "Jordan: Demographic and Health Survey 2002."

———. 2004. "Egypt: Demographic and Health Survey 2003."

———. 2006. "Egypt: Demographic and Health Survey 2005."

———. 2007. "Pakistan Demographic and Health Survey 2006–7." Preliminary report, National Institute for Population Studies, Measure DHS, and Macro International.

Mejri, S., A. B. Salah, H. Triki, N. B. Alaya, A. Djebbi, and K. Dellagi. 2005. "Contrasting Patterns of Hepatitis C Virus Infection in Two Regions from Tunisia." *J Med Virol* 76: 185–93.

Ministry of Health and Medical Education of Iran. 2006. "Treatment and Medical Education." Islamic Republic of Iran HIV/AIDS situation and response analysis.

Mirmomen, S., S. M. Alavian, S. M., B. Hajarizadeh, J. Kafaee, B. Yektaparast, M. J. Zahedi, A. A. Azami, M. M. Hosseini, A. R. Faridi, K. Davari, and B. Hajibeigi. 2006. "Epidemiology of Hepatitis B, Hepatitis C, and Human Immunodeficiency Virus Infections in Patients with Beta-Thalassemia in Iran: A Multicenter Study." *Arch Iran Med* 9: 319–23.

Mishwar. 2008. "An Integrated Bio-Behavioral Surveillance Study among Four Vulnerable Groups in Lebanon: Men Who Have Sex with Men; Prisoners; Commercial Sex Workers and Intravenous Drug Users." Final report.

Mohamed, M. K., M. Abdel-Hamid, M. N. Mikhail, F. Abdel-Aziz, A. Medhat, L. S. Magder, A. D. Fix, and G. T. Strickland. 2005. "Intrafamilial Transmission of Hepatitis C in Egypt." *Hepatology* 42: 683–87.

Mohamed, M. K., M. H. Hussein, A. A. Massoud, M. M. Rakhaa, S. Shoeir, A. A. Aoun, and M. Aboul Naser. 1996a. "Study of the Risk Factors for Viral Hepatitis C Infection among Egyptians Applying for Work Abroad." *J Egypt Public Health Assoc* 71: 113–47.

Mohamed, M. K., L. S. Magder, M. Abdel-Hamid, M. El-Daly, N. N. Mikhail, F. Abdel-Aziz, A. Medhat, V. Thiers, and G. T. Strickland. 2006. "Transmission of Hepatitis C Virus between Parents and Children." *Am J Trop Med Hyg* 75: 16–20.

Mohamed, M. K., M. Rakhaa, S. Shoeir, and M. Saber. 1996b. "Viral Hepatitis C Infection among Egyptians the Magnitude of the Problem: Epidemiological and Laboratory Approach." *J Egypt Public Health Assoc* 71: 79–111.

Mohammad Alizadeh, A. H., S. M. Alavian, K. Jafari, and N. Yazdi. 2003. "Prevalence of Hbs Ag, Hc Ab & Hiv Ab in the Addict Prisoners of Hammadan Prison (Iran, 1998)." *Journal of Research in Medical Sciences* 7: 311–13.

Mohammadi, M. R., K. Mohammad, F. K. Farahani, S. Alikhani, M. Zare, F. R. Tehrani, A. Ramezankhani, and F. Alaeddini. 2006. "Reproductive Knowledge, Attitudes and Behavior among Adolescent Males in Tehran, Iran." *Int Fam Plan Perspect* 32: 35–44.

Mohsen, A. M. 1998. "Assessment and Upgrading of Knowledge and Attitudes among Nurses and University Graduates towards AIDS." *J Egypt Public Health Assoc* 73: 433–48.

Montazeri, A. 2005. "AIDS Knowledge and Attitudes in Iran: Results from a Population-Based Survey in Tehran." *Patient Educ Couns* 57: 199–203.

Morocco MOH (Ministry of Health). 2007. *Surveillance sentinelle du VIH, résultats 2006 et tendances de la séro-prévalence du VIH.*

Moukeh, G., R. Yacoub, F. Fahdi, S. Rastam, and S. Albitar. 2009. "Epidemiology of Hemodialysis Patients in Aleppo City." *Saudi J Kidney Dis Transpl* 20: 140–46.

Mudawi, H. M., H. M. Smith, S. A. Rahoud, I. A. Fletcher, A. M. Babikir, O. K. Saeed, and S. S. Fedail. 2007. "Epidemiology of HCV Infection in Gezira State of Central Sudan." *J Med Virol* 79: 383–85.

Mujeeb, S. A., K. Aamir, and K. Mehmood. 2006. "Seroprevalence of HBV, HCV and HIV Infections among College Going First Time Voluntary Blood Donors." *J Pak Med Assoc* 56: S24–25.

Mujeeb, S. A., and A. Hafeez. 1993. "Prevalence and Pattern of HIV Infection in Karachi." *J Pak Med Assoc* 43: 2–4.

Mujeeb, S. A., Y. Khatri, and R. Khanani. 1998. "Frequency of Parenteral Exposure and Seroprevalence of HBV, HCV, and HIV among Operation Room Personnel." *J Hosp Infect* 38: 133–37.

Mujeeb, S. A., and M. S. Pearce. 2008. "Temporal Trends in Hepatitis B and C Infection in Family Blood Donors from Interior Sindh, Pakistan." *BMC Infect Dis* 8: 43.

Mutlu, B., M. Meric, and A. Willke. 2004. "Seroprevalence of Hepatitis B and C Virus, Human Immunodeficiency Virus and Syphilis in the Blood Donors." *Mikrobiyol Bul* 38: 445–48.

Mutter, R. C., R. M. Grimes, and D. Labarthe. 1994. "Evidence of Intraprison Spread of HIV Infection." *Arch Intern Med* 154: 793–95.

Nafeh, M. A., A. Medhat, M. Shehata, N. N. Mikhail, Y. Swifee, M. Abdel-Hamid, S. Watts, A. D. Fix, G. T. Strickland, W. Anwar, and I. Sallam. 2000. "Hepatitis C in a Community in Upper Egypt: I. Cross-Sectional Survey." *Am J Trop Med Hyg* 63: 236–41.

Najmi, R. S. 1998. "Awareness of Health Care Personnel about Preventive Aspects of HIV Infection/AIDS and Their Practices and Attitudes concerning Such Patients." *J Pak Med Assoc* 48: 367–70.

Nakhaee, F. H. 2002. "Prisoners' Knowledge of HIV/AIDS and Its Prevention in Kerman, Islamic Republic of Iran." *East Mediterr Health J* 8: 725–31.

Nakhaie, S., and E. Talachian. 2003. "Prevalence and Characteristic of Liver Involvement in Thalassemia Patients with HCV in Ali-Asghar Children Hospital, Tehran, Iran (Farsi)." *Journal of Iranian University Medical Science* 37: 799–806.

Nassirimanesh, B. 2002. "Proceedings of the Abstract for the Fourth National Harm Reduction Conference." Seattle, USA.

NEJM (*New England Journal of Medicine*). 2008. "Violence-Related Mortality in Iraq from 2002–2006." *N Engl J Med* 359: 431–34.

Njoh, J., and S. Zimmo. 1997. "Prevalence of Antibodies to Hepatitis C Virus in Drug-Dependent Patients in Jeddah, Saudi Arabia" *East Afr Med J* 74: 89–91.

Nobakht, Haghighi A., M. R. Zali, and A. Nowroozi. 2001. "Hepatitis C Antibody and Related Risk Factors in Hemodialysis Patients in Iran. *J Am Soc Nephrology* 12: 233A.

NSNAC (New Sudan AIDS Council), and UNAIDS (United Nations Joint Program on HIV/AIDS). 2006. *HIV/AIDS Integrated Report South Sudan, 2004–2005.* With United Nations General Assembly Special Session on HIV/AIDS Declaration of Commitment.

Nur, Y. A., J. Groen, A. M. Elmi, A. Ott, and A. D. Osterhaus. 2000. "Prevalence of Serum Antibodies against Bloodborne and Sexually Transmitted Agents in Selected Groups in Somalia." *Epidemiol Infect* 124: 137–41.

O'Grady, M. 2004. WFP Consultant Visit to Djibouti Report, 30 July.

Ocak, S., N. Duran, H. Kaya, and I. Emir. 2006. "Seroprevalence of Hepatitis C in Patients with Type 2 Diabetes Mellitus and Non-Diabetic on Haemodialysis." *Int J Clin Pract* 60: 670–74.

Othman, B. M., and F. S. Monem. 2001. "Prevalence of Hepatitis C Virus Antibodies among Health Care Workers in Damascus, Syria." *Saudi Med J* 22: 603–5.

———. 2002. "Prevalence of Hepatitis C Virus Antibodies among Intravenous Drug Abusers and Prostitutes in Damascus, Syria." *Saudi Med J* 23: 393–95.

Ozsoy, M. F., O. Oncul, S. Cavuslu, A. Erdemoglu, G. Emekdas, and A. Pahsa. 2003. "Seroprevalences of Hepatitis B and C among Health Care Workers in Turkey." *J Viral Hepat* 10: 150–56.

Pakistan AIDS Prevention Society. 1992–93. "Project Report on Sexual Behavior/Practices of International Travellers to Areas with High Prevalence of HIV Infection." Karachi, Pakistan.

Pakistan National AIDS Control Program. 2005a. *HIV Second Generation Surveillance in Pakistan.* National Report Round 1. Ministry of Health, Pakistan, and Canada-Pakistan HIV/AIDS Surveillance Project.

————. 2005b. *National Study of Reproductive Tract and Sexually Transmitted Infections. Survey of High Risk Groups in Lahore and Karachi.* Ministry of Health, Pakistan.

————. 2005c. "Report of the Pilot Study in Karachi & Rawalpindi." Ministry of Health Canada-Pakistan HIV/AIDS Surveillance Project, Integrated Biological & Behavioural Surveillance 2004–5.

————. 2006–7. *HIV Second Generation Surveillance in Pakistan.* National Report Round II. Ministry of Health, Pakistan, and Canada-Pakistan HIV/AIDS Surveillance Project.

————. 2008. *HIV Second Generation Surveillance in Pakistan.* National Report Round III. Ministry of Health, Pakistan, Canada-Pakistan HIV/AIDS Surveillance Project.

Parker, S. P., H. I. Khan, and W. D. Cubitt. 1999. "Detection of Antibodies to Hepatitis C Virus in Dried Blood Spot Samples from Mothers and Their Offspring in Lahore, Pakistan." *J Clin Microbiol* 37: 2061–63.

Petro-Nustas, W. 2000. "University Students' Knowledge of AIDS." *Int J Nurs Stud* 37: 423–33.

Petro-Nustas, W., A. Kulwicki, and A. F. Zumout. 2002. "Students' Knowledge, Attitudes, and Beliefs about AIDS: A Cross-Cultural Study." *J Transcult Nurs* 13: 118–25.

PFPPA (Palestinian Family Planning and Protection Association). 2005. "Assessment of Palestinian Students' Knowledge about AIDS and Their Attitudes toward the AIDS Patient." Jerusalem, Palestine.

Plummer, F. A., L. J. D'Costa, H. Nsanze, J. Dylewski, P. Karasira, and A. R. Ronald. 1983. "Epidemiology of Chancroid and Haemophilus Ducreyi in Nairobi, Kenya." *Lancet* 2: 1293–95.

Pourshams, A., R. Malekzadeh, A. Monavvari, M. R. Akbari, A. Mohamadkhani, S. Yarahmadi, N. Seddighi, M. Mohamadnejad, M. Sotoudeh, and A. Madjlessi. 2005. "Prevalence and Etiology of Persistently Elevated Alanine Aminotransferase Levels in Healthy Iranian Blood Donors." *Journal of Gastroenterology and Hepatology* 20: 229–33.

Qadi, A. A., H. Tamim, G. Ameen, A. Bu-Ali, S. Al-Arrayed, N. A. Fawaz, and W. Y. Almawi. 2004. "Hepatitis B and Hepatitis C Virus Prevalence among Dialysis Patients in Bahrain and Saudi Arabia: A Survey by Serologic and Molecular Methods." *Am J Infect Control* 32: 493–95.

Qatar National TB Programme. 2006. "TB Facts and Figures of Qatar." Hamad Medical Corporation.

Quadan, A. 2002. "Prevalence of Anti Hepatitis C Virus among the Hospital Populations in Jordan." *New Microbiol* 25: 269–73.

Quinti, I., D. el-Salman, M. K. Monier, B. G. Hackbart, M. S. Darwish, D. el-Zamiaty, R. Paganelli, F. Pandolfi, and R. R. Arthur. 1997. "HCV Infection in Egyptian Patients with Acute Hepatitis." *Dig Dis Sci* 42: 2017–23.

Quinti, I., E. Renganathan, E. El Ghazzawi, M. Divizia, G. Sawaf, S. Awad, A. Pana, and G. Rocchi. 1995. "Seroprevalence of HIV and HCV Infections in Alexandria, Egypt." *Zentralbl Bakteriol* 283: 239–44.

Rady, A. 2005. "Knowledge, Attitudes and Prevalence of Condom Use among Female Sex Workers in Lebanon: Behavioral Surveillance Study." UNFPA.

Rahbar, A. R., S. Rooholamini, and K. Khoshnood. 2004. "Prevalence of HIV Infection and Other Blood-Borne Infections in Incarcerated and Non-Incarcerated Injection Drug Users (IDUs) in Mashhad, Iran." *International Journal of Drug Policy* 15: 151–55.

Raheel, H., F. White, M. M. Kadir, and Z. Fatmi. 2007. "Knowledge and Beliefs of Adolescents regarding Sexually Transmitted Infections and HIV/AIDS in a Rural District in Pakistan." *J Pak Med Assoc* 57: 8–11.

Rais-Jalali, G., and P. Khajehdehi. 1999. "Anti-HCV Seropositivity among Haemodialysis Patients of Iranian Origin." *Nephrol Dial Transplant* (European Renal Association–European Dialysis and Transplant Association; ERA-EDTA): 2055–56.

Raja, N. S., and K. A. Janjua. 2008. "Epidemiology of Hepatitis C Virus Infection in Pakistan." *J Microbiol Immunol Infect* 41: 4–8.

Raja, Y., and A. Farhan. 2005. "Knowledge and Attitude of 10th and 11th Grade Students towards HIV/AIDS in Aden Governorate." Republic of Yemen.

Ramia, S., J. Mokhbat, A. Sibai, S. Klayme, and R. Naman. 2004. "Exposure Rates to Hepatitis C and G Virus Infections among HIV-Infected Patients: Evidence of Efficient Transmission of HGV by the Sexual Route." *Int J STD AIDS* 15: 463–66.

Raza, M. I., A. Afifi, A. J. Choudhry, and H. I. Khan. 1998. "Knowledge, Attitude and Behaviour towards AIDS among Educated Youth in Lahore, Pakistan." *J Pak Med Assoc* 48: 179–82.

Raziq, F., N. Alam, and L. Ali. 1993. "Serosurveillance of HIV Infection." *Pakistan Journal of Pathology*.

Razzaghi, E. M., A. R. Movaghar, T. C. Green, and K. Khoshnood. 2006. "Profiles of Risk: A Qualitative Study of Injecting Drug Users in Tehran, Iran." *Harm Reduct J* 3: 12.

Refaat, A. 2004. "Practice and Awareness of Health Risk Behaviour among Egyptian University Students." *East Mediterr Health J* 10: 72–81.

Rehan, N. 2006. "Profile of Men Suffering from Sexually Transmitted Infections in Pakistan." *J Pak Med Assoc* 56: S60–65.

Renganathan, E., I. Quinti, E. El Ghazzawi, O. Kader, I. El Sherbini, F. Gamil, and G. Rocchi. 1995. "Absence of HIV-1 and HIV-2 Infection in Different Populations from Alexandria, Egypt." *Eur J Epidemiol* 11: 711–12.

Rezvan, H., H. Abolghassemi, and S. A. Kafiabad. 2007. "Transfusion-Transmitted Infections among Multi-transfused Patients in Iran: A Review." *Transfus Med* 17: 425–33.

Rezvan, H., J. Ahmadi, M. Farhadi, and S. Taroyan. 1994. "A Preliminary Study on the Prevalence of Anti-HCV amongst Healthy Blood Donors in Iran." *Vox Sang* 67: 100.

Rizvi, T. J., and H. Fatima. 2003. "Frequency of Hepatitis C in Obstetric Cases." *J Coll Physicians Surg Pak* 13: 688–90.

Rodier, G. R., J. P. Sevre, G. Binson, G. C. Gray, S. Said, and P. Gravier. 1993. "Clinical Features Associated with HIV-1 Infection in Adult Patients Diagnosed with Tuberculosis in Djibouti, Horn of Africa." *Trans R Soc Trop Med Hyg* 87: 676–77.

Ryan, C. A., A. Zidouh, L. E. Manhart, R. Selka, M. Xia, M. Moloney-Kitts, J. Mahjour, M. Krone, B. N. Courtois, G. Dallabetta, and K. K. Holmes. 1998. "Reproductive Tract Infections in Primary Healthcare, Family Planning, and Dermatovenereology Clinics: Evaluation of Syndromic Management in Morocco." *Sex Transm Infect* 74 Suppl 1: S95–105.

Sakarya, S., S. Oncu, B. Ozturk, and S. Oncu. 2004. "Effect of Preventive Applications on Prevalence of Hepatitis B Virus and Hepatitis C Virus Infections in West Turkey." *Saudi Med J* 25: 1070–72.

Salama, I. I., N. K. Kotb, S. A. Hemeda, and F. Zaki. 1998. "HIV/AIDS Knowledge and Attitudes among Alcohol and Drug Abusers in Egypt." *J Egypt Public Health Assoc* 73: 479–500.

Saleh, E., W. McFarland, G. Rutherford, J. Mandel, M. El-Shazaly, and T. Coates. 2000. "Sentinel Surveillance for HIV and Markers for High Risk Behaviors among STD Clinic Attendees in Alexandria, Egypt." XIII International AIDS Conference, Durban, South Africa, Poster MoPeC2398.

Saleh, M. G., L. M. Pereira, C. J. Tibbs, M. Ziu, M. O. al-Fituri, R. Williams, and I. G. McFarlane. 1994. "High Prevalence of Hepatitis C Virus in the Normal Libyan Population." *Trans R Soc Trop Med Hyg* 88: 292–94.

Sallam, S. A., A. A. Mahfouz, W. Alakija, and R. A. al-Erian. 1995. "Continuing Medical Education Needs regarding AIDS among Egyptian Physicians in Alexandria, Egypt and in the Asir Region, Saudi Arabia." *AIDS Care* 7: 49–54.

Samimi-Rad, K., and B. Shahbaz. 2007. "Hepatitis C Virus Genotypes among Patients with Thalassemia and Inherited Bleeding Disorders in Markazi Province, Iran." *Haemophilia* 13: 156–63.

Savaser, S. 2003. "Knowledge and Attitudes of High School Students about AIDS: A Turkish Perspective." *Public Health Nurs* 20: 71–79.

Saxena, A. K., and B. R. Panhotra. 2004. "The Vulnerability of Middle-Aged and Elderly Patients to Hepatitis C Virus Infection in a High-Prevalence Hospital-Based Hemodialysis Setting." *J Am Geriatr Soc* 52: 242–46.

Schroeter, A. L., R. H. Turner, J. B. Lucas, and W. J. Brown. 1971. "Therapy for Incubating Syphilis: Effectiveness of Gonorrhea Treatment." *JAMA* 218: 711–13.

Scott, D. A., A. L. Corwin, N. T. Constantine, M. A. Omar, A. Guled, M. Yusef, C. R. Roberts, and D. M. Watts. 1991. "Low Prevalence of Human Immunodeficiency Virus-1 (HIV-1), HIV-2, and Human T Cell Lymphotropic Virus-1 Infection in Somalia." *American Journal of Tropical Medicine and Hygiene* 45: 653.

Sekkat, S., N. Kamal, B. Benali, H. Fellah, K. Amazian, A. Bourquia, A. El Kholti, and A. Benslimane. 2008. "Prevalence of Anti-HCV Antibodies and Seroconversion Incidence in Five Haemodialysis Units in Morocco." *Nephrol Ther* 4: 105–10.

Selcuk, H., M. Kanbay, M. Korkmaz, G. Gur, A. Akcay, H. Arslan, N. Ozdemir, U. Yilmaz, and S. Boyacioglu. 2006. "Distribution of HCV Genotypes in Patients with End-Stage Renal Disease according to Type of Dialysis Treatment." *Dig Dis Sci* 51: 1420–25.

Sellami, A., M. Kharfi, S. Youssef, M. Zghal, B. Fazaa, I. Mokhtar, and M. R. Kamoun. 2003. "Epidemiologic Profile of Sexually Transmitted Diseases (STD) through a Specialized Consultation of STD." *Tunis Med* 81: 162–66.

Semnani, S., G. Roshandel, N. Abdolahi, S. Besharat, A. A. Keshtkar, H. Joshaghani, A. Moradi, K. Kalavi, A. Jabbari, M. J. Kabir, S. A. Hosseini, S. M. Sedaqat, A. Danesh, and D. Roshandel. 2007. "Hepatitis B/C Virus Co-Infection in Iran: A Seroepidemiological Study." *Turk J Gastroenterol* 18: 20–21.

Shaikh, F., D., S. A. Khan, M. W. Ross, and R. M. Grimes. 2007. "Knowledge and Attitudes of Pakistani Medical Students towards HIV-Positive and/or AIDS Patients." *Psychol Health Med* 12: 7–17.

Shaikh, M. A., and S. Assad. 2001. "Adolescent's Knowledge about AIDS—Perspective from Islamabad." *J Pak Med Assoc* 51: 194–95.

Shama, M., L. E. Fiala, and M. A. Abbas. 2002. "HIV/AIDS Perceptions and Risky Behaviors in Squatter Areas in Cairo, Egypt." *J Egypt Public Health Assoc* 77: 173–200.

Sharifi-Mood, B., R. Alavi-Naini, M. Salehi, M. Hashemi, and F. Rakhshani. 2006. "Spectrum of Clinical Disease in a Series of Hospitalized HIV-Infected Patients from Southeast of Iran." *Saudi Med J* 27: 1362–66.

Sharifi-Mood, B., P. Eshghi, E. Sanei-Moghaddam, and M. Hashemi. 2007. "Hepatitis B and C Virus Infections in Patients with Hemophilia in Zahedan, Southeast Iran." *Saudi Med J* 28: 1516–19.

Shebl, F. M., S. S. El-Kamary, D. A. Saleh, M. Abdel-Hamid, N. Mikhail, A. Allam, H. El-Arabi, I. Elhenawy, S. El-Kafrawy, M. El-Daly, S. Selim, A. A. El-Wahab, M. Mostafa, S. Sharaf, M. Hashem, S. Heyward, O. C. Stine, L. S. Magder, S. Stoszek, and G. T. Strickland. 2009. "Prospective Cohort Study of Mother-to-Infant Infection and Clearance of Hepatitis C in Rural Egyptian Villages." *J Med Virol* 81: 1024–31.

Sheikh, N. S., A. S. Sheikh, Rafi-u-Shan, and A. A. Sheikh. 2003. "Awareness of HIV and AIDS among Fishermen in Coastal Areas of Balochistan." *J Coll Physicians Surg Pak* 13: 192–94.

Shemer-Avni, Y., Z. el Astal, O. Kemper, K. J. el Najjar, A. Yaari, N. Hanuka, M. Margalith, and E. Sikuler. 1998. "Hepatitis C Virus Infection and Genotypes in Southern Israel and the Gaza Strip." *J Med Virol* 56: 230–33.

Sherafat-Kazemzadeh, R., S. Shahraz, H. Mohaghegh-Shalmani, T. Ghaziani, L. Feghahati, Z. Mohammad-Reza, and M. Mohraz. 2003. "Iranian Persons Living with HIV/AIDS Unveil the Epidemic of Stigma: An Overview of Patients' Attitudes towards the Disease and Community in First GIPA Gathering in Tehran." *Archives of Iranian Medicine* 6.

Shidrawi, R., M. Ali Al-Huraibi, M. Ahmad Al-Haimi, R. Dayton, and I. M. Murray-Lyon. 2004. "Seroprevalence of Markers of Viral Hepatitis in Yemeni Healthcare Workers." *J Med Virol* 73: 562–65.

Shobokshi, O. A., F. E. Serebour, A. Z. Al-Drees, A. H. Mitwalli, A. Qahtani, and L. I. Skakni. 2003. "Hepatitis C Virus Seroprevalence Rate among Saudis." *Saudi Med J* 24 Suppl 2: S81–86.

Shrestha, P. N. 1996. "HIV/AIDS Surveillance in the Eastern Mediterranean Region." *Eastern Mediterranean Health Journal* 2: 82–89.

Siddiqi, S., S. A. Majeed, and M. Saeed Khan. 1995. "Knowledge, Attitude and Practice Survey of Acquired Immune Deficiency Syndrome (AIDS) among Paramedicals in a Tertiary Care Hospital in Pakistan." *J Pak Med Assoc* 45: 200–2.

Sit, D., A. K. Kadiroglu, H. Kayabasi, M. E. Yilmaz, and V. Goral. 2007. "Seroprevalence of Hepatitis B and C Viruses in Patients with Chronic Kidney Disease in the Predialysis Stage at a University Hospital in Turkey." *Intervirology* 50: 133–37.

Slama, H., N. Mojaat, R. Dahri, and K. Boukef. 1991. "Epidemiologic Study of Anti-HCV Antibodies in Tunisian Blood Donors." *Rev Fr Transfus Hemobiol* 34: 459–64.

SNAP (Sudan National AIDS Programme). 2006. "HIV Sentinel Surveillance among Tuberculosis Patients in Sudan." Federal Ministry of Health, General Directorate of Preventive Medicine, SNAP.

———. 2008. "Update on the HIV Situation in Sudan." PowerPoint presenation.

SNAP (Sudan National AIDS Programme), NSNAC (New Sudan National AIDS Council), and UNAIDS (United Nations Joint Progamme on HIV/AIDS). 2006. "Scaling-up HIV/AIDS Response in Sudan." "National Consultation on the Road towards Universal Access to Prevention, Treatment, Care and Support." February.

SNAP (Sudan National AIDS Programme), and UNAIDS. 2006. "HIV/AIDS Integrated Report North Sudan, 2004–2005 (Draft)." With United Nations General Assembly Special Session on HIV/AIDS Declaration of Commitment.

SNAP (Sudan National AIDS Programme), UNICEF (United Nations Children's Fund), and UNAIDS. 2005. "Baseline Study on Knowledge, Attitudes, and Practices on Sexual Behaviors and HIV/AIDS Prevention amongst Young People in Selected States in Sudan." HIV/AIDS KAPB Report. Projects and Research Department (AFROCENTER Group).

Somaliland Ministry of Health and Labour. 2007. *Somaliland 2007 HIV/Syphilis Seroprevalence Survey, A Technical Report.* Ministry of Health and Labour in collaboration with the WHO, UNAIDS, UNICEF/GFATM, and SOLNAC.

Sonmez, M., O. Bektas, M. Yilmaz, A. Durmus, E. Akdogan, M. Topbas, M. Erturk, E. Ovali, and S. B. Omay. 2007. "The Relation of Lymphoma and Hepatitis B Virus/Hepatitis C Virus Infections in the Region of East Black Sea, Turkey." *Tumori* 93: 536–39.

Soskolne, V., and S. Maayan. 1998. "HIV Knowledge, Beliefs and Sexual Behavior of Male Heterosexual Drug Users and Non-Drug Users Attending an HIV Testing Clinic in Israel." *Isr J Psychiatry Relat Sci* 35: 307–17.

Stoszek, S. K., M. Abdel-Hamid, S. Narooz, M. El Daly, D. A. Saleh, N. Mikhail, E. Kassem, Y. Hawash, S. El Kafrawy, A. Said, M. El Batanony, F. M. Shebl, M. Sayed, S. Sharaf, A. D. Fix, and G. T. Strickland. 2006. "Prevalence of and Risk Factors for Hepatitis C in Rural Pregnant Egyptian Women." *Trans R Soc Trop Med Hyg* 100: 102–7.

Sudan Government of National Unity. 2007. *United Nations National Integrated Annual Action Plan 2007.* United Nations.

Sudan MOH (Ministry of Health). 2005. *Sudan National HIV/AIDS Surveillance Unit, Annual Report.* Khartoum.

Sudan National AIDS Control Program. 1999. 1999 report. Khartoum: Federal Ministry of Health.

———. 2005. *Sentinel Sero-Survailance—2005 Data.* Annual Newsletter.

Sudan National HIV/AIDS Control Program. 2004. *HIV/AIDS/STIs Prevalence, Knowledge, Attitude, Practices and Risk Factors among University Students and Military Personnel.* Federal Ministry of Health, Khartoum.

Sultan, F., T. Mehmood, and M. T. Mahmood. 2007. "Infectious Pathogens in Volunteer and Replacement Blood Donors in Pakistan: A Ten-Year Experience." *Int J Infect Dis* 11: 407–12.

Syria Mental Health Directorate. 2008. "Assessment of HIV Risk and Sero-Prevalence among Drug Users in Greater Damascus." Programme SNA, Syrian Ministry of Health, UNODC, UNAIDS.

Syria National AIDS Programme. 2004. "HIV/AIDS Female Sex Workers KABP Survey in Syria."

Tabarsi, P., S. M. Mirsaeidi, M. Amiri, S. D. Mansouri, M. R. Masjedi, and A. A. Velayati. 2008. "Clinical and Laboratory Profile of Patients with Tuberculosis/HIV Coinfection at a National Referral Centre: A Case Series." *East Mediterr Health J* 14: 283–91.

Tahan, V., C. Karaca, B. Yildirim, A. Bozbas, R. Ozaras, K. Demir, E. Avsar, A. Mert, F. Besisik, S. Kaymakoglu, H. Senturk, Y. Cakaloglu, C. Kalayci, A. Okten, and N. Tozun. 2005. "Sexual Transmission of HCV between Spouses." *Am J Gastroenterol* 100: 821–24.

Talaie, H., S. H. Shadnia, A. Okazi, A. Pajouhmand, H. Hasanian, and H. Arianpoor. 2007. "The Prevalence of Hepatitis B, Hepatitis C and HIV Infections in Non-IV Drug Opioid Poisoned Patients in Tehran, Iran." *Pak J Biol Sci* 10: 220–24.

Tamim, H., N. Irani-Hakime, J. P. Aoun, S. Khoury, H. Samaha, and W. Y. Almawi. 2001. "Seroprevalence of Hepatitis C Virus (HCV) Infection among Blood Donors: A Hospital-Based Study." *Transfus Apher Sci* 24: 29–5.

Tanaka, Y., S. Agha, N. Saudy, F. Kurbanov, E. Orito, T. Kato, M. Abo-Zeid, M. Khalaf, Y. Miyakawa, and M. Mizokami. 2004. "Exponential Spread of Hepatitis C Virus Genotype 4a in Egypt." *J Mol Evol* 58: 191–95.

Tariq, W. U. Z., I. A. Malik, Z. U. Hassan, A. Hannan, and M. Ahmen. 1993. "Epidemiology of HIV Infection in Northern Pakistan." *Pakistan J Path* 4: 111–14.

Tavoosi, A., A. Zaferani, A. Enzevaei, P. Tajik, and Z. Ahmadinezhad. 2004. "Knowledge and Attitude towards HIV/AIDS among Iranian Students." *BMC Public Health* 4: 17.

Taziki, O., and F. Espahbodi. 2008. "Prevalence of Hepatitis C Virus Infection in Hemodialysis Patients." *Saudi J Kidney Dis Transpl* 19: 475–78.

Tehrani, F. R., and H. Malek-Afzalip. 2008. "Knowledge, Attitudes and Practices concerning HIV/AIDS among Iranian At-Risk Sub-Populations." *Eastern Mediterranean Health Journal* 14.

Tekay, F., and E. Ozbek. 2006. "Short Communication: Hepatitis B, Hepatitis C and Human Immuno-deficiency Virus Seropositivities in Women Admitted to Sanliurfa Gynecology and Obstetrics Hospital." *Mikrobiyol Bul* 40: 369–73.

Todd, C. S., A. M. Abed, S. A. Strathdee, P. T. Scott, B. A. Botros, N. Safi, and K. C. Earhart. 2007. "HIV, Hepatitis C, and Hepatitis B Infections and Associated Risk Behavior in Injection Drug Users, Kabul, Afghanistan." *Emerg Infect Dis* 13: 1327–31.

Todd, C. S., M. Ahmadzai, F. Atiqzai, S. Miller, J. M. Smith, S. A. Ghazanfar, and S. A. Strathdee. 2008. "Seroprevalence and Correlates of HIV, Syphilis, and Hepatitis B and C Virus among Intrapartum Patients in Kabul, Afghanistan." *BMC Infect Dis* 8: 119.

Todd, C. S., M. Ahmadzai, F. Atiqzai, J. M. Smith, S. Miller, P. Azfar, H. Siddiqui, S. A. Ghazanfar, and S. A. Strathdee. 2009. "Prevalence and Correlates of HIV, Syphilis, and Hepatitis Knowledge among Intrapartum Patients and Health Care Providers in Kabul, Afghanistan." *AIDS Care* 21: 109–17.

Tompkins, M., L. Smith, K. Jones, and S. Swindells. 2006. "HIV Education Needs among Sudanese Immigrants and Refugees in the Midwestern United States." *AIDS Behav* 10: 319–23.

Torabi, S. A., K. Abed-Ashtiani, R. Dehkhoda, A. N. Moghadam, M. K. Bahram, R. Dolatkhah, J. Babaei, and N. Taheri. 2006. "Prevalence of Hepatitis B, C and HIV in Hemophiliac Patients of East Azerbaijan in 2004." *Blood* 2: 291–99.

Triki, H., N. Said, A. Ben Salah, A. Arrouji, F. Ben Ahmed, A. Bouguerra, S. Hmida, R. Dhahri, and K. Dellagi. 1997. "Seroepidemiology of Hepatitis B, C and Delta Viruses in Tunisia." *Trans R Soc Trop Med Hyg* 91: 11–14.

UNAIDS (United Nations Joint Programme on HIV/AIDS). 2006. "Epidemiological Fact Sheets on HIV/AIDS and Sexually Transmitted Diseases." Somalia.

———. 2007a. *AIDS Epidemic Update.* Geneva. http://www.unaids.org.

———. 2007b. UNAIDS/WHO Global HIV/AIDS Online Database.

———. 2007c. "Key Findings on HIV Status in the West Bank and Gaza." Working document, Regional Support Team for the Middle East and North Africa.

———. 2008. "Notes on AIDS in the Middle East and North Africa." RST MENA.

UNAIDS, and WHO (World Health Organization). 2005. *AIDS Epidemic Update 2005.* Geneva.

Ungan, M., and H. Yaman. 2003. "AIDS Knowledge and Educational Needs of Technical University Students in Turkey." *Patient Educ Couns* 51: 163–67.

UNHCR. 2006–7a. *HIV Sentinel Surveillance among Antenatal Clients and STI Patients.* Dadaab Refugee Camps, Kenya.

———. 2006–7b. *HIV Sentinel Surveillance among Conflict Affected Populations.* Kakuma Refugee Camp—Refugees and Host Nationals, Great Lakes Initiative on HIV/AIDS.

———. 2007. "HIV Behavioural Surveillance Survey Juba Municipality, South Sudan." United Nations High Commissioner for Refugees.

Unknown. 2006. "HIV Risk among Heroin and Injecting Drug Users in Muscat, Oman." Quantitative Survey. Preliminary Data.

Unknown. "Rapport de l'enquête nationale de séro-surveillance sentinelle du VIH et de la syphilis en Algérie 2004–2005."

Unknown. "Statut de la réponse nationale: Caractéristiques de l'épidémie des IST/VIH/SIDA." Algeria.

UNODCP (United Nations Office for Drug Control and Crime Prevention), and UNAIDS (UN Joint Programme on HIV/AIDS). 1999. "Baseline Study of the Relationship between Injecting Drug Use, HIV and Hepatitis C among Male Injecting Drug Users in Lahore."

Vahdani, P., S. M. Hosseini-Moghaddam, L. Gachkar, and K. Sharafi. 2006. "Prevalence of Hepatitis B, Hepatitis C, Human Immunodeficiency Virus, and Syphilis among Street Children Residing in Southern Tehran, Iran." *Arch Iran Med* 9: 153–55.

van Egmond, K., A. J. Naeem, H. Verstraelen, M. Bosmans, P. Claeys, and M. Temmerman. 2004. "Reproductive Health in Afghanistan: Results of a Knowledge, Attitudes and Practices Survey among Afghan Women in Kabul." *Disasters* 28: 269–82.

Waked, I. A., S. M. Saleh, M. S. Moustafa, A. A. Raouf, D. L. Thomas, and G. T. Strickland. 1995. "High Prevalence of Hepatitis C in Egyptian Patients with Chronic Liver Disease." *Gut* 37: 105–7.

Watts, D. M., N. T. Constantine, M. F. Sheba, M. Kamal, J. D. Callahan, and M. E. Kilpatrick. 1993. "Prevalence of HIV Infection and AIDS in Egypt over Four Years of Surveillance (1986–1990)." *J Trop Med Hyg* 96: 113–17.

Watts, D. M., A. L. Corwin, M. A. Omar, and K. C. Hyams. 1994. "Low Risk of Sexual Transmission of Hepatitis C Virus in Somalia." *Trans R Soc Trop Med Hyg* 88: 55–56.

WHO (World Health Organization). 2002. "HIV/AIDS Epidemiological Surveillance Report for the WHO African Region 2002 Update."

———. 2004. *The 2004 First National Second Generation HIV/AIDS/STI Sentinel Surveillance Survey, Somalia: A Technical Report.*

———. 2005. "Summary Country Profile for HIV/AIDS Treatment Scale-Up." Djibouti.

WHO/EMRO (Eastern Mediterranean Region Office). 2000. "Presentation of WHO Somalia's Experience in Supporting the National Response." Somalia. Regional Consultation towards Improving HIV/AIDS & STD Surveillance in the Countries of EMRO, Beirut, Lebanon, Oct 30–Nov 2.

———. 2004. "Best Practice in HIV/AIDS Prevention and Care for Injecting Drug Abusers: The Triangular Clinic in Kermanshah, Islamic Republic of Iran."

———. 2007. "HIV/AIDS Surveillance in Low Level and Concentrated HIV Epidemics: A Technical Guide for Countries in the WHO Eastern Mediterranean Region."

WHO (World Health Organization), UNICEF (United Nations Children's Fund), and UNAIDS (United Nations Joint Programe on HIV/AIDS). 2006a. "Epidemiological Facts Sheets on HIV/AIDS and Sexually Transmitted Infections." Algeria.

———. 2006b. "Epidemiological Facts Sheets on HIV/AIDS and Sexually Transmitted Infections." Bahrain.

———. 2006c. "Epidemiological Facts Sheets on HIV/AIDS and Sexually Transmitted Infections." Djibouti.

———. 2006d. "Epidemiological Facts Sheets on HIV/AIDS and Sexually Transmitted Infections." Egypt.

———. 2006e. "Epidemiological Facts Sheets on HIV/AIDS and Sexually Transmitted Infections." Iraq.

———. 2006f. "Epidemiological Facts Sheets on HIV/AIDS and Sexually Transmitted Infections." Iran.

———. 2006g. "Epidemiological Facts Sheets on HIV/AIDS and Sexually Transmitted Infections." Jordan.

———. 2006h. "Epidemiological Facts Sheets on HIV/AIDS and Sexually Transmitted Infections." Kuwait.

———. 2006i. "Epidemiological Facts Sheets on HIV/AIDS and Sexually Transmitted Infections." Lebanon.

———. 2006j. "Epidemiological Facts Sheets on HIV/AIDS and Sexually Transmitted Infections." Libya, Arab Jamahiriya.

———. 2006k. "Epidemiological Facts Sheets on HIV/AIDS and Sexually Transmitted Infections." Morocco.

———. 2006l. "Epidemiological Facts Sheets on HIV/AIDS and Sexually Transmitted Infections." Oman.

———. 2006m. "Epidemiological Facts Sheets on HIV/AIDS and Sexually Transmitted Infections." Pakistan.

———. 2006n. "Epidemiological Facts Sheets on HIV/AIDS and Sexually Transmitted Infections." Qatar.

———. 2006o. "Epidemiological Facts Sheets on HIV/AIDS and Sexually Transmitted Infections." Somalia.

———. 2006p. "Epidemiological Facts Sheets on HIV/AIDS and Sexually Transmitted Infections." Sudan.

———. 2006q. "Epidemiological Facts Sheets on HIV/AIDS and Sexually Transmitted Infections." Syrian Arab Republic.

———. 2006r. "Epidemiological Facts Sheets on HIV/AIDS and Sexually Transmitted Infections." Tunisia.

———. 2006s. "Epidemiological Facts Sheets on HIV/AIDS and Sexually Transmitted Infections." Yemen.

Winer, R. L., S. K. Lee, J. P. Hughes, D. E. Adam, N. B. Kiviat, and L. A. Koutsky. 2003. "Genital Human Papillomavirus Infection: Incidence and Risk Factors in a Cohort of Female University Students." *Am J Epidemiol* 157: 218–26.

Winter, J. 1996. "Where the Imams Play Their Part." *AIDS Anal Afr* 6: 1–2.

World Bank. 2008. "Mapping and Situation Assessment of Key Populations at High Risk of HIV in Three Cities of Afghanistan." Human Development Sector, South Asia Region (SAR) AIDS Team, World Bank.

Yakaryilmaz, F., O. A. Gurbuz, S. Guliter, A. Mert, Y. Songur, T. Karakan, and H. Keles. 2006. "Prevalence of Occult Hepatitis B and Hepatitis C Virus Infections in Turkish Hemodialysis Patients." *Ren Fail* 28: 729–35.

Yazdi, C. A., K. Aschbacher, A. Arvantaj, H. M. Naser, E. Abdollahi, A. Asadi, M. Mousavi, M. R. Narmani, M. Kianpishe, F. Nicfallah, and A. K. Moghadam. 2006. "Knowledge, Attitudes and Sources of Information regarding HIV/AIDS in Iranian Adolescents." *AIDS Care* 18: 1004–10.

Yemen National TB Programme. 2006. "TB Facts and Figures of Yemen." NTCP, Ministry of Health.

Yildirim, B., S. Barut, Y. Bulut, G. Yenisehirli, M. Ozdemir, I. Cetin, I. Etikan, A. Akbas, O. Atis, H. Ozyurt, and S. Sahin. 2009. "Seroprevalence of Hepatitis B and C Viruses in the Province of Tokat in the Black Sea Region of Turkey: A Population-Based Study." *Turk J Gastroenterol* 20: 27–30.

Yorke, J. A., H. W. Hethcote, and A. Nold. 1978. "Dynamics and Control of the Transmission of Gonorrhea." *Sex Transm Dis* 5: 51–56.

Yousif, M. E. A. 2006. *Health Education Programme among Female Sex Workers in Wad Medani Town-Gezira State.* Final report.

Zafar, T., H. Brahmbhatt, G. Imam, S. ul Hassan, and S. A. Strathdee. 2003. "HIV Knowledge and Risk Behaviors among Pakistani and Afghani Drug Users in Quetta, Pakistan." *J Acquir Immune Defic Syndr* 32: 394–98.

Zahraoui-Mehadji, M., M. Z. Baakrim, S. Laraqui, O. Laraqui, Y. El Kabouss, C. Verger, A. Caubet, and C. H. Laraqui. 2004. "Infectious Risks Associated with Blood Exposure for Traditional Barbers and Their Customers in Morocco." *Sante* 14: 211–16.

Zali, M. R., R. Aghazadeh, A. Nowroozi, and H. Amir-Rasouly. 2001. "Anti-HCV Antibody among Iranian IV Drug Users: Is It a Serious Problem?" *Arch Iranian Med* 4: 115–19.

Zamani, S., M. Kihara, M. M. Gouya, M. Vazirian, M. Ono-Kihara, E. M. Razzaghi, and S. Ichikawa. 2005. "Prevalence of and Factors Associated with HIV-1 Infection among Drug Users Visiting Treatment Centers in Tehran, Iran." *AIDS* 19: 709–16.

Zamani, S., G. M. Mehdi, M. Ono-Kihara, S. Ichikawa, and M. Kuhara. 2007. "Shared Drug Injection Inside Prison as a Potent Associated Factor for Acquisition of HIV Infection: Implication for Harm Reduction Interventions in Correctional Settings." *Journal of AIDS Research* 9: 217–22.

Zidouh, A. Unknown. "VIH/SIDA et infections sexuellement transmissibles: connaissance et attitudes."

Index

Boxes, figures, and tables are indicated by *b*, *f*, and *t*, respectively.

A

abortions, unsafe, 169, 170*f*
abuse
  of FSWs, 43, 46
  of migrant women, 134
  of prisoners, 125
  of refugee women, 141*b*
  of street children, 138–39
  of women in general population, 70
Afghanistan
  ART in, 207, 208
  availability of drugs in, 16
  condom use in, 102*t*, 103*t*
  as covered country, 6
  emergency situations in, 133
  FSWs in, 47, 48, 50, 51, 53, 202
  general population and HIV in, 66*t*, 68*t*, 70
  HCV in different population groups, 232*t*
  HPV and cervical cancer in, 157*t*
  IDUs in, 11, 12*t*, 14*t*, 15*t*, 16, 17, 18*t*, 21, 22*t*, 123, 124, 135, 137, 200, 201
  knowledge of HIV/AIDS in, 109, 112, 113, 239*t*, 242*t*
  migrant population, 133, 135, 136
  molecular epidemiology in, 93
  MSM in, 34
  origins and evolution of HIV in, 180
  overlapping risks in, 206
  parenteral transmission other than IDU, 88
  PLHIV, estimated numbers of, 221*t*
  potential bridging populations in, 59, 60
  prevention efforts, 209
  prevention efforts in, 200, 201, 202, 207
  prisoners in, 121*t*, 124
  refugees and IDPs, 136, 137, 138
  status of current epidemic in, 184*t*
  STIs/STDs, 163*t*, 165, 209
  TB and HIV in, 228*t*
  vulnerable populations in, 189
  youth and HIV in, 129, 132

Africa. *See* HIV/AIDS in MENA region; sub-Saharan Africa
AIDs in MENA. *See* HIV/AIDS in MENA region
alcohol consumption by FSWs and their clients, 49
Algeria
  civil society organizations and NGOs in, 216
  condoms, access to, 203
  as covered country, 6
  FSWs in, 44*t*, 168, 202, 229*t*
  general population and HIV in, 66*t*, 68*t*, 69–70, 72, 73
  HCV in different population groups, 232*t*
  HPV and cervical cancer in, 157*t*, 158*f*, 159*t*
  IDUs in, 11, 12*t*, 15*t*, 18*t*, 21, 22*t*, 124, 229*t*
  marriage in, 128
  molecular epidemiology in, 92, 93
  MSM in, 201, 229*t*
  overlapping risks in, 206
  PLHIV, associations of, 206
  PLHIV, estimated numbers of, 221*t*
  polygamy in, 72
  pregnant women, prevalence of HIV among, 229*t*
  prevention efforts in, 201, 202
  prisoners in, 121*t*, 124
  response programs, expanding coverage of, 205
  status of current epidemic in, 184*t*
  STIs/STDs, 163*t*, 167*t*, 168, 226*t*, 229*t*
  TB and HIV in, 228*t*, 229*t*
  transmission modes in, 86*t*
  VCT services in, 204, 226*t*
  women, premarital sex as leading cause of suicide of, 73
anal sex
  FSWs, 48, 50, 52, 54
  MSM, 32, 33, 34, 35, 37, 39
  as transmission mode, 85
  youth and HIV, 128
anemia, hemolytic, 179

antenatal clinic (ANC) attendees and other pregnant
    women. *See also* mother-to-child transmission
  bacterial STIs, 168
  case notification surveillance reports, 82–84, 83*f*
  FSWs, 47
  general population, prevalence of HIV in, 65,
    66–67*t*, 71, 72
  HSV-2 incidence, 152, 154
  migrants, 134
  point-prevalence surveys, 229–32*t*
  refugees and IDPs, 138
  studies and surveys, 181
antiretroviral therapy (ART), 200, 203, 207–9, 208*f*,
    208*t*, 214
antischistosomal therapy, 89
Ar-Razi psychiatric hospital, Morocco, 201
Arab Republic of Egypt. *See* Egypt, Arab Republic of
armed forces, as potential bridging population. *See*
    potential bridging populations
ART (antiretroviral therapy), 200, 203, 207–9, 208*f*,
    208*t*, 214
Asia. *See also* East Asia and Pacific; Eastern Europe
    and Central Asia; South Asia
  FSWs, 52
  HSV-2 in, 155*t*
  parenteral transmission in, 91
  priority and bridging populations, HIV
    concentrated in, 5
  youth and HIV in, 132
Association Tunisienne de Lutte contre le SIDA
    (ATLS), 202
attitudes toward PLHIV, 110–11, 113, 245–47*t*
Azerbaijan, HPV and cervical cancer in, 157

B

Bahrain
  as covered country, 6
  FSWs in, 229*t*
  HCV in different population groups, 232*t*
  HPV and cervical cancer in, 157*t*, 159*t*
  IDUs in, 11, 12*t*, 15*t*, 229*t*
  knowledge of HIV/AIDS in, 232*t*
  MSM in, 229*t*
  origins and evolution of HIV in, 179
  parenteral transmission other than IDU, 90*t*
  PLHIV, estimated numbers of, 221*t*
  prevalence of HIV, 224*t*
  prevention efforts, 209, 210
  prisoners in, 121*t*
  status of current epidemic in, 184*t*
  STIs/STDs, 209, 210, 229*t*
  TB and HIV in, 229*t*
Bangladesh
  civil society organizations and NGOs in, 216
  HSV-2 in, 153*t*

migrant population, 134, 136
  MSM in, 34
banthas, 33
barbers, HCV prevalence among, 91
behavioral surveillance, increasing and expanding,
    213–14
bibliographies, 8–10
  condom use, 113–18
  current status and future potential, 191–97
  epidemiological factors, 94–100
  FSWs, 54–58
  general population and HIV, 75–80
  IDUs, 25–29
  knowledge of HIV/AIDS, 113–18
  MSM, 39–41
  potential bridging populations, 62–63
  proxy markers of risk behavior, 170–78
  responses to HIV in MENA, 210–12
  strategic recommendations, 218–19
  vulnerable populations, 141–49
blood and blood products
  case notification surveillance reports, 82–84, 83*f*
  general population, prevalence of HIV in, 65,
    68–69*t*
  IDUs providing, 21
  MSM providing, 35
  origins of HIV in MENA and, 179–81
  parenteral transmission other than IDU,
    88–92, 90*t*
  safety and screening programs, 180, 207
  STIs/STDs, 165
  as transmission mode, 86–87*t*
blood letting, traditional practices of, 89
Brazil, HPV and cervical cancer in, 161
bridging populations. *See* potential bridging
    populations

C

Cameroon, molecular epidemiology of
    HIV/AIDS in, 93
care and treatment of HIV/AIDS patients, 206*f*,
    207–9, 208*t*
Caribbean. *See* Latin America and Caribbean
case notification surveillance reports, 82–84,
    83*f*, 186
casual sex
  in general population, 70
  of refugees and IDPs, 137
  in youth populations, 129–31
Central America. *See* Latin America and Caribbean
Central Asia. *See* Eastern Europe and Central Asia
cervical cancer and HPV, 69–70, 72, 132, 156–62,
    157*t*, 158*f*, 159*t*, 160*f*, 161*f*, 222*t*
cervical lesions, noncancerous, in young women, 132
chancroid, 168, 222*t*

chastity houses, 71

chavas, 33

China, truck driver network in, 61

chlamydia, 162–69, 167–68*t*, 169*f*, 222*t. See also*
    sexually transmitted infections (STIs) and
    diseases (STDs) other than HIV

circumcision
    female genital mutilation, 74
    male, 4, 54, 62, 73–75, 160, 187, 190

civil society organizations, 201, 205–7, 215–16

clean needle programs, 201, 215

clinic attendees. *See* antenatal clinic (ANC) attendees and
    other pregnant women; sexually transmitted
    disease (STD) clinic attendees; voluntary
    counseling and testing (VCT) attendees

commercial sex. *See* sex workers

conceptual framework of HIV/AIDS in MENA
    region, 3–6, 4–6*f*, 182–85, 185*f*

condom use, 101–9
    accessibility of condoms, 101–8, 203–4
    actual condom use, 101, 103–8*t*, 108
    bibliography, 113–18
    conclusions regarding, 108–9
    by FSWs, 50–51, 101, 108
    general knowledge regarding, 101–9, 102–3*t*
    in general population, 70
    by IDUs, 21, 22–24*t*
    by MSM, 36–37, 101, 108
    prevention programs, 202, 203–4
    prisoners, 125
    refugees and IDPs, 137
    by street children, 139
    youth and HIV, 130–31

conflicts and postconflict situations, 133

crisis situations, 133

cultural issues
    desirability bias, 5–6
    as protective factors, 187–88
    status of HIV in MENA and, 2–3
    vulnerability due to cultural change, 2

cupping, 89

current status and future potential, 179–97
    bibliography, 191–97
    dynamics of current disease in conceptual
        framework, 185*f*
    expansion of HIV in MENA, 189–91, 190*f*
    knowledge of HIV and, 189
    number of current infections, 186
    origins and evolution of epidemic in MENA, 179–82
    overlap among priority groups, 188*f*
    prevalence of HIV, 186–87
    progress in controlling, 186
    protective factors, 187–88
    response to epidemic, 199–212. *See also* responses
        to HIV in MENA

status of current epidemic, 184*t*

typology of disease in different regions, 182–83

vulnerable populations, 188–89

D

Dar el Amal, 202

Demographic and Health Survey (DHS) reports, 7

desirability bias, 5–6

divorced women, sexual risk behaviors of, 70, 71

Djibouti
    ART in, 208*t*, 209
    attitudes toward PLHIV in, 245*t*
    civil society organizations and NGOs in, 216
    condom use in, 103*t*
    as covered country, 6
    female circumcision/genital mutilation in, 74
    FSWs in, 43, 44*t*, 47, 53, 54, 129, 202, 229*t*
    general population and HIV in, 65*t*, 66*t*, 68*t*, 69,
        70, 74
    HCV in different population groups, 232*t*
    HPV and cervical cancer in, 157*t*
    HSV-2 in, 153*t*
    IDUs in, 185, 229*t*
    knowledge of HIV/AIDS in, 109–10, 131, 239*t*, 244*t*
    molecular epidemiology in, 92, 93
    MSM in, 229*t*
    origins and evolution of HIV in, 181
    PLHIV, associations of, 206
    PLHIV, estimated numbers of, 221*t*
    potential bridging populations in, 59, 60, 62
    pregnant women, prevalence of HIV among, 229*t*
    prevalence of HIV in, 180, 187, 224*t*
    prevention efforts in, 202, 207, 209, 210
    prisoners in, 121*t*
    status of current epidemic in, 184*t*
    STIs/STDs, 81, 163*t*, 166*t*, 167*t*, 168, 209, 210,
        226*t*, 229*t*
    TB and HIV in, 228*t*, 229*t*
    typology of disease in, 183
    unsafe abortions in, 169
    VCT clinics and attendees, 81, 204, 226*t*
    youth and HIV in, 129–30, 131

domestic violence. *See* abuse

drug resistance monitoring, 209

E

East Asia and Pacific. *See also* Asia
    IDUs in, 16
    MSM, 31
    unsafe abortions in, 170*f*

Eastern Europe and Central Asia. *See also* Asia
    HSV-2 in, 155*t*
    IDUs, prevalence of, 14
    truck driver network, 61
    unsafe abortions in, 170*f*
    youth and HIV in, 126

G

gay men. *See* men who have sex with men

gender issues

female genital mutilation, 74

FSWs. *See* female sex workers

HPV and cervical cancer rates, male sexual behavior mainly affecting, 159

IDUs, female, 16, 52–53, 54

intergenerational sex, 61, 73

knowledge of HIV/AIDS, gender differentials in, 111–12

migrant populations, 134, 135

MSM. *See* men who have sex with men

premarital sex as leading cause of suicide for women, 73

prevalence of HIV by gender, 84–85

prisoners, female, having sex with guards, 125

risk behavior, men more likely to engage in, 61, 73, 84–85

transgender individuals, 31, 33, 35, 36, 37, 38, 61, 202

vulnerability factors exacerbated by, 2, 61

vulnerability of sexual partners/spouses, 188–89

widowed and divorced women, sexual risk behaviors of, 70, 71

young single women, large cohort of, 127–28

general population, 65–80

bibliography, 75–80

casual sex, 70

in conceptual framework, 3–4, 4*f*, 5*f*

conclusions regarding, 74–75

condom use, 70

extramarital sex, 69, 70–71

female genital mutilation in, 74

FSWs, contact with, 69, 70

male circumcision in, 73–75

nontraditional marriages, 71–72

polygamy, 69–70, 71, 72–73

premarital sex, 70, 71, 73

prevalence of HIV among, 65–69*t*, 187

risk behavior of, 69–73, 74

status of current epidemic, 184*t*

STIs/STDs, 69–74

genital herpes (herpes simplex virus type 2 or HSV-2), 132, 152–56, 153*t*, 154*f*, 155*t*

glass cupping, 89

Global Fund to Fight AIDS, Tuberculosis and Malaria (GFATM), 202, 203, 207

gonorrhea, 162–69, 166*t*, 169*f*, 222*t*. *See also* sexually transmitted infections (STIs) and diseases (STDs) other than HIV

government organized NGOs (GONGOs), 216

group of sustainable transmission (GST), 4

guest workers. *See* migrants

gurus (pimps) for *hijras,* 35

H

harm reduction as aim for priority populations, 217

HBV (Hepatitis B), 88, 89, 90, 91, 179

HCV. *See* Hepatitis C

health care in MENA, vulnerability factors arising from, 2

health care workers (HCWs)

hemodialysis, universal blood precautions in, 89

PLHIV, attitudes toward, 110

Helem (NGO), 201, 216

hemodialysis patients, 88, 89, 90*t*, 91

hemolytic anemia, 179

Hepatitis B (HBV), 88, 89, 90, 91, 179

Hepatitis C (HCV)

IDUs

MSM and, 38

as proxy marker of HIV risk among, 13, 14*t*

need to study, 3

parenteral transmission other than IDU, 88–92, 179

prevalence in MENA, 14*t*, 232–38*t*

in prison population, 120

research priorities, 214

surveillance practices, 213, 214

herpes simplex virus type 1 (HSV-1), 154

herpes simplex virus type 2 (HSV-2), or genital herpes, 132, 152–56, 153*t*, 154*f*, 155*t*, 214, 222*t*

heterogeneity of risk, 3–4, 4*f*, 5*f*

heterosexual sex, as transmission mode, 85, 86–87*t*

High Risk Corridor Initiative, 216

hijamah (traditional medical practices), 89

hijras, 31, 33, 35, 36, 37, 38, 60, 168, 202

HIV/AIDS in MENA region, 1–10

bibliographies. *See* bibliographies

as bloodborne pathogen. *See entries at* blood

case notification surveillance reports, 82–84, 83*f*, 186

conceptual framework, 3–6, 4–6*f*, 182–85, 185*f*

condom use, 101–9. *See also* condom use

countries covered, 6. *See also specific countries*

current status and future potential, 179–97. *See also* current status and future potential

epidemiological data for, 1, 7–8

exogenous HIV exposures, 85–87, 180, 182

FSWs, 43–58. *See also* female sex workers

gender issues related to. *See* gender issues

in general population, 65–80. *See also* general population

IDUs, 15–29. *See also* injecting drug users

knowledge about HIV/AIDS, 109–13

knowledge of HIV/AIDS. *See also* knowledge about HIV/AIDS

limitations of study, 8

literature review, 6–7, 222–23

integrated biobehavioral surveillance surveys (IBBSS), 214

intergenerational sex, 61, 73

internally displaced persons (IDPs). *See* refugees and IDPs

International Agency for Research on Cancer (IARC), 7

International Centre for Prison Studies (ICPS), 7

International Organization for Migration (IOM), 7, 133

Iran, Islamic Republic of

  ART in, 208*t*, 209

  attitudes toward PLHIV in, 245*t*

  availability of drugs in, 16

  case notification surveillance reports, 83–84

  civil society organizations and NGOs in, 216

  condom use in, 102*t*, 104*t*, 108

  as covered country, 6

  FSWs in, 44*t*, 47, 48–49, 50, 51, 52, 53, 182, 202, 230*t*

  general population and HIV in, 65*t*, 66*t*, 68*t*, 70, 71

  harm reduction approach in, 215, 217

  HCV in different population groups, 234–35*t*

  HPV and cervical cancer in, 157*t*, 159*t*, 161

  HSV-2 in, 152, 153*t*

  IDUs in, 11, 12*t*, 14*t*, 15*t*, 16, 17, 18*t*, 19, 20, 21, 22*t*, 38, 52, 123, 124, 125, 135, 182, 185, 199, 200, 201, 214, 230*t*

  knowledge of HIV/AIDS in, 109, 110, 111, 112, 113, 131, 239*t*, 242*t*, 244*t*, 247*t*

  marriage, age at, 127

  migrant population, 135

  molecular epidemiology in, 92–93

  MSM in, 33, 34, 36, 37, 38, 182, 188, 230*t*

  nontraditional marriage in, 71, 72

  origins and evolution of HIV in, 179, 182

  overlapping risks in, 206

  parenteral transmission other than IDU, 88, 90*t*, 91

  PLHIV, estimated numbers of, 221*t*

  PMTCT services, 209

  potential bridging populations in, 60, 60*t*

  pregnant women, prevalence of HIV among, 230*t*

  prevalence of HIV in, 180, 224*t*

  prevention efforts in, 199, 200, 201, 202, 203, 207, 209, 210

  prisoners in, 120, 121*t*, 123, 124, 125, 126, 128

  refugees and IDPs, 136, 137, 138

  STIs/STDs, 81, 129, 163*t*, 165, 166*t*, 167*t*, 168, 210, 226*t*, 230*t*

  street children in, 139

  tattooing by prisoners, 125

  TB and HIV in, 228*t*, 230*t*

  transmission modes in, 85, 86*t*

  VCT clinic attendees, 81, 226*t*

  youth and HIV in, 128, 129, 130, 131, 132, 203

Iranian National Center for Addiction Studies (INCAS), 201

Iraq

  ART in, 208

  as covered country, 6

  emergency situations in, 133

  FSWs in, 230*t*

  HCV in different population groups, 235*t*

  HPV and cervical cancer in, 157*t*, 158

  IDUs in, 12*t*, 15*t*, 230*t*

  knowledge of HIV/AIDS in, 239*t*

  MSM in, 230*t*

  PLHIV, estimated numbers of, 221*t*

  pregnant women, prevalence of HIV among, 230*t*

  prevention efforts in, 207, 210

  prisoners in, 121*t*

  refugees and IDPs, 136, 141*b*

  sexual trafficking, 46

  status of current epidemic in, 184*t*

  STIs/STDs, 210, 230*t*

  TB and HIV in, 228*t*, 230*t*

  vulnerable populations in, 189

Islam and HIV/AIDS, 110, 111, 113, 187–88, 217

Islamic Republic of Iran. *See* Iran, Islamic Republic of

Israel. *See also* West Bank and Gaza

  as covered country, 6

  exogenous exposures of West Bank and Gaza residents in, 180

  HPV and cervical cancer in, 157*t*, 158*f*

  HSV-2 in, 153*t*

  PLHIV, estimated numbers of, 221*t*

J

jawaz al misyar, 72

"jerking," 21

Joint United Nations Programme on HIV/AIDS. *See* UNAIDS

Jordan

  attitudes toward PLHIV in, 245*t*

  civil society organizations and NGOs in, 216

  condom use in, 102*t*, 104*t*, 108, 203

  as covered country, 6

  DHS reports, 7

  exogenous HIV exposures, 85, 180

  FSWs in, 48, 202, 230*t*

  general population and HIV in, 68*t*, 72

  HCV in different population groups, 235*t*

  HPV and cervical cancer in, 157*t*, 158, 159*t*

  HSV-2 in, 152–54

  IDUs in, 12*t*, 15*t*, 230*t*

  knowledge of HIV/AIDS in, 110, 111, 112, 239*t*, 242*t*, 244*t*

  marriage in, 72, 127, 128

  migrant population, 133, 134, 135

future expansion of HIV in, 189

general population and HIV in, 68*t*, 70

HCV in different population groups, 235–36*t*

HPV and cervical cancer in, 157*t*, 158*f*, 159*t*, 160, 161

HSV-2 in, 153*t*

IDUs in, 11, 12–13*t*, 13, 14*t*, 15*t*, 16, 17–21, 18*t*, 23*t*, 24, 38, 52, 87, 123, 185, 186–87, 201, 232*t*

knowledge of HIV/AIDS in, 109, 111, 240*t*, 242*t*, 244*t*, 247*t*

migrant population, 134–35, 136

molecular epidemiology in, 93

MSM in, 31, 32*t*, 33, 34–35, 36, 37, 38, 128–29, 188, 202, 231*t*

origins and evolution of HIV in, 180

parenteral transmission other than IDU, 88, 90, 90*t*, 91

PLHIV, estimated numbers of, 221*t*

PMTCT services, 209

potential bridging populations in, 59, 60–61, 60*t*

pregnant women, prevalence of HIV among, 231*t*

prevalence of HIV in, 181, 186–87, 225*t*

prevention efforts in, 200, 201, 202, 207, 209, 210

prisoners in, 122*t*, 123

refugees and IDPs, 136, 137

status of current epidemic in, 184*t*

STIs/STDs, 81, 164*t*, 166*t*, 167*t*, 168, 210, 227*t*, 231*t*

street children in, 139

TB and HIV in, 228*t*, 231*t*

transmission modes in, 86*t*

VCT clinic attendees, 81, 227*t*

youth and HIV in, 128–29

Palestinian refugees, 127, 136. *See also* Israel; West Bank and Gaza

Pap smears, 132, 160–61

parenteral transmission other than IDU, 88–92, 90*t*. *See also* entries at blood

people living with HIV (PLHIV)

attitudes toward, 110–11, 113, 245–47*t*

care and treatment, 206*f*, 207–9, 208*t*

estimated numbers by country, 221*t*

knowledge of HIV status, 208

migrants, 136

response efforts, involvement in, 205–7

sexual partners of. *See under* potential bridging populations

stigma and discrimination against, 210

strategic recommendation to rely on, 215–16

Persepolis (NGO), 216

Philippines, migrant workers from, 134, 136

phlebotomy, traditional practices of, 89

physical abuse. *See* abuse

pimps

FSWs, 45, 47

hijras, 35

PITC (provider-initiated testing and counseling), 205

PLHIV. *See* people living with HIV

PMTCT (prevention of mother-to-child transmission) services, 138, 209

point-prevalence surveys, 7–8, 82, 224–38*t*

polygamy, 69–70, 71, 72–73

Population Reference Bureau (PRB), 7

postconflict situations, 133

potential bridging populations, 59–63

bibliography, 62–63

in conceptual framework, 3–4, 4*f*, 5*f*

conclusions regarding, 62

defined, 59

prevalence of HIV among, 59–60, 60*t*

research on, 59–63

risk behavior of, 60–61

sexual partners, 61–62

case notification surveillance reports, 82–84, 83*f*

of FSWs, 47–49

of IDUs, 20–21

of MSM, 34, 37

STIs/STDs, 60, 62

studies and surveys, 181

surveillance of, 213–14

youth as, 126

PRB (Population Reference Bureau), 7

pregnancy. *See* antenatal clinic (ANC) attendees and other pregnant women

premarital sex

in general population, 70, 71, 73

migrants and, 135

refugees and IDPs, 137

youth involvement in, 127, 129–31

prevention of HIV. *See* responses to HIV in MENA

prevention of mother-to-child transmission (PMTCT) services, 138, 209

primary stage of infection, 217

priority populations. *See also* female sex workers; injecting drug users; men who have sex with men

behavioral surveillance, increasing and expanding, 213–14

case notification surveillance reports, 82

in conceptual framework, 5

current status and future potential, 182–83, 185*f*, 186, 188*f*

focused prevention programs for, 200–203

harm reduction as aim for, 217

law enforcement approach to HIV control, avoiding, 215

overlapping risks, 188*f*, 206

STI/STD prevention programs, importance of, 210

weak surveillance systems for, 87

prisoners, 119–26
    case notification surveillance reports, 82–84, 83f
    conclusions regarding, 125–26
    condom use, 125
    female prisoners having sex with guards, 125
    IDUs and drug use generally, 91, 119–20, 123–25, 128
    imprisonment as risk factor, 123
    knowledge of HIV/AIDS, 109, 112, 113
    as migrants, 134
    MSM, 33, 125
    parenteral transmission other than IDU, 91
    prevalence of HIV among, 120, 121–22t
    rates of imprisonment in MENA, 120, 121–22t
    risk behaviors, 120–25
    sexually risky behavior in and out of prison, 125
    studies and surveys, 181
    tattooing, 125
    as vulnerable population, 119–20
    youth and HIV, 128
prostitution. *See* sex workers
protective factors, 187–88
provider-initiated testing and counseling (PITC), 205
proxy markers of risk behavior, 151–78
    bacterial STIs (syphilis, gonorrhea, and
        chlamydia), 162–69, 163–68t, 169f
    bibliography, 170–78
    conclusions regarding, 169–70
    HPV and cervical cancer, 69–70, 72, 132, 156–62,
        157t, 158f, 159t, 160f, 161f
    HSV-2, 132, 152–56, 153t, 154f, 155t
    unsafe abortions, 169, 170f
    validity of reported risk behavior, verifying, 151–52

Q

Qatar
    as covered country, 6
    general population and HIV in, 68t
    HPV and cervical cancer in, 157t
    IDUs in, 15t, 231t
    marriage in, 128
    migrant population, 135
    origins and evolution of HIV in, 179
    parenteral transmission other than IDU, 90t
    PLHIV, estimated numbers of, 221t
    prisoners in, 122t
    status of current epidemic in, 184t
    STIs/STDs, 164t, 231t
    TB and HIV in, 228t, 231t
    transmission modes in, 86t

R

R_0, concept of, 4–5, 5f
rape. *See* abuse
recommendations regarding HIV in MENA. *See*
        strategic recommendations

refugees and IDPs, 136–38
    conclusions regarding, 138
    data sets covering, 7
    FSWs and, 48, 141b
    high numbers in MENA, 2
    IDUs, 137
    knowledge of HIV/AIDS, 112, 137
    numbers of, 136
    Palestinian refugees, 127, 136
    in polygamous marriages, 71, 72
    prevalence of HIV among, 138
    risk behavior, 137–38
    studies and surveys, 181
    typology of disease in southern Sudan and, 183
    vulnerability of, 137
religion and HIV/AIDS, 110, 111, 113, 187–88, 217
remittances from migrant populations, 133
renal dialysis, 89
Republic of Yemen. *See* Yemen, Republic of
research for evidence-based policy, 214–15
responses to HIV in MENA, 199–212
    access to prevention programs, 203–4
    bibliography, 210–12
    blood safety and screening efforts, 180, 207
    care and treatment, 206f, 207–9, 208t
    civil society organizations, involvement of, 201,
        205–7, 215–16
    conclusions regarding, 210
    expanding coverage for, 205
    FSWs and MSWs, prevention programs for, 202
    IDUs, prevention programs for, 200–201
    M&E systems, 206–7
    MSM, prevention programs for, 201–2
    NGOs, involvement of, 200–202, 204–7, 210,
        215–16
    outreach efforts, 207
    PLHIV, involvement of, 205–7, 215–16
    PMTCT services, 138, 209
    progress in prevention programs, 203
    scope and scale of prevention programs, 199–200
    STIs/STDs, 209–10
    strategic focus on prevention, 216–17
    testing and counseling, 204–5, 214. *See also*
        voluntary counseling and testing (VCT)
        attendees
    translating evidence into programs, 206–7
    youth, prevention programs for, 203
risk and risk behavior
    of FSWs, 48–53
    of general population, 69–73, 74
    heterogeneity and sustainability of, 3–5, 4–6f
    of IDUs, 16–21, 18t, 22–24t
    law enforcement approach to HIV control,
        avoiding, 215
    men more likely to engage in, 61, 73, 84–85

of migrants, 135
of MSM, 33–38
perception of risk from HIV, 109–10, 131
of potential bridging populations, 60–61
priority populations, overlapping risks among, 188*f*, 206
of prisoners, 120–25
proxy markers of, 151–78. *See also* proxy markers of risk behavior
of refugees and IDPs, 137–38
research priorities, 214
of street children, 139
VCT and STD clinic attendees, 81
of youth, 128–32
rural/urban
knowledge of HIV/AIDS, 112
migration between, 134
Russian Federation/former Soviet Union
IDUs in, 17, 214
migrant FSWs in United Arab Emirates, 135
surveillance efforts in, 214
truck driver network, 61

S

sailors, as potential bridging population. *See* potential bridging populations
Saudi Arabia
attitudes toward PLHIV in, 246*t*
as covered country, 6
FSWs in, 43, 52
general population and HIV in, 68*t*
HCV in different population groups, 236–37*t*
HPV and cervical cancer in, 157*t*, 158, 159*t*, 160
HSV-2 in, 154
IDUs in, 13*t*, 14*t*, 15*t*
knowledge of HIV/AIDS in, 109, 113, 240*t*, 242*t*, 244*t*
marriage, age at, 127
migrant population, 133, 135
molecular epidemiology in, 93
origins and evolution of HIV in, 179, 180
parenteral transmission other than IDU, 89, 90*t*
PLHIV, estimated numbers of, 221*t*
prevalence of HIV in, 181, 225*t*
prevention efforts in, 207, 210
spouses, vulnerability of, 188–89
status of current epidemic in, 184*t*
STIs/STDs, 167*t*, 168, 210
TB and HIV in, 228*t*
transmission modes in, 85, 87*t*
vulnerability of women to HIV infection in, 61
youth and HIV in, 132
scientific research for evidence-based policy, 214–15
seafarers, as potential bridging population. *See* potential bridging populations

security approach to HIV control, avoiding, 215
sex workers
female. *See* female sex workers
hijras, 31, 33, 35, 36, 37, 38, 60, 168
MSWs, 34–36, 60, 128–29, 202
prevention programs for, 202
street children as, 33, 46, 138–39
sexual abuse. *See* abuse
sexual identity in MENA, fluidity of, 32–33
sexual issues. *See* gender issues
sexual partners
HPV and cervical cancer rates, 159, 160*f*
of potential bridging populations. *See under* potential bridging populations
vulnerability of, 188–89
sexual trafficking, 46, 134
sexually risky behavior. *See* risk and risk behavior
sexually transmitted disease (STD) clinic attendees
case notification surveillance reports, 82–84, 83*f*
chancroid, 168
FSWs, 51–52, 202
general population, 71, 72, 73
HSV-2 incidence, 155
as migrants, 134, 135
potential bridging populations, 60
prevalence of HIV among, 81–82, 181, 226–27*t*, 229–32*t*
prevention efforts, 202, 203
studies and surveys, 181
sexually transmitted infections (STIs) and diseases (STDs) other than HIV
bacterial STIs, 162–69, 163–68*t*, 169*f*
chancroid, 168, 222*t*
chlamydia, 162–69, 167–68*t*, 169*f*, 222*t*
epidemiological characteristics of different STIs/STDs, 222*t*
FSWs and, 48, 50, 51–52, 53, 81
in general population, 69–74
gonorrhea, 162–69, 166*t*, 169*f*, 222*t*
heterogeneity of risk, 4
HPV and cervical cancer, 69–70, 72, 132, 156–62, 157*t*, 158*f*, 159*t*, 160*f*, 161*f*, 222*t*
HSV-2, 132, 152–56, 153*t*, 154*f*, 155*t*, 214, 222*t*
IDUs, sexually risky behavior of, 21
intergenerational sex and, 73
knowledge of, 112
literature review, criteria for, 222–23
migrants, 133, 136
MSM and, 31, 33, 39
need to study, 3, 7
nontraditional marriage, associated with, 72
polygamy and, 72–73
potential bridging populations and, 60, 62
prevention efforts, 209–10
research priorities, 214

Tunisia (*continued*)
    mobile populations in, 133
    molecular epidemiology in, 93
    MSM in, 34, 36, 37, 38, 201, 204
    origins and evolution of HIV in, 180
    parenteral transmission other than IDU, 90*t*
    PLHIV, estimated numbers of, 221*t*
    pregnant women, prevalence of HIV among, 232*t*
    prevention efforts in, 200, 201, 202, 203, 204, 207
    prisoners in, 122*t*
    status of current epidemic in, 184*t*
    STIs/STDs, 129, 226*t*, 232*t*
    TB and HIV in, 229*t*, 232*t*
    transmission modes in, 87*t*
    youth and HIV in, 127, 128, 129, 131, 203
Turkey
    attitudes toward PLHIV in, 246*t*
    condom use in, 108*t*
    as covered country, 6
    FSWs in, 45*t*
    general population and HIV in, 69*t*
    HCV in different population groups, 237–38*t*
    HPV and cervical cancer in, 157*t*, 159*t*
    HSV-2 in, 153*t*, 154
    IDUs in, 13*t*, 15*t*
    knowledge of HIV/AIDS in, 111, 241*t*, 243*t*,
        245*t*, 247*t*
    parenteral transmission other than IDU, 91
    PLHIV, estimated numbers of, 221*t*
    prevalence of HIV, 225*t*
    prevalence of HIV in, 181
    STIs/STDs, 132, 165*t*, 166*t*, 168*t*
    women, premarital sex as leading cause of
        suicide of, 73
    youth and HIV in, 131, 132
typology
    in core MENA region, 182–83
    in subregion with considerable prevalence
        (Djibouti, Somalia, and Southern Sudan), 183

U
Uganda
    molecular epidemiology in, 92, 93
    refugees and IDPs, 138
    youth and HIV in, 126
UNAIDS (Joint United Nations Programme on
        HIV/AIDS)
    ART, use of, 207
    covered countries, 6
    data limitations, 8
    epidemiological fact sheets, 82
    on epidemiology of AIDS in MENA, 1
    literature review, 7
    prevention programs for FSWs, 202

unemployment rates
    migration fueled by, 134
    youth in MENA, 127
UNHCR (Office of the UN High Commissioner for
        Refugees), 7
UNICEF (United Nations Children's Fund), 7
uniformed personnel, as potential bridging
        population. *See* potential bridging populations
United Arab Emirates
    attitudes toward PLHIV in, 246*t*
    as covered country, 6
    FSWs, 135
    HPV and cervical cancer in, 157*t*
    HSV-2 in, 153*t*
    IDUs in, 15*t*
    knowledge of HIV/AIDS in, 241*t*, 243*t*, 245*t*
    migrant population, 135, 136
    origins and evolution of HIV in, 180
    PLHIV, estimated numbers of, 221*t*
    polygamy in, 72
    prevention efforts in, 207
    prisoners in, 122*t*
    status of current epidemic in, 184*t*
    STIs/STDs, 168*t*
United Kingdom, availability of drugs in, 16
United Nations Children's Fund (UNICEF), 7
United Nations High Commissioner for Refugees
        (UNHCR), 136, 141*b*
United Nations Joint Programme on HIV/AIDS.
        See UNAIDS
United Nations Office on Drugs and Crime
        (UNODC), 7, 16
United Nations Relief and Works Agency for Palestine
        Refugees in the Near East (UNRWA), 136
United States
    availability of drugs in, 16
    bacterial STIs in, 168
    IDUs in, 15, 16, 17
    prison population in, 120
UNODC (United Nations Office on Drugs and Crime), 16
UNRWA (United Nations Relief and Works Agency
        for Palestine Refugees in the Near East), 136
unsafe abortions, 169, 170*f*
urban/rural
    knowledge of HIV/AIDS, 112
    migration between, 134
'*urfi* marriage (clandestine marriage), 71–72

V
vaccination against HPV, 161–62
voluntary counseling and testing (VCT) attendees,
        204–5
    case notification surveillance reports, 82–84, 83*f*
    FSWs and, 48, 81, 202

Eco-Audit

Environmental Benefits Statement

The World Bank is committed to preserving endangered forests and natural resources. The Office of the Publisher has chosen to print *Characterizing the HIV/AIDS Epidemic in the Middle East and North Africa* on recycled paper with 50 percent postconsumer fiber in accordance with the recommended standards for paper usage set by the Green Press Initiative, a nonprofit program supporting publishers in using fiber that is not sourced from endangered forests. For more information, visit www.greenpressinitiative.org.

Saved:
- 16 trees
- 5 million Btu of total energy
- 1,568 lb. of net greenhouse gases
- 7,553 gal. of waste water
- 459 lb. of solid waste

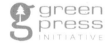